REGULATORY FUNCTIONS OF INTERFERONS

ANNALS OF THE NEW YORK ACADEMY OF SCIENCES
Volume 350

REGULATORY FUNCTIONS OF INTERFERONS

Edited by Jan Vilček, Ion Gresser, and Thomas C. Merigan

The New York Academy of Sciences
New York, New York
1980

Library of Congress Cataloging in Publication Data

Main entry under title:

Regulatory functions of interferons.

(Annals of the New York Academy of Sciences; v. 350)
Papers presented at a conference sponsored by the New York Academy of Sciences, held Oct. 23–26, 1979.
Includes index.
1. Interferons—Physiological effect—Congresses. 2. Immune response—Regulation—Congresses. I. Vilček, J., 1933– II. Gresser, Ion. III. Merigan, Thomas C. IV. New York Academy of Sciences. V. Series:

New York Academy of Sciences. Annals; v. 350.
[DNLM: 1. Interferon—Congresses. W1 AN626YL v. 350 / QW 800 R344 1979]
Q11.N5 vol. 350 [QR187.5] 500s [615.07'9]
80-25207

SP
Printed in the United States of America
ISBN 0-89766-089-7 (cloth)
ISBN 0-89766-090-0 (paper)

ANNALS OF THE NEW YORK ACADEMY OF SCIENCES
VOLUME 350
October 23, 1980

REGULATORY FUNCTIONS OF INTERFERONS*

Editors and Conference Chairmen
Jan Vilček, Ion Gresser, and Thomas C. Merigan

CONTENTS

*This series of papers is the result of a conference entitled Regulatory Functions of Interferons held October 23–26, 1979 by The New York Academy of Sciences.

Part III. Interferons as Lymphokines

Part IV. Mechanisms of Cell Growth Inhibitory and Antitumor Action; Genetics of the Interferon System

Part V. Regulatory Effects of Interferons in Various Cells

Part VI. Purification and Properties of Interferons

Part VII. Molecular Mechanisms of Interferon Action

Part VIII. Antiviral Mechanisms: Studies at the Cellular Level

Poster Papers

Financial assistance was received from:

- ABBOTT LABORATORIES
- AMERICAN CYANAMID COMPANY
- BEHRING INSTITUT
- BURROUGHS WELLCOME CO.
- CUTTER LABORATORIES, INC.
- E. I. DU PONT DE NEMOURS & COMPANY
- ENDO LABORATORIES, INC.
- ERNST-BOEHRINGER-INSTITUT FÜR ARZNEIMITTELFORSCHUNG
- FLOW LABORATORIES, INC.
- HOFFMANN-LA ROCHE INC.
- LILLY RESEARCH LABORATORIES
- MCNEIL LABORATORIES
- MERCK SHARP & DOHME RESEARCH LABORATORIES
- MERRELL-NATIONAL LABORATORIES
- MILES LABORATORIES, INC.
- NATIONAL INSTITUTE OF ALLERGY AND INFECTIOUS DISEASES
- NATIONAL SCIENCE FOUNDATION
- ORTHO PHARMACEUTICAL CORPORATION
- PFIZER CENTRAL RESEARCH
- P-L BIOCHEMICALS, INC.
- DR. RENTSCHLER ARZNEIMITTEL GMBH & CO.
- REVLON HEALTH CARE GROUP
- SANDOZ FORSCHUNGSINSTITUT
- SCHERING CORPORATION
- G. D. SEARLE & CO.
- SYNTEX USA, INC.
- TORAY INDUSTRIES, INC.
- THE UPJOHN COMPANY
- USV PHARMACEUTICAL CORPORATION
- WARNER-LAMBERT COMPANY
- WINTHROP LABORATORIES
- WYETH LABORATORIES

OPENING REMARKS

Jan Vilček

Department of Microbiology
New York University School of Medicine
New York, New York 10016

I would like to welcome you on behalf of the three co-chairmen—Ion Gresser, Tom Merigan and myself. The program is the result of preparations that stretched over a period of about 18 months. In the process of assembling this most impressive program we relied on the judgment and advise of many colleagues. This is the appropriate time to express our thanks to those of you in the audience who provided us with very valuable help.

Let me say just a few words about the guiding philosophy of this meeting. In the last few years interferon research has grown tremendously in scope and significance. Until quite recently there were perhaps a couple of hundred active investigators throughout the world—most of them virologists by training. This has changed dramatically as interferon has become a household expression among immunologists and oncologists, cell geneticists and molecular biologists, protein chemists and gene cloners. In preparing the program of this conference we strived to stress the new frontiers of interferon research at the expense of more traditional aspects.

In order to allow for thorough analysis of some new areas we had to limit the scope of this conference even further. For instance, clinical trials with interferon are not covered, despite the broad interest in this work. However, many of the papers will be relevant to clinical applications of interferon. Specifically, throughout this conference we shall be asking the question: "What is the rational basis for clinical trials with interferon?"

Even though we limited the scope of the conference, we were still faced with the difficult task of selecting speakers from a large pool of potential candidates. Unfortunately, many outstanding investigators could not be included in the program. In making the choices we had to rely on information available to us at the time of scheduling. Human judgment is always subjective as well as error-prone, and we must apologize to all who would have deserved to be included but were not, particularly to our younger colleagues. The alternative would have been to have a vastly overcrowded program with insufficient time for thorough analysis. I would like to emphasize that the Poster Session is part and parcel of this conference, with much exciting, new information to emerge from this forum. Unfortunately, because of space limitations, we were also forced to restrict the number of posters.

When we were preparing the program of this conference about a year ago, we were hoping that despite our careful planning some element of scientific surprise would emerge from this meeting. It so appears that our wishes reached sympathetic ears on Olympus. (Or perhaps it was somewhere else?) I would not dare to spoil the fun by revealing too many surprises prematurely. However, I have heard rumors that the partial amino acid sequences of three different interferons might be revealed for the first time in just about 51 hours from now. Let's all be surprised.

Judging from the number of participants this conference should be most successful. In fact we had grossly underestimated the number of people likely to attend. The conference room can seat a little over 500 people and we fervently hope to accommodate everyone. As a result of our inadequate planning a number of participants experienced difficulties with hotel reservations. We were simply unprepared for this most enthusiastic response.

Alick Isaacs would be both amazed and delighted to see how from its modest beginnings interferon research has grown to be important in so many varied fields of scientific activity. What a pity that Alick cannot be with us today!

This conference could not take place without the support of many individuals and organizations. Generous financial assistance was obtained from the National Institute of Allergy and Infectious Diseases, the National Science Foundation, and from as many as 30 private organizations. The staff of the New York Academy of Sciences provided able organizational support. We wish you all a most productive stay at the conference. And if you have any time left, enjoy the Indian summer in the Big Apple!

IMMUNOREGULATORY ACTION OF TYPE I INTERFERON IN THE MOUSE*

Edward De Maeyer and Jaqueline De Maeyer-Guignard

Institut Curie
Université de Paris-Sud
91405 Orsay, France

INTRODUCTION

The regulation of the immune response is highly complex, involving interaction of different lymphocyte populations and their subsets and collaboration of lymphocytes and macrophages, either through direct cell-to-cell contact or through the release of soluble mediators such as lymphokines, monokines, or antigen-specific suppressor substances.[1] Not everything by definition capable of influencing immunity also participates in its regulation, and a substance can have immunomodulating effects without being a normal component of an immune reaction.[2] Several immunomodulating effects have been attributed to interferon,[3,4] and however interesting and important these may be, this does not necessarily imply that interferon participates in the regulation of the immune response.

In this communication we summarize evidence indicating that interferon (IF) not only can influence cell-mediated immunity (CMI), but is actually part of the regulatory mechanism of delayed hypersensitivity (DH) with at least one viral antigen. Our work deals exclusively with the effects of type I interferon, and we have not yet investigated the effect on CMI of type II interferon, although this would be most interesting. As a reminder, type II interferon is a lymphokine made by antigen-sensitized cells, whereas the synthesis of type I interferon, as a result of viral infection, does not imply any previous contact of the host with the same virus.

EVIDENCE THAT INTERFERON CAN INFLUENCE DELAYED HYPERSENSITIVITY IN THE MOUSE

We have previously presented evidence that exogenous interferon, that is IF prepared in tissue culture and then inoculated into the animal, can influence both the afferent and efferent pathways of DH in the mouse. Endogenous IF, that is IF synthesized by the animal as a result of virus infection, acts similarly. These effects of interferon were found by studying expression and sensitization to several antigens, and are summarized in FIGURE 1.

Effect on Expression

When mice sensitized to picryl chloride, sheep red blood cells (SRBC) or Newcastle disease virus (NDV), are challenged with the antigen, interferon

*Supported by the CNRS (AI 00031858), the Ligue Nationale Française contre le Cancer and the Fondation pour la Recherche Médicale. The pleasant collaboration with D.W. Bailey of the Jackson Laboratory at Bar Harbor, ME is gratefully acknowledged.

0077-8923/80/0350-0001 $01.75/0 © 1980, NYAS

decreases or completely inhibits the reaction. This inhibitory effect is dose-dependent and, for example, 10^6 units given systemically a few hours before footpad challenge of BALB/c mice sensitized with SRBC, completely inhibits footpad swelling measured 24 and 48 hours later.[5,6]

Effect on Sensitization

The effect of interferon on sensitization is dependent on the timing of interferon administration. As reported previously, when administered to mice 24 hours *before* immunization, IF can inhibit sensitization, either to SRBC or NDV.[6,7] This timing is crucial, since, as observed recently, when given a few hours *after* the antigen interferon enhances sensitization. For example, administration of 10^6 units i.v. to C57BL/6 mice, a few hours after immunization with $10^{4.3}$ SRBC, significantly enhances footpad swelling in animals challenged 4 days later. Thus, interferon can have opposite effects on sensitization, depending on the time it acts.

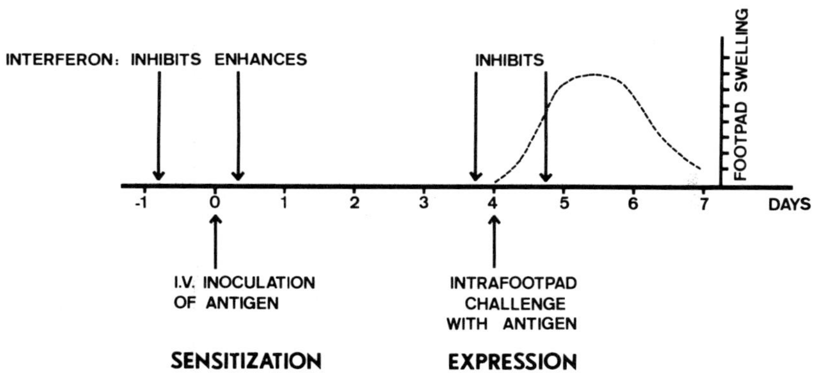

FIGURE 1. A schematic overview of the effects of exogenous interferon on sensitization or expression of delayed hypersensitivity in the mouse.

Evidence That Interferon Itself Is Responsible for These Different Effects on Delayed Hypersensitivity

Until recently, mouse interferon had not been purified to homogeneity, and there remained some legitimate doubt as to whether the nonantiviral effects, including those on the immune system, were due to interferon itself. In collaboration with I. Gresser and M. Tovey, we have recently shown that electrophoretically pure mouse interferon does have many of the varied biological effects previously described with crude or partially purified interferon preparations, including the effects on delayed hypersensitivity in the mouse.[8,9] The latter finding is important for the interpretation of the results presented in this paper, since it establishes beyond any reasonable doubt that we are indeed dealing with effects of interferon, and not of other substances contaminating interferon preparations or induced *in vivo* concomitantly with interferon.

Search for an Experimental System Allowing an Approach to the Question of Regulation

Interferon then is capable of influencing the afferent and efferent pathways of DH to picryl chloride, SRBC or NDV, but i.v. or i.p. inoculation of exogenous interferon into a mouse before or after injection of sheep red blood cells does not mirror a physiological situation, and hence does not allow for any extrapolation as to a possible contribution or intervention of interferon in the establishment or expression of DH. Moreover, interferon is not even induced by SRBC in the mouse. (We could not detect any antiviral activity in the serum of mice at various times after primary or secondary inoculation of SRBC.) Two conclusions can be drawn from the experiments summarized above: (1) type I IF has immunomodulating properties; (2) the presence of interferon as a result of viral infection can affect delayed hypersensitivity to other, unrelated antigens, as shown by the effect on SRBC DH in If-1^l and If-1^h NDV-infected mice.[5] Nevertheless, these immunopharmacological actions of interferon raise the possibility of an immunophysiological activity as well. In this respect, two pertinent questions arise:

(1) Does interferon, produced as a result of viral infection, influence the establishment of CMI to the interferon-inducing virus, and if this is the case,

(2) can this influence be called a regulatory effect?

This problem was approached by studying DH to NDV in If-1^l and If-1^h mice, and the results will be presented here in some detail. Concerning the If-1 locus itself, the reader is referred to the original publications and to a recent more general review on If-loci in the mouse.[10–12]

The If-1 system was chosen because it specifically and exclusively (within the limits of the viruses tested, obviously) influences interferon levels induced by NDV and not by other viruses. Therefore, several control experiments in which the role of interferon can be specifically examined become possible. If-1 has two alleles, l and h, and If-1^h mice, after i.v. inoculation, produce about 10 times more circulating interferon than If-1^l mice. BALB/c mice are If-1^l and C57BL/6 If-1^h. These two mouse strains have been chosen for our experiments because seven recombinant inbred and many congenic lines, derived from them by D.W. Bailey, are available.[13] Of these, the congenic B6.C-H-28^c-If-1^l line is of particular interest since the c allele at H-28 together with the l allele at If-1 was introduced into the C57BL/6 background.[11] This strain has been useful for studying the effect of NDV-induced interferon on cell-mediated immunity.

To study CMI to NDV, we have developed a test for measuring DH to this virus, based upon the footpad swelling test first described by Gray and Jennings[14] and extensively studied by Crowle[15] and by Lagrange and Mackanness.[16] A number of criteria were applied to ensure that the test is specific for NDV and truly measures delayed hypersensitivity. This test consists of sensitization through i.v. inoculation of virus; no other route of sensitizing has been investigated. Five days later the sensitized animals receive an inoculation of the same virus into the left hind footpad, and footpad swelling is then measured, with calipers, at different intervals: swelling is expressed as the difference in footpad thickness between the inoculated and the uninoculated hind footpad. A period of 5 days between sensitization and challenge was adopted because testing at daily intervals after sensitization of different groups of mice has shown that the maximal reaction occurs if the animals are challenged on day 5. Also determined was the optimal amount of NDV (expressed in PFU measured in chick embryo fibroblasts), used to sensitize and to challenge. Optimal results are obtained by using 5×10^6 PFU, suspended in 0.2 ml of PBS, for sensitization and for footpad challenge by using 1 × 10^7 PFU in 50 μl. A higher dose of NDV was not tested. Lower doses of virus gave proportionally less reaction than the highest dose tested, and subsequently adopted routinely. The specificity of the reaction measured 24 and 48 hours after footpad challenge was ascertained by sensitizing mice with various control preparations, followed by challenge with NDV, and also by sensitizing with NDV and challenging with different control preparations. As summarized in FIGURE 2, the footpad swelling measured 48 hours after challenge is specifically provoked by a reaction to the injected NDV.

Anatomo-pathological examination of the footpads 24 and 72 hours after challenge, revealed massive infiltration first by polynuclears followed by monocytes and macrophages.

DELAYED HYPERSENSITIVITY TO NEWCASTLE DISEASE VIRUS IN BALB/c AND C57BL/6 MICE AND GENETIC ANALYSIS

When footpad swelling of NDV-sensitized BALB/c and C57BL/6 mice is compared, the 24-hour reaction is quite similar in both strains, although slightly but not significantly higher in C57BL/6 mice. However, at 48 hours, there is no longer any appreciable swelling in BALB/c mice, whereas the reaction of C57BL/6 mice is at least as pronounced as at 24 hours, and even at 72 hours C57BL/6 mice still have significant swelling (FIGURE 3). In fact, when 48-hour measurements are plotted for C57BL/6 and BALB/c mice, the latter appear as nonresponders, and for all further genetic analysis and comparison of different generations and strains, the 48-hour measurements will be used. The difference between BALB/c and C57BL/6 is not due to the fact that optimal conditions for sensitization and timing of challenge are different for these two strains, since experiments on timing and dosage of antigen have ruled out differences in that area. One cannot ascribe the poor response of BALB/c to a general incapacity of these mice to mount a more pronounced DH reaction, since when BALB/c and

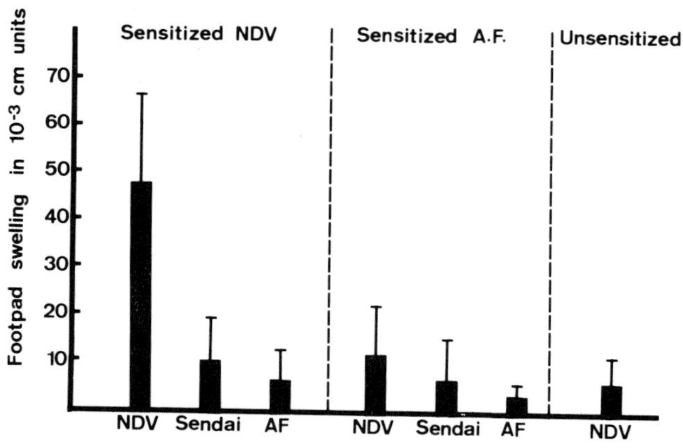

FIGURE 2. Evidence that the footpad swelling in mice is specific for Newcastle disease virus. Groups consisting of 6 C57BL/6 mice each were inoculated intravenously with a suspension of egg-grown NDV or of allantoic fluid, at a 1/15 dilution in phosphate-buffered saline. Five days later the mice were challenged into their footpads either with NDV, Sendai virus, or allantoic fluid. Average 48-hr footpad swelling ± S.D. is given.

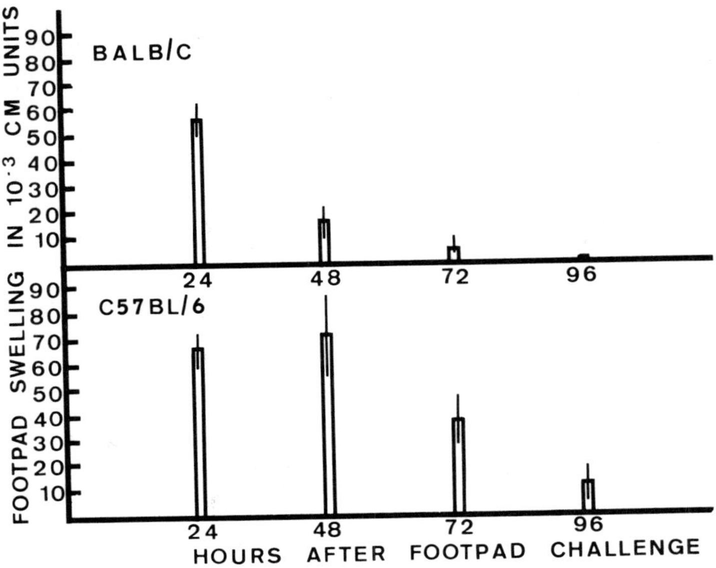

FIGURE 3. Expression of DH to NDV when challenged 5 days after sensitization. Mean 48-hr footpad swelling in BALB/c versus C57BL/6 mice. There were six mice per group and the animals were 3 months old.

C57BL/6 mice are compared for DH to SRBC, using a similar footpad swelling test, both strains react identically. The possibility that the enhanced reaction of C57BL/6 to NDV is related to the high interferon production of this strain when this virus is inoculated was therefore considered. Large amounts of interferon appear in the circulation after i.v. inoculation of NDV and, in view of the fact that interferon, given a few hours *after* the antigen, stimulates sensitization, as shown in experiments with SRBC, it seemed possible that the higher interferon production in C57BL/6 mice was responsible for their enhanced footpad reaction. This possibility received experimental support when the congenic B6.C-H-28^c If-1^l strain was compared with its C57BL/6 If-1^h inbred partner.

DH to NDV in the If-1^l congenic mice is much more of BALB/c than of C57BL/6 type, since at 48 hours very little footpad swelling remains (TABLE 1), which strongly suggests that the allele at If-1 influences the degree of DH to NDV, possibly by enhancing sensitization in If-1^h animals. However, since the congenic strains used differ from C57BL/6 by more than the allele at the If-1 locus, even the results in the congenic lines, however suggestive, are no definite proof for an involvement of interferon. Therefore, additional evidence was sought by giving extra interferon on the one hand, and by using anti-interferon serum or globulin on the other hand. The low reaction of B6.C-H-28^c If-1^l mice can be significantly enhanced if these animals receive exogenous interferon 3 and 6 hours after sensitization, in an attempt to mimic the high interferon levels of C57BL/6 mice. This result shows that, as is the case for SRBC, sensitization to NDV can be stimulated by interferon, and that by giving additional interferon to a low interferon producer a cumulative effect of endogenous and exogenous interferon is obtained. The converse experiment is carried out by treating mice

TABLE 1

FORTY-EIGHT HOUR FOOTPAD SWELLING IN PARENTAL AND CONGENIC STRAINS*

	C57BL/6	BALB/c	B6.C-H-28^c-If-1^1
Number of mice	21	18	23
Average footpad swelling	61	10	16
S.D.	21	10	13

*All mice were sensitized with 5×10^6 PFU of NDV, and challenged into their footpads five days later.

with anti-interferon goat serum or globulin, 15 minutes after sensitization with NDV, with the purpose of neutralizing as much as possible of the interferon induced by the virus. This treatment results in a significant decrease in footpad reaction when the animals are challenged five days later, and compared to untreated mice or mice that have received control goat serum or control goat globulin (FIGURE 4). In a control experiment, using SRBC instead of NDV as antigen, it was shown that anti-interferon serum or globulin has no effect on

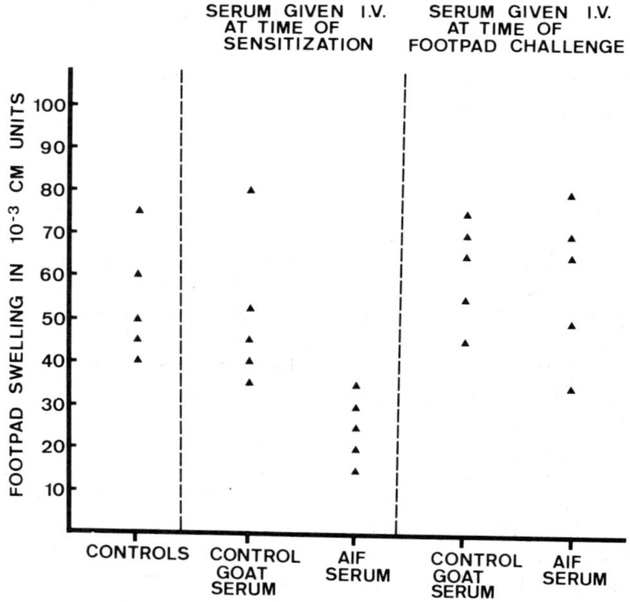

FIGURE 4. Effect of AIF serum on sensitization and expression of DH to NDV in C57BL/6 mice. Five groups consisting each of five 3-month-old male C57BL/6 mice were sensitized to NDV. Fifteen minutes after inoculation of the virus, the mice of one group received an i.v. inoculation of 0.15 ml of goat anti-interferon serum, titering 1/500,000 when measured against 4 units of mouse interferon (AIF). A second group received 0.15 ml i.v. of a control goat serum. Five days later, just before footpad challenge, a third group received also 0.15 ml of anti-interferon serum, and a fourth group 0.15 ml of control goat serum. Footpad swelling was measured 24 and 48 hours later, and, as can be seen from the figure, was only significantly inhibited in the group that received the AIF serum right after sensitization.

sensitization with SRBC, indicating that in the case of NDV the effect is obtained through the anti-interferon action and not through some other effect on sensitization in general.

The fact that giving additional interferon after virus inoculation augments DH, whereas inhibiting the action of interferon produced as a result of virus inoculation decreases DH, strengthens the conclusion arrived at in the congenic strains and provides further evidence for an involvement of interferon in sensitization to NDV. This permits the conclusion that the decreased DH in the B6.C-H-28^c If-1^l congenic strain can be ascribed to the fact that this strain carries the l allele of If-1, unlike the C57BL/6 strain. Further evidence is obtained by comparing DH to Sendai virus in these same two strains. Circulating interferon production with this virus is identical both in B57BL/6 and B6.C-H-28^c since other loci, different from If-1, are involved in the quantitative control of interferon induction by Sendai virus.[10] When DH to Sendai is measured, no difference between C57BL/6 and B6.C-H-28^c If-1^l is observed.

Evidence That Loci Other Than If-1 Are Also Involved in Determining the Degree of Delayed Hypersensitivity to Newcastle Disease Virus

When DH to NDV is examined in the seven RI strains derived from BALB/c and C57BL/6, none of the strains reacts like C57BL/6, and the reaction in all seven strains, even in the three that are If-1^h, is much closer to BALB/c (Table 2).

Table 2

Forty-Eight Hour Footpad Swelling in Parental and Recombinant Inbred Lines

	BALB/c	C57BL/6	CXBD	CXBE	CXBG	CXBH	CXBI	CXBJ	CXBK
Allele at If-1	l	h	l	l	h	h	l	l	h
Number of mice	18	21	15	17	15	18	21	13	11
Average footpad swelling	10	61	9	8	11	10	17	17	30
S.D.	10	21	8	8	12	7	16	15	22

This means that, in addition to If-1, other loci, present in the C57BL/6 background, are required for high DH to develop. This is further borne out by studying segregation of If-1 and DH to NDV in F2 and F1 × C57BL backcross progeny. To type the mice for the allele at If-1 a blood sample is taken 8 hours after i.v. sensitization with NDV for measurement of interferon levels. Five days later, the same animals are challenged in their footpads and 48-hour footpad swelling is measured.

Out of 117 F2 progeny, only 4 have DH reactions comparable to C57BL/6 values, which indicates that several genes are involved in the inheritance of this C57BL/6 trait. This is confirmed by the results of the F1 × C57BL/6 backcross. Out of 43 progeny, only 6 have DH of a magnitude comparable to the mean C57BL/6 value, again indicating the multiple factorial inheritance of this trait. The high responders for DH all are If-1^h as determined from their interferon levels measured after sensitization, but obviously, many If-1^h progeny do not have high DH values. The result confirms the observations in RI strains, and shows that although the h allele at If-1 is a necessary condition for high DH to develop, it is not sufficient by itself, and several other genes present in the C57BL/6 background are involved. Preliminary evidence indicates that one or several of these determine susceptibility to interferon action both on the afferent and efferent pathway of DH. C57BL/6 mice are more susceptible than are BALB/c mice to the sensitization-enhancement effect of interferon, as shown by experiments in which mice of both strains are sensitized with suboptimal amounts of SRBC, followed by an intravenous inoculation of interferon (FIGURE 5). On the contrary, C57BL/6 mice are less susceptible to the sensitization-depressing effect of interferon, as shown in experiments in which animals of both strains received an identical amount of interferon, intravenously, followed a few hours later by sensitization with SRBC. B6.C-H-28^c If-1^l mice in both respects behave like C57BL/6, indicating that the genes responsible for this difference in susceptibility to interferon *action* are not linked to H-28 or If-1.

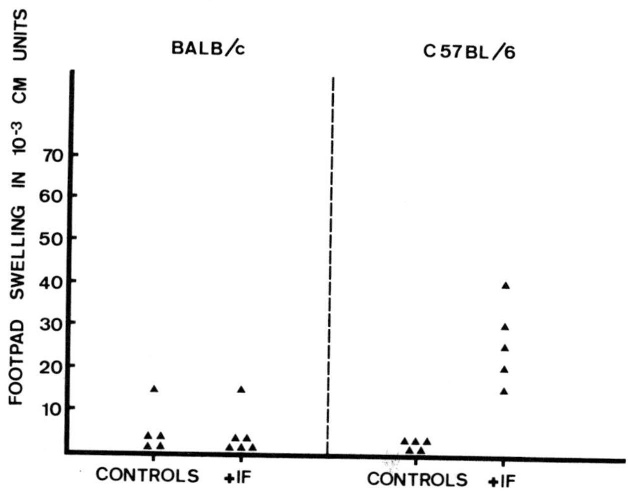

FIGURE 5. Effect of interferon on sensitization with subminimal dose of SRBC (48-hr reaction). Female 3-month-old BALB/c and C57BL/6 mice were sensitized i.v. with $10^{4.3}$ SRBC. Three hours after sensitization, one group of each strain received an i.v. inoculation of 1 ml of interferon titering 10^5 units/0.2 ml (+ IF). Intrafootpad challenge was administered 4 days later. The figure represents the 48-hr footpad swelling. Each triangle corresponds to the individual value obtained for one mouse.

DISCUSSION

Type I interferon can affect both afferent and efferent pathways of DH to antigens of viral and nonviral origin, which by itself does not signify that it is a normal component of the DH reaction. Indeed type I interferon is mainly, though not exclusively, induced by viruses and most antigens do not trigger its production.

From our results and those of others, it appears that type I interferon is an immunomodulator, without antigen-specificity; a distinguishing characteristic of this immunomodulator is that it can be made by practically any cell of the organism. Unlike type II interferon or lymphokines in general, type I interferon does not require for its synthesis previous contact of the host with the virus, nor is this a specialized function of T or B cells. When infected by a virus or in the presence of dsRNA, most cells are capable of producing type I interferon and they can thus directly affect the activity of the specialized cells of the immune system; type I interferon is a message that various body cells can use for influencing the activity of the immune system.

DH is one parameter of CMI, and its essential effector cells are T cells. We now have to ask the question how interferon either depresses or stimulates T-cell activity, depending on whether it acts before or after sensitization. The cell multiplication inhibitory effect of IF, as witnessed for example by inhibition of blast formation *in vivo*[17] could explain the inhibition of sensitization that is observed when interferon is given 24 hours before the antigen, since upon antigenic stimulation, T-cell progenitors within lymphoid tissue transform into blast cells, divide and give rise to progeny with effector function.[18] More difficult to explain is the stimulation of sensitization occurring when interferon is administered *after* the antigen; inhibition of formation of specific suppressor cells can be envisaged, if one wants to cling to the anti-blastogenic effect of interferon as the sole mechanism, that explains it all. Although suppressor T cells have been mainly described in the control of antibody formation, there is some evidence that cells of the Te subclass (Ly 1,2,3) also contribute to the regulation of cellular immunity.[19]

Whatever the mechanism, these effects of interferon on DH can be called immunopharmacological, since they are obtained by treating animals with interferon in a situation where normally there is no interferon production, such as sensitization to SRBC. However, the results obtained in the NDV-inoculated animals, in which the effect of endogenous, NDV-induced, interferon on DH to NDV is examined, provide evidence for an immunophysiological role for type I interferon as well. It is clear that type I interferon induced by NDV influences the establishment of DH to this virus by stimulating sensitization; in its turn the level of interferon synthesis directly determines the intensity of DH, since on a C57BL/6 background, the presence of the h or the l allele at If-1 determines the intensity and duration of DH. How this stimulation takes place is presently a matter of conjecture; it may be due to inhibition of suppressor cell formation, as discussed above. This will be studied using *in vivo* cell transfer experiments and by *in vitro* experiments using NDV-infected target cells as in the systems developed by Kozinowski *et al.* for Sendai virus.[19,20] There are several other examples of enhancement of activity after interferon treatment. Interferon can stimulate various *in vitro* activities of lymphocytes and macrophages such as toxicity for target cells of T cells and of NK cells[21,22] and phagocytosis by macrophages.[23] In this respect, the observations of Manejias *et al.* are particularly relevant to our work, since these authors observed that the presence of the h allele at If-1 was instrumental in stimulating macrophage activity after the i.v. inoculation of NDV into mice.[24]

In many respects, If-1 can be considered to function as an immune response locus, specific for NDV and regulating the level of DH. However, the simple correlation that high IF production means high DH and low IF production low DH does not hold, as shown by the results obtained in RI strains and the F2 and backcross generations. When DH to NDV is measured in the seven RI strains, and in F2 and backgross progeny, it is evident that segregation between If-1 and high or low DH is possible, and that high interferon production alone is not sufficient to stimulate DH. Other genes, present in the C57BL/6 background are involved in determining the effect of interferon on DH, and only when they are present in the combination found in C57BL/6 does interferon have its maximal stimulatory effect on DH. This is furthermore borne out by the fact that exogenous interferon, when given after sensitization with an antigen such as SRBC, stimulates sensitization more in C57BL/6 than in BALB/c.

The segregational analysis of If-1 and DH in F2 and backcross mice indicates that several genes are involved in determining the level of response to interferon, since in only a few of these animals did the presence of the h allele stimulate DH to a level comparable to that of C57BL/6.

Summary

The effect of type I interferon production on immunity to the interferon-inducing virus was examined using the Newcastle disease virus (NDV)-mouse model and comparing If-1^h and If-1^l animals. The degree of cell-mediated immunity, as measured by delayed hypersensitivity (DH) to NDV, was influenced by the levels of interferon produced. Anti-interferon globulin given immediately after immunization decreased sensitization to NDV, whereas additional, exogenous, interferon, given to low interferon producers, stimulated sensitization to NDV. The alleles at the If-1 locus influenced the extent of DH to NDV, in that If-1^h mice developed much stronger DH than did If-1^l mice. However, results from recombinant inbred strains, F_2 and backcross generations showed that for high interferon production to stimulate DH to NDV, other genes, present in the C57BL/6 background but as yet not characterized, are required. Thus DH to NDV is determined on the one hand by the alleles at If-1, influencing interferon production, and on the other hand by a combination of several genes affecting the interaction of interferon with cells of the immune system.

References

1. Sercarz, E., L. A. Herzenberg & C. F. Fox, Eds. 1977. Immune System: Genetics and Regulation. Academic Press, Inc. New York.
2. Waksman, B. H. 1979. Adjuvants and immune regulation by lymphoid cells. Springer Seminars in Immunopathol. **2:** 5–33.
3. Epstein, L. B. 1977. The effects of interferons on the immune response in vitro and in vivo. *In* Interferons and Their Actions. W. Stewart II, Ed.: 92–132, CRC Press. Cleveland.
4. De Maeyer, E. & J. De Maeyer-Guignard. 1980. Interferons and the immune system. *In* The Immune System: Function and Therapy of Dysfunction. G. Doria and A. Eshkol, Eds.: 213–225. Academic Press. New York.
5. De Maeyer, E., J. De Maeyer-Guignard & M. Vandeputte. 1975. Inhibition by interferon of delayed-type hypersensitivity in the mouse. Proc. Nat. Acad. Sci. USA **72:** 1753–1757.
6. De Maeyer, E. 1976. Interferon and delayed-type hypersensitivity to a viral antigen. J. Infect. Dis. **133:** A63–A65.
7. De Maeyer-Guignard, J., A. Cachard & E. De Maeyer. 1975. Delayed-type hypersensitivity to sheep red blood cells: Inhibition of sensitization by interferon. Science **190:** 574–576.
8. Gresser, I., J. De Maeyer-Guignard, M. G. Tovey & E. De Maeyer. 1979. Electrophoretically pure mouse interferon exerts multiple biologic effects. Proc. Nat. Acad. Sci. USA **76:** 5308–5312.
9. De Maeyer, E. & J. De Maeyer-Guignard. Effects of interferon on sensitization and

expression of delayed hypersensitivity in the mouse. *In* Proceedings of the Second International Lymphokine Workshop. A. de Weck and M. Landy, Eds. In press.

10. De Maeyer, E. & J. De Maeyer-Guignard. 1969. Gene with quantitative effect on circulating interferon induced by Newcastle disease virus. J. Virol. **3:** 506–512.
11. De Maeyer, E., J. De Maeyer-Guignard & D. W. Bailey. 1975. Effect of mouse genotype on interferon production. Lines congenic at the If-1 locus. Immunogenetics **1:** 438–445.
12. De Maeyer, E. & J. De Maeyer-Guignard. 1979. Considerations on mouse genes influencing interferon production and action. *In* Interferon 1979. I. Gresser, Ed.: 75–99. Academic Press. London.
13. Bailey, D. W. 1971. Recombinant inbred-strains: An aid to finding identity, linkage and function of histocompatibility and other genes. Transplantation **11:** 325–327.
14. Gray, D. F. & P. A. Jennings. 1955. Allergy in Experimental Mouse Tuberculosis. Am. Rev. Tuberc. **72:** 171–195.
15. Crowle, A. J. 1975. Delayed hypersensitivity in the mouse. Adv. Immunol. **20:** 197–264.
16. Lagrange, P. H., G. B. Mackaness & T. E. Miller. 1974. Influence of dose and route of antigen injection on the immunological induction of T cells. J. Exp. Med. **139:** 528–542.
17. Lindahl, P., P. Leary & I. Gresser. 1972. Interferon inhibits DNA synthesis induced in mouse lymphocyte suspensions by phytohaemagglutinin or by allogeneic cells. Nature New Biol. **237:** 120–121.
18. Cantor, H. & E. Boyse. 1977. Regulation of the immune response by T cell subclasses. *In* Contemporary Topics in Immunobiology. O. Stutman, Ed. Vol. **7:** 47–67. Plenum Press. New York.
19. Gething, M. J., U. Koszinowski & M. Waterfield. 1978. Fusion of Sendai virus with the target cell membrane is required for T cell cytotoxocity. Nature **274:** 689–691.
20. Koszinowski, U. H. & M. M. Simon. 1979. Generation of virus specific tytotoxic T cells in vitro. I. Induction conditions of primary and secondary Sendai virus specific cytotoxic T cells. Eur. J. Immunol. **9:** 715–722.
21. Lindahl, P., P. Leary & I. Gresser. 1972. Enhancement by interferon of the specific toxicity of sensitized lymphocytes. Proc. Nat. Acad. Sci. USA **69:** 721–725.
22. Gidlund, M., A. Orn, H. Wigzell, A. Senik & I. Gresser. 1978. Enhanced NK cell activity in mice injected with interferon and interferon inducers. Nature **273:** 759–761.
23. Rabinovitch, M., R. E. Manejias, M. Russo & E. E. Abbey. 1977. Increased spreading of macrophages from mice treated with interferon inducers. Cell. Immunol. **29:** 86–95.
24. Manejias, R. E., S. I. Hamburg & M. Rabinovitch. 1978. Serum interferon and phagocytic activity of macrophages in recombinant inbred mice inoculated with Newcastle disease virus. Cell. Immunol. **38:** 209–213.

INTERFERON-INDUCED DISEASE IN MICE AND RATS*

Ion Gresser,† Liliane Morel-Maroger,‡ Yves Rivière,§
Jean-Claude Guillon,§ and Michael G. Tovey†

†Institut de Recherches Scientifiques sur le Cancer
94800 Villejuif, France

‡Hôpital Tenon
Paris, France 75020

§Institut Pasteur
Paris, France 75724

David Woodrow, John C. Sloper, and Jill Moss

Charing Cross Hospital
London W6 8RF England

Interferon is a potent antiviral protein. There are abundant experimental data indicating that the production of interferon in the course of viral infections is an integral part of the host response; and interferon treatment of animals and (recently) man is associated with prophylactic and therapeutic antiviral effects. For many years most investigators believed that interferon inhibited viral multiplication within the cell without affecting host cell metabolism or function. It is now widely accepted however that interferon can also affect cell division and function both in cell culture and in the animal. If this is so, we might expect to find instances in which too much interferon, instead of being beneficial, might even prove inimical to the host. This is the subject of our presentation.

When newborn mice were inoculated daily from birth subcutaneously or intraperitonealy with potent mouse interferon preparations¶ there was a progressive inhibition of growth in the first week of life; the mean weight of interferon-treated mice was 60 to 80% of the weight of control inoculated litter mates. When interferon treatment was continued for the next few days, *all* of the interferon-treated mice died (TABLE 1A).[1] At autopsy, the most striking abnormality was a pale grey liver. Light microscopic examination revealed a marked steatosis, large areas of cell degeneration, and necrosis without any inflammatory reaction (FIGURE 1). The only other abnormalities on light microscopic examination were some diminution of the cortical region of the thymus in some mice, and poorly differentiated germinal follicles in the spleens of most mice. No renal lesions were present. Examination of liver sections under the electron microscope showed a marked accumulation of fat in hepatocytes. No viral particles were observed.[1]

In these experiments, interferon treatment proved lethal only when begun on the day of birth and continued daily for the first week of life. When treatment was initiated on day 6 and continued daily for 14 days, mice grew normally and liver lesions were not observed. The effect of interferon on newborn mice

*This work was aided by grants from the Direction de Recherches et Etudes Techniques (78-34-210), the Institut National de la Santé et de la Recherche Médicale (ATP 44-76-76, 78-82/15, 47-77, 78-94).

¶.05 ml of interferon having a titer of 8×10^{-5} reference units.

0077-8923/80/0350-0012 $01.75/0 © 1980, NYAS

TABLE 1

EFFECTS OF TREATMENT OF SUCKLING MICE WITH MOUSE INTERFERON

			Injected with				
	Mouse Strain	Number of* Experiments	Mouse† Interferon	Control Preparation	Inactivated Mouse Interferon	Human Interferon	Uninoculated
A. Lethality of mouse interferon preparations (Daily interferon treatment continued)	Swiss	5	107/107‡	0/52	0/15	0/23	0/142
	C_3H	1	15/15	0/30	0/15	NT	0/18
B. Development of glomerulonephritis§ (Daily interferon treatment stopped at day 6 to 8)	Swiss	9	60/60¶	0/50	0/18	1/18	2/65
	C_3H	1	13/17	—	—	—	0/13

*For experimental details see references 1 and 2.
†Mice injected daily subcutaneously with 0.05 ml of a C-243 cell interferon preparation (titer 3.2×10^{-6} reference units).
‡Number of mice deal/total number of mice injected. Mean day of death = 11 days.
§Results pooled – mice sacrificed between 20 and 274 days of life.
¶No. of mice with histological confirmation of glomerulonephritis per total number of mice killed.

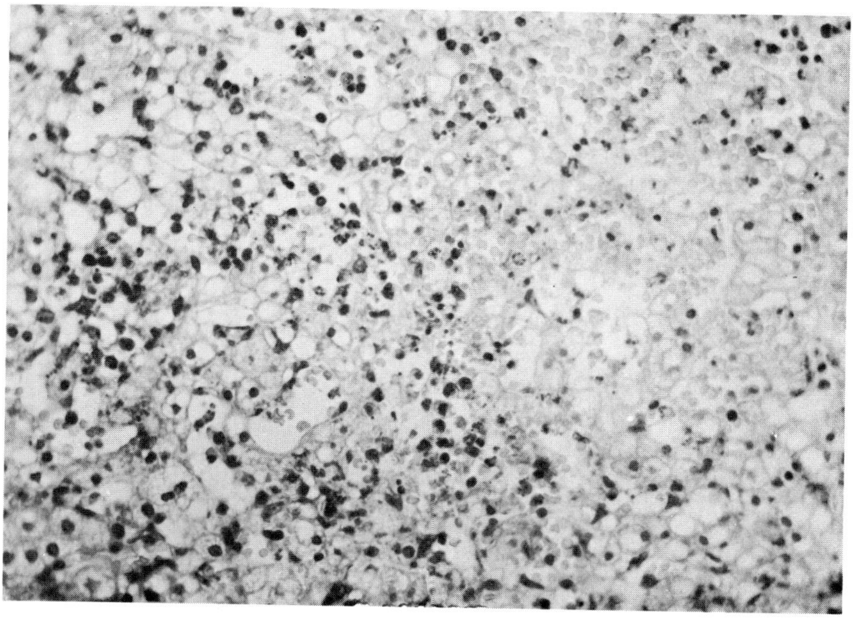

FIGURE 1. Section of liver of 9-day-old Swiss mouse treated with a highly purified mouse C-243 cell interferon preparation (titer 1.2×10^{-7}) showing marked steatosis and necrosis.

depended therefore not only on the amount of interferon administered but also on the immaturity of the host.[1]

What happened to these mice when interferon treatment, begun at birth, was stopped on the seventh day of life (a time when steatosis and discrete foci of liver cell necrosis were present)? The majority of these mice appeared to recover and they gained weight. However, in the ensuing months a number of these mice died. At autopsy, although the liver and other organs appeared normal, the kidneys were pale and the surface was granular. Histologic examination revealed a severe glomerulonephritis (TABLE 1B).[2] The kidney pathology can be summarized as follows: In "early" lesions (30th day) the glomeruli appeared moderately enlarged with some thickening of the mesangium, some segmental foci of mesangial proliferation, and some thickening of capillary loops. By immunofluorescence there were focal and segmental granular deposits of IgG, IgM, and C3 in the mesangial spaces and along some glomerular basement membranes (GBM). Subsequently, the lesions were more conspicuous with hyalinization of glomerular tufts (with epithelial crescents and voluminous subendothelial deposits) (FIGURE 2). In well advanced disease, virtually all glomeruli were sclerotic and there was extensive sclerosis and diffuse atrophy of tubules. By immunofluorescence there were coarse granular deposits of IgG, IgM, and C3 along the GBM.[2]

Although glomerular lesions were first seen by light microscopy towards the 3rd week of life, electron microscopic examination of the kidneys of interferon-treated mice at 8 days of life showed a marked thickening of the glomerular basement membrane, involving mainly the lamina rara interna and characterized by lacunae containing coarse granules, fibrillary material, and finely granular electron-dense deposits.[3]

We should emphasize at this point that under our experimental conditions *all* Swiss and C3H mice treated with potent interferon preparations have shown the liver lesions described above, and *all* Swiss mice treated for the first week of life developed glomerulonephritis (TABLE 1). These syndromes have been seen in *all* strains of mice tested and also in axenic and nude mice.

These experiments had been carried out with partially purified interferon preparations having a specific activity of 10^7 reference units per mg protein. Mice were injected with approximately 50 μg of protein per day. Control preparations consisting of mock mouse interferon preparations, heated or periodate-inactivated mouse interferon preparations, or human interferon preparations did not induce disease in mice. All these preparations contained comparable amounts of protein.

Nevertheless, we wanted to determine the effect of even more purified mouse interferon preparations. Recently, we have tested highly purified mouse interferon prepared by Dr. Michel Aguet in our laboratory using methods developed by De Maeyer-Guignard *et al.*[4,5] This material had a specific activity of 0.5 to 1×10^9 units per mg of protein. After electrophoresis in polyacrylamide gels in SDS, and staining with Coomassie Blue, only three bands corresponding to molecular weights of 35,000, 28,000 and 22,000 were observed. Biological activity of interferon was found only in eluates of gel slices corresponding to these bands. We injected newborn mice with 25 μl of interferon (containing 500 nanograms of protein). We also tested the original partially purified interferon (having a

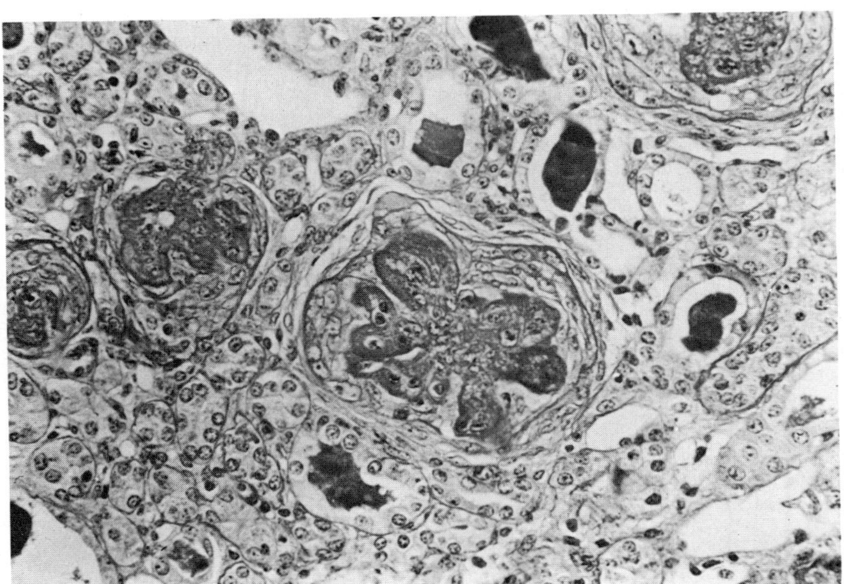

FIGURE 2. Kidney of a 36-day-old Swiss mouse treated for the first 8 days of life with a highly purified mouse C-243 cell interferon preparation (titer 1.2×10^{-7}). Note marked sclerosis of glomeruli with crescent formation.

comparable titer) and preparations containing the major contaminants collected during the purification procedures. Only partially and highly purified interferons inhibited mouse growth, delayed maturation of different organs, induced liver lesions, caused death, and induced glomerulonephritis (FIGURES 1,2). I believe therefore that there is no longer any doubt that interferon itself is the responsible factor in inducing these lesions.

Furthermore, this phenomenon is not confined to mice. When newborn rats were injected with rat interferon preparations (but not mouse or human interferon preparations) there was also a clear-cut inhibition of growth (FIGURE 3), delay in the maturation of several different organs, and the late development of glomerulonephritis.[6] Liver lesions were not observed, however.

The experiments discussed so far have concerned the use of exogenous interferon. I want now to discuss with you some of the effects of endogenous interferon induced in newborn mice by lymphocytic choriomeningitis (LCM) virus. When newborn mice of most strains were injected at birth with this virus, they grew poorly, and after the eighth day began to die. The only histological lesions observed were in the liver, which showed steatosis and focal or diffuse necrosis. Mice surviving this acute episode, subsequently developed glomerulonephritis. In other words, the syndromes induced in mice with LCM virus were identical to those induced by treatment of mice with interferon (TABLE 2). To explain this similarity of syndromes we proposed two hypotheses[8]: (1) interferon was lethal for suckling mice because it activated a latent virus (such as LCM virus) or (2) some of the manifestations of LCM virus disease in suckling mice were in fact due to endogenous interferon induced by the virus. We found no evidence to support hypothesis (1) because neither LCM virus nor mouse hepatitis virus nor any other infectious agent was recovered from the liver and kidneys of interferon-treated suckling mice.[1] We therefore turned our attention to the second hypothesis. First, we found that despite previous reports to the contrary, LCM virus induced large amounts of interferon in suckling and adult mice.[7,8] We then injected newborn mice with LCM virus and a potent sheep antiglobulin to mouse interferon.[8] Injection of this immunoglobulin neutralized the endogenous interferon and resulted in a 100-fold increase in the serum LCM virus titer. Despite this marked increase in circulating virus, anti-interferon

TABLE 2

SIMILARITY IN SYNDROMES INDUCED IN SUCKLING MICE BY INTERFERON AND LCM VIRUS

Time	Clinical Findings	Injected with: Mouse Interferon	Injected with: LCM Virus	Comments
Early 2–3 weeks	Decreased weight gain	+	+	Similar curves of weight gain
	Delay in maturation of several organs	+	+	
	Liver cell steatosis leading to necrosis	+	+	Similar histology
	Mortality	+	+	
Late >1 month	Glomerulonephritis	+	+	Similar histology Deposits of C3, IgG along GBM

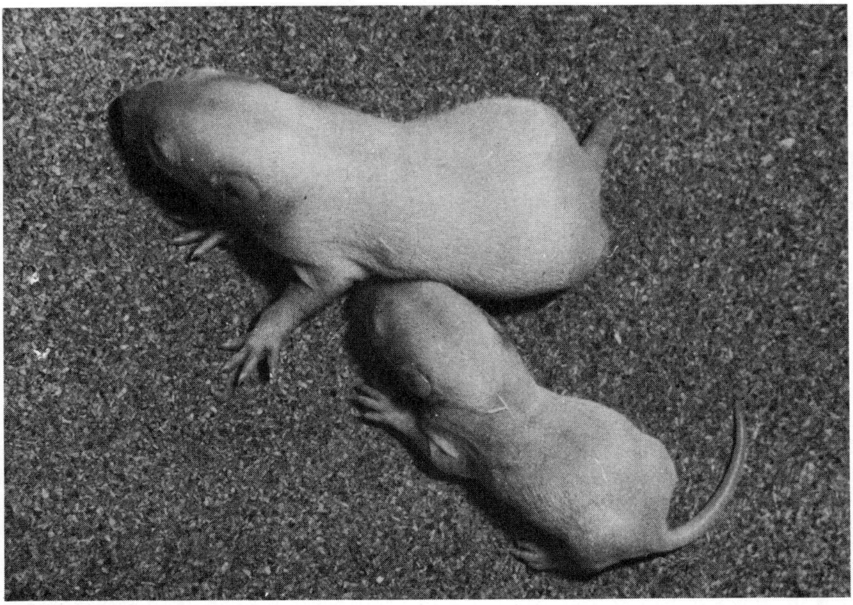

FIGURE 3. Nine-day-old suckling rats from the same litter. Above, rat inoculated daily with 0.1 ml i.p. of PBS (the tail was cut at birth to distinguish it from the interferon-treated rat). Below, suckling rat inoculated daily with a rat interferon preparation titering 1.6×10^{-6}.

globulin-treated mice grew normally, showed no liver lesions, and the incidence of death was much decreased.[8] Furthermore, injection of this anti-interferon antibody also markedly inhibited the appearance of glomerulonephritis characteristic of late LCM virus disease.[9] LCM virus was present in the blood and kidneys of these mice in amounts comparable to control virus-infected mice developing glomerulonephritis.[9]

The lethality of LCM virus for suckling mice varies with the mouse strain. We have some preliminary evidence that the genetic control of susceptibility or resistance is determined not by the extent of virus multiplication but by the amount of interferon produced. Thus, in some strains of suckling mice infected at birth with LCM virus, large amounts of interferon are produced for several days; the mice develop liver lesions and die. In another strain of mouse, although the virus multiplies to the same high titers, less interferon is produced and for a shorter period of time, and these mice survive. Subsequently, these mice show only minimal glomerulonephritis (although glomerulonephritis can be induced in this strain of mouse when they are inoculated in the first week of life with enough interferon).

We believe this ensemble of results shows that the presence of both exogenous or endogenous interferon in large quantities in an immature animal can be harmful. Furthermore, this brief exposure to interferon at a critical period of rapid growth and maturation can be an important factor in the development of disease that only becomes manifest later in life. Space does not permit me to discuss the possible mechanisms of action of interferon in inducing disease. Discussion of the various possibilities may be found in the references cited.[1-3,6,8,9] I should like instead to emphasize several points that I feel are important:

It might be argued that these effects are observed by administering large amounts of interferon to a newborn mouse or rat, or by injecting an immature animal with an esoteric virus, and therefore that these findings are perhaps of little relevance to human pathology. In a recent editorial in the *New England Journal of Medicine*,[10] Dr. F. Rosen quotes a statement of William Harvey (1651) which I offer as a partial reply:

> Nature is nowhere accustomed more openly to display her secret mysteries than in cases where she shows traces of her workings apart from the beaten path; nor is there any better way to advance the proper practice of medicine than to give our minds to the discovery of the usual law of Nature by careful investigation of cases of rarer forms of disease. For it has been found, in almost all things, that what they contain of useful or applicable nature is hardly perceived unless we are deprived of them, or they become deranged in some way.

Thus, we may ask whether there are other instances in which interferon may be in part responsible for disease. Virelizier and Allison have shown that C3H and A2G strain mice can become carriers of mouse hepatitis virus (MHV-3) and develop a progressive neurological disease lasting for weeks or months.[11] These virus carrier mice also showed a chronic interferonemia,[12] and thus the possibility exists that interferon may be exerting untoward effects in some of these mice.

Interferon does not cross the placental barrier in mice[13] and I believe for a very good reason. Pregnant animals can contract virus infections and produce circulating interferon. If interferon crossed the placenta, it might well affect the developing embryo. But what about a virus that crosses the placenta and infects the embryo? Is it possible that the embryotoxic effects ascribed to rubella virus, for example, may be related to interferon induced in the embryo itself? In other words, is it possible that cellular lesions considered heretofore as being caused by the virus are in fact caused by host substances (such as interferon) induced by the infectious agent? Recently, Hooks, Notkins and coworkers found immune interferon in the sera of patients with systemic lupus erythematosus, rheumatoid arthritis, scleroderma, and Sjögren's syndrome.[14] Serial serum samples showed a good correlation between interferon titers and disease activity, and these investigators suggested that the production of interferon might contribute to immunological aberrations in auto-immune disease.[14]

In case these speculations might be misunderstood, I should like to emphasize however that I do not feel that the results presented herein constitute an argument against the use of interferon in patients. Over the years, we have pleaded long and hard the potential clinical usefulness of exogenous interferon.[15] I have been too often witness in the past 15 years to interferon's therapeutic efficacy in viral and neoplastic diseases of mice, not to believe that comparable results would be obtained in man, were it properly used. I have also been witness to its extraordinary activity—and to the varied effects interferon exerts on cells.[16] In some instances, interferon inhibits specialized cellular functions and in other instances it enhances cellular functions.[16,17] Factors such as the amount of interferon and time of treatment can determine the biological effects observed. Aside from the theoretical interest, these considerations are of utmost importance in determining how to use interferon in patients. Our results emphasize that we are dealing with a most potent substance—and as with hormones—use of interferon must be based on knowledge of its effects and if possible of its mode of action.

Summary

Treatment of newborn mice with potent mouse interferon preparations resulted in an acute "early" syndrome characterized by inhibition of growth, delay in maturation of several organs, diffuse liver cell necrosis and death. When interferon treatment was discontinued at 1 week of life, mice appeared to recover, but subsequently developed a progressive glomerulonephritis ("late syndrome").

Treatment of newborn rats with potent rat interferon preparations also resulted in inhibition of growth, delay in maturation, and the subsequent development of glomerulonephritis.

After infection at birth with lymphocytic choriomeningitis (LCM) virus, most strains of mice developed a similar acute early syndrome and surviving mice subsequently developed glomerulonephritis. We postulated that the endogenous interferon induced by LCM virus early in life was partially responsible for these syndromes. Administration of a potent anti-mouse interferon serum to LCM virus-infected mice neutralized the circulating endogenous interferon and inhibited the development of both the early and late syndromes.

Our results suggest that large amounts of exogenous or endogenous interferon at a crucial stage of rapid growth or development of mice and rats can induce lesions in several different organs. Some lesions (i.e. the kidney) only become apparent weeks or even months after exposure to interferon.

References

1. Gresser, I., M. G. Tovey, C. Maury & I. Chouroulinkov. 1975. Lethality of interferon preparations for new-born mice. Nature **258:** 76–78.
2. Gresser, I., L. Morel-Maroger, C. Maury, M. G. Tovey & F. Pontillon. 1976. Progressive glomerulonephritis in mice treated with interferon preparations at birth. Nature **263:** 420–422.
3. Morel-Maroger, L., J. C. Sloper, J. Vinter, D. Woodrow & I. Gresser. 1978. Lab. Invest. **39:** 513–522.
4. Sipe, J. D., J. De Maeyer, B. Fauconnier & E. De Maeyer 1973. Purification of mouse interferon by affinity chromatography on a solid-base immunoadsorbent. Proc. Nat. Acad. Sci. USA **70:** 1037–1040.
5. De Maeyer, J., M. G. Tovey, I. Gresser & E. De Maeyer. 1978. Purification of mouse interferon by sequential affinity chromatography on poly(U)-and antibody-agarose columns. Nature **271:** 622–625.
6. Gresser, I., L. Morel-Maroger, F. Chatelet, C. Maury, M. G. Tovey, M-T. Bandu, J. Buywid & M. Delauche. 1979. Delay in growth and the development of nephritis in rats treated with interferon preparations in the neonatal period. Am. J. Pathol. **95:** 329–346.
7. Riviere, Y. & M-T. Bandu. 1977. Induction d'interféron par le virus de la chorioméningite lymphocytaire chez la souris. Ann. Microbiol. (Institut Pasteur) **128A:** 323–329.
8. Riviere, Y., I. Gresser, J-C. Guillon & M. G. Tovey. 1977. Inhibition by anti-interferon serum of lymphocytic choriomeningitis virus disease in suckling mice. Proc. Nat. Acad. Sci. USA **74:** 2135–2139.

9. GRESSER, I., L. MOREL-MAROGER, P. VERROUST, Y. RIVIERE & J-C. GUILLON. 1978. Anti-interferon globulin inhibits the development of glomerulonephritis in mice infected at birth with lymphocytic choriomeningitis virus. Proc. Nat. Acad. Sci. USA **75:** 3413–3416.
10. ROSEN, F. S. 1979. Lead exposure among children—a reassessment. New Engl. J. Med. **300:** 732–.
11. VIRELIZIER, J-L., A. D. DAYAN & A. C. ALLISON. 1975. Neuropathological effects of persistent infection of the mouse by mouse hepatitis virus (MHV-3). Infect. Immun. **12:** 1127–1140.
12. VIRELIZIER, J-L., A-M. VIRELIZIER & A. C. ALLISON. 1976. The role of circulating interferon in the modifications of immune responsiveness by mouse hepatitis virus (MHV-3). J. Immunol. **117:** 748–753.
13. GRESSER, I. (Unpublished observations).
14. HOOKS, J. J., H. M. MOUTSOPOULOS, S. A. GEIS, N. I. STAHL, J. L. DECKER & A. L. NOTKINS. 1979. Immune interferon in the circulation of patients with autoimmune disease. New Engl. J. Med. **301:** 5–8.
15. GRESSER, I. 1971. *In* Third International Symposium on Medical and Applied Virology. M. Sanders & M. Schaeffer, Eds.: 416–429. Reprinted *from* Viruses Affecting Man and Animals. W. H. Green. St. Louis, MO.
16. GRESSER, I. 1977. On the varied biologic effects of interferon. Cell. Immunol. **34:** 406–415.
17. GRESSER, I. & M. G. TOVEY. 1978. Antitumor effects of interferon. Biochem. Biophys. Acta **516:** 231–247.

THE ROLE OF INTERFERON IN IMMEDIATE HYPERSENSITIVITY AND AUTOIMMUNE DISEASES

John J. Hooks,* Haralampos M. Moutsopoulos,† and
Abner Louis Notkins*

**Laboratory of Oral Medicine and*
†Clinical Immunology Section
National Institute of Dental Research
National Institutes of Health
Bethesda, Maryland 20205

INTRODUCTION

During the past decade, it has become apparent that interferon can affect a variety of biological activities, including immune functions.[1-3] Moreover, we now know that there are at least two types of interferon. Type I or standard interferon is produced by both nonlymphoid and lymphoid cells in response to viruses, polynucleotides and endotoxin.[4] Type II or immune interferon is a lymphokine that sensitized lymphocytes produce in response to specific antigens and antigen-antibody complexes.[5-9] In this report, we review some of our recent findings on two aspects of the immunoregulatory actions of interferon: (1) the enhancement of IgE-mediated histamine release (immediate hypersensitivity); and (2) the presence of interferon in the circulation of patients with autoimmune diseases.

INTERFERON IN IMMEDIATE HYPERSENSITIVITY

Clinical studies dating back almost 40 years have suggested that upper respiratory tract infections can precipitate or potentiate attacks of bronchial asthma.[10-13] On the basis of these clinical observations, we decided to investigate the role of viruses in allergic reactions.

The release of histamine from basophils of allergic individuals after stimulation with ragweed antigen E or anti-IgE is a reliable *in vitro* model for immediate hypersensitivity reactions.[14] A schematic representation of the release of histamine and other mediators from basophils is shown in FIGURE 1. The host's exposure to allergen can trigger the lymphocytes (plasma cells) to produce allergen-specific IgE antibodies. These IgE antibodies bind to receptors on the surface of peripheral blood basophils. The interaction between the allergen and IgE on the cell surface results in the bridging of IgE molecules. This reaction initiates a series of events resulting in the release of the pharmacological mediators of anaphylaxis (e.g., histamine, serotinin, slow reacting substance of anaphylaxis and eosinophil chemotactic factor).

The *in vitro* assay system for histamine release that we used involved incubating human peripheral blood leukocytes with serial dilutions of a stimulant (ragweed antigen E or anti-human IgE), and the percent of histamine release was determined by an automated fluorometric technique.[10,14] First, we asked whether viruses can induce basophils to release histamine. Our initial experiments demonstrated that viruses did not directly cause the release of histamine; that is, leukocyte cultures incubated with viruses (HSV, influenza or adenovirus), but

0077-8923/80/0350-0021 $01.75/0

not exposed to ragweed antigen, failed to release histamine. Next, we asked whether viruses could influence IgE-mediated release of histamine. Leukocytes were incubated with infectious viruses or control media for 24 hours and then the cells were challenged with anti-IgE for 45 minutes and the amount of histamine released into the supernatant fluids was determined. The results of a typical experiment with the cells from one individual are shown in FIGURE 2. Leukocytes that had been treated with HSV, influenza or adenovirus showed enhanced histamine release when exposed to anti-IgE ($p < 0.001$).

Additional studies demonstrated that UV-inactivated viruses enhanced IgE-mediated histamine release as efficiently as live viruses. Because enhancement of histamine release did not require virus replication, we next tested the

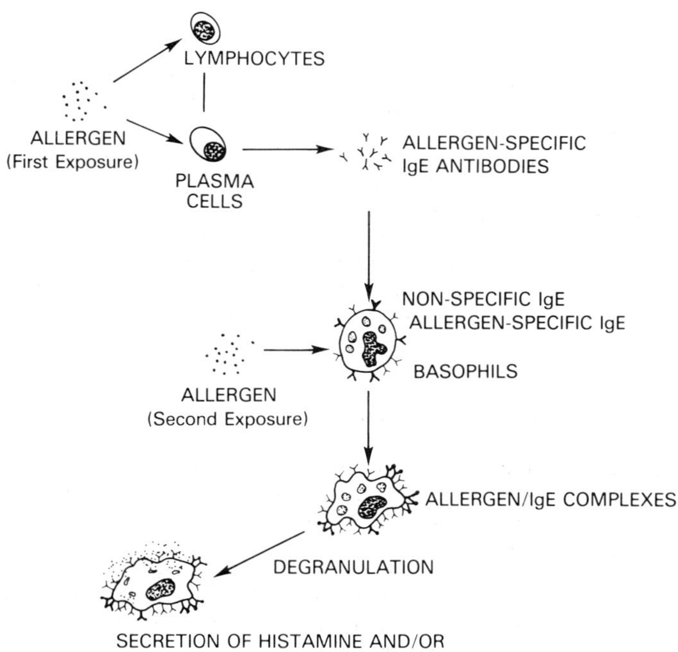

FIGURE 1. Schema of specific allergen-induced histamine release.

possibility that the increase might be caused by virus-induced interferon. We found that there is a temporal relationship between the capacity of viruses to augment IgE-mediated histamine release and the induction of interferon. Additional studies showed that the increase of histamine release was in fact due to interferon induced by viruses. As is seen in TABLE 1, the antiviral and the histamine-release enhancing activities of interferon preparations could not be dissociated. Moreover, an induction period and new RNA synthesis were required for interferon to exert its effect.[15]

Because interferon is produced by immune lymphocytes in response to specific antigens, we next studied the effect of specific antigen stimulation.[16] In

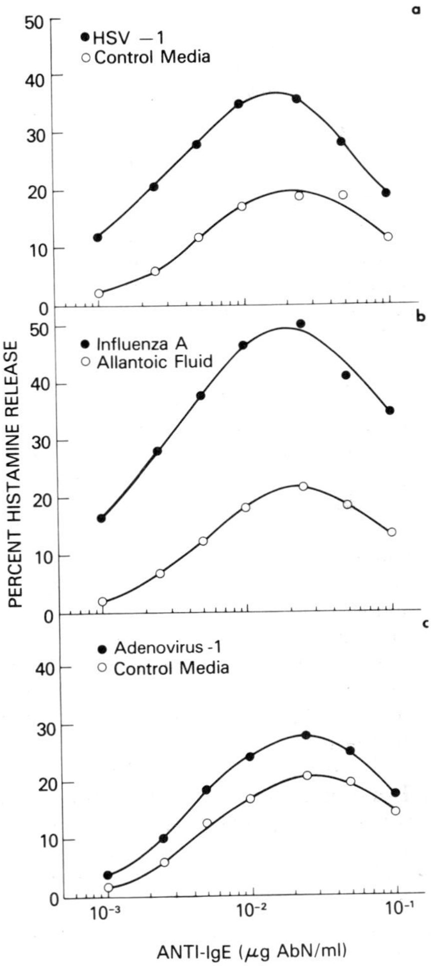

FIGURE 2. Enhanced IgE-mediated release of histamine from leukocytes incubated with infectious viruses. Leukocytes were incubated for 24 hr with HSV-1, influenza A, or Adeno-1. The cells were then washed and the amount of histamine released after challenge with different concentrations of anti-IgE was determined.

TABLE 1

EFFECT OF VARIOUS TREATMENTS OF INTERFERON ON BOTH ANTIVIRAL AND HISTAMINE-ENHANCING ACTIVITY

	Effect on	
Treatment	Antiviral Activity	Histamine-enhancing Activity
Ultracentrifugation	None	None
Dialysis (pH 7.2)	None	None
Heat	None	None
Trypsin	Inhibited	Inhibited
Anti-interferon sera	Inhibited	Inhibited
Actinomycin-D	Inhibited	Inhibited

TABLE 2

INTERFERON PRODUCTION AND ENHANCEMENT OF IgE-MEDIATED HISTAMINE RELEASE FOLLOWING INCUBATION OF LEUKOCYTES WITH PPD*

Donor Cells	Antigen	Interferon Production	Enhanced IgE-Mediated Histamine Release
BCG negative	PPD	No	No
BCG positive	PPD	Yes	Yes

*Peripheral blood leukocytes from BCG-positive donors and BCG-negative donors were incubated with PPD. After a 24 to 48-hour incubation period, the supernatant fluids were assayed for interferon activity and the cells were challenged with antigen E and the amount of histamine released was measured.

brief, we incubated cells from BCG-positive and BCG-negative donors with PPD and looked for the production of interferon and the enhancement of IgE-mediated histamine release. We found that when leukocytes from BCG-positive donors are first incubated with PPD and then challenged with antigen E, histamine release increases. In contrast, when leukocytes from BCG-negative donors are incubated with PPD and then challenged with antigen E, there is no enhancement of histamine release (TABLE 2). Examination of the supernatant fluids from BCG-positive leukocyte cultures stimulated with PPD showed that the presence of immune interferon correlated with the increased release of histamine. These studies demonstrate that the antigen-specific stimulation of leukocytes results in the release of soluble mediators, lymphokines, that are capable of enhancing IgE-mediated histamine release. This finding suggests that one of the factors involved in this enhancement of histamine release is immune interferon.[16]

The demonstration that both type I and type II interferon can enhance IgE-mediated release of histamine suggests that interferon may be one of the co-factors responsible for precipitating or potentiating attacks of bronchial asthma during upper respiratory tract infections. However, the mechanism by which interferon exerts this effect is not clear. In preparations of human leukocytes, histamine is present only in basophils. Moreover, these cells have specific receptors for IgE. The release of histamine is a multistep process known to be triggered by the binding of allergen or anti-IgE to IgE molecules on the basophil surface. The subsequent steps in the release mechanism are complex, energy-requiring reactions that involve Ca^{++}, cyclic nucleotide, esterase activation, and microtubular and microfilament functions.[17-19] Localization of the precise site along the histamine release pathway at which interferon acts may provide new insight into how interferon exerts its antiviral and other regulating effects.

AUTOIMMUNE DISEASES AND INTERFERON

Interferon is produced in response to specific antigens, mitogens or antigen-antibody complexes. This fact suggested to us that interferon also might be produced in patients with autoimmune diseases.[20] Aberrations in immunological regulation may cause autoimmunity, or the activation of the immune system against constituents of one's own body.

To investigate the possibility that interferon is produced in the autoimmune host, we measured serum levels of interferon in patients with autoimmune diseases such as systemic lupus erythematosus, rheumatoid arthritis, scleroderma, and Sjögren's syndrome. Systemic lupus erythematosus is a multisystemic, chronic inflammatory disease characterized by immunological abnormalities such as hypergammaglobulinemia, autoantibodies, immune complexes, depressed blastogenesis, depressed functioning of suppressor T-cell and circulating activated B lymphocytes.[21,22] Rheumatoid arthritis, scleroderma, and Sjögren's syndrome are three additional collagen vascular disorders that are autoimmune in nature and show some of the immunological aberrations seen in systemic lupus erythematosus.

We detected interferon ($\geq$16 U per ml) more frequently in the sera of patients with these autoimmune diseases than in the sera of healthy sex- and age-matched controls (TABLE 3).[20] Interferon was present in the sera of 50% of patients with systemic lupus erythematosus, 50% with rheumatoid arthritis, 60% with scleroderma, and 27% with Sjögren's syndrome. The highest levels of interferon (32 to 512 units/ml) were found in patients with active systemic lupus erythematosus.

Characterization of Interferon

Proof that the antiviral activity in the serum was interferon was demonstrated by the capacity of serum samples to inhibit the replication of vesicular stomatitis virus (VSV) and encephalomyocarditis virus (EMC) in cultures of human cell lines but not in cultures of mouse cells. Moreover, the serum samples were not toxic for human cells; an induction period was required for development of the antiviral state; pretreatment of cells with cycloheximide inhibited the development of the antiviral state; incubation of serum samples with VSV did not result in viral neutralization; and the antiviral activity was destroyed by trypsin. Since type II interferon is inactivated by treatment at pH 2, whereas type I is resistant to

TABLE 3

INTERFERON IN SERA OF PATIENTS WITH AUTOIMMUNE DISEASE*

Serum Source	Interferon: No. Positive / No. Tested	Interferon: % Positive
Systemic lupus erythematosus	18/36	50
Rheumatoid arthritis	5/10	50
Scleroderma	6/10	60
Sjögren's syndrome	4/15	27
Aphthous stomatitis	0/13	0
Normal	1/34	3

*Human-amnion (WISH) cells in 35 mm petri plates were used to assay for interferon. The antiviral activity expressed in interferon units per milliliter was calculated as the reciprocal of the highest dilution of serum (tested in 1 ml volume) that reduced the number of vesicular stomatitis virus plaques by 50%. Sera sometimes produced a nonspecific depression of virus plaques when tested at a dilution of 1 to 4. Sera that failed to show antiviral activity at a dilution of 1 to 8 were recorded as zero. Sera that contained antiviral activity at a dilution of 1 to 16 or higher were considered positive.

TABLE 4

EFFECT OF pH ON INTERFERON ACTIVITY

Serum Source	Treatment* pH 7.2†	pH 2.0
	(Interferon U/ml)	
Systemic lupus erythematosus		
1	32	8
2	128	8
5	32	16
10	32	0
11	512	64
Rheumatoid arthritis		
1	32	0
2	16	0
Type I interferon‡	400	400

*Serum samples were dialyzed at pH 2.0 for 24 hr, neutralized by dialysis at pH 7.2 for 24 hr and then tested for interferon activity.

†The interferon titer in serum samples dialyzed at pH 7.2 was the same as in untreated samples.

‡Lymphoblastoid interferon.

such treatment, seven sera were tested at pH 2 (TABLE 4). Dialysis at this low pH completely or partially destroyed the antiviral activity. In contrast, the antiviral activity of type I interferon was not destroyed by dialysis at pH 2. On the basis of these studies, we conclude that the interferon in the serum of six of the seven patients was primarily type II, or immune interferon.

Relationship Between Interferon and Disease Activity

Because patients with systemic lupus erythematosus had the highest levels of interferon and have easily recognizable flare-ups and remissions, we separated these patients into groups with and without active clinical disease. Systemic lupus erythematosus was considered active when clinical findings such as arthritis, nephritis, serositis, myositis, cerebritis or widespread cutaneous lesions were associated with either low levels of the third component of complement (C_3) or high levels of antibody to DNA. We found interferon in the sera of 79% of

TABLE 5

INTERFERON IN SERA OF SYSTEMIC LUPUS ERYTHEMATOSUS PATIENTS*

Sera Source	Interferon (U/ml) 0	8	16	32	≥64	No. Positive / No. Tested	% Positive
Systemic lupus erythematosus	12	6	1	15	2	18/36	50
Inactive	12	2	0	3	0	3/17	17
Active	0	4	1	12	2	15/19	79

*Tests were performed as described in TABLE 3. A serum was considered positive if the interferon titer was equal to or greater than 16 U/ml.

patients with active systemic lupus erythematosus but in only 17% of those in remission (TABLE 5).

These results suggested a relationship between the presence of interferon and clinical disease activity. To further elucidate this relationship, we obtained serial serum samples from 9 patients with systemic lupus erythematosus and tested these sera for interferon. The first five patients showed clinically active disease at some time during the study (FIGURE 3). Moreover, these five patients had elevated levels of antibody to DNA throughout the study. Serum C_3 levels were often low when the patients were symptomatic. Patient 2, however, did not always demonstrate this correlation with C_3. When symptomatic, patients 1 to 4

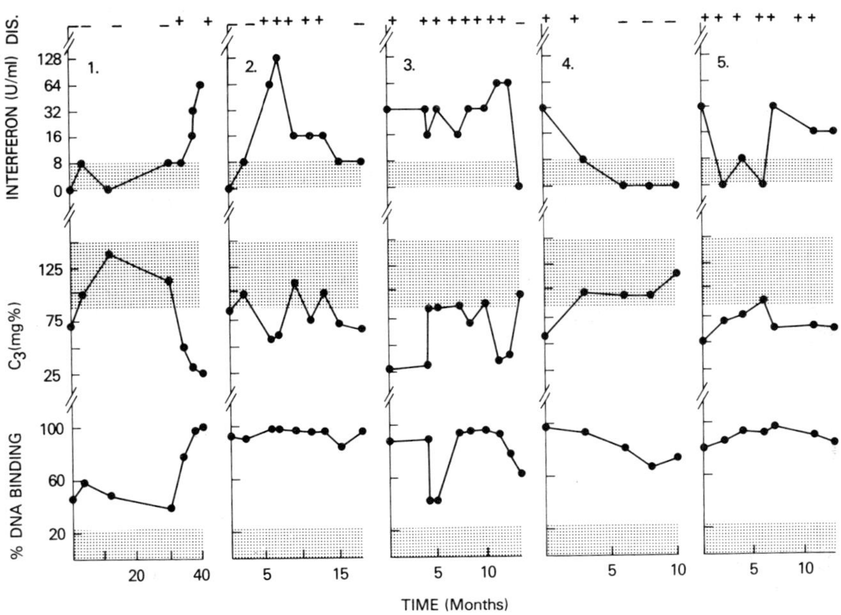

FIGURE 3. Comparison of disease activity with interferon, C_3, and DNA binding in serial serum specimens from five patients with active systemic lupus erythematosus.

had interferon levels ranging from 16 to 128 U per ml. Although patient 5 had clinically active disease throughout the study, only four of seven serum samples contained interferon (16 to 32 U per ml). When patients were free of clinically active disease, we detected normal levels of interferon in the circulation (i.e., 8 U per ml or lower).

In patients 6 to 9 (FIGURE 4), the disease was clinically inactive throughout the observation period despite a moderate increase of antibody to DNA in three of them. C_3 levels were within the normal range. Interferon was rarely detected and never at levels above 8 U per ml.

Antibody to double-stranded DNA and decreased serum C_3 levels are both recognized laboratory measurements of disease activity in systemic lupus erythematosus. Our studies showed that clinical disease activity correlated with interferon activity and with antibody to DNA and low levels of C_3 in the serum. Serum interferon correlated positively with antibody to DNA and negatively with serum levels of C_3 ($p < 0.005$). The striking correlation with disease activity, in fact, raises the possibility that interferon levels may be as good an index of such activity as the current laboratory measures. Interferon did not correlate with renal insufficiency, and was not observed in three patients with lupus who had renal insufficiency and clinically inactive disease. Moreover, no relation was found between drug treatment regimens and interferon titers.

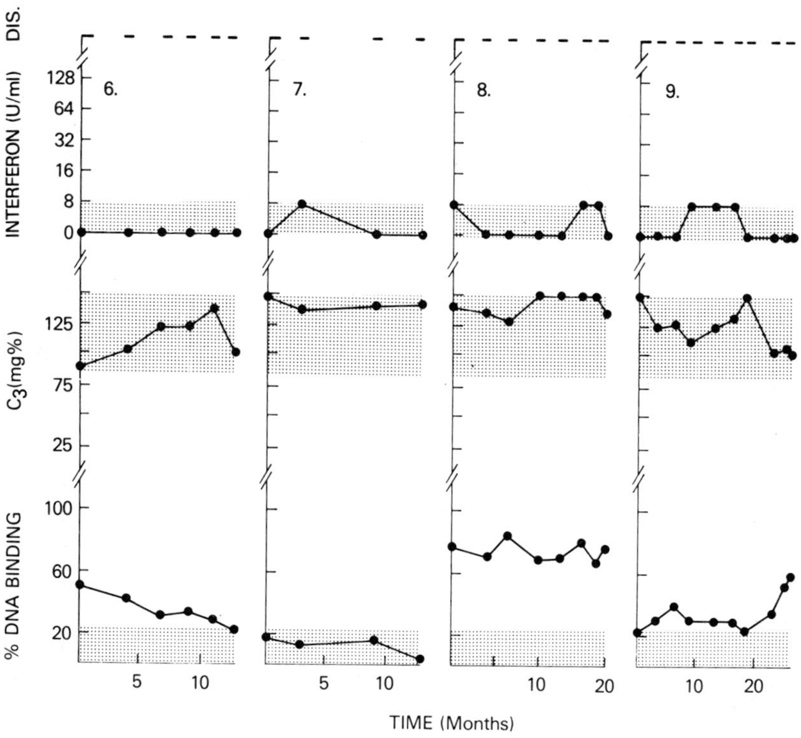

FIGURE 4. Comparison of disease activity with interferon, C_3, and DNA binding in serial serum specimens from four patients with inactive systemic lupus erythematosus.

To follow more closely the interferon levels, we tested sera collected every other day from an untreated patient with active systemic lupus erythematosus. The data in FIGURE 5 show that circulating interferon was constantly present during the patient's first 16 days of hospitalization. This observation is noteworthy because the half-life of type I interferon in the circulation is short. Although the half-life of type II interferon has not been tested, it is known that the half-life of type I is two to four hours.[23] Thus, the continuous presence of interferon in active disease suggests that it is being produced by activated immune cells.

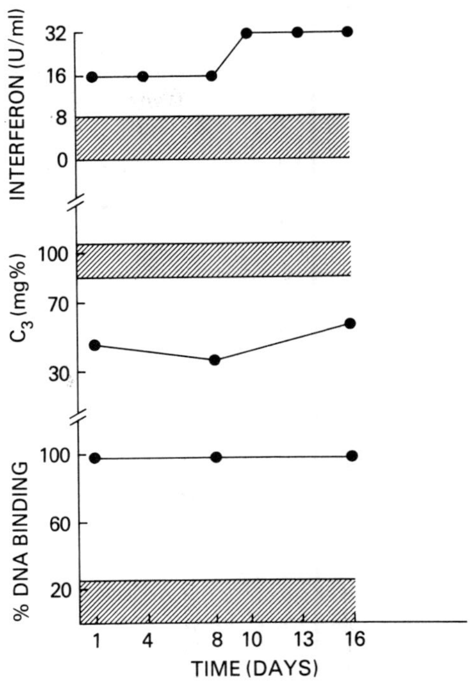

FIGURE 5. Interferon, C_3, and DNA binding in serial serum specimens from an untreated patient with active systemic lupus erythematosus.

ROLE OF INTERFERON IN SYSTEMIC LUPUS ERYTHEMATOSUS

Autoantibodies and antigen-antibody complexes are found in the circulation of patients with systemic lupus erythematosus.[21,22] It is entirely possible that these host antigens, immune complexes and anti-lymphocyte antibodies can stimulate the patients' leukocytes to produce type II interferon and other lymphokines. The role interferon plays in systemic lupus erythematosus is unknown. However, experimental studies suggest that interferon can alter immune functions (TABLE

TABLE 6

COMPARISON OF IMMUNOLOGICAL ABERRATIONS IN SYSTEMIC LUPUS ERYTHEMATOSUS PATIENTS AND CHANGES EXPERIMENTALLY PRODUCED IN ANIMALS AND IN CELL CULTURES BY INTERFERON

Immune Response	SLE Patients	Treatment with Interferon
Antibody synthesis	Enhanced	Enhanced or depressed
Delayed-type hypersensitivity	Decreased	Decreased
Lymphocyte blastogenesis	Decreased	Decreased
Serum complement	Decreased	Decreased
Immune complex glomerulonephritis	Present	Enhanced
Viral infections	Uncertain	Decreased

6). Under certain circumstances it can suppress both humoral and cell-mediated immunity.[23] Under other circumstances, interferon can enhance antibody production, macrophage phagocytosis and lymphocyte cytotoxicity.[2,3] Possibly, some of the immunological aberrations associated with systemic lupus erythematosus, such as hypergammaglobulinemia, autoantibodies, immune complexes, depressed lymphocyte blastogenesis, decreased suppressor T-cell activity and activated B-cell activity may, in part, be mediated by circulating immune interferon.

Furthermore, inoculating neonatal mice or rats with interferon can result in impaired growth, liver cell degeneration and death.[28] Inoculation of these animals for the first week of life can lead to the subsequent development of a progressive and lethal glomerulonephritis.[29] Other studies have shown that when mice are infected at birth with lymphocytic choriomeningitis (LCM) virus, some of the surviving mice develop glomerulonephritis later in life. Gresser and coworkers found that antibody to interferon inhibits this glomerulonephritis. This finding suggests that some of the deleterious effects of LCM virus are actually caused by interferon produced in response to the viral infection.[30] Further, the autoimmune disease in New Zealand black mice, which is a good model of systemic lupus erythematosus, can be accelerated by the administration of interferon.[31] These studies in animals also support the idea that interferon may contribute to some of the manifestations of systemic lupus erythematosus.

Nevertheless, interferon is an important host defense against many viral infections, including herpes zoster.[32] Reactivation of herpes zoster occurs more frequently among patients with systemic lupus erythematosus than among normal individuals. This is probably due to immunosuppression that occurs either as a result of the disease process or secondary to therapeutic agents, such as corticosteroids and cytotoxic drugs. Paradoxically, a recent report states that this virus infection occurs less frequently in patients with active systemic lupus erythematosus than in those with inactive disease.[33] This observation might be explained by the presence of interferon in the blood of those with active disease. Thus, the production of interferon during the host's immunological response to one disease may protect the host from contracting a second (e.g., viral) disease.

Summary

We have presented evidence showing that interferon can enhance the IgE-mediated release of histamine. We have also shown that immune interferon is present in the circulation of patients with certain autoimmune diseases. Furthermore, there is a positive correlation between active systemic lupus erythematosus and interferon levels. Systemic lupus erythematosus is characterized by immune hyperactivity. The continuous presence of type II, immune interferon in the circulation of these patients may, on one hand, contribute to the immunological aberrations, while on the other hand, protect against viral infections. At the present time we are looking for interferon in the circulation of patients with other autoimmune disorders.

References

1. Stewart, W. E., III, Ed. 1979. The Interferon system. Springer-Verlag. New York.
2. Gresser, I. 1977. On the varied biologic effects of interferon. Cell. Immunol. **34:** 406–415.

3. JOHNSON, H. M. & S. BARON. 1977. Evaluation of effects of interferon and interferon inducers on the immune response. Pharmacol. Ther. (A) **1:** 349–367.
4. BARON, S. & F. DIAZANI. 1977. General considerations of the interferon system. Tex. Rep. Biol. Med. **35:** 1–10.
5. WHEELOCK, E. F. 1965. Interferon-like virus-inhibition induced in human leukocytes by phytohemagglutinin. Sci. **149:** 310–311.
6. GREEN, J. A., S. R. COOPERBAND & S. KIBRICK. 1969. Immune specific induction of interferon production in cultures of human blood lymphocytes. Sci. **164:** 1415–1417.
7. YOUNGER, J. S. & S. B. SALVIN. 1973. Production and properties of migration inhibitory factor and interferon in the circulation of mice with delayed hypersensitivity. J. Immunol. **111:** 1914–1922.
8. VALLE, M. J., G. W. JORDAN, S. HAAHR & T. C. MERIGAN. 1975. Characteristics of immune interferon produced by human lymphocyte cultures compared to other human interferons. J. Immunol. **115:** 230–233.
9. FUJIBAYASHI, T., J. J. HOOKS & A. L. NOTKINS. 1975. Production of interferon by immune lymphocytes exposed to herpes simplex virus-antibody complexes. J. Immunol. **115:** 1191–1193.
10. IDA, S., J. J. HOOKS, R. P. SIRAGANIAN & A. L. NOTKINS. 1977. Enhancement of IgE-mediated histamine release from human basophils by viruses: Role of interferon. J. Exp. Med. **145:** 892–906.
11. McINTOSH, K., E. F. ELLIS, L. S. HOFFMAN, T. G. LYBASS, J. J. ELLER & V. A. FULGINITI. 1973. The association of viral and bacterial respiratory infections with exacerbations of wheezing in young asthmatic children. J. Pediatr. **82:** 578–590.
12. HUHTI, E., T. MOKKA, J. NIKOSKELAINEN & P. HALONEN. 1974. Association of viral and mycoplasma infections with exacerbations of asthma. Ann. Allergy **33:** 145–149.
13. MINOR, T. E., E. C. DICK, A. N. DEMEO, J. J. OUELLETTE, M. COHEN & C. E. REED. 1974. Viruses as precipitants of asthmatic attacks in children. JAMA **227:** 292–298.
14. SIRAGANIAN, R. P. 1976. Histamine release and assay methods for the study of human allergy. *In* Manual of Clinical Immunology. N. R. Rose & H. Friedman, Eds. Chapter **80:** 603–615. Am. Soc. Microbiol.
15. HERNANDEZ-ASENSIO, M., J. J. HOOKS, S. IDA, R. P. SIRAGANIAN & A. L. NOTKINS. 1979. Interferon-induced enhancement of IgE-mediated histamine release from human basophils requires RNA synthesis. J. Immunol. **122:** 1601–1603.
16. IDA, S., J. J. HOOKS, R. P. SIRAGANIAN & A. L. NOTKINS. 1980. Enhancement of IgE-mediated histamine release from human basophils by immune-specific lymphokines. Clin. Exp. Immunol. In press.
17. AUSTEN, K. F. 1974. Reaction mechanisms in the release of mediators of immediate hypersensitivity from human lung tissue. Fed. Proc. **33:** 2256–2262.
18. KALINER, M. & K. F. AUSTEN. 1975. Immunologic release of chemical mediators from human tissues. Ann. Rev. Pharmacol. **15:** 177–189.
19. ISHIZAKA, T. & K. ISHIZAKA. 1975. Biology of immunoglobulin E. Prog. Allergy **19:** 60–121.
20. HOOKS, J. J., H. M. MOUTSOPOULOS, S. A. GEIS, N. I. STAHL, J. L. DECKER & A. L. NOTKINS. 1979. Immune interferon in the circulation of patients with autoimmune disease. N. Engl. J. Med. **301:** 5–8.
21. DECKER, J. L., A. D. STEINBERG, M. E. GERSHWIN, W. E. SEAMAN, J. H. KLIPPEL, P. H. PLOTZ & S. A. PAGET. 1975. Systemic lupus erythematosus: Contrasts and comparisons. Ann. Intern. Med. **82:** 391–404.
22. FAUCI, A. S., A. D. STEINBERG, B. F. HAYNES & G. WHALEN. 1978. Immunoregulatory aberrations in systemic lupus erythematosis. J. Immunol. **121:** 1473–1479.
23. JORDAN, G. W., R. P. FRIED & T. C. MERIGAN. 1974. Administration of human leukocyte interferon in herpes zoster. I. Safety, circulating antiviral activity, and host responses to infection. J. Infect. Dis. **130** (1): 56–62.
24. SONNENFELD, G., A. D. MANDEL & T. C. MERIGAN. 1978. Time and dosage dependence of immunoenhancement by murine type II interferon preparations. Cell. Immunol. **40:** 285–293.
25. STRANNEGÅRD, O., I. LARSSON, E. LUNDGREN, H. MIORNER & H. PERSSON. 1978.

Modulation of immune responses in newborn and adult mice by interferon. Infect. Immun. **20** (2): 334–339.

26. GRESSER, I. 1977. On the mechanisms of the antitumor effects of interferon. Tex. Rep. Biol. Med. **35:** 394–398.
27. TRINCHIERI, G. & D. SANTOLI. 1978. Anti-viral activity induced by culturing lymphocytes with tumor-derived or virus-transformed cells. J. Exp. Med. **147:** 1314–1333.
28. GRESSER, I., M. TOVEY, C. MAURY & I. CHOUROULINKOV. 1975. Lethality of interferon preparations for newborn mice. Nature **258:** 76–78.
29. GRESSER, I., L. MOREL-MAROGER, C. MAURY, M. G. TOVEY & F. PONTILLON. 1976. Progressive glomerulonephritis in mice treated with interferon preparations at birth. Nature **263:** 420–422.
30. RIVIERE, Y., I. GRESSER, J. C. GUILLON & M. G. TOVEY. 1977. Inhibition by anti-interferon serum of lymphocytic choriomeningitis virus disease in suckling mice. Proc. Nat. Acad. Sci. USA **74:** 2135–2139.
31. HEREMANS, H., A. BILLIAU, A. COLOMBATTI, J. HILGERS & P. DESOMER. 1978. Interferon treatment of NZB mice: Accelerated progression of autoimmune disease. Infect. Immun. **21**(3): 925–930.
32. GALASSO, G. J. & J. K. DUNNICK. 1977. Interferon, an antiviral drug for use in man. Tex. Rep. Biol. Med. **35:** 478–485.
33. MOUTSOPOULOS, H. M., J. D. GALLAGHER, J. L. DECKER & A. D. STEINBERG. 1978. Herpes zoster in patients with systemic lupus erythematosus. Arth. Rheum. **21:** 798-802.

IMMUNE MODULATING EFFECTS OF POLY ICLC

Hilton B. Levy,* E. Lvovsky,* F. Riley,* D. Harrington,†
A. Anderson,† J. Moe,† J. Hilfenhaus,‡ and E. Stephen†

**National Institute of Allergy and Infectious Diseases*
National Institutes of Health,
Bethesda, Maryland 20014

†USAMRIID
Ft. Detrick, Maryland 21701

‡Behringeverke
Marburg, West Germany

This presentation will compare immune modulation brought about by interferon with those brought about by interferon inducers, particularly double-stranded RNA. If the only effect of the interferon inducer was the induction of interferon, then we would expect that interferon and its inducers would have the same effect in any given immune phenomenon, be it no effect, enhancement or inhibition. The fact that inducers can elicit a higher level of circulating interferon *in vivo* than is readily obtainable by administering exogenous interferon might modify this expectation in that large amounts of interferon might act differently from small amounts of interferon. However, within this limitation, interferon inducers might be expected to act like interferon. Indeed, there are many instances where this is the case. You will hear of them during this session. One such is the enhancement of natural killer cell activity by interferon and by poly I·poly C.[1]

There are some rather clear-cut differences also between the effects of interferon and poly I·poly C. Drs. McNeil and Fleming have reported that interferon blocks the action of a glycoprotein-stimulating factor that stimulates the production in soft agar of granulocyte-macrophage colonies, whereas poly I·poly C, both *in vivo* and *in vitro*, stimulate such activity.[2] That is, even though poly I·poly C leads to the production of interferon, which is a colony-inhibiting substance, the stimulating activity of the double-stranded RNA itself overcomes such inhibition.

Two groups, at least, have found differences between poly I·poly C and interferon on the graft-versus-host (GvH) reaction, with poly I · poly C enhancing GvH reaction and interferon either inhibiting or having no effect.[3,4] Unfortunately in most other areas of immune regulation, direct comparison is not readily made. While both poly I · poly C and the stabilized derivative of poly I · poly C with polylysine and carboxymethylcellulose (poly ICLC) have been tested for their effect on immunity and antibody formation, as has interferon, the several projects have been done by different people in different laboratories using different antigens and different techniques. Mostly, interferon, both the virus-induced type and immune interferon, has been inhibitory to antibody production, while poly I · poly C and its derivatives have been stimulatory.

Rather than dwell further on these comparisons, I would like to present data that show that the primate-effective interferon inducer, poly I · poly C, complexed with polylysine and carboxymethylcellulose is an effective enhancer of immune reactivity when given with certain weakly effective vaccines.

0077-8923/80/0350-0033 $01.75/0 © 1980, NYAS

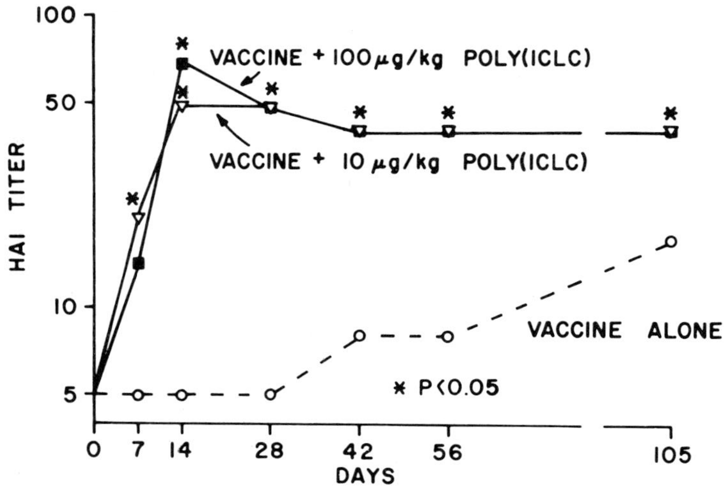

FIGURE 1. Effect of one injection of poly ICLC on HAI antibody production by young Rhesus monkeys in response to a subunit vaccine to swine flu (200 CCA units). (Four monkeys per group)

Monovalent influenza virus subunit vaccine designated A/swine X-53, prepared from A/NJ/76 (New Jersey, Swine) is only moderate to weakly effective when given as a single dose to young people. When the vaccine was given to monkeys simultaneously with one dose of poly ICLC, HAI antibody titers in the serum were detectable earlier and rose to higher levels than in monkeys receiving vaccine alone. Four monkeys were used per group, each receiving 200 CCA units.

The adjuvant activity of poly ICLC was particularly pronounced in young monkeys, where as little as 10 μg of drug per kg of body weight was effective, as seen in FIGURE 1. This level of poly ICLC does not induce detectable levels of serum interferon, and no fever was produced.[5]

Analogous results were obtained in monkeys using inactivated Venezuelan Equine Encephalomyelitis virus vaccine.[6] FIGURE 2 shows some of the data. It can be seen that antibody levels in serum were boosted about 40-fold after primary immunization when one compares levels attained after administration of vaccine along with poly ICLC with that attained with vaccine alone, and perhaps 200-fold after a secondary immunization. There was no alteration in the progression of IgM and IgG development. At the peak of antibody levels, most of the antibody was IgG. Polylysine complexed to carboxymethylcellulose without poly I · poly C had no adjuvant action.

A polysaccharide vaccine made from *Hemophilus influenzae* is a poor vaccine in very young children, where the disease threat is maximum. The vaccine is also poor in young monkeys. TABLE 1 shows this.[7] The data presented are normalized values, obtained by radioimmune assays done by Dr. Porter Anderson. The value of 100 was assigned in each case to the amount of radioactivity found prior to immunization. The vaccine alone caused a minimum boost, but when given with poly ICLC there was a more pronounced boost.

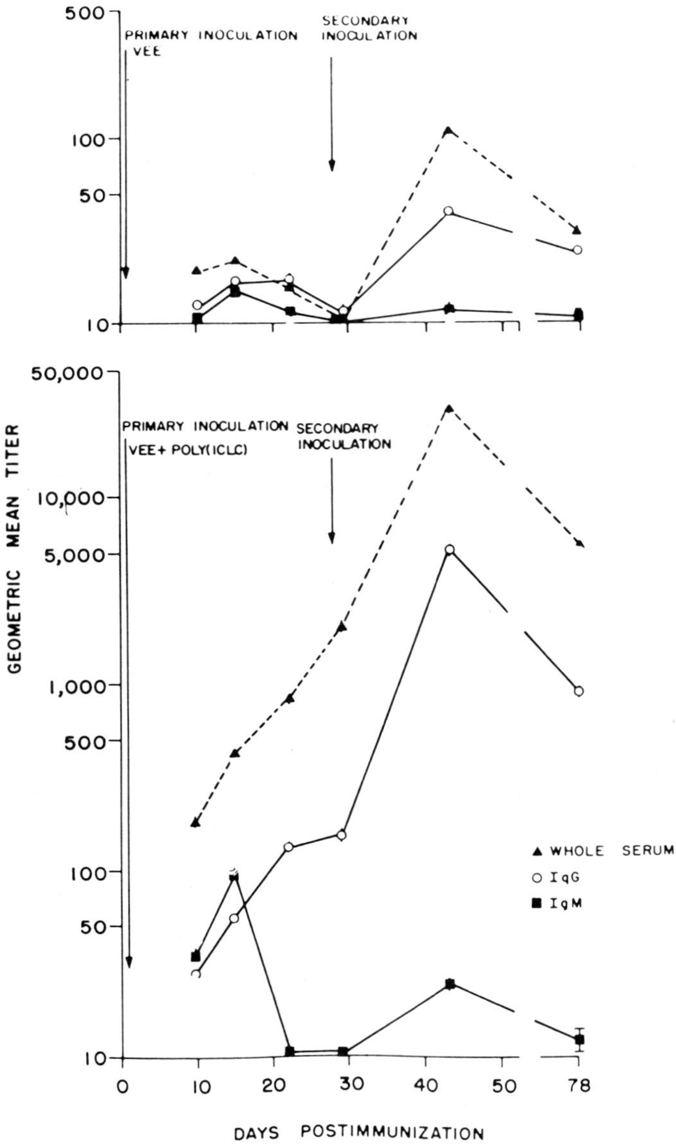

FIGURE 2. Effect of poly ICLC (200 μg/kg body weight) on antibody production by Rhesus monkeys in response to Venezuelan equine encephalomyelitis (VEE) virus vaccine (strain tc-83). (Four monkeys per group)

TABLE 1

EFFECT OF ADJUVANTS ON RESPONSE TO *HEMOPHILUS INFLUENZAE* VACCINE*

Treatment	Pre	Antibody Levels, (normalized ng/ml) Day 18	Day 25	Day 32
Vaccine dose	100	114	124	143
PICLC + (1 mg/kg) Vaccine	100	564	435	300
PAULC	100	191	166	166

*Comparison of effects of poly ICLC and polyadenylic-polyuridylic acid-polylysine carboxymethylcellulose on antibody production by Rhesus monkeys in response to a polysaccharide vaccine for *Hemophilus influenzae*.

TABLE 2

EFFECT OF LOW DOSES OF POLY ICLC ON ANTIBODY PRODUCTION BY RHESUS MONKEYS IN RESPONSE TO A POLYSACCHARIDE VACCINE FOR *HEMOPHILUS INFLUENZAE*

Treatment	Pre	Day 7	Day 14	Day 20	Day 28	Day 34	Day 42
Vaccine	100	590	348	286	225	187	113
Vaccine + poly ICLC, 0.3 mg/kg	100	5643	5040	3340	2063	2162	780
Vaccine + poly ICLC, 0.03 mg/kg	100	6589	3904	1884	1132	839	721

TABLE 3

EFFECTS OF ADJUVANTS ON SURVIVAL OF VACCINATED MICE*

Treatment: Vaccine		Treatment: Adjuvant	Dose/kg	% Survivors Day 35 (N = 16)
Vaccine	+	Poly (ICLC)	20 μg	50
			100 μg	50
			200 μg	13
Saline	+	Poly (ICLC)	200 μg	6
Vaccine	+	Freund's complete adjuvant		6
Saline	+	Freund's complete adjuvant		6
Vaccine	+	Freund's incomplete adjuvant		6
Saline	+	Freund's incomplete adjuvant		0
Vaccine controls				19
Saline controls				0

*Effects of one dose of poly ICLC, Freund's complete adjuvant, or Freund's incomplete adjuvant plus vaccine vs. Rift Valley Fever (Zagazig) virus on survival of mice challenged on day 14 postimmunization with 750 PFU virulent virus.

Polyadenylic · polyuridylic acid complexed to CMC and polylysine was not so effective as poly ICLC.

TABLE 2 show another experiment of the same type where the dose of poly ICLC was reduced.[7] There was no statistical difference between the two doses. In three experiments there was no effect of poly ICLC on platelets, total and differential leucocytes, packed cell volume, erythrocyte sedimentation rate, serum urea nitrogen, total and direct bilirubin, glutamicoxalacetic transaminase, latic dehydrogenase, alkaline phosphatase, and creatinine.

In an experiment using a different type of endpoint, it was shown that poly ICLC, given together with a vaccine versus Rift Valley fever (RVF) virus, increased the survival of mice subsequently challenged with live RVF virus.[8] TABLE 3 shows the increased survival rates of mice given poly ICLC and vaccine, as compared with those found in mice immunized with vaccine alone.

The last of these adjuvant effects that I will mention deals with observations made with Joachim Hilfenhaus, using an envelope antigen made from herpes virus.[9] In these experiments, both antibody levels and survival after subsequent

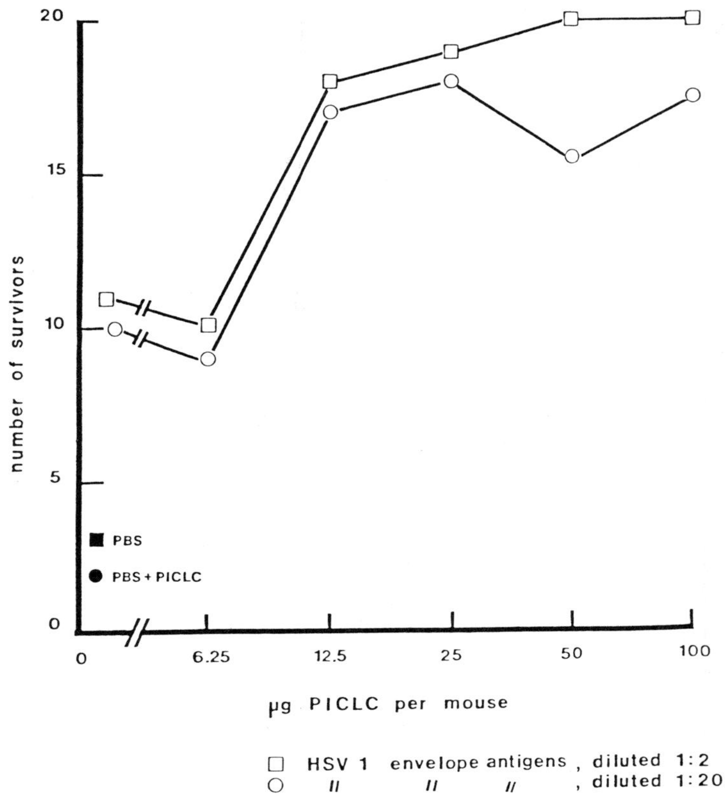

FIGURE 3. Effect of poly ICLC given with envelope antigen from herpes virus on survival in mice against subsequent challenge with live virus.

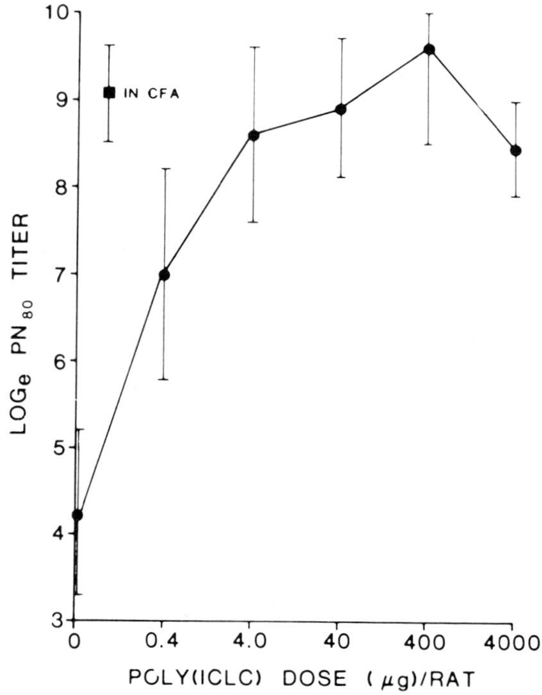

FIGURE 4. Effect of poly ICLC on antibody production by rats in respose to Venezuelan equine encephalomyelitis virus vaccine.

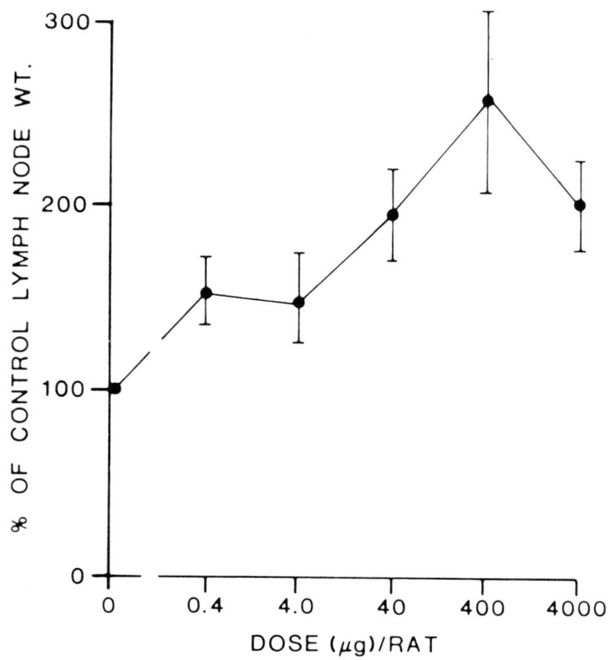

FIGURE 5. Effect of dose of poly ICLC given along with VEE virus vaccine on weight of lymph nodes draining the site of injection.

challenge with whole virus were measured. Both these aspects of immunity were enhanced when the envelope antigen was administered with poly ICLC. FIGURE 3 summarizes some of the data.

Dr. Arthur Anderson has done some experiments in rats that shed some light on physiological changes associated with administration of antigens plus poly ICLC.[10]

FIGURE 4 shows that antibody response by rats to Venezuelan equine encephalomyletis vaccine is augmented by poly ICLC as it is in monkeys.

FIGURE 5 relates that the weight of the nodes draining the area where the poly ICLC was injected increases as the dose of drug increases. With 40 μg/rat there is an increase of 100 percent.

FIGURE 6 shows that the number of small lymphocytes in the high venules of

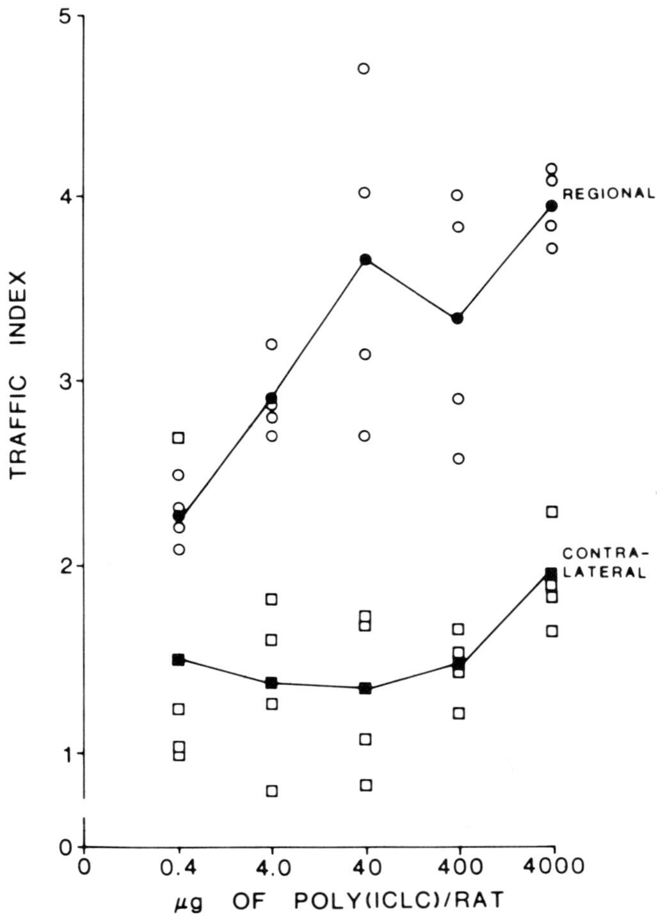

FIGURE 6. The lymphocyte migration index in the high venules of the paracortex of the nodes mentioned in FIGURE 5.

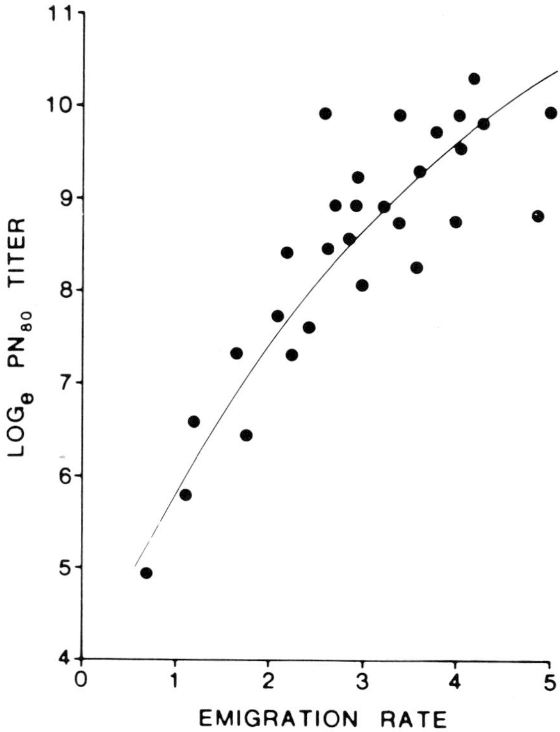

FIGURE 7. Correlation of the number of lymphocytes in the paracortex of nodes 2 days after injection, with antibody levels 28 days after infection.

the paracortex of these nodes increases with the dose of poly ICLC within 24–48 hours after injection.

Finally, to complete the picture, FIGURE 7 shows that in individual rats the number of small lymphocytes in the paracortex at 2 days relates to the antibody level in that animal at 28 days.

It is therefore apparent that, somehow, injection of poly ICLC increases the size of the node, this increase in size is associated with an increase in small lymphocytes, which are cells capable of producing antibody, and the increase in number of these lymphocytes is related to the increase in antibody production.

One other thing should be mentioned, because it ties in in ways that seem related. Poly ICLC is a good radioprotective agent.[11] Mice given poly ICLC can tolerate and recover from a significantly higher level of x-irradiation than mice not given the inducer. This protection and recovery is associated with an increase in the number of growing stem-cell colonies in spleen and marrow. Which brings us back to where we started, namely, that double-stranded RNA does seem to enhance growth of certain white cells, which is a different effect from that seen with interferon.

REFERENCES

1. DJEU, J. Y., J. A. HEINBAUGH, H. T. HOLDEN & R. B. HERBERMAN. 1979. Augmentation of mouse natural killer cell activity by interferon and interferon inducers. J. Immunol. **122:** 175–181.
2. MCNEILL, T. A., Z. W. A. FLEMING & D. J. MCCANCE. 1972. Interferon and hemopoietic colony inhibitor responses to poly I · poly C in rabbits and hamsters. Immunology **22:** 711–721.
3. CANTOR, H., R. ASOFSKY & H. B. LEVY. 1970. The effect of polyinosinic polyadenylic acid upon graft vs host activity in BALB/c mice. J. Immunol. **104:** 1035.
4. DE MAEYER, E. & J. DE MAEYER-GUIGNARD. 1977. Effect of interferon on cell mediated immunity. Tex. Rep. Biol. Med. **35:** 370–374.
5. STEPHEN, E. L., D. E. HILMAS, J. A. MANGIAFICO & H. B. LEVY. 1977. Swine influenza virus vaccine; potentiation of antibody response in Rhesus monkeys. Science **197:** 1289–1290.
6. HARRINGTON, D. L., C. L. CRABBS, D. E. HILMAS, J. R. BROWN, C. A. HIGBEE, F. E. COLE Jr. & H. B. LEVY. 1979. Adjuvant effects of low doses of a nuclease resistant derivative of polyinosinic polycytidylic acid on antibody responses of monkeys to inactivated Venezuelan Equine Encephalomyelitis virus vaccine. Infect. Immun. **24:** 60–166.
7. LEVY, H. B., E. STEPHEN & D. HARRINGTON. Unpublished observations.
8. HARRINGTON. D., E. STEPHEN, J. PETERS & H. B. LEVY. Unpublished observations.
9. HILFENHAUS, J. & H. B. LEVY. Unpublished observations.
10. ANDERSON, A. O., J. A. REYNOLDS & D. G. HARRINGTON. 1979. Immunomodulating effect of polynucleotides on lymphocyte traffic and antiviral immunity. Proceedings of Symposium on Potentiation of Immune Response to Vaccines. J. Infect. Dis. In press.
11. LVOVSKY, E., W. B. BAZE D. E. HILMAS & H. B. LEVY. 1977. Radiation damage and the interferon system. Tex. Rep. Biol. Med. **35:** 388–393.

INTERFERON, NK CELLS AND PERSISTENT VIRUS INFECTION*

Nagahiro Minato, Lola Reid, Andrew Neighbour, Barry R. Bloom, and John Holland†

Departments of Microbiology and Immunology
Pharmacology and Pathology
Albert Einstein College of Medicine
Bronx, New York 10461

†Department of Biology
University of California, San Diego
La Jolla, California 92093

Persistent viral infections present an immunological paradox in that the viruses manage to survive in a host which has generated appropriate immune responses to protect it from the acute phase of viral infection. It is clear that antibodies serve primarily to neutralize viruses prior to infection of cells and to restrict their spread in the acutely infected host but have little activity in eliminating already existent persistent infections.[1,2] In at least some cases antibodies may be involved in maintenance of the persistent viral state.[3,4] A great deal of work over the past several years has indicated that specifically immune cytotoxic T lymphocytes have a critical role in providing resistance against acute viral infections, and do so in a histocompatibility-restricted fashion.[5] The existence of persistent viral infections in man, and slow viral diseases thought to be caused by them, indicate that these two lines of defense are insufficient to prevent or eliminate persistent viral infections in at least some hosts, and immunological mechanisms effective against persistently infected cells remain unclear.

Rejection of Virus Persistently Infected (PI) Tumor Cells by Nude Mice

While congenically athymic nude mice have been widely used to study tumorigenicity of a variety of human and animal neoplasms, nude mice are not totally immunodeficient and many tumors fail to grow in the nude mouse.[6,7] Over the past several years we have studied the mechanisms of resistance of nude mice to tumor cells persistently infected with a variety of viruses, since this provides a system in which mechanisms of natural immunity largely independent of antibody and T-cell function can be studied.

As few as 10–100 HeLa or BHK cells will produce tumors in 3 weeks in 100% of BALB/c nu/nu mice. However, when these cells are rendered persistently infected with a variety of RNA viruses including vesicular stomatitis virus, mumps, influenza, and measles, and doses up to 10^4 PI tumor cells are inoculated subcutaneously into nude mice, no evidence of tumor growth is seen; when

*Supported by United States Public Health Service Grants AI 07118, AI 10702, AI 09807, AI 19627 and CA 1330, and Grant RG 1006 from the National Multiple Sclerosis Society.

0077-8923/80/0350-0042 $01.75/0 © 1980, NYAS

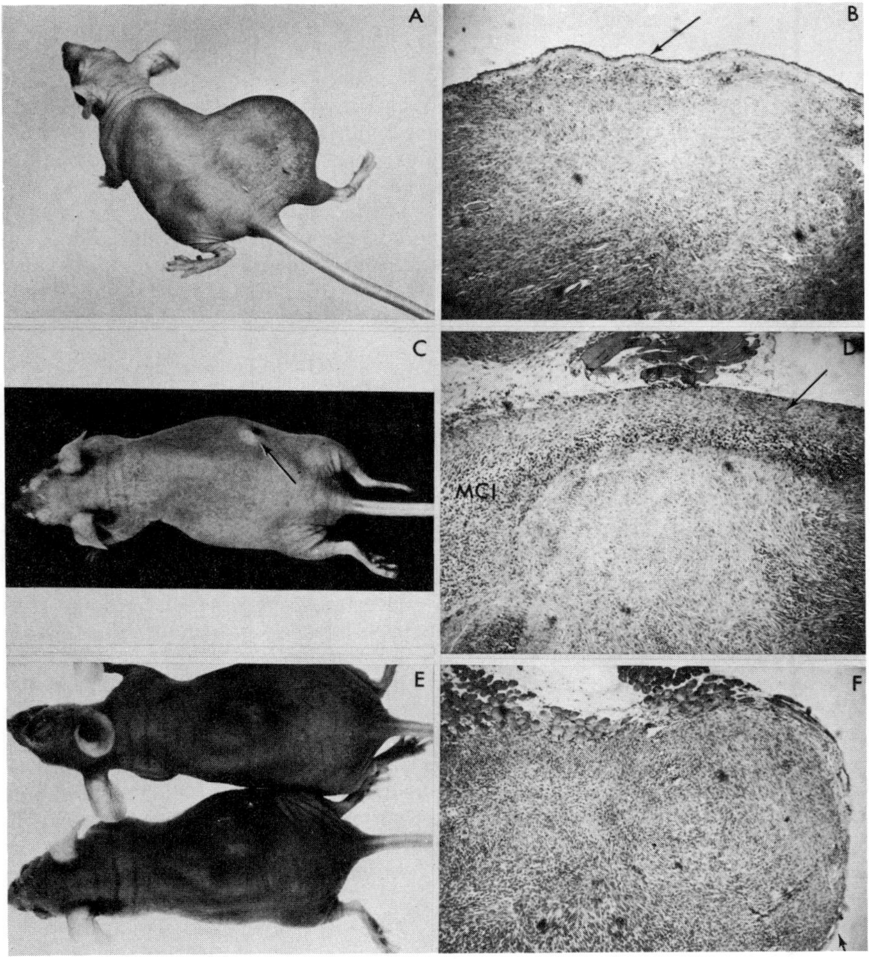

FIGURE 1. Neoplasms in BALB/c nude mice injected with BHK21 or BHK-VSV cells.

A. The mouse was inoculated with 10^6 BHK21 cells subcutaneously. A tumor formed which was initially palpable by 10 days, and the animal was moribund with the tumor by 6 weeks. **B.** Histological section of a tumor produced in a nude mouse injected with 10^6 BHK 21 cells. Note the thin but distinct fibrous capsule (arrow) infiltrated with a small population of mononuclear cells. The 8-μm paraffin section was stained with hematoxylin and eosin. Magnification: $\times$ 80. **C.** The mouse was inoculated with 10^6 BHK-VSV cells subcutaneously. The small neoplasm noted on the right side of the mouse (arrow) developed by the fourth week after inoculation and persisted in this "benign" form for more than 6 months. **D.** Section from a nodule produced in a nude mouse injected with 10^6 BHK-VSV cells. Similar results were obtained from tumors from injections with other virus PI tumor cell lines. Note the thick fibrous capsule (arrow) and the mononuclear infiltrate surrounding the tumor cells. Magnification: $\times$ 160. **E.** The mice were irradiated with 600 rads of ^{135}Ce and subsequently injected with 10^6 BHK-VSV cells 12 days after irradiation. The tumors were palpable within 2 weeks and the mice were moribund with the tumors by 6 weeks. **F.** Section of a tumor produced in an irradiated nude mouse injected with 10^6 BHK-VSV cells. The capsule surrounding the tumor was thin (arrow) and could be seen only with Masson's trichrome stain. Note the deficiency in the mononuclear cell infiltrate in the capsule. The paraffin section was stained with Masson's trichrome. Magnification: $\times$ 80. (From Minato *et al.*[9] Used with permission of the publishers of *J. Exp. Med.*)

10^4–10^7 PI cells are injected, nodules appear that do not develop into tumors.[8,9] The *in vitro* growth rates of the persistently infected cells cannot be distinguished from those of the uninfected cells. These findings are illustrated in FIGURE 1. Biopsies of the nodules indicated a marked round cell infiltration of the nodules produced by virus PI tumor cells, with only slight infiltration of the uninfected parental tumor cell sites. That the failure of the nodules containing persistently infected tumor cells to develop into tumors is a function of an active process of resistance of the nude mouse host was indicated by the observation that treatment of nude mice with gamma irradiation rendered them all susceptible to tumor growth.

THE ROLE OF NATURAL KILLER CELLS IN RESISTANCE TO PERSISTENTLY INFECTED TUMOR CELLS

The mechanism of resistance to virus PI tumor cells by nude mice was investigated by studying *in vitro* cytoxic activity of spleen cells derived from normal nude mice against uninfected or virus PI tumor cell lines. The results using both persistently infected HeLa cells and BHK cells are illustrated in TABLE 1. The results of over 50 experiments have indicated that while uninfected BHK or HeLa cells are not subject to spontaneous cytotoxicity *in vitro*, the same cells persistently infected with a variety of viruses are lysed to various degrees within 9 hours *in vitro*.[9]

A number of selective enrichment and depletion procedures were applied to spleen cells from nude mice in order to characterize the cytotoxic effector cell, and a summary of the characteristics is given in TABLE 2. Under conditions in which conventional anti-Thy 1.2 antiserum + complement abolished over 90% of an *in vitro* Con A response, the spontaneous cytotoxicity of nude mouse spleen cells for HeLa-measles was unaffected. Similarly passage over nylon wood or treatment with anti-Ig + complement were without effect. By these criteria, the effector cell cannot be considered a conventional B cell, T cell, or macrophage.

TABLE 1

SELECTIVE SPONTANEOUS CYTOTOXICITY OF NORMAL MOUSE SPLEEN CELLS *IN VITRO* AGAINST VIRUS PERSISTENTLY INFECTED TUMOR CELLS

	Target Cells	*In Vitro* Cytotoxicity by Spleen Cells from: BALB/c nu/nu	CBA/J
		%	%
A.*	HeLa	3.5	14.0
	HeLa-measles	26.0	56.5
	HeLa-mumps	26.3	52.5
	HeLa-VSV	27.6	49.6
B.†	BHK 21	2.0	
	BHK 21-mumps	21.5	N.T.
	BHK 21-VSV	58.0	
C.*	LU 106		7.0
	LU 106-measles	N.T.	38.9
	LU 106-CDV		27.9

*Percent specific ^{51}Cr-release, A/T = 100:1.
†Percent reduction of the incorporated [^{3}H] uridine, A/T = 100:1.

TABLE 2

CHARACTERISTICS OF NK CELLS IN THE NUDE MOUSE

I. Effector cell	
Nonadherent to plastic	Thy 1.2 (30% $^{+}$, 70% $^{-}$)
Nonphagocytic	Ly 5.1^{+}
Surface Ig^{-}	asialo-G_{M1}
Ly 1^{-}	
Ly 2,3^{-}	
II. Strain Distribution	
Level of NK Activity and Level of IF Production by Virus P I Tumor Cells	
Low	A/J; AKR; be/be
Intermediate	C57B1/6; BALB/c; DBA
High	CBA; C3H; nu/nu > nu/+ = +/+

Thus the effector cell in nude mouse spleen capable of lysing virus PI cell lines had the characteristics generally associated with natural killer (NK) cells. In addition it is positive for another T-cell marker, the Ly 5 antigen[10] to be discussed below. Of particular interest was the finding that using two treatments of a monoclonal anti-Thy 1.2 + complement, the cytotoxic activity was consistently reduced by 30–35%, consistent with recent reports of Herberman *et al.*[11] using a leukemia target-cell system.

NONSPECIFIC INDUCTION OF NK CELL ACTIVITY

The cytotoxic activity of spleen cells from mice that had been inoculated *in vivo* with either PI or uninfected cell lines was examined to ascertain whether any increase in specific cytotoxic activity for the inducing cell line was found. BHK, BHK-mumps or BHK-VSV cell lines were injected subcutaneously into age-matched (6 weeks) nude mice, and after various intervals, the cytotoxic activity of spleen cells was assayed on HeLa-measles as targets. In this situation, the target differed from the inducing cell both by the nature of the virus involved and the nature of the target cell itself. The results illustrated in FIGURE 2 indicate a significant increase in cytotoxic activity over controls was observed in nude mice previously infected with essentially any of the virus PI cell lines. The augmentation of cytotoxic activity was detected as early as 2 days after inoculation and remained at high levels for at least 35 days, differing in this regard from the augmentation seen in conventional mice, which waned after 7 days. No augmented cytotoxic activity was observed with spleen cells from nude mice which had been inoculated with uninfected tumor cells; in fact, there was significant and reproducible depression in NK activity in these mice as compared to normal control nude mice. These results clearly demonstrated that inoculation with virus PI cell lines nonspecifically enhanced NK activity for both specific or irrelevant virus PI targets.

THE ROLE OF INTERFERON IN THE ACTIVATION OF NK CELLS

The nonspecific augmentation induced by any virus PI tumor cell in NK activity suggested that a humoral factor might be released *in vivo* which had the

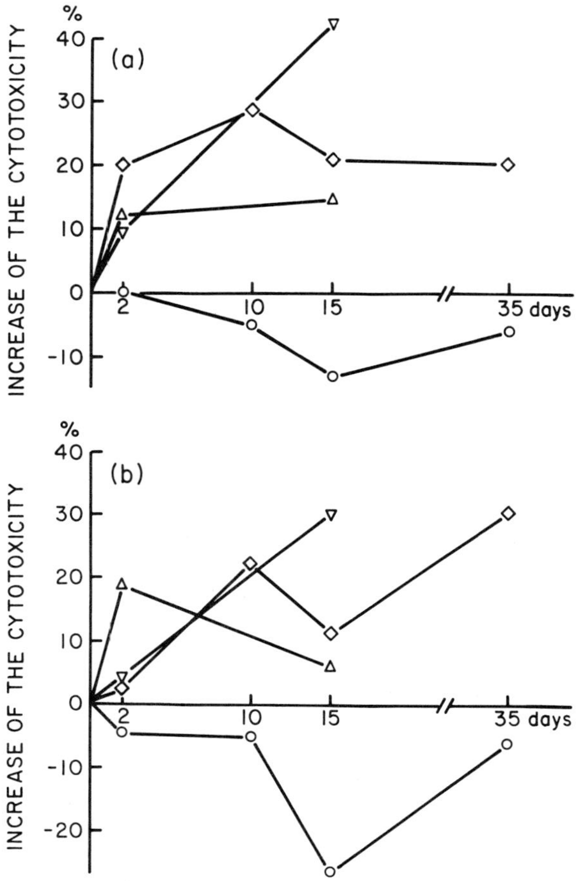

FIGURE 2. Normal BALB/c nude mice (6 to 10 weeks old) were injected with 10^6 of BHK (○), BHK-mumps (◇), BHK-VSV (△), or with BHK-VSV-P (▽) cells subcutaneously. Two, 10, 15, and 35 days later, the mice were killed and the NK activity of the spleen cells were assayed *in vitro* using HeLa-measles cells as a target. In each case, the NK activity of the normal nude mice spleen cells was also assayed as a control. The result is expressed as the increase of the cytotoxicity over the control; (% cytotoxicity of the tumor-injected nude spleen cells)-(% cytotoxicity of the normal nude spleen cells.) (a) 100:1 A/T ratio; (b) 50:1 A/T ratio.

capability of nonspecifically activating NK cells. It had previously been shown by several laboratories that interferon (IF) and interferon inducers served nonspecifically to augment NK activity.[12–14,17] Experiments were designed to test the role of interferon in augmenting NK cell activity *in vitro*. In the first instance, coculture of spleen cells from normal nude mice with a variety of PI cells caused a release of detectable, although relatively small, amounts of IF in the culture medium (TABLE 3), while uninfected tumor cells were ineffective at inducing *in vitro* production of interferon. When normal nude mouse spleen cells were incubated for 0.5–3 hours with supernatants of uninfected or infected cells, and

TABLE 3

SELECTIVE INTERFERON PRODUCTION BY NORMAL MOUSE SPLEEN CELLS *IN VITRO* IN RESPONSE TO VIRUS PERSISTENTLY INFECTED TUMOR CELLS.

Mixed Lymphocyte Tumor Cell Cultures		IF Titer in the 24-hr Culture Supernates
Spleen Cells	Tumor Cells	
		Units
BALB/c nu/nu	none	<2
	HeLa	<2
	HeLa-measles	64
	HeLa-mumps	16
	HeLa-VSV	16
CBA/J	HeLa	<2
	HeLa-measles	512
	HeLa-VSV	128
None	HeLa-measles	<2

the cytotoxic activity measured, a consistent augmentation of NK activity was seen by spleen cells that had been incubated in culture supernatants of virus PI cell lines. Thus, supernatants of mixed lymphocyte-PI tumor cell cultures contained a soluble factor capable of augmenting NK activity (TABLE 4). When goat anti-mouse leukocyte interferon generously provided by Dr. Ion Gresser was added to the supernatants of the mixed lymphocyte-PI tumor culture, the augmenting activity was eliminated. Finally, highly purified mouse interferon,[15] generously provided by Dr. Peter Lengyel, with a specific activity of 2×10^9 U/mg produced a similar augmentation. We conclude that interferon is responsible for the nonspecific augmentation of NK activity because: (1) there is a parallel between the ability of virus PI cell lines to augment NK activity *in vitro* and their ability to induce detectable levels of interferon; (2) the effect is abolished by antibodies against mouse interferon; and (3) similar augmentation is produced by authentic purified mouse interferon.

TABLE 4

EVIDENCE THAT THE AUGMENTATION IN NK ACTIVITY BY VIRUS PI CELLS IS MEDIATED THROUGH INTERFERON

Pretreatment of Spleen Cells	Specific ^{51}Cr Release from HeLa-Measles (CBA/J spleen effector cells)
	%
I. Medium	19.4
(HeLa-Ms + spleen cells) MLTC supernatant	28.1
(HeLa-Ms + spleen cells) MLTC supernatant + AIF†	17.2
HeLa-Ms culture supernatant alone	21.8
II. Medium	19.0
Purified mouse EAT-interferon*	28.2

*EAT-Interferon, kindly provided by Dr. Peter Lengyel, had a specific activity of 2×10^9 units/mg, and was used at a final concentration of 1,500 units.

†AIF = anti-interferon serum.

Mechanism of Augmentation of NK Cell Activity by Interferon

It is widely assumed that interferon acts directly on NK cells to "activate" them, although there is no evidence on this point. An alternative view would be that interferon acted on precursors to NK cells initiating its differentiation to functional effector cells. We have designed experiments to clarify the role of interferon in regulating NK activity.

One of the characteristics of the effector cell capable of lysing virus PI tumor cell lines, as indicated above, is the display of the Ly 5 surface marker.[19] In conventional mice, Ly 5 is found on both T cells and NK cells, but in the nude mouse it serves usefully as a specific marker for NK cells. Using this marker, it was possible to examine whether interferon exerted a regulatory influence directly on Ly 5^+ NK cells. As illustrated in Figure 3, treatment of nude mouse spleen cells with anti-Ly 5 + C reduced their NK activity. When these anti-Ly 5-depleted spleens were treated for 3 hours with purified mouse interferon, there was an almost complete restoration of NK activity.[16] This result umambiguously demonstrates that interferon has the capability of acting on an Ly 5^- cell which lacks demonstrable NK activity and converting it, within a short time, into an Ly 5^+ functional NK cell. The final experiment demonstrated that in the process of converting the Ly 5^- inactive precursor into a functional NK cell, after only 3 hours of incubation with interferon, the resulting effector cells all exhibited the Ly 5^+ surface marker. It has not been possible to design an experiment to rule out the possibility that interferon may also act directly on Ly 5^+ NK cells with effector activity. Thus, the function of interferon as an immunoregulatory molecule in this system seems to be to promote the differentiation of an inactive precursor into a fully effective Ly 5^+ NK cell.

The Effect of Anti-Interferon Antibodies *in Vivo*

Because of the parallel between susceptibility to NK cytotoxicity *in vitro* and failure of virus PI tumor cell lines to grow *in vivo,* we have inferred that NK cells are responsible for rejection of these PI tumor cells *in vivo.* If interferon serves to regulate the development of NK cells, one would predict that elimination of IF *in*

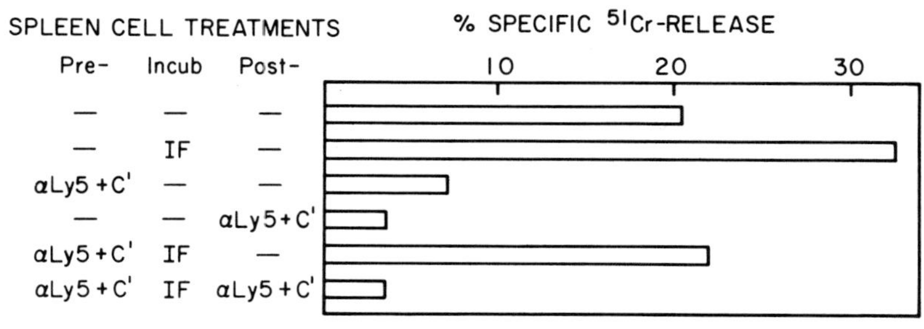

Figure 3. Normal nude mouse spleen cells were treated with medium or anti-Ly 5.1 plus C′ (step 1). The cells were washed, and incubated with medium or purified mouse interferon (1,500 u) for 1 hr at 37°C in 5% CO_2 incubator (step 2). The cells were then washed, and again treated with medium or anti-Ly 5.1 plus C′ (step 3). After final wash, the NK activity of these treated cells was assayed on HeLa-measles cells at A/T ratio 100:1 at 10 hr, using ^{51}Cr-release assay.

TABLE 5
EFFECT OF ANTI-INTERFERON SERUM ON GROWTH OF BHK-MUMPS IN ATHYMIC NUDE MICE

Treatment	Cell Line	Seeding Density	No. Mice with Neoplasms / No. Mice Inoculated
Normal rabbit serum	BHK21	10^6	9/9
Anti-interferon	BHK21	10^6	9/9
Normal rabbit serum	BHK-Mumps	10^6	2/11*
Anti-interferon	BHK-Mumps	10^6	12/12

*All mice were sacrificed 12 days after inoculation. Neoplasms formed in two of the mice injected with BHK-Mumps. By histopathology these neoplasms showed encapsulation and lymphocytic infiltration, typical traits of the "benign nodules" described previously. Confirmation of their "benign" form, however, would have required maintenance of the mice for some months.

vivo would block the development of NK cells capable of rejecting the virus PI tumor cells *in vivo*. Consequently, nude mice were treated with small samples of goat or rabbit anti-mouse IF serum, kindly provided by Drs. Ion Gresser and Kurt Paucker, respectively. They were then challenged with 10^6 virus PI tumor cells. The results of representative experiments are shown in TABLE 5. Even as little as one dose of 0.1 ml of anti-interferon serum permitted the growth of the virus PI tumor cells in the nude mouse, in contrast to control nude mice, untreated with anti-interferon, which once again restricted the growth of the tumor and formed only nodules. While these experiments must be expanded, they strongly suggest that the induction of interferon *in vivo* by the virus PI cell lines is responsible for the restriction of their growth in nude mice. Since the tumors are of human and hamster origin, and IF acts in a generally species-specific fashion, we infer that the regulation of the virus PI tumors *in vivo* occurred through the mediation of NK cells.

RELEVANCE OF INTERFERON AND NK CELLS IN PERSISTENT VIRUS INFECTIONS OF MAN

A number of chronic diseases of man are thought to be caused by persistent virus infection. Among these may be included subacute sclerosing panencephalitis, (SSPE), multiple sclerosis, systemic lupus erythematosis, and some forms of cancer. With the exception of SSPE, the nature of the etiologic agent in most cases remains unestablished. If interferon and NK cells played roles in man similar to those described in the model system of the nude mouse, one might anticipate that this system would provide a significant host defense mechanism against persistent virus infection. Indeed, since the above disease states have a relatively low prevalence, at least compared to the frequency of individuals recovering from acute virus infections, it may well be that this system does provide effective resistance against virus persistence in man. Therefore, it is necessary to provide some explanation for the persistence of viruses in those individuals with slow virus diseases. A number of possibilities can be envisaged: (1) a resistance of persistently infected cells to the cytolytic activity of NK cells; (2) a failure to produce interferon to the persisting virus or persistently infected cells; or (3) an absence of or failure to develop NK cells.

Clearly not all tumor cells are sensitive to killing by NK cells.[13] In the nude mouse model, we have reported previously the development of a variant of BHK-VSV cells by serial passage through nude mice which is persistently infected and yet grows in the nude mouse.[9] We have shown that these cells are excellent inducers of NK-cell augmentation *in vivo* and interferon *in vivo* and *in vitro*. Their growth *in vivo* appears to be attributable to a remarkable resistance to the cytolytic effect of NK cells, suggesting that virus or cell variants that are resistant to NK-cell killing can arise under immunological selection. Recent studies of Holland *et al.*[17] indicate that the property of resistance to natural immunity by these variants is controlled by the viral mutant, which persists and can be transferred by isolated virus as to parental BHK tumor cells.

In exploring the second alternative, we have examined the possibility of a defective cell-mediated immune response to viruses or virus PI cell lines in patients with putative persistent viral diseases, specifically multiple sclerosis and lupus erythematosis. Our initial observation indicated that while normal individuals whose lymphocytes were exposed for three days to measles antigen produced a suppressive activity on Con A-stimulated autochthonous cells, those

TABLE 6

DECREASED INTERFERON PRODUCTION BY LYMPHOCYTES FROM PATIENTS WITH MULTIPLE SCLEROSIS AND SYSTEMIC LUPUS ERYTHEMATOSIS

Donor Groups	Measles-induced IF (units/ml)	"Non-Responders"*
Normals	177 ± 38	7/44
Multiple sclerosis	27 ± 9 ($p < .01$)†	16/36 ($p < .01$)‡
Systemic lupus erythematosis	27 ± 11 ($p < .01$)†	5/11 ($p < .01$)‡

*Number of donors/total number tested producing less than the mean − 2 standard deviations of the titer of interferon produced by normals.

†Significant difference from normal donors, Student's t-test, $\log_{10}$ transformed data.

‡Significant difference from normal donors, χ^2 test.

from patients with multiple sclerosis were markedly deficient in this suppressive response.[18] Because of a correlation between the suppression of the T-cell response *in vitro* and the antiviral activity in those same cultures, we established that the *in vitro* suppression in normal individuals was mediated by interferon. There was a significant diminution in interferon production by lymphocytes of patients with multiple sclerosis upon exposure either to killed measles virus or killed Newcastle disease virus relative to normal individuals (TABLE 6). Recently, examination of lymphocytes from patients with lupus erythematosis revealed a similar defect. Under the conditions of study, the interferon is produced by a cell lacking conventional markers for B cells, T cells, and macrophages, and the type of interferon that is produced by normal controls but diminished in the patients is pH 2-stable, and neutralized by anti-leukocyte interferon serum, so it thus appears to be type I leukocyte interferon. These studies suggest that there is a defect in interferon production in patients with persistent viral infections which could represent a predisposing factor to disease. Studies are underway to characterize whether the primary deficiency is in a failure to produce interferon, or in the general functioning of NK cells in these patients.

CONCLUSION

While as few as 10–100 HeLa or BHK cells invariably produce tumors in nude mice, the same tumor cells persistently infected (PI) with measles, mumps, VSV, influenza or rabies viruses fail to do so, even when as many as 10^7 virus PI tumor cells are inoculated. The tumors either fail to grow or remain only as small nodules infiltrated with lymphocytes. The resistance of the nude mouse to virus PI tumor cells is an active process and abolished by irradiation.

Spleen cells from normal nude mice spontaneously lyse virus persistently infected tumor cells *in vitro*, but not the uninfected parental HeLa or BHK tumor cells. The cell responsible for cytotoxicity *in vitro* is not a conventional, T cell, B cell, or macrophage, but has characteristics of natural killer (NK) cells. However, while fewer than 2% of spleen cells in nude mice are lysed by monoclonal anti-Thy 1.2 + C, 30% of the NK activity on virus PI tumor cell targets is reproducibly eliminated by treatment with this monoclonal reagent. In addition, all of the NK activity is eliminated by treatment with anti-Ly 5.1 + C, indicating that in the nude mouse, Ly 5 surface antigen serves as a useful marker for NK cells.

Challenge of nude mice with any virus PI tumor cell induces an augmentation in the NK activity of spleens, not only for the homologous PI tumor cell but also for other susceptible NK targets. No augmentation of NK activity is seen when nude mice are inoculated with parental tumor cells. These results suggested that the augmentation in NK activity was mediated by a humoral factor stimulated by virus PI cells, and that the most likely such factor would be interferon.

Treatment of nude mouse spleen cells with culture supernatants containing mouse leukocyte or fibroblast interferon, or with small amounts (10^3–10^4 U) of chemically purified mouse interferon for periods as brief as 1–3 hours significantly augmented the degree of cytotoxicity on virus PI target cells *in vitro*. The augmenting effect was abrogated by treatment with anti-mouse interferon serum. These experiments confirm that interferon exerts a significant immunoregulatory role on NK activity.

Two hypotheses on the mode of action in interferon were considered: (1) that interferon acts on existing NK cells and augments their activity; (2) that interferon acts on a precursor to NK cells, regulating its differentiation into functional effector cells. Treatment of nude mouse spleen cells with anti-Ly 5.1 + C abrogated essentially all NK activity. Treatment of anti Ly 5-depleted spleen cells with purified interferon resulted in regeneration of significant levels of NK activity within 3 hours. All of the regenerated NK activity was susceptible to killing with anti-Ly 5 serum + C. These results formally demonstrate that interferon can act on Ly 5^- precursor to NK cells and initiate their differentiation into Ly 5^+ NK effector cells.

In order to establish that the killing of virus PI tumor cells by NK cells *in vitro* reflected the mechanism of resistance to the virus PI tumor cells *in vivo*, nude mice were treated with anti-IF antibodies and challenged with virus PI tumor cells. Preliminary results indicate that anti-interferon antibodies abrogated the ability of nude mice to reject the virus PI tumor cell lines.

If interferon and NK cells represent important mechanisms for resistance to persistent virus infection in man, one might predict that patients suffering from diseases thought to be caused by persistent virus infection would demonstrate some deficiency in the interferon-NK system. Lymphocytes from patients with multiple sclerosis or systemic lupus erythematosis were studied for their ability to produce interferon upon exposure to killed virus *in vitro*. The mean titer of interferon produced by lymphocytes from patients with multiple sclerosis or systemic lupus erythematosis challenged *in vitro* with killed measles or NDV was reduced by more than 75%. The results suggest that a defect in interferon production, and possibly NK cells, might be a predisposing factor to these diseases.

Acknowledgments

We are deeply indebted to Drs. Ion Gresser and Kurt Paucker for making anti-mouse interferon sera available to use for these studies, and to Dr. Peter Lengyel for generously providing chemically pure mouse interferon. We are grateful to Drs. John Holland and Charlotte Jones for providing the virus persistently infected tumor cell lines used in this work. We are grateful to Dr. Harvey Cantor for generously providing anti-Ly5 serum and for helpful discussion.

References

1. Bloom, B. R. & B. Rager-Zisman. 1975. *In* Viral Immunology and Immunopathology. A. L. Notkins, Ed: 113. Academic Press. New York.
2. Allison, A. C. & W. H. Burns. 1972. *In* Immunogenicity. F. Borek, Ed.: 155. North Holland. Amsterdam.
3. Stevens, J. C. & M. L. Cooke. 1974. J. Immunol. **113:** 1685.
4. Porter, D. D. 1975. *In* Viral Immunology and Immunopathology. A. L. Notkins, Ed.: 189. Academic Press. New York.
5. Zinkernagel, R. M. 1978. Immunol. Revs. **42:** 224.
6. Reid, L. & S. Shin. 1978. *In* The Nude Mouse in Experimental and Clinical Research. J. Fogh & B. Giovanella, Eds.: 313. Academic Press. New York.
7. Stutman, O. 1978. *In* The Nude Mouse in Experimental and Clinical Research. J. Fogh & B. Giovanella, Eds.: 411. Academic Press. New York.
8. Reid, L., C. Jones, & J. Holland. 1974. J. Gen. Virol. **42:** 609.
9. Minato, N., B. R. Bloom, C. Jones, J. Holland & L. Reid. 1979. J. Exp. Med. **149:** 1117.
10. Cantor, H., M. Kasai, F. W. Shen, J. C. LeClerc & L. Glincher. 1979. Immunol. Revs. **44:** 1.
11. Herberman, R. B., M. E. Nunn & H. T. Holden. 1978. J. Immunol. **121:** 304.
12. Gidlund, M., A. Orn, H. Wigzell, A. Senik & I. Gresser. 1978. Nature **237:** 759.
13. Trinchieri, G., D. Santoli, R. R. Dec & B. B. Knowles. 1978. J. Exp. Med. **147:** 1299.
14. Santoli, D. & H. Koprowski. 1979. Immunol. Revs. **44:** 125.
15. Cabrer, B., H. Taira, R. J. Braeze, T. D. Kempe, K. Williams, E. Stattery, W. H. Konigsberg & P. Lengyel. 1979. J. Biol. Chem. **254:** 3681.
16. Minato, N., L. Reid, H. Cantor, P. Lengyel & B. R. Bloom. J. Exp. Med. In press.
17. Herberman, R. R., J. R. Ortaldo, & G. D. Bonnard. 1979. Nature **277:** 221.
18. Neighbour, P. A. & B. R. Bloom. 1979. Proc. Nat. Acad. Sci. USA **76:** 476.
19. Kasai, M., J. C. Leclerg, H. W. Shan, & H. Cantor. Immunogenetics. In press.

PART II. REGULATORY EFFECTS OF INTERFERONS IN LYMPHOCYTES AND MACROPHAGES

REGULATORY EFFECTS OF INTERFERONS IN LYMPHOCYTES AND MACROPHAGES INTRODUCTORY REMARKS

Hans Wigzell

Department of Immunology
Biomedical Centre, Uppsala University
75123 Uppsala, Sweden

Time has amply proved the wisdom of the two discoverers of interferon, Isaacs and Lindenmann, in their denotation of the substance(s) originally found to be inhibitory for viral replication. It has thus become increasingly clear that interferon has a very broad field of action in addition to its antiviral function, involving cellular functions within but also outside the immune system. In this section we will deal with the ability of interferon to regulate the functional properties of lymphocytes and macrophages. It has been known for many years that interferon could enhance or inhibit antibody formation depending on the actual experimental conditions, thus indicating an effect on the B-lymphocyte system.[1,2]

This activity of interferon will not be discussed here, but the session will deal rather with the striking enhancement of aggressive, cell-mediated activities by the presence of interferon. The effector cells participating in such inhibitory or lytic functions constitute a mixed population, including cells with relatively nonspecific activities such as macrophages, cells intermediate with regard to selectivity, like natural killer (NK) cells, as well as highly specific killer T lymphocytes. Interferon has been shown to be a potent enhancing agent for all these cell types or their functional systems. It has been known since the work of Gresser and Lindahl that interferon has a stimulating function in killer T-cell systems, perhaps through its striking ability to increase the density of the major histocompatibility complex antigens on the target cells.[3] This ability has been reported to be relatively select for MHC molecules compared to other surface structures[4] and should result in a denser, more avidly binding surface for the MHC-restricted killer T cells.[5] But killer T lymphocytes appear rather late in the immune response, and interferon is known to be produced before the first appearance of cytolytic T cells. It was thus not surprising (if one would follow the dangerous line of logic) that interferon could also in an efficient manner activate macrophages and NK cells more rapidly, that is, in a matter of hours subsequent to viral or other infections.

Macrophages are known to either be aggressive "on their own," which could help during the early, comparatively nonspecific phase, whereas specific immune T cells when called into action may also "arm" as well as activate macrophages. Interferon is known to be able to activate macrophages as well as T cells.[6,7]

The third cell type to be dealt with during the coming session is the NK cell. This cell type has a distinct specificity pattern with yet no firm evidence as to the expression of clonally derived, antigen-specific receptors.[8] Its activity has been known for some time to be under regulation by various agents, and it is now well proven that interferon is the major regulatory substance *in vivo* for NK-cell activity.[9] These cytolytic cells have no requirement for the presence of MHC antigens on the target surface and can thus fill the gap left by the killer T cells for MHC-negative target cells, e.g., teratoma cells. Interferon would seem to act directly on these NK cells (or their precursors) leading to a rapid increase in the lytic potential of this cell group *in vivo*. As NK cell levels can be shown to be nicely correlated *in vivo* with resistance to tumor grafts in several animal systems,[10,11] it is not surprising that the long-known s.c. host component participating in the generation of interferon-induced tumor resistance[12,13] is now hypothesized by several workers to be caused by such NK cells.

In short, interferon is a major enhancing agent for cell-mediated reactions of an aggressive nature. Which function is most efficiently regulated by what interferon and how this regulation takes place will no doubt be a prime target for intense research activities in the near future.

References

1. Gisler, R. H., P. Lindahl & I. Gresser. 1974. Effects of interferon on antibody synthesis *in vitro*. J. Immunol. **113:** 438–444.
2. Johnson, H. M. 1977. Effect of interferon on antibody formation. Texas Reports Biol. Med. **35:** 357–369.
3. Lindahl, P., I. Gresser, P. Leary & M. Tovey. 1976. Interferon treatment of mice: Enhanced expression of histocompatibility antigens on lymphoid cells. Proc. Nat. Acad. Sci. USA **73:** 1284–1287.
4. Vignaux, F. & I. Gresser. 1977. Differential effect of interferon on the expression of H-2K, H-2D and Ia antigens on mouse lymphocytes. J. Immunol. **118:** 721–723.
5. Doherty, P. C., R. V. Blanden & R. M. Zinkernagel. 1976. Specificity of virus-immune effector T cells for H-2K or H-2D compatible interactions: Implications for H-2 antigen diversity. Transplant. Rev. **29:** 89–104.
6. Huang, H. 1977. Effect of interferon on phagocytosis. Texas Reports Biol. Med. **35:** 350–355.
7. Lindahl, P., P. Leary & I. Gresser. 1972. Enhancement by interferon of the specific cytotoxicity of sensitized lymphocytes. Proc. Nat. Acad. Sci. USA **69:** 721–725.
8. Kiessling, R. & H. Wigzell. 1979. An analysis of the murine NK cell as to structure, function and biological relevance. Immunol. Rev. **44:** 165–208.
9. Gidlund, M., A. Örn, H. Wigzell, A. Senik & I. Gresser. 1978. Enhanced NK cell activity in mice injected with interferon and interferon inducers. Nature **273:** 759–760.
10. Kiessling, R., G. Petranyi, G. Klein & H. Wigzell. 1975. Genetic variation of *in vitro* cytolytic activity and *in vivo* rejection potential of non-immunized semisyngeneic mice against a mouse lymphoma line. Int. J. Cancer **15:** 933–940.
11. Haller, O., M. Hansson, R. Kiessling & H. Wigzell. 1977. Non-conventional natural killer cells may play a decisive role in providing resistance against syngeneic tumor cells *in vivo*. Nature **270:** 609–611.
12. Gresser, I., I. Maury & D. Brouty-Boye. 1972. Mechanism of antitumor effect of interferon in mice. Nature **239:** 167–168.
13. Schellekems, H., W. Weimar, K. Cantell & L. Stitz. 1979. Antiviral effects of interferon *in vivo* may be mediated by the host. Nature **278:** 742.

INTERFERON MODULATION OF NATURAL KILLER CELL ACTIVITY*

Bice Perussia,† Daniela Santoli, and Giorgio Trinchieri

The Wistar Institute of Anatomy and Biology
Philadelphia, Pennsylvania 19104

In addition to their antiviral and anticellular activities, interferons (IF) appear to have a regulatory effect on immune functions. Interferons suppress lymphocyte proliferation in response to mitogens and antigens,[1] suppress graft-versus-host reactions,[2] inhibit or enhance (depending on the experimental protocol), antibody formation,[3-5] enhance the generation of specific cytotoxic T lymphocytes,[6,7] and increase the phagocytic and cytotoxic activity of macrophages.[8,9]

We have shown[10-15] IF to have a complex modulatory effect on the spontaneous cytotoxicity mediated by lymphocytes (FIGURE 1). Peripheral blood lymphocytes obtained from normal donors in the absence of disease or of any known or deliberate sensitization, are spontaneously cytotoxic *in vitro*.[16,17] In humans, this cytotoxic activity is mediated by effector lymphocytes, commonly referred to as natural killer (NK) cells. These cells are characterized by the presence of surface receptors for the Fc fragment of IgG immunoglobulins and by the absence of complement receptors and surface immunoglobulins. Both subpopulations of lymphocytes, obtained after separation according to their ability to form rosettes with sheep erythrocytes, contain NK cells.[18,19] Although antibodies do not seem to play any role in the cytotoxicity of NK cells, Fc receptors might be actively involved in the mechanism of lysis. This is suggested by the fact that Fc-receptor modulation induced by immune complexes results in inactivation of cytotoxic activity.[20]

Antiviral activity with the characteristics of type I (viral) IF is rapidly released from lymphocytes when they are cultured with most tumor-derived or virus-infected cell lines.[10,11] Most of the target cells that are commonly used for testing of NK-cell activity have been demonstrated to be inducers of IF. The mechanism of IF induction is still not understood, but the ability of cell lines to induce IF correlates with their tumor origin or transformation with certain viruses; normal fibroblast strains do not induce IF. The induction of IF under these conditions appears to be nonimmunological; it is induced in lymphocytes obtained from any healthy donor with no requirement for previous sensitization. Induction is not dependent on allogeneic differences between lymphocytes and inducer cell line; IF production is observed in mixed cultures of autologous or syngeneic cells. As judged by surface markers, the lymphocytes responsible for IF production in the mixed cultures belong to the same cell populations which mediate NK activity.

Interferons strongly affect both the activity of effector NK cells and the susceptibility of their target cells to lysis.[12-15] The effects on the two partners of the cytotoxic reaction are, however, paradoxically opposite: the cytotoxicity of NK

*Supported, in part, by United States Public Health Service Research Grants CA-20833, CA-10815 from the National Cancer Institute, and NS-11036 from the National Institute of Neurologic and Communicative Diseases and Strokes, and by the National Multiple Sclerosis Society.

†Recipient of a fellowship from the University of Milano (Italy).

0077-8923/80/0350-0055 $01.75/0 © 1980, NYAS

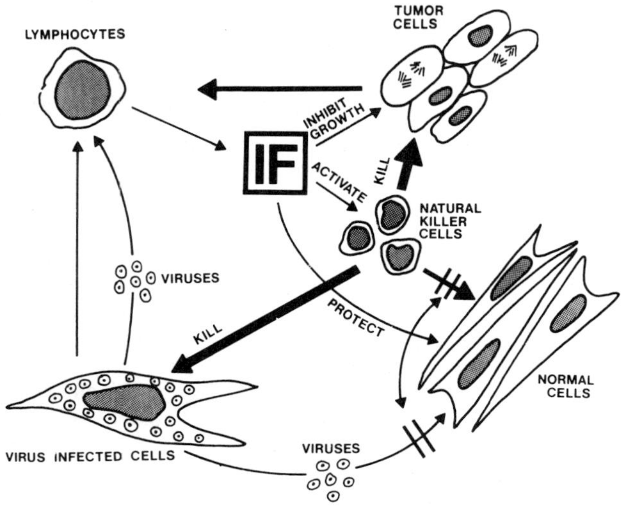

FIGURE 1. Model for the effects of interferon (IF) on NK cell activity *in vitro*. Viruses, virus-infected cells, most tumor-derived cell lines, and other IF inducers stimulate lymphocytes to produce IF. Interferon inhibits growth of rapidly dividing cells, inhibits viral replication in susceptible cells and enhances the NK cell activity. NK cells lyse any target cell lines nonspecifically. Interferon, however, renders normal cells (fibroblasts) and some tumor cell lines resistant to lysis by NK cells, whereas virus-infected cells and most tumor-derived cell lines are not protected.

cells is increased severalfold, while the susceptibility of target cells to lysis is drastically reduced or abolished by IF treatment. The enhancing effect of IF on NK cells is nonspecific; treated lymphocytes, although more active, show the same pattern of reactivity on a panel of target cell lines as untreated lymphocytes. On the other hand, the protective effect on target cells is selective; IF render normal fibroblasts almost completely resistant to lysis, while virus-infected cells and most tumor-derived cell lines are poorly or not protected. During *in vitro* assays of NK activity against IF-inducing target cells, the endogenous IF produced in the culture affects the observed cytotoxicity: after 4 hours of incubation, concomitant with the appearance of antiviral activity in the supernatant of the mixed cultures, an enhancement of cytotoxic activity of NK cells becomes demonstrable. Interferons, by stimulating nonspecific cytotoxic cells and by protecting normal cells from lysis, might act *in vivo* by rendering the NK cell system an inducible defense mechanism against tumor and virus-infected cells.

The enhancing effect of IF on NK activity can be readily demonstrated and quantitated by preincubating lymphocytes in the presence of known IF preparations and then testing them in a cytotoxic assay not affected by the production of endogenous IF, i.e., performing a short-term assay (less than 4 hr) and/or using target cell lines unable to induce IF. The IF produced in the mixed culture of lymphocytes and cell lines, the first one demonstrated to increase NK activity, has the molecular and biological characteristics of virus-induced type I leukocyte IF. All three known types of human IF (fibroblast and leukocyte types I and II[21] IF) increase the human NK-cell activity (see FIGURE 2a) and induce target-cell resistance to lysis (FIGURE 2b) to a similar extent. The use of electrophoretically homogeneous leukocyte IF in different laboratories[22,23] has clearly shown that the same molecules in IF preparations are responsible for both the antiviral activity and the enhancing effect on cytotoxicity. The enhancing effect of IF on NK cells can also be demonstrated by incubating lymphocytes with IF inducers such as viruses and inducer cell lines. Increase of cytotoxicity is observed after only a few hours of incubation at 37°C, but reaches the maximum level when lymphocytes have been preincubated with IF or IF inducers for 24–48 hours. Interferons appear to bind to lymphocytes independently of temperature, and the presence of IF is required for only a few minutes; however, subsequent incubation at 37°C, and active cellular protein and RNA synthesis are necessary in order to detect the enhancing effect.[23]

These data show that IF act by inducing complex metabolic alterations in the effector cells. Interferons do not simply provide a bridge between effector and target cells, as suggested in the case of IgG induction of antibody-dependent cell-mediated cytotoxicity[24] and in the case of mitogen induction of lysis of nonspecific target cells during the efferent phase of T-cell-mediated cytotoxicity.[25] Interferons can act either at the single effector cell level or by recruiting

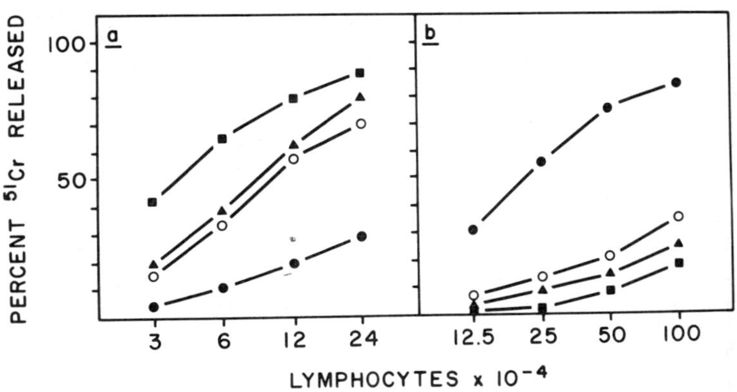

FIGURE 2. Effect of IF in enhancing NK cell cytotoxicity (a) and in protecting their target cells (b).

(a) Peripheral blood lymphocytes (5 × 10^6 cell/ml in RPMI 1640 supplemented with 10% fetal bovine serum) were incubated 18 hr at 37°C in the presence of 1,000 antiviral units/ml of human fibroblast IF (partially purified, kindly provided by Dr. A. Billiau, Leuven, Belgium), 1,000 U/ml of leukocyte type I (from Newcastle disease virus-induced human lymphocytes) or 250 U/ml of leukocyte type II (supernatant from secondary human mixed lymphocyte cultures at the second day after restimulation. NK cell-mediated cytotoxicity was tested at different effector-to-target cell ratios against human rhabdomyosarcoma-derived cells in a 4-hr ^{51}Cr release assay.[12] ●——●, lymphocytes preincubated in medium; ○——○, lymphocytes preincubated with leukocyte type I IF; ▲——▲, fibroblast IF; ■——■, leukocyte type II IF.

(b) Fetal skin fibroblasts, preincubated 18 hr at 37°C in medium or in the presence of the three different types of IF described above, were tested as target cells using human peripheral blood lymphocytes pretreated with 1,000 U/ml of human fibroblast IF as effector cells, in a 18-hr ^{51}Cr release assay.[12] ●——●, target cells preincubated in medium; ○——○, target cells preincubated with leukocyte type I IF; ▲——▲, fibroblast IF, and ■——■, leukocyte type II IF.

previously inactive cytotoxic cells. Interferons are able to enhance the cytotoxicity only of the lymphocyte subpopulations that originally contain NK activity. Lymphocyte subpopulations that do not contain NK cells (B cells, Fc-receptor negative "null" cells and IgG-Fc-receptor negative T cells) do not acquire cytotoxic activity upon exposure to IF. Saksela *et al.*[26] have demonstrated, however, that once active NK cells are removed by absorption on bead-attached fetal fibroblasts, a cell population is obtained devoid of NK activity. However, "pre-NK" cells can be demonstrated in this population since after treatment with IF the cytotoxic activity is again demonstrated.

Do IF induce activation of NK cells by facilitating effector-target recognition or by increasing the activity of cellular factors involved in the cytolytic mechanism of cytotoxicity? Some clarification on this point may be derived by comparing the effect of IF on the activity of NK cells and of the effector "killer" (K) cells responsible for antibody-dependent, cell-mediated cytotoxicity. K and NK cells are contained in the same lymphocyte subpopulations,[19] and it has been suggested that the same effector cell, although through a different mechanism of recognition, mediates both spontaneous and antibody-dependent cytotoxicity. Interferons have a differentiated effect on these two types of cytotoxic activity: NK-cell activity is enhanced in *in vitro* experiments up to 20-fold whereas K activity is either nonmodified[12,13,22] or increased only two or three times, depending on the experimental conditions.[23,27] The target cells used for testing K-cell activity are, to various extents, also susceptible to NK activity. Treatment of lymphocytes with IF activates NK cells and may result in an increase in the background of spontaneous cytotoxicity against unsensitized target cells. As a consequence, an apparent increase in the cytotoxicity of antibody-coated target cells is often observed. When target cells that are very susceptible to NK activity, e.g., human fibroblasts, are used, the increase in spontaneous cytotoxicity may mask the antibody-dependent cytotoxicity and therefore unsensitized and antibody-coated target cells are killed to a similar extent. In view of the possibility that both spontaneous and antibody-dependent cytotoxicity are mediated by the same cell, these data could suggest that IF is acting on NK cells at the recognition level, facilitating the contact between effector and target cells. In the presence of IgG antibodies on the target cells, the binding would be almost optimal because of the high affinity of the IgG-Fc receptors present on the effector cells. A further enhancing effect of IF would then be marginal. Interferons also mediate protection of target cells by acting at the recognition level as it has been shown by competition experiments. In this case there is a blocking effect.[12] Alternatively, IF could act by increasing the rate of killing, allowing each effector cell to lyse a higher number of target cells in the same time interval. In antibody-dependent, cell-mediated cytotoxicity an inactivation of the effector cells, due to a modification of the Fc receptors,[20] probably occurs after the first round of lysis. An effect of IF on the rate of cytotoxicity would then be difficult to detect. The limited increase in cytotoxicity sometimes observed[26] could be due to an additional effect on recruitment of "pre-NK" cells.

Interferons could affect NK cytotoxicity at the recognition level by modifying the membrane properties of effector cells (e.g., surface charge or mobility) or by affecting the expression of receptors involved in the target cell recognition by NK cells. Several investigators have shown cell surface alteration to result from the action of IF.

Treatment of L cells with IF resulted in an increased membrane negative charge.[28] The ability to bind the hormone thyrotropin and the cholera toxin was also altered in membranes from interferon-treated cells.[29,30] In addition, IF treatment of cells releasing RNA tumor viruses resulted in decreased virus yield and accumulation of virus particles on membranes, with an inhibitory mechanism which may be related to IF-induced alteration in the plasma membranes.[31,32] Interferon treatment of mouse lymphocytes resulted in an increase in the buoyant density of the plasma membranes and increased concentration of two major glycoproteins.[33] The expression of H-2 antigens was enhanced by IF treatment by a factor of two- to fourfold in the mouse lymphoid line L1210,[34] mouse thymocytes, and spleen cells.[35,36] The expression of θ or Ia antigens on those cells was, however, not increased. Interferon treatment of mouse lymphocytes also resulted in an increase in specific antigen-binding cells, an increase that was specifically inhibited by anti-H-2 but not anti-Ia sera.[36]

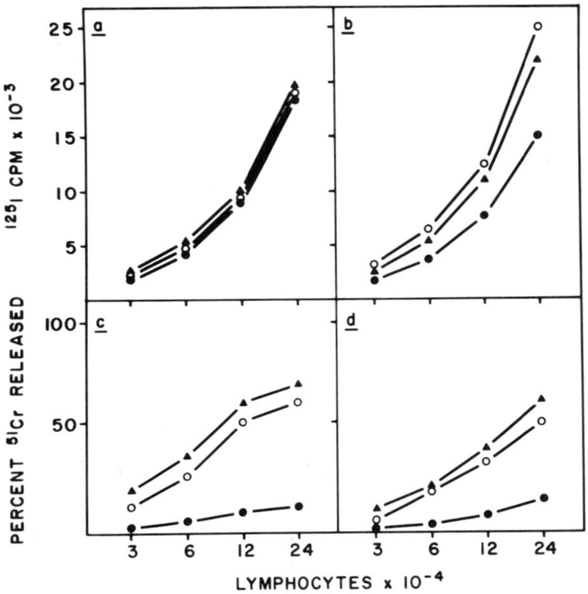

FIGURE 3. Effect of IF on the expression of HLA antigens on lymphocytes and on NK-cell cytotoxicity.

Lymphocytes from two donors were incubated with medium or 1,000 U/ml of leukocyte type I or fibroblast IF. After an 18-hr incubation at 37°C, the lymphocytes were tested for their ability to bind monoclonal anti-HLA antibodies (a,b) and to mediate spontaneous cytotoxicity (c,d). W6/32 monoclonal antibodies (γ_{2a}), specific for the products of the A, B, and C loci of the HLA complex, were originally produced in the laboratory of Dr. C. Milstein (Cambridge, England)[38] and obtained as an ascites fluid. Antibodies were purified by affinity chromatography on a protein A-Sepharose column and directly labeled with ^{125}I by the chloramine T method. 0.5 μg of labeled immunoglobulins have been used for each triplicate experimental point, the cells washed after 1 hr incubation at room temperature and cell bound radioactivity measured in a well-type γ counter. NK cell activity was measured in a 4-hr ^{51}Cr-release assay using a human rhabdomyosarcoma-derived cell line as target cells.[12] Parts a and c refer to the data obtained with one donor, b and d with the other donor.

●——●, lymphocytes incubated in medium; ○——○, lymphocytes incubated with leukocyte type I IF; and ▲——▲, with fibroblast IF.

Treatment of human lymphocytes with IF induced an increase in the expression of HLA antigens and of the associated β-2 microglobulin, but not of surface IgM or human T-cell antigens.[37] We have been investigating the possible correlation between the effect of IF on lymphocyte cytotoxicity and on the expression of surface antigens. Monoclonal antibodies, produced by somatic cell hybrids obtained by fusion of spleen cells of mice immunized with human lymphocytes and a mouse myeloma cell line, and specific for human lymphocyte surface antigens have been utilized. The purified antibodies were directly labeled with ^{125}I and tested in excess of antibody to obtain a linear correlation between the number of molecules (counts) bound and the number of cells tested. The assay of lymphocytes treated with IF using monoclonal antibodies of different specificity confirmed the increase in the expression of HLA and β-2 microglobulin. The same effect was obtained with the three types of human IF. Reagents specific for Dr antigens, surface immunoglobulins and other surface glycoproteins were also used, but no enhancing effect of IF was observed on the expression of these antigens either on purified preparations of peripheral blood lymphocytes or on thymocytes. The binding of anti-HLA monoclonal antibodies was increased up to three to four times in all the preparations of human thymocytes when they were incubated for several hours in the presence of IF. The effect on peripheral blood lymphocytes was less evident, with a maximum twofold increase. Interferon-treated lymphocytes have also been analyzed at the single cell level by cytofluorimetry. No change in the average size of the cells was detected by light scattering analysis, whereas the increase in the expression of HLA antigens, when analyzed by fluorescent antibodies, was observed in all the cells. The increase in the expression of HLA antigens induced by IF in peripheral blood lymphocytes from different donors showed individual variability, as also reported by Heron *et al.*[37] FIGURE 3 reports the data obtained with lymphocytes from two donors: lymphocytes from one donor displayed an increase of almost twofold in their ability to bind anti-HLA antibodies after treatment with either leukocyte or fibroblast IF; under the same conditions lymphocytes from the other donor showed no increase. When the NK activity of the two cell preparations was tested, IF induced a similar enhancement of cytotoxicity in both of them. This lack of correlation between enhanced expression of HLA antigens and augmentation of cytotoxicity was observed in repeated experiments and would argue against a direct role of the increased expression of histocompatibility antigens in the cytotoxic reactions of NK cells. The possibility that the IF-induced enhancement of cytotoxicity is mediated through a modulation of the expression of other surface structures or through a nonspecific modification of membrane properties will be further investigated.

REFERENCES

1. LINDAHL-MAGNUSSON, P., P. LEARY & I. GRESSER. 1972. Interferon inhibits DNA synthesis induced in mouse lymphocyte suspensions by phytohaemagglutinin or by allogeneic cells. Nature New Biol. **237:** 120.
2. CEROTTINI, J.C., K.T. BRUNNER, P. LINDAHL & I. GRESSER. 1973. Inhibitory effect of interferon preparations and inducers on the multiplication of transplanted allogeneic spleen cells and syngenic bone marrow cells. Nature New Biol. **242:** 152.
3. GISLER, R. H., P. LINDAHL & I. GRESSER. 1974. Effect of interferon on antibody synthesis *in vitro*. J. Immunol. **113:** 438.
4. BRAUN, W. & H. B. LEVY. 1972. Interferon preparations as modifiers of the immune response. Proc. Soc. Exp. Biol. Med. **141:** 769.

5. JOHNSON, H. & S. BARON. 1976. The nature of the suppressive effect of interferon and interferon inducer on the *in vitro* immune response. Cell Immunol. **25:** 106.
6. LINDAHL, P., P. LEARY & I. GRESSER. 1972. Enhancement by interferon of the specific cytotoxicity of sensitized lymphocytes. Proc. Nat. Acad. Sci. USA **69:** 721.
7. HERON, I., K. BERG & K. CANTELL. 1976. Regulatory effect of interferon on T cells *in vitro*. J. Immunol. **117:** 1370.
8. HUANG, K. Y., R. M. DONAHOE, F. B. GORDON & H. R. DRESSLER. 1971. Enhancement of phagocytosis by interferon-containing preparations. Infect. Immun. **4:** 581.
9. DONAHOE, R. M. & K. Y. HUANG. 1976. Interferon preparations enhance phagocytosis *in vivo*. Infect. Immun. **13:** 1250.
10. TRINCHEIRI, G., D. SANTOLI & B. KNOWLES. 1977. Tumor cell lines induce interferon in human lymphocytes. Nature **270:** 611.
11. TRINCHIERI, G., D. SANTOLI, R. R. DEE & B. B. KNOWLES. 1978. Antiviral activity induced by culturing lymphocytes with tumor-derived or virus-transformed cells. Identification of the antiviral activity as interferon and characterization of the human effector lymphocyte subpopulation. J. Exp. Med. **147:** 1299.
12. TRINCHIERI, G. & D. SANTOLI. 1978. Antiviral activity induced by culturing lymphocytes with tumor-derived or virus-transformed cells. Enhancement of human natural killer cell activity by interferon and antagonistic inhibition of susceptibility of target cells to lysis. J. Exp. Med. **147:** 1314.
13. TRINCHIERI, G., D. SANTOLI & H. KOPROWSKI. 1978. Spontaneous cell-mediated cytotoxicity in humans. Role of interferon and immunoglobulins. J. Immunol. **120:** 1849.
14. SANTOLI, D., G. TRINCHIERI & F. S. LIEF. 1978. Cell-mediated cytotoxicity against virus-infected target cells in humans. I. Characterization of the effector lymphocyte. J. Immunol. **121:** 526.
15. SANTOLI, D., G. TRINCHIERI & H. KOPROWSKI. 1978. Cell-mediated cytotoxicity in humans against virus-infected target cells. II. Interferon induction and activation of natural killer cells. J. Immunol. **121:** 532.
16. JONDAL, M. & H. PROSS. 1975. Surface markers on human B and T lymphocytes. VI. Cytotoxicity against cell lines as a functional marker for lymphocyte subpopulations. Int. J. Cancer **15:** 596.
17. PETER, H. J., J. PAVIE-FISHER, W. FRIDMAN, C. AUBERT, J. P. CESARINI, R. ROUBIN & F. KOURILSKY. 1975. Cell-mediated cytotoxicity *in vitro* of human lymphocytes against a tissue culture melanoma cell line. J. Immunol. **115:** 39.
18. WEST, W. H., G. B. CANNON, H. D. KAY, G. D. BONNARD & R. B. HERBERMAN. 1977. Natural cytotoxic reactivity of human lymphocytes against a myeloid cell line: Characterization of the effector cells. J. Immunol. **118:** 355.
19. SANTOLI, D., G. TRINCHIERI, L. MORETTA, C. M. ZMIJEWSKI & H. KOPROWSKI. 1978. Spontaneous cell-mediated cytotoxicity in humans. Distribution and characterization of the effector cell. Clin. Exp. Immunol. **33:** 309.
20. PERUSSIA, B., G. TRINCHIERI & J. C. CEROTTINI. 1979. Functional studies of Fc receptor-bearing human lymphocytes: Effect of treatment with proteolytic enzymes. J. Immunol. **123:** 681.
21. YOUNGNER, J. S. & S. B. SALVIN. 1973. Production and properties of migration inhibitory factor and interferon in the circulation of mice with delayed hypersensitivity. J. Immunol. **111:** 1914.
22. HERON, I., M. HOKLAND, A. MOLLER-LARSEN & K. BERG. 1979. The effect of interferon on lymphocyte-mediated effector cell functions: Selective enhancement of natural killer cells. Cellular Immunol. **42:** 185.
23. HERBERMAN, R. B., J. R. ORTALDO, J. Y. DJEU, H. T. HOLDEN, J. JETT, N. P. LANG & S. PESTKA. 1980. Role of interferon in regulation of cytotoxicity by natural killer cells and macrophages. This annal.
24. PERLMANN, P. & G. HOLM. 1969. Cytotoxic effect of lymphoid cells *in vitro*. Adv. Immunol. **11:** 117.
25. CEROTTINI, J. C. & K. T. BRUNNER. 1974. Cell-mediated cytotoxicity, allograft rejection and tumor immunity. Adv. Immunol. **18:** 67.
26. SAKSELA, E., T. TIMONEN & K. CANTELL. 1979. Human natural killer cell activity is

augmented by interferon via recruitment of 'pre-NK' cells. Scand. J. Immunol. **10:** 257.
27. HERBERMAN, R. B., J. R. ORTALDO & G. D. BONNARD. 1979. Augmentation by interferon of human natural and antibody-dependent cell-mediated cytotoxicity. Nature **277:** 221.
28. KNIGHT, R. E., JR. & B. D. KORANT. 1977. A cell surface alteration in mouse L cells induced by interferon. Biochem. Biophys. Res. Commun. **74:** 707.
29. FRIEDMAN, R. M. & L. D. KOHN. 1976. Cholera toxin inhibits interferon action. Biochem. Biophys. Res. Commun. **70:** 1078.
30. KOHN, L. D., R. M. FRIEDMAN, J. M. HOLMES & G. LEE. 1976. Use of thyrotropin and cholera toxin to probe the mechanism by which interferon mediates its antiviral activity. Proc. Nat. Acad. Sci. USA **73:** 3695.
31. CHANG, E. H., S. J. MIMS, T. J. TRICHE & R. M. FRIEDMAN. 1977. Interferon inhibits mouse leukemia virus release: An electron microscopy study. J. Gen. Virol. **34:** 363.
32. BILLIAU, A., H. HEREMANS, P. T. ALLEN, J. DEMAYER-GUIGNARD & P. DESOMER. 1976. Trapping of oncornavirus particles at the surface of interferon-treated cells. Virology **73:** 537.
33. CHANG, E. H., F. T. JAY & R. M. FRIEDMAN. 1978. Physical, morphological, and biochemical alterations in the membrane of AKR mouse cells after interferon treatment. Proc. Nat. Acad. Sci. USA **75:** 1859.
34. LINDAHL, P., P. LEARY & I. GRESSER. 1973. Enhancement by interferon of the expression of surface antigens on murine leukemia L1210 cells. Proc. Nat. Acad. Sci. USA **70:** 2785.
35. LINDAHL, P., P. LEARY & I. GRESSER. 1974. Enhancement of expression of histocompatibility antigens of mouse lymphoid cells by interferon *in vitro*. Eur. J. Immunol. **4:** 779.
36. LONAI, P. & L. STEINMAN. 1977. Physiological regulation of antigen binding to T cells: Role of a soluble macrophage factor and of interferon. Proc. Nat. Acad. Sci. USA **74:** 5662.
37. HERON, I., M. HOKLAND & K. BERG. 1978. Enhanced expression of beta-2 microglobulin and HLA antigens on human lymphoid cells by interferon. Proc. Nat. Acad. Sci. USA **75:** 6215.
38. BARNSTABLE, C. J., W. F. BODMER, G. BROWN, G. GALFRÉ, C. MILSTEIN, A. F. WILLIAMS & A. ZIEGLER. 1978. Production of monoclonal antibodies to group A erythrocytes, HLA and other human cell surface antigens—new tools for genetic analysis. Cell **14:** 9.

ROLE OF INTERFERON IN REGULATION OF CYTOTOXICITY BY NATURAL KILLER CELLS AND MACROPHAGES

Ronald B. Herberman,* John R. Ortaldo,* Julie Y. Djeu,† Howard T. Holden,* James Jett,* Nicholas P. Lang,* Menachem Rubinstein,‡ and Sidney Pestka‡

**Laboratory of Immunodiagnosis*
National Cancer Institute
Bethesda, Maryland 20205

†Bureau of Biologics
Bethesda, Maryland 20205

‡Roche Institute of Molecular Biology
Nutley, New Jersey 07110

A principal effector of natural cell-mediated cytotoxicity against tumors has been found to be a particular subpopulation of lymphocytes that have been termed natural killer (NK) cells.[1] An area of substantial interest has been the factors influencing the levels of NK activity. Although there is some evidence for a role of genetic factors in the relative levels of reactivity among different strains of rodents,[2,3] or among human donors,[4] this does not account for the characteristic age-related changes in NK activity of rodents. Young mice and rats, between 5 and 8 weeks of age, have high NK activity, whereas little or no activity is usually found in animals older than 12 weeks.

Augmentation of NK Activity by Interferon

Some clues regarding regulation of activity were obtained when it was found that inoculation of NK-susceptible target cells, viruses, or bacterial adjuvants such as BCG or *Corynebacterium parvum* caused a rapid increase in cytotoxicity by cells with characteristics of NK cells.[5,6] When it was found that rat NK activity could also be boosted by poly I:C,[7] a potent interferon (IF) inducer, the possible mediation of the boosting by IF was seriously considered. The peak of the augmentation of NK activity by a variety of agents in mice[5,8] was found to be very similar to that previously found for the peak levels of circulating IF in response to the same agents. A variety of murine oncogenic and nononcogenic viruses (murine sarcoma virus, lymphocytic choriomeningitis virus, mouse hepatitis virus, Sendai virus, mouse adenovirus, mouse cytomegalovirus) and other viruses (e.g., influenza A) was found to have peak effects on NK activity at 2–4 days after inoculation. Similarly, peak boosting of NK by tumor cells,[5] *Corynebacterium parvum*,[5] BCG,[6] and pyran copolymer[9] was seen at about 3 days. In contrast, endotoxin boosted within 3–6 hr[8] and poly I:C within 12–18 hr.[8] We have measured serum IF levels in mice treated with each of these boosting agents and have found elevated levels to be closely associated with augmentation of cytotoxicity. In addition to observing this with known IF-inducers, NK-susceptible target cells were shown to be potent inducers of IF.[10] The tumor cell-induced

0077-8923/80/0350-0063 $01.75/0 © 1980, NYAS

IF was found to be labile at low pH and required a relatively prolonged period for induction of viral resistance, and thus appeared to be type II or immune IF, although it was neutralized by anti-type I IF.[10] As further and more direct evidence for the role of IF in augmenting NK activity in mice, inoculation of crude or purified virus-induced type I IF (10^4 units) was shown to boost cytotoxicity within 3 hr.[8,11]

After overcoming some of the problems associated with *in vitro* lability of mouse NK activity, we have also been able to incubate mouse spleen cells with poly I:C or IF (minimal dose, 10^3 units) and produce rapid augmentation of NK activity and these effects were inhibited by anti-IF.[8] Recent studies have indicated that incubation of spleen cells with IF for less than 1 min at 37°C or 0°C, followed by washing, resulted in substantial boosting of cytotoxicity in the 4-hr ^{51}Cr release cytotoxicity assay. This indicates that binding of IF to the cell surface and/or triggering of the NK cells occurs very rapidly and that the further processes required for augmentation of reactivity can occur during the course of the assay.

Boosting by IF or IF-inducers has been particularly noticeable in mice older than 12 weeks of age, whose spontaneous levels of NK activity had already declined to negligible levels. The degree of boosting *in vitro* by IF has varied substantially among strains, with high NK strains being more sensitive to boosting.[12] This suggests that the differences in NK activity among strains of mice may be due, at least in part, to differential susceptibility to IF, produced by various *in vivo* stimuli.

A similar stimulatory role of IF for human NK cell activity has been demonstrated. We have been able to confirm the suggestive evidence of Trinchieri and Santoli[13] by showing that three different preparations of partially purified IF (1×10^6–3×10^7 units/mg protein), from fibroblasts as well as from leukocytes or a lymphoblastoid cell line, could boost the NK activity of most normal human donors.[14] We initially observed that exposure of lymphocytes to IF for 1 hr caused significantly increased activity in about half of the donors, and longer exposure gave somewhat more consistent results.[14] In more recent studies with lymphocytes from donors known to be susceptible to boosting by IF, incubation with IF for 5 min or less, at 4°C, 22°C or 37°C, followed by washing, was found to be sufficient for boosting.[15] As in the mouse studies, the boosting effects by human IF could be abrogated by the addition of either of two different anti-IF preparations.[14] Boosting could also be blocked by pretreatment of the lymphocytes with ouabain,[15] an agent known to block the antiviral effects of IF.

Effects of Interferon on Various Types of Effector Cells

It has been of considerable interest to determine whether the ability of IF to augment cytotoxicity is restricted to NK cells or whether other effector cells could also be affected. We have therefore performed a series of experiments to examine the spectrum of activity of IF on various human effector cell populations. The results are summarized in TABLE 1. We have obtained evidence that cytotoxicity of K cells mediating antibody-dependent, cell-mediated cytotoxicity (ADCC),[14-16] and of monocytes[17] could be boosted by IF. In addition, some subpopulations of cells mediating cytotoxicity induced by the lectin, phytohemagglutinin, (LICC)[18] and the cytotoxicity of cultured cells against K-562 target cells could be boosted by IF.

TABLE 1

EFFECTS OF INTERFERON ON CYTOTOXIC REACTIVITY OF VARIOUS HUMAN EFFECTOR CELLS

Effector Cells	Effect
NK cells	Boost
E-RFC, FcR+*	Boost (relatively strong)
E−, FcR+	Boost (relatively weak)
K cells vs. variety of ab-coated targets (Chang, RBL-5, CRBC)	Boost
Monocytes	Boost
Lectin-induced cytotoxicity	
E-RFC, FcR−	Boost (relatively weak)
E-RFC, FcR+	Boost (very strong)
After MLC	
vs. K-562 target cells	Boost
vs. PHA blasts	No effect
Cultured T cells	
vs. K-562 target cells	Boost
vs. PHA blasts	No effect

*E-RFC, cells forming rosettes with sheep erythrocytes; E−, cells not forming rosettes with sheep erythrocytes; FcR+, cells with receptors for the Fc portion of IgG, and FcR−, cells lacking this receptor; CRBC, chicken erythrocytes.

The effects of IF on K-cell activity is a controversial issue. Although we previously reported[14] that human IF could augment ADCC, Trinchieri and his colleagues[13,19] reported negative results. One possible explanation was that different IF-containing preparations were used, with differing degrees of purity. To more definitively examine the role of IF in boosting of cytotoxic activity, we have performed experiments with pure human leukocyte IF.[20] As shown in TABLE 2, crude, partially purified fibroblast IF (HEM Research, Rockville, MD) and pure leukocyte IF induced substantial augmentation of ADCC activity against antibody-coated Chang cells, as well as NK activity against K-562 cells. The pure IF also augmented the cytolytic activity of human monocytes (TABLE 3).

Another possible explanation for our observations of an apparent boost of ADCC was that treatment with IF was actually augmenting the NK activity against the target cells and that this plus the antibody coating resulted in high levels of cytotoxicity. To resolve this, it was necessary to use target cells

TABLE 2

EFFECTS OF VARIOUS INTERFERON PREPARATIONS ON CYTOLYTIC ACTIVITY BY NK CELLS AND ON ANTIBODY-DEPENDENT, CELL-MEDIATED CYTOTOXICITY

IF Preparation	Cytolytic Activity (LU/10^7 cells) NK (K-562)	ADCC (Ab-Chang)	ADCC Control (Chang)	IF Titer (U/ml)
None	19.4	130	<1	<1
Fibroblast, partially purified	78	200	6	1000
Control preparation	22.5	155	<1	<1
Leukocyte, crude	93	303	5.7	950
Leukocyte, pure	92	242	1	1000

TABLE 3

EFFECTS OF PURE LEUKOCYTE INTERFERON ON CYTOLYTIC ACTIVITY OF NORMAL HUMAN MONOCYTES*

Expected Titer of IF (U/ml)	% Cytolysis		
	Untreated	Interferon	Control Preparation
333		35.7†	22.7
33		25.7†	20.3
0	18.2		

*Monocytes from a normal donor tested against TU5 target cells at an effector:target cell ratio of 30:1, in a 48-hr ^{3}H-thymidine release assay.

†Significantly above untreated control, $p < 0.01$.

completely resistant to lysis by human NK cells. We have therefore performed experiments with mouse tumor lines and chicken red blood cells (CRBC) as targets and some of these data are summarized in TABLE 4.

With the mouse lymphoma RBL-5, and with CRBC as targets, no cytotoxicity was seen in the absence of antibody-coating, yet a substantial increase in ADCC was observed. We had yet another opportunity to examine the effects of IF on ADCC when we observed that leukemic cells from a patient with T-cell chronic lymphocytic leukemia (T-CLL) had strong ADCC activity in the absence of detectable NK activity.[21] As shown in TABLE 5, ADCC activity of the leukemic cells was substantially augmented by IF. Taken together, our data strongly support the conclusion that cytotoxic activity by K cells, as well as by NK cells, is boosted by IF.

IF was also found to appreciably augment LICC against Chang target cells.[18] To further analyze this, peripheral blood mononuclear cells were fractionated into T cells forming rosettes with sheep erythrocytes (E-RFC) and into non-rosette-forming cells (E−). These populations were further divided according to presence (FcR+) or absence FcR−) of Fc receptors for IgG. As previously observed, most of the LICC activity was in the E-RFC, FcR− subpopulation (TABLE 6). When these cells were preincubated with IF, their activity was boosted to an appreciable extent. The E-RFC, FcR+ subpopulation, as well as the E− subpopulations, had little LICC activity. However, after exposure to IF, the E-RFC, FcR+ cells were very strongly boosted, attaining activity even higher than that of the main subpopulation of effector cells. In contrast, the E− cells acquired only low levels of LICC activity after treatment with IF. Thus, the E-RFC, FcR+ subpopulation stands out as the most sensitive to augmentation of LICC by IF.

Previous reports indicated that the reactivity of cytotoxic T cells from *in vivo*

TABLE 4

EFFECTS OF INTERFERON ON ADCC AGAINST VARIOUS TARGET CELLS

Treatment of Effector Cells	Cytotoxicity (LU/10^7 cells)						
	K-562	Chang	ab-Chang	RBL-5	ab-RBL-5	CRBC	ab-CRBC
None	76	<.1	21	<.1	79	<.1	149
IF, 1000 U, 1 hr	135	1	89	<.1	128	<.1	315

TABLE 5

EFFECTS OF INTERFERON ON ADCC BY CELLS FROM PATIENT WITH T-CLL

Effector Cells and Treatment	Cytotoxicity (LU/10^7 cells) K-562	Chang	ab-Chang
CLL patient			
Untreated	<.1	<.1	167
IF, 1000 U, 1 hr	<.1	<.1	597
Normal donor			
Untreated	40	<.1	33
IF, 1000 U, 1 hr	188	<.1	71

allosensitized mice could be boosted with IF.[22] However, the activity of human cytotoxic T cells, after sensitization *in vitro* in mixed lymphocyte cultures, was not boosted by IF.[23,24] One possible explanation for this apparent discrepancy is that cultured lymphocytes lose the ability to interact with or be stimulated by IF. Alternatively, the subpopulation of human T cells mediating the alloimmune cytotoxic reaction may not be sensitive to the effects of IF. To examine this issue, we have tested the cytotoxicity of human lymphocytes after one-way mixed lymphocyte culture against PHA-stimulated lymphocytes from the stimulator and also against K-562 cells, to measure NK-like activity[25] as well as specific cytotoxic T cells (TABLE 6). As previously reported,[23,24] reactivity of the immune T cells against PHA blasts was not affected by treatment with IF. In contrast, the NK-like activity against K-562 was appreciably increased. Similarly, the cytotoxicity of cultured T cells against K-562 was augmented by IF,[26] whereas reactivity against PHA blasts was unaffected. These results indicate that some lymphocytes that have been in culture for at least several days can respond well to IF. It is therefore more likely that the subpopulation of human effector cells mediating alloimmune cytotoxicity is resistant to augmentation by IF.

Taken together, the pattern of responsiveness to IF of human cytotoxic effector cells (TABLE 1) suggests that they can be classified as sensitive or resistant, depending on their cell surface characteristics and possibly their mechanism of cytotoxicity. It is of particular interest to note that effector cells bearing Fc receptors for IgG (i.e., NK cells, K cells, monocytes, and a subpopulation of LICC effector cells) are sensitive to augmentation by IF, whereas effectors lacking Fc

TABLE 6

EFFECT OF INTERFERON ON LECTIN-INDUCED CELL-MEDIATED CYTOTOXICITY (LICC) BY VARIOUS LYMPHOCYTE SUBPOPULATIONS

Effector Cell Population	Cytotoxicity (LU/10^7 cells)* Untreated	IF (1000 U, 1 hr)
E-RFC, FcR+	3	112
E-RFC, FcR−	20	84
E−, FcR+	<1	4
E−, FcR−	<1	7

*4-hr ^{51}Cr release assay against Chang target cells, in presence of 2 μg/ml PHA. In the absence of PHA, little or no lysis was seen in any of the groups. Results given are the means from 4 experiments.

receptors were either unaffected (alloimmune cytotoxic T cells) or affected to a lesser extent (the main subpopulation mediating LICC). The reasons for this apparent association between responsiveness to IF and Fc receptors are not clear and need to be investigated.

There have been some interesting differences noted for the conditions required for IF to boost various effector cells. To obtain consistent augmentation of human NK- and K-cell activities, 100 units of IF/ml have been sufficient and sometimes even 10 units have been effective. For augmentation of human monocyte cytolytic activity, 200–400 units of IF/ml have usually been required, and stronger boosting has been seen with 1,000 units. A more striking difference has been related to the time required for binding of IF and/or activation. As noted above, maximal boosting of mouse and human NK cell activity can be seen after preincubation of the effector cells for 1–5 min, even at 4°C, and washing before testing in the cytotoxicity assay.[15] In contrast, preincubation of human monocytes with IF for 1 hr has had little effect, and only modest boosting was seen after preincubation for 18 hr at 37°C.[17] Optimal boosting by IF of monocyte-mediated cytolysis has required the presence of IF during the assay.

Effects of Metabolic Inhibitors and Anti-Interferon on Spontaneous and Boosted NK Activity

To better understand the mechanism of NK activity and its regulation by IF, we have studied the effects of various metabolic inhibitors and anti-IF on spontaneous mouse and human NK activity and on boosting of activity by IF. Treatment of mouse NK cells with inhibitors of DNA, RNA or protein synthesis or with anti-IF has not affected their spontaneous activity.[27] In contrast, boosting of mouse NK activity by IF was completely blocked by inhibitors of RNA or protein synthesis and by anti-IF. For several hours after IF treatment, the boosted activity remains dependent on RNA and protein synthesis. Thereafter the boosted state becomes stable and cannot be reversed by these inhibitors. Based on these results, we have formulated a model for augmentation of mouse NK activity by IF (Figure 1). The proposed sequence of events is quite similar to those described for the activation by IF of cellular resistance to virus infection, which has been shown to be dependent on a transient period of new messenger RNA and protein synthesis.[28] Also shown on the Figure is the ability of prostaglandins E_1 and E_2 to inhibit spontaneous and boosted NK activity,[29] indicating that NK activity may be subject to negative as well as positive regulation.

Table 7

Effect of Interferon on Cytotoxicity of Lymphocytes After Mixed Lymphocyte Culture

Donor	Treatment of Effector Cells	Cytotoxicity ($LU/10^7$ cells): K-562	Cytotoxicity ($LU/10^7$ cells): PHA Blasts of Stimulator
HP	none	12.8	288
	IF, 1000 U, 1 hr	84.2	312
DT	none	22.8	399
	IF, 1000 U, 1 hr	51.3	411

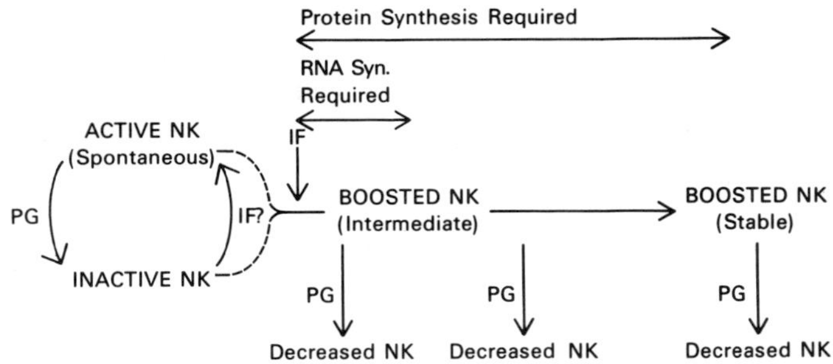

FIGURE 1. Model for regulation of mouse NK activity. Interferon (IF) appears to be responsible for augmentation of spontaneous NK activity to the "boosted NK" state. It remains unclear, as indicated in the left side of the model, whether IF acts on inactive precursors of NK cells or whether it augments the reactivity of already spontaneously activated NK cells. During the early period of boosting, RNA and protein synthesis is required, as indicated by the ability of the appropriate inhibitors to block or reverse augmentation. After 4–6 hr for RNA synthesis, and approximately 18 hr for protein synthesis, the boosted NK state becomes stable and is no longer affected by the metabolic inhibitors. Prostaglandins E_1 or E_2 (PG) have been found to inhibit both spontaneous and boosted NK activity and may be important negative regulatory factors.

When similar studies were performed with human NK cells, the effects of the various agents on boosting by IF were quite analogous.[30] However, some interesting differences were noted with spontaneous human NK activity. In contrast to mouse NK cells, the activity of human NK cells was strongly inhibited by pretreatment with protein synthesis inhibitors or with anti-IF. To explain these observations, we postulate that the levels of spontaneous human NK activity remain high in individuals over a wide age range because of continued endogenous *in vivo* production of IF. Spontaneous NK activity in man may represent recent boosting by IF and thus be susceptible to reversal by inhibitors of protein synthesis and anti-IF. Clearly, further studies will be needed to support this hypothesis.

STUDIES OF REGULATION OF NK ACTIVITY IN CANCER PATIENTS

NK activity has been found to be depressed in mice[31,32] and patients[33] bearing large tumors and some evidence has been obtained for a role of prostaglandins in producing this inhibition.[29] The depressed reactivity in tumor-bearing mice has been reversed, at least in part, by inoculation of lymphocytic choriomeningitis virus. A particularly important practical issue is how IF or IF-inducers might affect the levels of cytotoxicity of NK cells and other effector cells in cancer patients and thereby potentially alter host resistance against tumor growth. We have recently monitored the effects of BCG and *Corynebacterium parvum* inoculation on NK activity of cancer patients. In some recipients, a rapid rise in NK activity has been seen, with kinetics similar to that observed in mice. However, in other patients, these agents have induced depression of cytotoxic activity. These observations appear analogous to observations in mice that *C. parvum*[34] and other IF-inducers[35] can under some circumstances depress rather than augment NK activity. It will be very important to adequately understand the factors influencing the direction of regulatory effects on effector cell function induced by clinical immunotherapeutic agents. Such information should lead to more effective and rational approaches to immunotherapy of cancer.

References

1. Herberman, R. B. & H. T. Holden. 1978. Natural cell-mediated immunity. *In* Advances in Cancer Research. G. Klein & S. Weinhouse, Eds. Vol. **27:** 305–377. Academic Press. New York.
2. Kiessling, R., E. Klein & H. Wigzell. 1975. "Natural" killer cells in the mouse. I. Cytotoxic cells with specificity for mouse Moloney leukemia cells. Specificity and distribution according to genotype. Eur. J. Immunol. **5:** 112–117.
3. Oehler, J. R., L. R. Lindsay, M. E. Nunn & R. B. Herberman. 1978. Natural cell-mediated cytotoxicity in rats. I. Tissue and strain distribution, and demonstration of a membrane receptor for the Fc portion of IgG. Int. J. Cancer. **21:** 204–209.
4. Santoli, D., G. Trinchieri, C. M. Zmijewski & H. Koprowski. 1976. HLA-related control of spontaneous and antibody-dependent cell-mediated cytotoxic activity in humans. J. Immunol. **117:** 765–770.
5. Herberman, R. B., M. E. Nunn, H. T. Holden, S. Staal & J. Y. Djeu. 1977. Augmentation of natural cytotoxic reactivity of mouse lymphoid cells against syngeneic and allogeneic target cells. Int. J. Cancer **19:** 555–564.
6. Wolfe, S. A., D. E. Tracey & C. S. Henney. 1976. Induction of "natural killer" cells by BCG. Nature **262:** 584–586.
7. Oehler, J. R., L. R. Lindsay, M. E. Nunn, H. T. Holden & R. B. Herberman. 1978. Natural cell-mediated cytotoxicity in rats. II. *In vivo* augmentation of NK-cell activity. Int. J. Cancer **21:** 210–220.
8. Djeu, J. Y., J. A. Heinbaugh, H. T. Holden & R. B. Herberman. 1979. Augmentation of mouse natural killer cell activity by interferon and interferon inducers. J. Immunol. **122:** 178–181.
9. Santoni, A., P. Puccetti, C. Riccardi, R. B. Herberman & E. Bonmassar. 1979. Augmentation of natural killer activity by pyran copolymer in mice. Int. J. Cancer. **24:** 656–661.
10. Djeu, J. Y., K. Y. Huang, H. T. Holden & R. B. Herberman. 1980. Augmentation of mouse natural killer activity and induction of interferon by tumor cells. J. Exp. Med. **151:** 781–789.
11. Gidlund, M., A. Örn, H. Wigzell, A. Senik & I. Gresser. 1978. Enhanced NK cell activity in mice injected with interferon and interferon inducers. Nature **223:** 259–261.
12. Herberman, R. B., J. Y. Djeu, H. D. Kay, J. R. Ortaldo, C. Riccardi, G. D. Bonnard, H. T. Holden, R. Fagnani A. Santoni & P. Puccetti. 1979. Natural killer cells: Characteristics and regulation of activity. Immunol. Rev. **44:** 43–70.
13. Trinchieri, G. & D. Santoli. 1978. Anti-viral activity induced by culturing lymphocytes with tumor derived or virus-transformed cells. Enhancement of human natural killer cell activity by interferon and antagonistic inhibition of susceptibility of target cells to lysis. J. Exp. Med. **147:** 1314–1333.
14. Herberman, R. B., J. R. Ortaldo & G. D. Bonnard. 1979. Augmentation by interferon of human natural and antibody-dependent cell-mediated cytotoxicity. Nature **277:** 221–223.
15. Ortaldo, J. R., N. P. Lang & R. B. Herberman. Augmentation of human natural killer cell activity by interferon: Conditions required for boosting and characteristics of the effector cells. Submitted for publication.
16. Ortaldo, J. R., S. Pestka, B. Slease, M. Rubinstein & R. B. Herberman. 1980. Augmentation of human K cell activity with interferon. Scand J. Immunol. In press.
17. Jett, J. R., A. Mantovani & R. B. Herberman. 1980. Augmentation of human monocyte-mediated cytolysis by interferon. Cell. Immunol. In press.

18. LANG, N. P., G. D. BONNARD & R. B. HERBERMAN. Effects of interferon on human lectin-induced cell-mediated cytotoxicity. Submitted for publication.
19. TRINCHIERI, G., D. SANTOLI & H. KOPROWSKI. 1978. Spontaneous cell-mediated cytotoxicity in humans. Role of interferon and immunoglobulins. J. Immunol. **120:** 1849–1858.
20. RUBINSTEIN, M., S. RUBINSTEIN, P. C. FAMILLETTI, R. S. MILLER, A. A. WALDMAN & S. PESTKA. 1979. Human leukocyte interferon: Production, purification to homogeneity, and initial characterization. Proc. Nat. Acad. Sci. USA **76:** 640–644.
21. PANDOLFI, F., D. M. STRONG, R. B. SLEASE, M. L. SMITH, J. R. ORTALDO & R. B. HERBERMAN. 1980. Characterization of a suppressor T-cell chronic lymphocytic leukemia with ADCC but not NK activity. Blood. In press.
22. LINDAHL, P., P. LEARY & I. GRESSER. 1972. Enhancement by interferon of the specific cytotoxicity of sensitized lymphocytes. Proc. Nat. Acad. Sci. USA **69:** 721–725.
23. HERON, I., K. BERG & K. CANTELL. 1976. Regulatory effect of interferon on T cells *in vitro*. J. Immunol. **117:** 1370–1377.
24. ZARLING, J. M., J. SOSMAN, L. ESKRA, E. C. BORDEN, J. S. HOROSZEWICZ & W. A. CARTER. 1978. Enhancement of T cell cytotoxic responses by purified human fibroblast interferon. J. Immunol. **121:** 2002–2009.
25. SEELEY, J. K. & S. A. GOLUB. 1978. Studies on cytotoxicity generated in mixed lymphocyte cultures. I. Time course and target spectrum of several distinct concomitant cytotoxic activities. J. Immunol. **120:** 1415–1423.
26. LANG, N. P., J. R. ORTALDO & R. B. HERBERMAN. The effects of interferon, prostaglandins, and dibutyryl cyclic nucleotides on human cell-mediated cytotoxicity. Submitted for publication.
27. DJEU, J. Y., H. T. HOLDEN & R. B. HERBERMAN. Effects of metabolic inhibitors on spontaneous and interferon-boosted mouse natural killer cell activity. Submitted for publication.
28. BAGLIONE, C. 1979. Interferon-induced enzymatic activities and their role in the antiviral state. Cell **17:** 255–264.
29. HOLDEN, H. T., J. Y. DJEU, M. J. BRUNDA & R. B. HERBERMAN. 1980. Regulation of the activity of natural killer cells by interferon and prostaglandins. *In* Biochemical Characterization of Lymphokines. A. L. deWeck, F. Kristensen & M. Landy, Eds.: 369–373. Academic Press. New York.
30. ORTALDO, J. R., W. PHILLIPS & R. B. HERBERMAN. Effects of metabolic inhibitors on spontaneous and interferon-boosted human natural killer cell activity. Submitted for publication.
31. HERBERMAN, R. B., M. E. NUNN & D. H. LAVRIN. 1975. Natural cytotoxic reactivity of mouse lymphoid cells against syngeneic and allogeneic tumors. I. Distribution of reactivity and specificity. Int. J. Cancer **16:** 216–229.
32. BECKER, S. & E. KLEIN. 1977. Decreased "natural killer"-NK-effect in tumor bearing mice and its relation to the immunity against oncorna virus determined cell surface antigens. Eur. J. Immunol. **6:** 892–898.
33. PROSS, H. F. & M. G. BAINES. 1976. Spontaneous human lymphocytemediated cytotoxicity against tumor target cells. I. The effect of malignant disease. Int. J. Cancer **18:** 593–604.
34. OJO, E., O. HALLER, A. KIMURA & H. WIGZELL. 1978. An analysis of conditions allowing Corynebacterium parvum to cause either augmentation or inhibition of natural cytotoxicity against tumor cells. Int. J. Cancer **21:** 444–452.
35. PUCCETTI, P., A. SANTONI, C. RICCARDI, H. T. HOLDEN & R. B. HERBERMAN. 1979. Activation of mouse macrophages by pyran copolymer and role in augmentation of natural killer activity. Int. J. Cancer. **24:** 819–825.

MONONUCLEAR PHAGOCYTES: RESPONDERS TO AND PRODUCERS OF INTERFERON*

Solomon I. Hamburg, Howard B. Fleit, Jay C. Unkeless,† and Michel Rabinovitch

Department of Cell Biology
New York University School Medicine
New York, New York 10016

†The Rockefeller University
New York, New York 10021

Macrophages from animals subjected to inflammatory stimuli, infected with intracellular pathogens, or inoculated with killed microorganisms or with fractions from microorganisms display enhanced immunological and nonimmunological phagocytosis, as well as an increased ability to spread over inert substrates.[1]

We have previously shown that *in vivo* administration of interferon (IF) inducers such as Newcastle disease virus (NDV), polyinosinic-polycytidylic acid (poly I.C) or tilorone, enhances both Fc-mediated phagocytosis and the rapid spreading of peritoneal macrophages over inert substrates.[2,3] Correlative evidence indicated that the *in vivo* effects of IF inducers on macrophages were mediated by induced IF. Mice that carry alleles for high or low IF reponses to NDV demonstrated that the degree of macrophage spreading and phagocytosis segregated with the serum IF response.[3,4] Also, administration of anti-IF globulin reduced both the serum IF and the phagocytic enhancement induced by either NDV or tilorone.[5] Finally, homozygous nude mice inoculated with NDV displayed reduced serum IF titers and macrophage phagocytosis when compared with their heterozygous littermates, and T-cell administration prior to NDV administration restored both responses in the nude animals.[6] The evidence, reviewed in more detail elsewhere,[7] confirms and extends the findings of Huang,[8] of enhanced pinocytic uptake of colloidal carbon by macrophages stimulated *in vivo* with NDV or *in vitro* with IF-rich preparations.

The results presented here provide direct evidence for the role of IF in the enhancement of Fc-mediated phagocytosis by macrophages. Macrophages cultivated *in vitro* with IF-rich preparations display enhanced phagocytosis of IgG-coated erythrocytes. The stimulation of phagocytosis does not appear to be mediated by increased numbers of detectable Fc receptors but requires protein and RNA synthesis. Inflammatory macrophages can also be stimulated by IF *in vitro*. In addition, experiments are described on the production of IF by bone marrow-derived macrophage cultures induced with poly I.C, NDV, or a lipopolysaccharide.

*This work was supported by Grants I-T 32-6M 07308 (to SIH), GMO 7238-04 (to HBF), AI 14603 (to JCU), and AI 10969 (to MR) from the National Institutes of Health.

0077-8923/80/0350-0072 $01.75/0 © 1980, NYAS

In Vitro Stimulation of Macrophages by Interferon Preparations

Unstimulated resident macrophages were obtained from mice by peritoneal lavage. The suspensions were allowed to adhere onto glass coverslips, which were then rinsed to remove nonadherent cells. Macrophages were cultivated overnight in the presence of 5% heat-inactivated rat serum and used the next day in all experiments. The experimental protocol involved incubation of the cultures with IF-rich or control preparations and evaluation of their phagocytic response using sheep erythrocytes opsonized with limiting amounts of rabbit anti-sheep erythroycte IgG (EA). The percentage of macrophages ingesting four or more EA, as determined by phase contrast microscopy was used as the criterion for enhanced phagocytic activity. The concentration of IgG used for opsonization was such that less than 20% of control macrophages ingested four or more EA. The microscopic appearance of the cultivated cells before and after phagocytosis is shown in FIGURE 1, a & b. The macrophages are well spread, show membrane ruffling and are phagocytic.

Precultivation of the adherent cell population resulted in an almost entirely pure macrophage population (>99%). Thus it is unlikely that contaminating lymphocytes mediated the stimulation of the macrophages by IF-preparations. However, both the initial attachment to a foreign substrate and cultivation in the presence of fetal bovine serum can stimulate the phagocytic activity of macrophages. While nonelicited macrophages did not thrive in serum-free medium, we found that mouse or rat sera were less stimulatory than the commonly used fetal calf or calf sera.

Incubating macrophages with IF preparations resulted in a significant increase in the phagocytic activity of macrophages (FIGURE 2) as compared to that of control cells (FIGURE lb). In the initial experiments serum from female Swiss Webster mice inoculated intravenously with NDV 6 hours prior to sacrifice was used as the source of IF. As shown in FIGURE 3, incubation of the cultures for 4 hours with 5% mouse serum containing approximately 500 U/ml IF significantly stimulated macrophage phagocytosis. In contrast, macrophages incubated with 5% normal mouse serum displayed only a minor enhancement of phagocytic activity.

In succeeding experiments we examined the phagocytic enhancement induced by a semipurfied IF preparation, kindly provided by Dr. Eugene Sulkowksi (Roswell Park Memorial Institute, Buffalo, NY). The IF was induced in L cells with NDV and purified on metal-chelate columns to a specific activity of 2×10^7 U/mg protein.[9]

The results of time course studies indicated that doses of 50, 100, or 500 U/ml IF enhanced macrophage phagocytosis by 4 hours, but that only the highest dose continued to increase the number of macrophages recruited into the stimulated population (FIGURE 4). FIGURE 5 presents the results of a dose-response experiment in which macrophages were incubated with different concentrations of IF for 8 hours and evaluated for phagocytosis of EA. A linear phagocytic response was obtained between 5 and 100 U/ml IF. Additional IF did not further increase the percentage of macrophages ingesting EA and there was a nonsignificant rise in the phagocytosis of EA by macrophages cultivated with the IF diluent, 0.1% bovine serum albumin in phosphate buffered saline (PBS).

Stimulation of phagocytosis was also obtained after 8 hours incubation of macrophages with a highly purified mouse IF preparation (sp. act. of 2.4×10^9

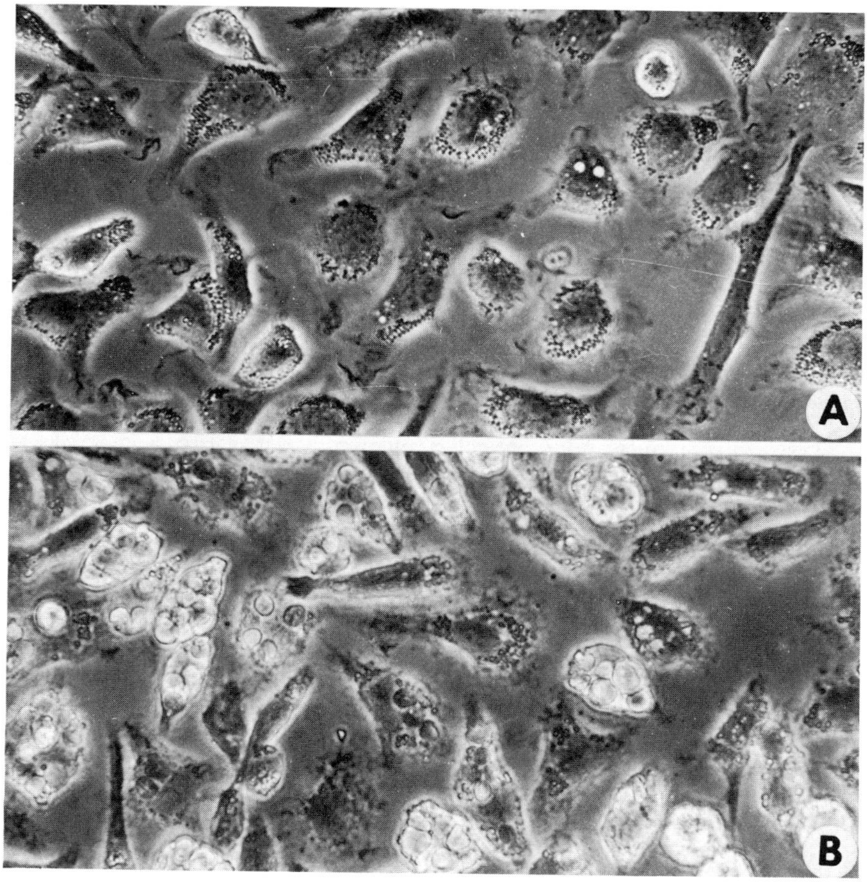

FIGURE 1. Cultivated macrophages (A) with or (B) without phagocytosis of EA. Macrophages were plated at a density of 2×10^5 cells/12 mm diameter coverslip and cultivated for 24 hr in serumless media (Neuman and Tytell, Gibco) containing 5% heat-inactivated rat serum with penicillin and streptomycin. The cells were overlaid with sheep erythrocytes opsonized with 1000 molecules of anti-sheep erythrocyte IgG/cell and incubated for 30 min at 37°C. The externally bound erythrocytes were lysed with hypotonic saline in order to allow the internalized erythrocytes to be counted by phase contrast microscopy.

U/mg protein;[10] kindly provided by Dr. Jacqueline DeMaeyer-Guignard, Institut du Radium, Faculté des Sciences, Orsay, France).

Since the induction of the antiviral state only requires a short single pulse of IF,[11] we determined whether a pulse of IF is also sufficient to enhance the uptake of EA. Macrophages were cultivated for various periods of time in the presence of 100 U/ml IF or control diluent, the medium was removed, the cells washed and new medium previously conditioned by macrophages, was added back to the cultures. At 8 hours of incubation the macrophages were tested for their phagocytic activity. The results, presented in FIGURE 6, indicate that a 1-hour pulse of IF followed by incubation in IF-free medium was necessary and

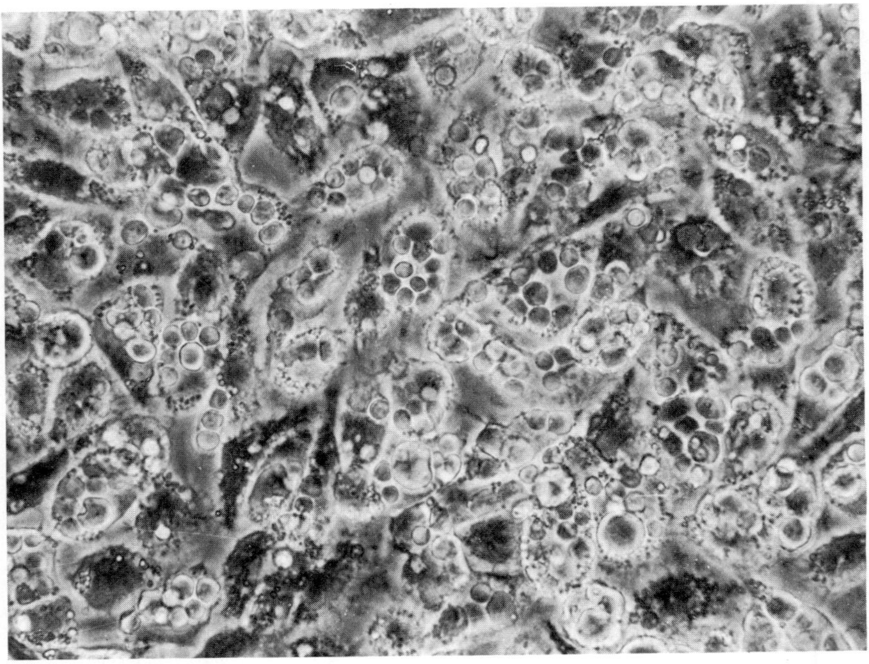

FIGURE 2. Phagocytosis of EA by macrophages incubated with interferon. Cultivated macrophages were incubated with 100 U/ml IF for 8 hr and overlaid with EA as in FIGURE 1.

FIGURE 3. Time course of macrophage phagocytic response to mouse serum containing interferon activity. *Abscissa:* Time. *Ordinate:* Percent ingestion of four or more EA. Cultivated macrophages were incubated in media containing mouse sera from animals given NDV 6 hours prior to sacrifice such that the final IF activity was 500 U/ml (*open circles*) or control mouse sera (*closed circles*). At various times of incubation the phagocytic activity was assayed by overlaying EA as in FIGURE 1. The percentage of macrophages ingesting four or more EA was determined microscopically by counting 200 cells per coverslip. All points are an average of quadruplicate determinations.

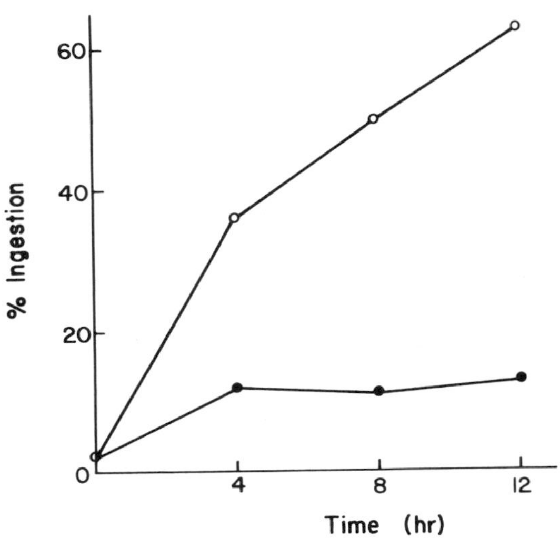

sufficient for maximal enhancement of phagocytosis. Again, a proportion of the macrophages did not respond to IF under the conditions of the experiment.

Ribonucleic Acid and Protein Synthesis Requirements for the Interferon-mediated Enhancement of Macrophage Phagocytosis

The antiviral activity of IF requires both RNA and protein synthesis.[12-15] Thus it is important to determine whether the acquisition of the antiviral state and of enhanced phagocytosis have similar requirements for macromolecular synthesis.

Reversible inhibitors were used in these studies, since continuous inhibition of either RNA or protein synthesis over 8 hours was found to depress phagocytosis by macrophages[16] (unpublished observations). Accordingly, the RNA inhibitor

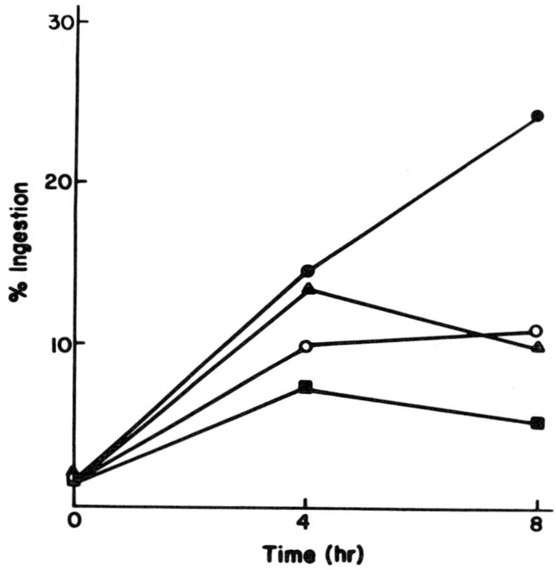

FIGURE 4. Time course of macrophage phagocytic response to purified interferon. *Abscissa:* Time. *Ordinate:* Percent ingestion of four or more EA. Cultivated macrophages were incubated with either 50 U/ml (*open circles*), 100 U/ml (*closed triangles*) or 500 U/ml (*closed circles*) interferon or control buffer (*closed squares*) and assayed for their phagocytic activity at 4 and 8 hr as in FIGURE 3. All points are an average of quadruplicate determinations.

camptothecin, and the protein synthesis inhibitor pactamycin were used to examine these requirements for IF-induced enhancement of phagocytosis.

Cultivated macrophages were preincubated with either camptothecin or pactamycin prior to the addition of 200 U/ml IF or the control diluent. After a 1-hour pulse of IF, the medium containing the inhibitor and IF or control diluent was removed, the cells were washed and incubated in fresh medium. At the end of 8 hours the macrophages were tested for their phagocytic activity. As positive controls, cultures were also continuously incubated with IF during the 8-hour period.

The results of typical experiments with pactamycin or camptothecin are presented in FIGURES 7 and 8, respectively. A 1-hour pulse of IF was found to stimulate the phagocytosis of the macrophages to the same degree as continuous incubation. In contrast, in the presence of either inhibitor the stimulatory effect

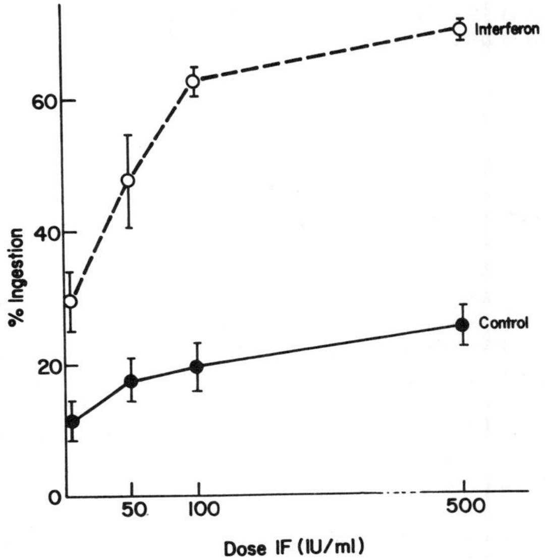

FIGURE 5. Response of macrophage phagocytosis to increasing doses of purified interferon. *Abscissa:* Dose IF. *Ordinate:* Percent ingestion of four or more EA. Cultivated macrophages were incubated for 8 hr with different concentrations of IF and assayed for their phagocytic activity as in FIGURE 3. IF (*open circles*), control (*closed circles*). Average ± S.E.M. of quadruplicate determinations.

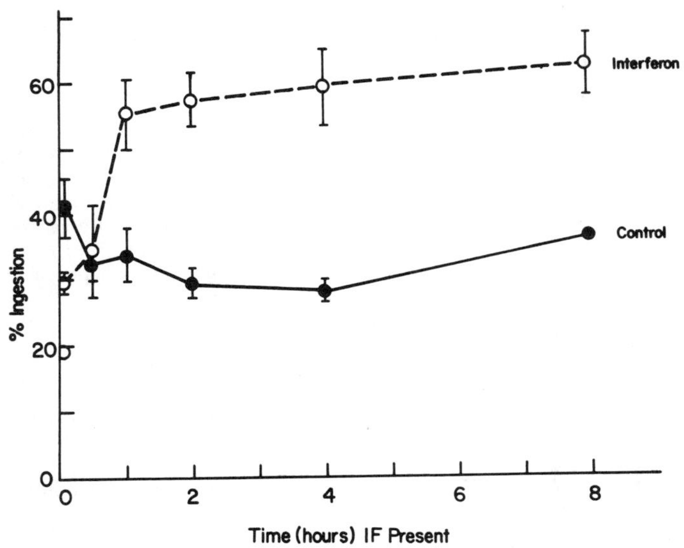

FIGURE 6. Duration of required macrophage exposure to interferon for phagocytic enhancement. *Abscissa:* Time IF present before media change. *Ordinate:* Percent ingestion of four or more EA. Cultivated macrophages were incubated with 100 U/ml purified IF for different lengths of time and assayed for phagocytic activity at 8 hr as in FIGURE 3. IF treated (*open circles*), control (*closed circles*). Average ± S.E.M. of quadruplicate determinations.

of IF was significantly decreased without any reduction in the phagocytic activity of control macrophages.

Fc Receptors in Interferon-treated Macrophages

Fc-mediated phagocytosis appears to involve primarily two steps: (1) attachment to the phagocyte's surface, mediated by the recognition of the Fc portion of IgG bound to the particle; and (2) ingestion, triggered by sequential recognition of the ligands on the surface of the particle, resulting in a localized cytoskeletal reorganization and formation of an endocytic vacuole.[17] Both steps require the Fc receptor located on the surface of the phagocytic cell.

The enhanced phagocytic activity of macrophages exposed to IF could be the result of IF effects on any of the steps involved in the endocytic process. Thus, binding of EA would be enhanced if more functional Fc receptors were available or if the avidity of the receptors for Fc were increased. Increased ingestion could result from metabolic changes; from changes in cytoskeletal elements, such as of the state of polymerization of actin; or from increased mobility of the Fc receptors in the plane of the membrane.[18]

There is evidence that there are at least two Fc receptors on the surface of macrophages.[19-22] FcRI is sensitive to proteolytic cleavage by trypsin and binds to the Fc region of IgG2a; in contrast, FcR II is trypsin-resistant and binds to either IgG1 or IgG2b. Both receptors bind rabbit IgG equally well.

Until recently the numbers of available Fc receptors could be evaluated only by indirect methods. However, with the availability of a hybridoma antibody against FcR II,[23] it is now possible to determine whether the enhancement of

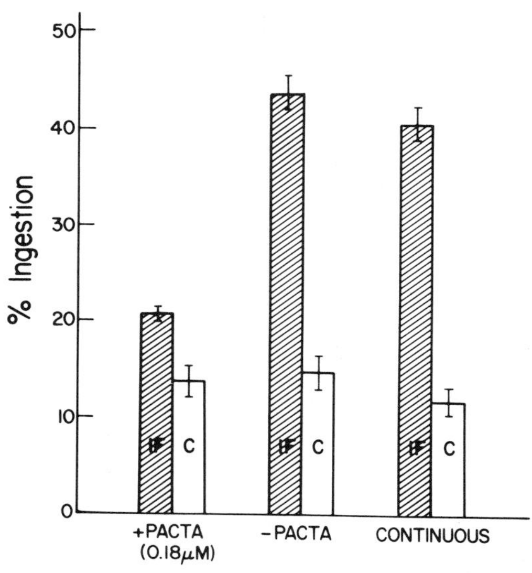

FIGURE 7. Inhibition of interferon-induced macrophage phagocytic enhancement by pactamycin. *Abscissa:* Treatments. *Ordinate:* Percent ingestion of four or more EA. Cultivated macrophages were preincubated for 1 hr in the presence of 0.18 μM pactamycin or control diluent followed by an additional 1-hr incubation with 200 U/ml IF (*cross-hatched bars*) or control buffer (*open bars*). The pactamycin and IF-containing media were removed, replaced with macrophage-conditioned media and incubated at 37°C for an additional 7 hr. Phagocytic activity was assayed as in FIGURE 3. Continuous incubation with IF or control buffer was also performed as positive controls. Average ± S.E.M., quadruplicate determinations per point.

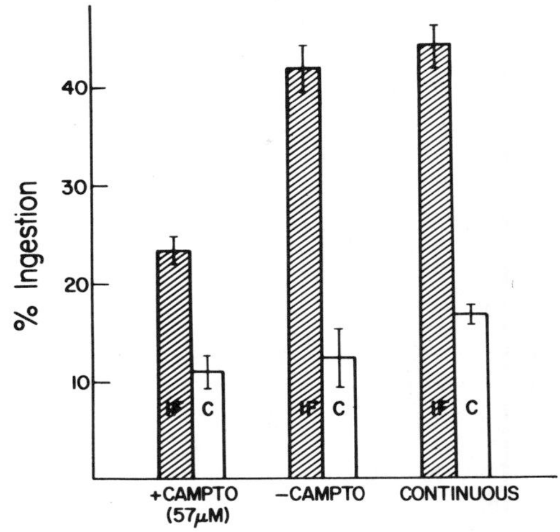

FIGURE 8. Inhibition of interferon-induced macrophage phagocytic enhancement by the ribonucleic acid synthesis inhibitor, camptothecin. *Abscissa:* Treatments. *Ordinate:* Percent ingestion of four or more EA. Cultivated macrophages were preincubated for 25 min in the presence of 57 μM camptothecin or control diluent followed by an additional 1-hr incubation with 200 U/ml IF (*cross-hatched bars*) or control buffer (*open bars*). The camptothecin and IF-containing media were removed and replaced with macrophage-conditioned media and incubated at 37°C for an additional 7 hr. Phagocytic activity was assayed as in FIGURE 3. Continuous incubation with IF or control buffer was also performed as positive controls. Average± S.E.M., quadruplicate determinations per point.

phagocytosis by IF is due to an increased availability of Fc II receptors on the surface of the macrophages. Our studies revealed no significant differences in the uptake of radioiodinated Fab fragments of the hybridoma antibody by macrophages treated with IF when compared to control macrophages. As shown in FIGURE 9, macrophages cultivated in the presence or absence of 200U/ml IF bound anti-FcR II ^{125}I-Fab fragments at similar rates when assayed at 4°C. As controls, L929B cells, known to lack Fc receptors[24] and coverslips without cells were used to determine background binding. Additional experiments using excess noniodinated Fab as a carrier indicated that by 5 minutes the binding was nearly saturated (data not shown) and that approximately 5×10^4 FcR II antibody-binding sites per cell were present on IF treated and control macrophages.

To exclude the possibility that the binding of the Fab at 4°C did not reflect the number of Fc receptors available at 37°C, binding studies were also performed at the higher temperature. The results of these experiments did not reveal any significant difference between IF-treated and control macrophages.

Previous studies have demonstrated[25,26] that the uptake of erythrocytes opsonized with rabbit antibody is unaffected by preliminary trypsinization of the macrophages. As FcR II is trypsin resistant, it appears that in our assay FcR II is primarily involved. The results support the conclusion that the phagocytic stimulation mediated by IF does not involve the synthesis of additional Fc receptors. However, since turnover of Fc receptors does occur, the possibility cannot be excluded that new more avid Fc receptors have been synthesized during the period between the addition of IF and the assay of the response. Nor can one exclude the possibility that IF induces new Fc receptors that bear an

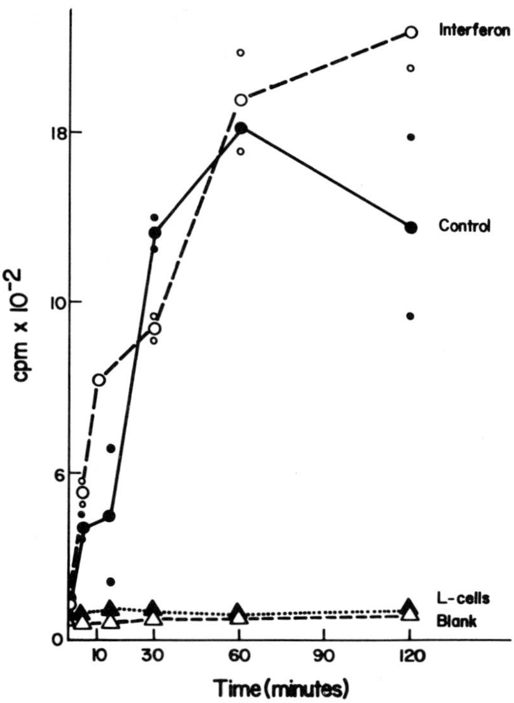

FIGURE 9. Kinetics of binding of a monoclonal anti-Fc II receptor antibody to interferon- or control-treated macrophages. *Abscissa:* Time. *Ordinate:* Counts per minute. Cultivated macrophages bound to coverslips, were incubated with 200 U/ml IF or control buffer for 8 hr and then overlaid with 300 μl of anti-FcRII ^{125}I–Fab for various time periods at 4°C. The coverslips were washed in PBS and the cpm determined in a gamma counter. IF, *open circles;* control, *closed circles;* L-cells, *closed triangles;* blank coverslips, *open triangles.*

antigenic determinant different from that recognized by the hybridoma antibody.

RESPONSE OF INFLAMMATORY OR LPS-STIMULATED MACROPHAGES TO INTERFERON *IN VITRO*

In addition to work with normal macrophages the phagocytic responses of *in vivo* prestimulated macrophages were also examined. Results from several laboratories indicated that macrophage activation for cytotoxicity may involve a series of steps. While the highly phagocytic inflammatory macrophage is not cytotoxic, it can acquire this ability when exposed to small concentrations of endotoxins, serum fractions or lymphocyte products[27–31] at concentrations that do not activate resting, noninflammatory cells. It was therefore of interest to determine whether inflammatory macrophages could still respond to IF *in vitro* with a further enhancement of phagocytosis.

Macrophages obtained from animals given either thioglycollate medium or proteose peptone, intraperitoneally, or LPS, subcutaneously, displayed a significant enhancement of their phagocytic activity over the ingestion of EA by macrophages from control mice. Cultivation of the inflammatory or stimulated macrophages in the presence of 500 U/ml of semipurified IF for 6-8 hours resulted in additional stimulation. In contrast, little if any further stimulation was obtained with macrophages from mice given IF inducers such as NDV or poly I.C prior to *in vitro* cultivation with IF. The results of these experiments are shown in FIGURE 10. The figure also indicates that the macrophages from animals that received the inducers had enhanced activity when compared to macrophages from control mice.

The enhancement of phagocytosis by IF was further examined with macrophages obtained 24 hours after administration of LPS. FIGURE 11 shows that macrophages prestimulated by LPS showed enhanced uptake of EA when compared to those from control animals given PBS alone. Further stimulation of phagocytosis was obtained when IF was present during the cultivation of either

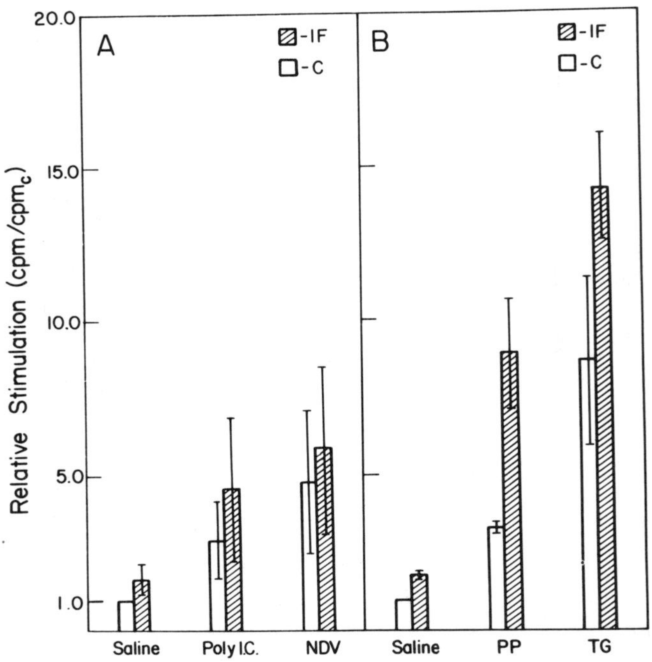

FIGURE 10. Relative *in vitro* phagocytic response to interferon of *in vivo* prestimulated macrophages. *Abscissa: In vivo* stimulator. *Ordinate:* Relative stimulation. Peritoneal macrophages were obtained from animals given either (A) NDV (1 × 10^8 PFU/ animal), poly I.C (100 ug/animal), or 0.25 ml PBS i.v. 24 hr prior to sacrifice; or (B) 10% proteose peptone, 3% thioglycollate broth, or 3.0 ml PBS i.p., 3 days prior to sacrifice. Macrophages were plated at a density of 3.5 × 10^5 cells/16 mm diameter well, incubated with 500 U/ml IF (*cross-hatched bars*) or control diluent (*open bars*) for 6–8 hr and overlaid with ^{51}Cr-labeled EA to assay phagocytic activity. After 30 min at 37°C, externally bound erythrocytes were lysed, the macrophages were washed and lysed with distilled water to solubilize the cell associated ^{51}Cr. The extracts were counted in a gamma counter. All counts are normalized relative to unstimulated macrophages. Average ± S.E.M., triplicate determinations.

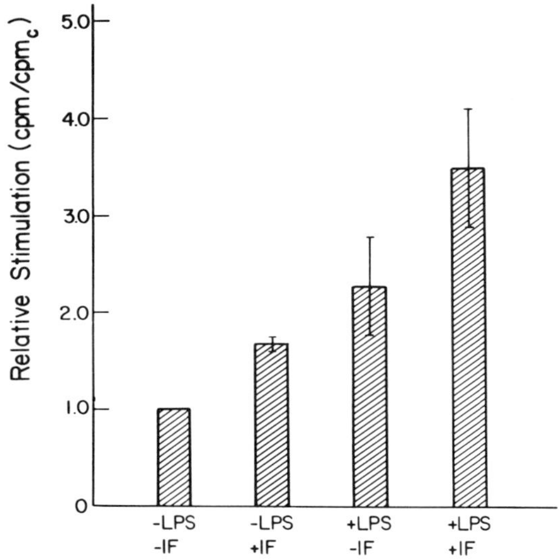

FIGURE 11. Relative stimulation of *in vivo* lipopolysaccharide-prestimulated macrophages by interferon *in vitro*. *Abscissa:* Top, LPS or control administered *in vivo;* bottom, presence or absence of IF in culture. Peritoneal macrophages were obtained from animals given 50 μg *S. abortus equi* lipopolysaccharide (Difco) or PBS subcutaneously 24 hr prior to sacrifice. The macrophages were then incubated with 500 U/ml IF or control buffer for 6 hr and assayed for phagocytosis as in FIGURE 10. Average ± S.E.M. eight determinations.

normal or prestimulated macrophages. The additional stimulation appeared to be additive.

Dose response studies revealed that both normal and LPS-stimulated macrophages responded similarly to a range of concentrations of IF (FIGURE 12). In addition, the time course of the responses to 500 U/ml IF was also similar for stimulated and for control macrophages (FIGURE 13).

Since the time course and dose responses of IF stimulation were similar in

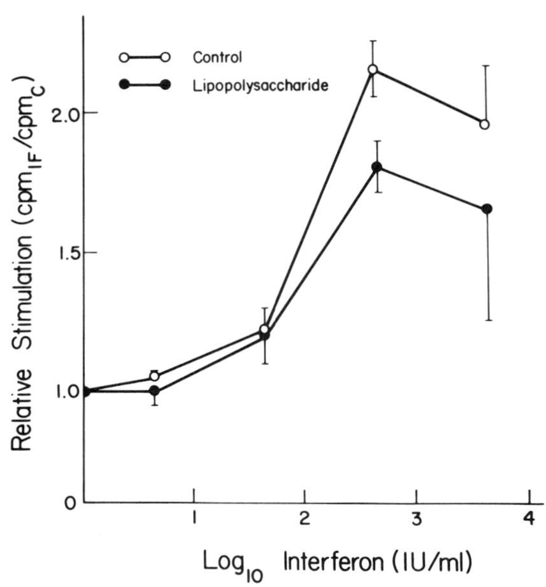

FIGURE 12. Comparison of the phagocytic response of normal or lipopolysaccharide-prestimulated macrophages to increasing concentrations of interferon. *Abscissa:* Log_{10} units per ml of interferon. *Ordinate:* Relative stimulation. Normal (0.25 ml PBS subcutaneously) or lipopolysaccharide (50 μg/animal subcutaneously) prestimulated macrophages were incubated with increasing concentrations of IF for 6 hr and assayed for phagocytic activity as in FIGURE 10. Average ± S.E.M., triplicate determinations. IF, *closed circles;* control, *open circles.*

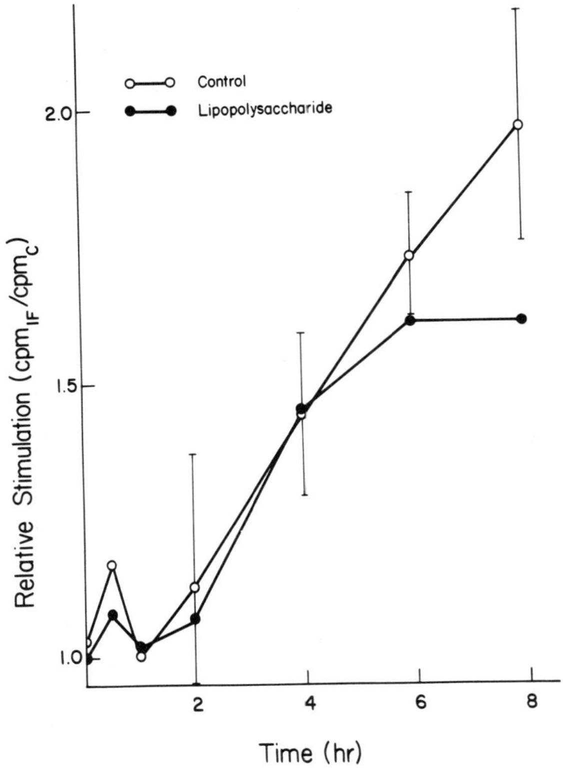

FIGURE 13. Comparison of time course of the response to interferon by fresh or lipopolysaccharide-prestimulated macrophages. *Abscissa:* Time. *Ordinate:* Relative stimulation. Normal (0.25 ml/animal PBS subcutaneously) or lipopolysaccharide (50 μg/animal subcutaneously) prestimulated macrophages were incubated with 500 U/ml IF or control diluent for various times and assayed for phagocytosis as in FIGURE 10. Average ± S.E.M., triplicate determinations. IF, *closed circles;* control, *open circles.*

macrophages from LPS-treated or control mice, it is probable that the effect of IF involves similar mechanisms in both cases.

INTERFERON PRODUCTION BY BONE MARROW MACROPHAGES

Peritoneal macrophages and monocyte-derived macrophages have been shown to produce IF when treated by viruses, double-stranded polyribonucleotides or lipopolysaccharides.[32-35] Cultivation of bone marrow cells in media containing colony-stimulating activity (CSA) provides large numbers of pure macrophages.[36,37] We have examined the production of IF by marrow-derived macrophages after induction by a lipopolysaccharide, poly I.C, or NDV. In addition to dose-response and time-course studies with these inducers, we have confirmed that the yield of macrophage-derived IF induced by LPS or poly I.C is increased at lower temperatures.[34]

Bone marrow cell suspensions from female Swiss Webster mice were plated in Dulbecco's Modified Eagle Medium (DMEM) with fetal calf serum (15%), horse serum (5%), and L-cell conditioned medium (30%) for CSA.[36] Between day 3 and day 6 the average doubling time was approximately 24 hours. After 7 days cultivation there were 1.0–3.0 × 10^6 adherent macrophages per flask. Adherent cells were confirmed to be macrophages since 98% phagocytized sheep erythrocytes opsonized with anti-sheep erythrocyte IgG.[2]

A summary of the results of eight experiments using lipopolysaccharide (*S. abortus equi*) as the IF inducer is shown in FIGURE 14A. At every dose of LPS, the IF titer was higher at 26°C than at 37°C. At 26°C an average of 2.45 ± 0.22 $\log_{10}$ U/ml IF were produced by marrow macrophages treated with 10 μg/ml LPS. In contrast, only 1.10 ± 0.39 $\log_{10}$ U/ml IF were produced at 37°C. The IF detected at 26°C without additional LPS was presumably induced by endotoxin present in the medium since polymyxin B sulfate (50 μg/ml) prevented the "spontaneous" production of IF (data not shown). Polymyxin B binds the lipid A moiety of LPS[38] and thereby inhibits the biological effects of endotoxins.[39]

Similar observations were made with poly I.C as inducer. FIGURE 14B demonstrates higher production of IF at 26°C at every dose of poly I.C. Significant IF titers were obtained with as little as 0.01 μg/ml poly I.C or 0.1 μg/ml LPS. It is of interest that the poly I.C used did not induce IF production by L cells or primary fibroblasts unless the concentration was increased 100-fold and DEAE dextran was added.

In contrast to the findings with LPS and poly I.C, there was no enhancing effect of temperature on the induction of IF by NDV. Indeed, FIGURE 14C shows that at an m.o.i. of 0.1 or 1.0 more IF was produced at 37°C than at 26°C.

Time course experiments were performed with either LPS or poly I.C as the inducers. IF titers were determined in cultures that had been in contact with LPS for various periods from 0-24 hours, at either 37°C or 26°C. At 37°C the maximum titer of IF was detected after 6-7 hours of incubation with LPS, after which there was a slight decline in the detectable IF titer (FIGURE 15A). There was a delay in the appearance of IF from cultures incubated at 26°C for the first 4 hours followed by a linear increase of the IF titer which peaked at 18 hours.

Essentially similar kinetics of appearance of IF were found with poly I.C as the inducer (FIGURE 15B). As was seen with LPS, the appearance of IF occurred rapidly at 37°C, reached a plateau by 6 hours and remained at this level. At 26°C there was again a lag in the appearance of IF until 4 hours; the maximal titer, approximately a log unit greater than that found in 37°C cultures, was reached by 8 hours.

Experiments using polymyxin B sulfate to inhibit the induction of IF by 10 μg/ml LPS (*S. abortus equi*) indicated that 50 μg/ml polymyxin B completely inhibited IF production. The polymyxin B had no effect on the IF synthetic capacity of marrow macrophages since incubation with 50 or 100 μg/ml polymyxin B had no effect on the IF titer induced by 10 μg/ml poly I.C. To determine the minimum time of incubation with LPS required for maximal IF production, marrow macrophage cultures were pulsed with 10 μg/ml LPS from 15 minutes to 3 hours. The media were removed, replaced with LPS-free media containing 50 μg/ml polymyxin B and incubated at 26°C. FIGURE 16 demonstrates that a 2-hour pulse of LPS was sufficient to produce maximum titers of IF when examined at 24 hours.

The physicochemical characteristics of the IF induced by LPS or poly I.C in bone marrow macrophages were also examined. Supernatants were removed from cultures after 24 hours and aliquots were treated at 56°C from 10-60

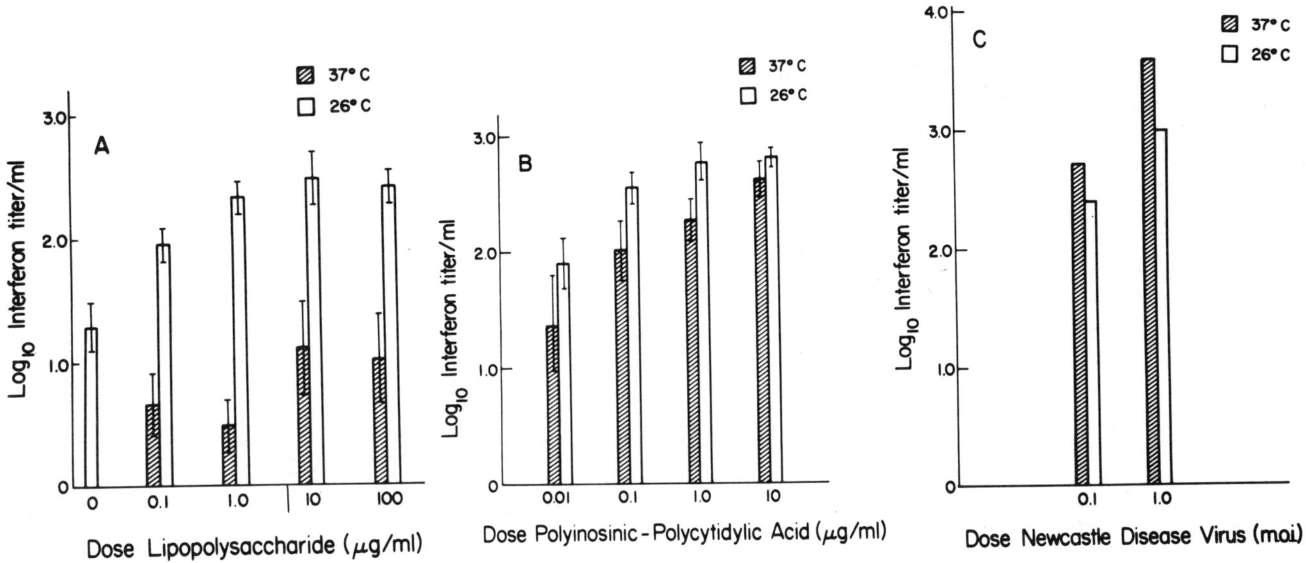

FIGURE 14. Dose response to interferon inducers by bone marrow-derived macrophage cultures. (A) Lipopolysaccharide. (B) Poly I.C. (C) Newcastle disease virus. *Abscissa:* Dose of inducer. *Ordinate:* Log_{10} units per ml of IF. Cultures were incubated with the inducer for 24 hr. NDV supernatants were collected and dialyzed against 0.05M glycine-HC1 pH2.2 for 24 hr then returned to pH 7.2 prior to titration. Average ± S.E.M. Eight or four determinations for LPS or poly I.C, respectively. NDV was performed once. 26°C cultures, *open bars;* 37°C, *cross-hatched bars.*

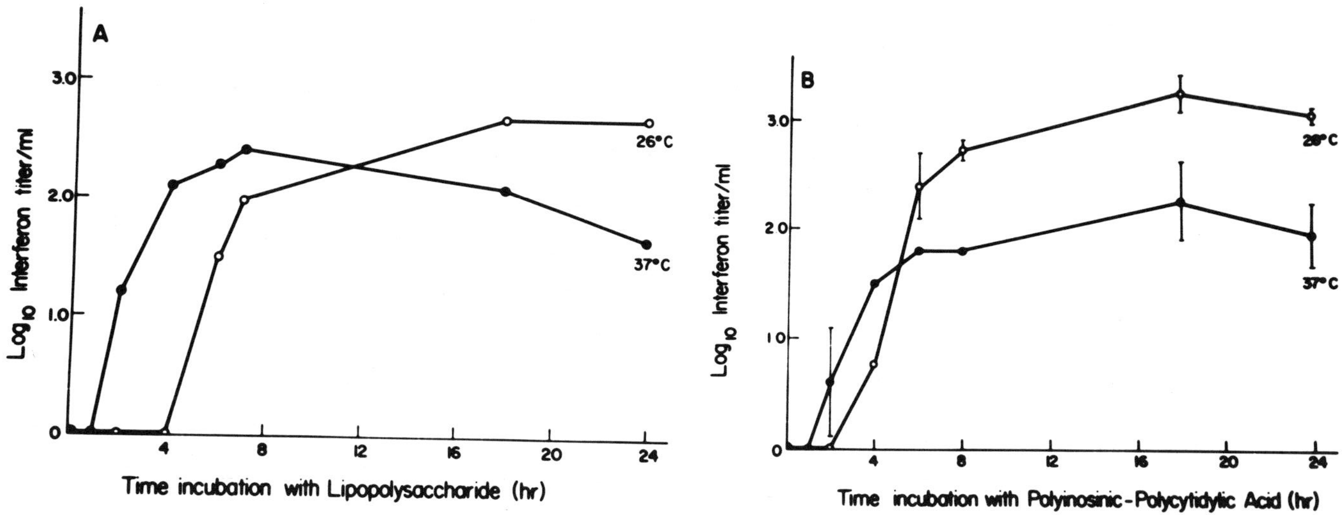

FIGURE 15. Time course of interferon production by bone marrow-derived macrophages. (A) Lipopolysaccharide. (B) Poly I.C. *Abscissa:* Time. *Ordinate:* Log_{10} units per ml of IF. Cultures were incubated with either 10 μg/ml LPS or poly I.C. 37°C cultures, *closed circles;* 26°C, *open circles.*

minutes, after which IF titers were determined. The IF activity was completely abolished by exposure to 56°C for 40 minutes. When samples were dialyzed against 0.05 M glycine-HCl pH 2.2 for 24 or 48 hours followed by dialysis against DMEM pH 7.2, there was only a slight loss of IF activity. LPS-induced IF was 2.07 $\log_{10}$ U/ml in controls and 1.87 $\log_{10}$ U/ml in pH 2.2-treated samples. Incubation of IF, induced by either LPS or poly I.C, with a sheep anti-type I IF globulin (supplied by Dr. I. Gresser, Institut de Recherches Scientifiques sur le Cancer, Villejuif, France),[40] completely inhibited the antiviral activity. Control globulin had no effect on the IF titer. These features are consistent with the characteristics of type I IF.

Thus, using bone marrow macrophages we have confirmed previous studies in which peritoneal macrophages were used to produce IF in response to LPS or

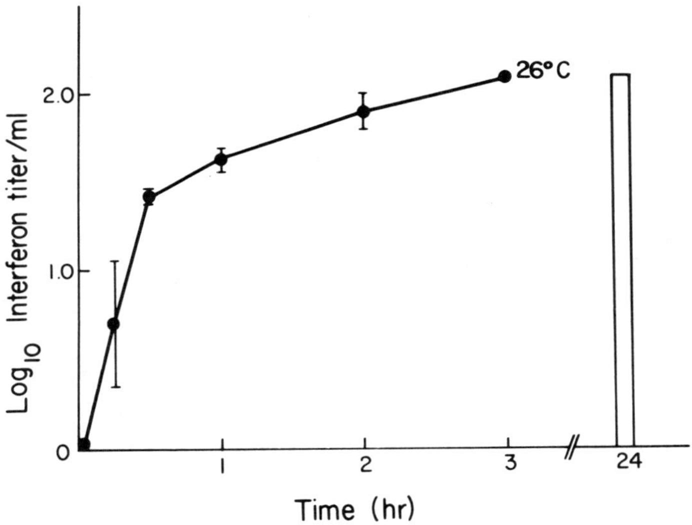

FIGURE 16. Duration of minimal exposure to LPS required for interferon production. *Abscissa:* Time. *Ordinate:* Log_{10} units per ml of IF. Cultures were incubated with 10 μg/ml LPS at 26°C. At various times LPS was removed and replaced with LPS-free media containing 50 μg/ml polymyxin B sulfate. Controls were incubated continuously with LPS for 24 hr (*open bar*).

poly I.C. In addition, we confirmed and extended the earlier observations of Lackovic[34] that the induction of IF by LPS or poly I.C is enhanced by decreased temperature. Our studies also emphasize the remarkable sensitivity of marrow macrophages to induction of IF by LPS, poly I.C. or NDV.

SUMMARY

We have provided evidence that *in vivo*-induced type I IF enhanced Fc-mediated particle uptake by mouse macrophages. Fc-mediated phagocytosis of opsonized erythrocytes by unelicited fresh or cultivated macrophages was stimulated by 4–8 hours of cultivation with 100 U/ml IF. A 1-hour pulse was sufficient when followed by incubation in IF-free medium. Pactamycin, a protein synthesis inhibitor, and camptothecin, an RNA synthesis inhibitor, blocked the stimulation of phagocytosis, indicating a requirement for macromolecular synthesis. Binding by the macrophages of a radioiodinated monoclonal antibody with anti-Fc receptor II specificity indicated that the stimulation of phagocytosis did not result from an increase in the numbers of available Fc receptors. Inflammatory macrophages, while more phagocytic than resting cells, could be further stimulated by IF *in vitro*, as could macrophages stimulated with LPS. In contrast, macrophages obtained from animals treated with IF inducers could not be further stimulated by IF. LPS-prestimulated and normal macrophages showed similar time-course and dose-response curves to IF, indicating that the probable mechanism of stimulation is similar in both types of cells.

Cultivated bone marrow-derived macrophages were found to be sensitive to IF induction by LPS, poly I.C, or NDV. The induction of IF by either LPS or poly I.C was greater at 26°C than at 37°C, while no such difference was found using NDV. A 2-hour pulse of LPS was sufficient to induce IF in marrow-derived macrophages. The induced IF activity was shown to be type I IF.

References

1. Cohn, Z. A. 1978. The activation of mononuclear phagocytes: Fact, fancy, and future. J. Immunol. **121:** 813–816.
2. Hamburg, S. I., R. E. Manejias & M. Rabinovitch. 1978. Macrophage activation: Ingestion of IgG-coated erythrocytes after administration of interferon inducers to mice. J. Exp. Med. **147:** 593–598.
3. Rabinovitch, M., R. E. Manejias, M. Russo & E. E. Abbey. 1977. Increased spreading of macrophages from mice treated with interferon inducers. Cell. Immunol. **29:** 86–95.
4. Manejias, R. E., S. I. Hamburg & M. Rabinovitch. 1978. Serum interferon and phagocytic activity of macrophages in recombinant inbred mice inoculated with Newcastle disease virus. Cell. Immunol. **38:** 209–213.
5. Rabinovitch, M. & R. E. Manejias. 1978. Anti-interferon globulin inhibits macrophage phagocytic enchancement in vivo by tilorone or Newcastle disease virus. Cell. Immunol. **39:** 402–406.
6. Hamburg, S. I., G. H. Cassell & M. Rabinovitch. 1980. Relationship between enhanced macrophage phagocytic activity and the induction of interferon by Newcastle disease virus in mice. J. Immunol. **124:** 1360–1364.
7. Rabinovitch, M. & S. I. Hamburg. 1979. Macrophage activation by interferon and interferon inducers. *In* Proceedings of the Third Conference on Mononuclear Phagocytes. R. van Furth, Ed. Martinus Nijhoff Publishers B. V. The Hague, the Netherlands. In press.
8. Huang, K. 1977. Effect of interferon on phagocytosis. *In* Texas Reports on Biology and Medicine. S. Baron and F. Dianzani, Eds. Vol. **35:** 350–356. University of Texas Medical Branch. Galveston, Tx.
9. Vastola, K., W. von Muenchhausen, D. Oleszek & E. Sulkowski. Personal communication, March 1979.
10. De Maeyer-Guignard, J., M. G. Tovey, I. Gresser & E. De Maeyer 1978. Purification of mouse interferon by sequential affinity poly (U) and antibody agarose columns. Nature **271:** 622–625.
11. Friedman, R. M. 1967. Interferon binding: The first step in establishment of antiviral activity. Science **156:** 1760–1762.
12. Taylor, J. 1964. Inhibition of interferon by actinomycin. Biochem. Biophys. Res. Commun. **14:** 447–451.

13. FRIEDMAN, R. M. & J. A. SONNABEND. 1964. Inhibition of interferon action by p-fluorophenylalanine. Nature. **203:** 366–367.
14. RADKE, K. L., C. COLBY, J. R. KATES, H. M., KRIDER & D. M. PRESCOTT. 1974. Establishment and maintenance of interferon-induced antiviral state: Studies in enucleated cells. J. Virol. **13:** 623–630.
15. YOUNG, C. S. H., C. R. PRINGLE & E.A.C. FOLLET. 1975. Action of interferon in enucleated cells. J. Virol **15:** 428–429.
16. SCHUIT, K. 1979. Evidence for active protein synthesis in phagocytosis by human monocytes. J. Reticuloendothel. Soc. **26:** 31–34.
17. SILVERSTEIN, S. C., R. M. STEINMAN & Z. A. COHN. 1977. Endocytosis. Ann. Rev. Biochem. **46:** 669–722.
18. MICHL, J., M. M. PIECZONKA, J. C. UNKELESS & S. C. SILVERSTEIN. 1979. Effects of immobilized immune complexes on Fc and complement receptor function in resident and thioglycollate-elicited mouse peritoneal macrophages. J. Exp. Med. **150:** 607–621.
19. UNKELESS, J. C. & H. N. EISEN. 1975. Binding of monomeric immunoglobulin to Fc receptors of mouse macrophages. J. Exp. Med. **142:** 1520–1533.
20. UNKELESS, J. C. 1977. The presence of two Fc receptors on mouse macrophages; evidence for a variant cell line and differential trypsin sensitivity. J. Exp. Med. **145:** 931–947.
21. HEUSER, C. H., C. L. ANDERSON & H. M. GREY. 1977. Receptors for IgG: Subclass specificity of receptors on different mouse cell types and a definition of two distinct receptors on a mouse cell line. J. Exp. Med. **145:** 1316–1327.
22. DIAMOND, B., B. R. BLOOM & M. D. SCHARFF. 1978. The Fc receptors of primary and cultured phagocytic cells studied with homogenous antibodies. J. Immunol. **121:** 1329–1333.
23. UNKELESS, J. C. 1979. Characterization of a monoclonal antibody directed against mouse macrophage and lymphocyte Fc receptors. J. Exp. Med. **150:** 580–596.
24. RABINOVITCH, M. 1970. Phagocytic recognition. *In* Mononuclear Phagocytes. R. van Furth, Ed. Vol **1:** 299–315. Blackwell Scientific Publications. Oxford, England.
25. LAY, W. H. & V. NUSSENSWEIG. 1968. Receptors for complement on leukocytes. J. Exp. Med. **128:** 991–1007.
26. RABINOVITCH, M. 1968. Effect of antiserum on the attachment of modified erythrocytes to normal or to trypsinized macrophages. Proc. Soc. Exp. Biol. Med. **127:** 351–355.
27. RUSSELL, S. W., W. F. DOE & A. T. MCINTOSH. 1977. Functional characterization of a stable, noncytolytic stage of macrophage activation in tumors. J. Exp. Med. **146:** 1511–1519.
28. NATHAN, C. F. & R. K. ROOT. 1977. Hydrogen peroxide release from mouse peritoneal macrophages: Dependence of sequential activation and triggering. J. Exp. Med. **146:** 1648–1662.
29. HIBBS JR., J. B., R. R. TAINTOR, H. A. CHAPMAN JR. & J. B. WEINBERG. 1977. Macrophage tumor killing: Influence of the local environment. Science **197:** 270–282.
30. RUCO, L. P. & M. S. MELTZER. 1978. Macrophage activation for tumor cytotoxicity: Increased lymphokine responsiveness of peritoneal macrophages during acute inflammation. J. Immunol. **120:** 1054–1062.
31. CHAPMAN, H. A., JR. Z. VAVRIN & J. B. HIBBS, JR. 1979. Modulation of plasminogen activator secretion by activated macrophages: Influence of serum factors and correlation with tumoricidal potential. Proc. Nat. Acad. Sci. USA **76:** 3899–3903.
32. SMITH, T. J. & R. R. WAGNER. 1967. Rabbit macrophage interferon I. Conditions for biosynthesis by virus infected and uninfected cell. J. Exp. Med. **125:** 559–577.
33. KONO, Y. 1967. Rapid production of interferon in bovine leucocyte cultures. Proc. Soc. Exp. Biol. **124:** 155–160.
34. LACKOVIC, V., L. BORECKY, D. SIKL, L. MASLER & S. BAUER. 1967. The temperature requirement for interferon production in cells stimulated by Newcastle disease virus or microbial agents in vitro. Acta Virol. **11:** 500–505.
35. BORECKY, L., V. LACKOVIC & N. FUCHSBERGER. 1970. Comparison of interferon production in mouse leukocytes by statolon and a complexed polyribonucleotide (POLY I:POLY C). Acta Virol. **14:** 329–336.

36. LOHMANN-MATHES, M. L., B. KOLB & H. MEERPOHL. 1978. Susceptibility of malignant and normal target cells to the cytotoxic action of bone marrow macrophages activated in vitro with the macrophage cytotoxicity factor (MCF). Cell. Immunol. **41:** 231–239.
37. GOUD, T. J. L. M., C. SCHOTTE & R. van FURTH. 1975. Indentification and characterization of the monoblast in mononuclear phagocyte colonies grown in vitro. J. Exp. Med. **142:** 1180–1199.
38. MORRISON, D. C. & D. M. JACOBS. 1976. Binding of polymyxin B to the lipid A portion of bacterial lipopolysaccharide. Immunochemistry **13:** 813–818.
39. BANNATYNE, R. M., N. M. HARNETT, K. Y. LEE & W. D. BIGGAR. 1977. Inhibition of the biological effects of endotoxin on neutrophils by polymyxin B sulfate. J. Inf. Dis. **136:** 469–474.
40. GRESSER, I., M. G. TOVEY, M. T. BANDU, C. MAURY & D. BROUTY-BOYE. 1976. Role of interferon in the pathogenesis of virus diseases in mice as demonstrated by the use of anti-interferon serum. I. Rapid evolution of encephalomyocarditis virus infection. J. Exp. Med. **144:** 1305–1315.

INTERACTION OF INTERFERON, MACROPHAGE AND LYMPHOCYTE TUMORICIDAL ACTIVITY WITH PROSTAGLANDIN EFFECT

Michael A. Chirigos, Richard M. Schultz, and William A. Stylos

Virus and Disease Modification Section
Laboratory of Chemical Pharmacology
Division of Cancer Treatment, National Cancer Institute
Bethesda, Maryland 20205

Introduction

The vital role of mononuclear phagocytes in host defense against neoplasia, as well as infectious organisms, has been amply demonstrated. Little, however, is known concerning the ability of specific agents which are capable of modifying the functional activity of macrophages. There appears to be a close relationship between the ability of biological and synthetic agents to enhance host antitumor resistance and their capacity to activate macrophages. Increasing evidence suggests that the activated macrophage is a major effector of tumor surveillance, rather than the specifically immunologically active lymphocyte. It then becomes important to better understand the mechanisms by which these agents are involved in the pharmacological control of the macrophage system. By judiciously controlling macrophage activity to express a tumoricidal or tumor-stasis effect, through agents capable of enhancing this effect, it is possible to combine a tumor cytoreductive therapy with a macrophage-activating agent, thus enhancing tumor reduction.

Recent results indicate that fibroblast interferon or several interferon inducers have the capacity to activate macrophages to exert a tumoricidal activity. This report will present the current findings of our laboratory studies devoted to defining the mechanisms through which macrophages exert a tumoricidal effect and factors affecting this response.

Materials and Methods

Mice

Male $CD2F_1$ mice, 6 to 8 weeks old, were obtained from the Mammalian Genetics and Animal Production Section of the National Institutes of Health, Bethesda, MD. Mice were housed in plastic cages with air filter bonnets and given tap water and Purina laboratory chow *ad libitum*.

Drugs

Partially purified mouse L-cell interferon (specific activity 2×10^7 units/mg protein) was purchased from Dr. K. Paucker, Medical College of Pennsylvania, Philadelphia, PA. Interferon, induced by Newcastle disease virus and purified by affinity chromatography on anti-interferon globulin-sepharose, was found to be free of endotoxin contamination as measured by the Limulus amebocyte lysate assay. *Escherichia coli* LPS (0127:B8) was purchased from DIFCO Laboratories,

0077-8923/80/0350-0091 $01.75/0 © 1980, NYAS

Detroit, MI. Prostaglandins (PG) were generously provided by Dr. John Pike, Upjohn Co., Kalamazoo, MI. Concentrated solutions of PG were initially dissolved in 95% ethyl alcohol, and dilutions were made in Dulbecco's phosphate-buffered saline (PBS) (pH 7.2).

Leukemia Cell Cultures

MBL-2 lymphoblastic leukemia cells were maintained as suspension cultures in RPMI-1640 medium supplemented with 20% heat-inactivated (56 C, 30 min) fetal calf serum, 100 mg/ml gentamicin solution, 0.075% $NaHCO_3$ and 10 mM HEPES buffer (RPMI-FCS). Viability of the cells was determined by the trypan blue exclusion test.

Peritoneal Macrophages

Noninduced peritoneal macrophages were harvested from treated or normal control mice as previously described[1] and washed in RPMI-1640 medium, and approximately 4×10^5 macrophages were seeded into 16-mm wells on tissue culture Cluster[24] plates (Costar, Cambridge, MA) in 1.0 ml RPMI-FCS. The cultures were incubated for 90 min, and macrophage monolayers were washed thoroughly with jets of medium before use in experiments.

Macrophage Activation Assay

Our technique for measuring the ability of interferon to produce growth inhibitory macrophages has previously been described.[1] For *in vivo* activation, macrophages were harvested 24 hr after i.p. inoculation of interferon at 1×10^4 units/mouse. Prostaglandins tested for inhibitory activity were usually given i.p. simultaneously with the interferon stimulus. Treated macrophages in 16-mm wells were overlaid with 4×10^4 MBL-2 cells contained in 2.0 ml.

RPMI-FCS

The cultures were incubated at 37°C in an atmosphere of 5% CO_2 in air, and viable leukemia cells were counted with a hemacytometer after 48 hr. For *in vitro* activation, monolayers of macrophages in 16-mm wells were treated with partially purified interferon (lot #1835) at a final concentration of 1,000 units/ml culture medium. Agents tested for inhibitory activity on macrophage function were added in 100 μl aliquots to the macrophage cultures for a 2-hr period of incubation following the 16-hr interferon treatment at 37°C. Following the incubation period, the macrophage cultures were washed 3 times with medium to remove interferon and/or inhibitor, and the macrophages were overlaid with 4×10^4 MBL-2 lymphoblastic leukemia cells contained in 2 ml RPMI-FCS. All cultures were again incubated at 37°C in an atmosphere of 5% CO_2 in air, and viable leukemia cells were counted 48 hr after with a hemacytometer. The ratio of macrophages to target cells was approximately 10:1 at the beginning of each experiment. The percentage growth inhibition of MBL-2 cells due to macrophage-interferon interaction was calculated by comparison to MBL-2 cells growth in the presence of normal resting macrophages alone.

Results

Role of Interferon and Interferon Inducers in Macrophage Tumoricidal Activity

As we previously described,[1] L-cell interferon at doses greater than 1 unit/ml culture medium renders normal peritoneal macrophages cytotoxic for MBL-2 leukemia target cells. Results in FIGURE 1 show the cytostatic effect of macrophage exposed to increasing doses of interferon. No MBL-2 leukemic cells could be detected at the 2000 units ml interferon dose. When rabbit anti-interferon globulin, sufficient to neutralize approximately 250 units, was added to the macrophage:MBL-2 leukemic cell reaction culture at the same time as interferon, the ability of interferon to render macrophages cytotoxic was inhibited. The degree of neutralization of interferon titer corresponded to the inhibition of interferon-induced, macrophage-mediated cytotoxicity.

We have previously reported that several agents, particularly chemicals that possess polyanionic characteristics, render macrophages tumoricidal through direct exposure.[2] We postulated that this direct activation of macrophages by polyanions, may be mediated by the interferon produced by macrophages as a result of polyanion exposure. We thus tested whether anti-L-cell interferon globulin could negate macrophage activation by synthetic polyanions. The various macrophage-activating compounds were tested in optimal concentrations and added to macrophage cultures simultaneously with the anti-interferon

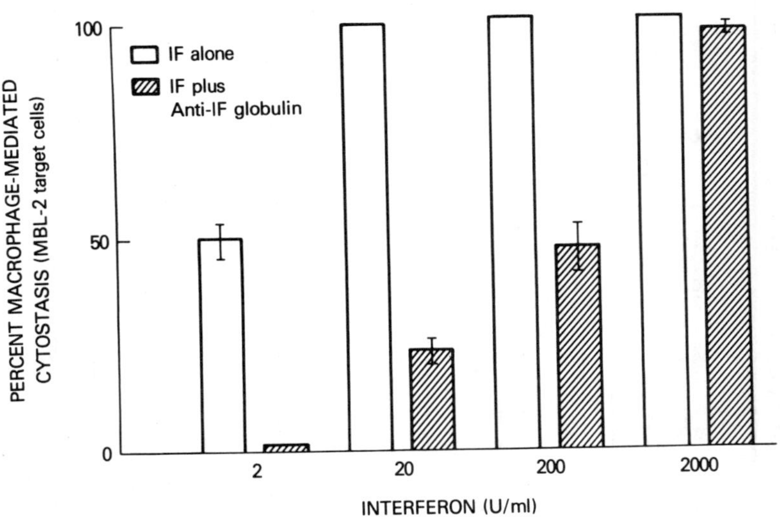

FIGURE 1. Ability of highly specific rabbit anti-L-cell interferon globulin to neutralize macrophage activation by L-cell interferon *in vitro*. Macrophage monolayers were exposed to varying concentrations of interferon in the presence or absence of anti-interferon globulin sufficient to neutralize approximately 250 units of interferon. Macrophage-mediated cytostatis of MBL-2 leukemia target cells was determined after 48 hr of incubation at 37°C. The bars represent the mean ± standard errors obtained from duplicate cultures.

globulin (FIGURE 2). The anti-interferon globulin completely neutralized the ability of BruPel, LPSw, poly (I):poly(C), and pyran copolymer to render macrophages cytotoxic. These agents are all inducers of a type I interferon. Control rabbit globulin did not significantly alter macrophage cytotoxic activity induced by these agents. Of particular interest was the inability of anti-interferon globulin to affect macrophage activation by concanavalin A-induced lymphokine, even when the lymphokine was added to suboptimal concentrations. It is worth noting that concanavalin A-induced lymphokine, which contains an antigenically unrelated interferon, was not neutralized by the anti-L-cell interferon globulin.

Role of Prostaglandins in Macrophage Tumoricidal Function

Recently we have provided experimental evidence that macrophage tumoricidal activity is a relative capability influenced by several opposing factors in the local environment, including prostaglandins of the E-series.[3,4] These findings suggest that host resistance to neoplasia may be compromised by elevated levels of PGE in the microenvironment of the tumor.[5] The observations that many tumors contain a high percentage of macrophages but continue to grow[6] supports the view that PGE may depress the tumoricidal activity of the activated macrophage.

When PGE_1 or PGE_2 was added to macrophage cultures simultaneously with interferon, the interferon induction of tumoricidal macrophages was markedly reduced (TABLE 1), although macrophages were observed to be activated as defined by morphological criteria and remained fully viable. Both PGE_1 and PGE_2 showed similar kinetics of inhibiting macrophage function. PGE_1 and PGE_2 at the 10^{-5} M concentrations caused 97 and 94% inhibition of tumoricidal

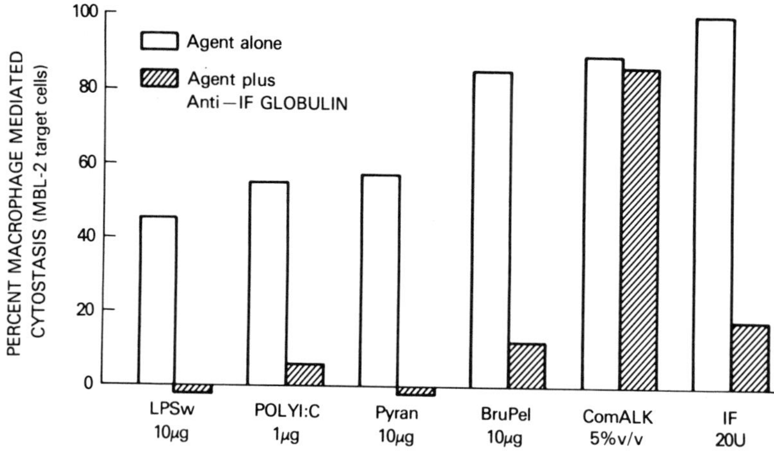

FIGURE 2. Ability of highly specific rabbit anti-L-cell interferon globulin to neutralize macrophage activation by L-cell interferon and various macrophage activators. Macrophage monolayers were exposed to diverse biological and synthetic agents, at doses indicated in the presence or absence of anti-interferon globulin sufficient to neutralize approximately 250 units of interferon. Macrophage-mediated cytostasis of MBL-2 leukemia target cells was determined after 48 hr of incubation at 37°C.

TABLE 1

EFFECT OF PROSTAGLANDINS ON MACROPHAGE TUMORICIDAL FUNCTIONS

Inhibitor	Concentration of Inhibitor with 1000 units/ml of Interferon (M)	Tumoricidal Activity (%)
None	None	62
PGE_1	10^{-5}	3
	10^{-6}	22
	10^{-7}	45
	10^{-8}	62
PGE_2	10^{-5}	6
	10^{-6}	28
	10^{-7}	40
	10^{-8}	52
PGE_2a	10^{-5}	56
	10^{-6}	55
	10^{-7}	56
	10^{-8}	59

*Prostaglandins were added simultaneously with interferon. Macrophage monolayers were then washed several times prior to the addition of target cells and tumoricidal function was assessed after 48 hr.

activity, respectively, compared to the interferon control value (62% tumoricidal activity). In contrast, $PGE_2\alpha$ was ineffective at all concentrations tested. Indomethacin, the prostaglandins or prostaglandin synthetase inhibitor, was without effect on resting macrophages.

In vivo administration of PGE_1 and PGE_2 at doses of 5 or 20 μg per mouse was also shown to significantly decrease the MBL-2 cytotoxcity in mice simultaneously injected with 1×10^4 units of interferon. PGA_1 or $PGE_2\alpha$ were without effect on interferon-stimulated macrophages. In studies designed to determine the effect of time of PGE_1 administration in relation to interferon inoculation, it was found that the suppressive effect of PGE_1 lasted for only 24 hr. Treatment with PGE_1, 48 hr prior to interferon, was without effect on interferon induction of macrophage cytotoxic activity.

Role of Cortiocosteroids and Other Pharmacological Agents in Macrophage Cytotoxic Function

Several compounds were evaluated as potential inhibitors of tumor cell cytostasis induced by interferon-treated macrophages. This study was instigated by the report that hydrocortisone possessed the capacity to block nonspecific macrophage-mediated cytotoxicity.[7] Peritoneal macrophages, harvested 24 hr after interferon treatment (1×10^4 units/animal), inhibited MBL-2 proliferation by 94%. Cortiocosteroids, administered i.p. at 1 to 100 mg/kg simultaneously with interferon, suppressed macrophage tumor killing in a dose-dependent fashion (TABLE 2). Dexamethasone almost completely nullified the ability of interferon-treated macrophages to inhibit MBL-2 tumor cell growth at the 10 and 100 mg/kg dose. A similar degree of suppression was attained when the cortocosteroids were also tested *in vitro* to assess their suppressive effect on interferon activation of macrophages.

TABLE 2

EFFECT OF *IN VIVO* CORTICOSTEROID ADMINISTRATION ON SUPPRESSION OF INTERFERON-INDUCED MACROPHAGE CYTOTOXIC FUNCTION

Inhibitor	Concentration of Inhibitor (mg/kg)*	Macrophage-mediated Cytostasis (%)
None	none†	94
Hydrocortisone	1	91
	10	78
	100	45
Prednisone	1	66
	10	55
	100	40
Dexamethasone	1	60
	10	15
	100	10

*Both interferon at 1×10^4 units/mouse and corticosteroids at the doses shown were administered i.p. and peritoneal macrophages were harvested 24 hr later. MBL-2 leukemia growth inhibition by treated macrophages was determined at 48 hr of incubation at 37°C from triplicate cultures.

†Control mice given interferon alone, 1×10^4 units/mouse.

In view of the widespread involvement of 3′5′-cyclic nucleotides in cellular regulatory processes and since prostaglandins of the E-series increase intracellular levels of cyclic AMP in macrophages, studies were undertaken to determine the effect of dibutyryl cyclic AMP and dibutyryl cyclic GMP on macrophage functional activity. As shown in TABLE 3, dibutyryl cyclic AMP inhibited the cytotoxic activity of interferon-treated macrophages in a dose dependent manner. The inhibition was significant in view of the 52% inhibition attained with interferon alone. In contrast, cyclic GMP did not markedly alter interferon-

TABLE 3

EFFECTS OF DIBUTYRYL CYCLIC AMP AND GMP ON TUMORICIDAL ACTIVITY OF INTERFERON-ACTIVATED MACROPHAGES

Cyclic Nucleotide	Concentration of Inhibitor (M)*	Inhibition of MBL-2 Cells (%)
None		52
Cyclic AMP	10^{-3}	23
	10^{-4}	35
	10^{-5}	45
	10^{-6}	50
Cyclic GMP	10^{-3}	58
	10^{-4}	53
	10^{-5}	54
	10^{-6}	52

*Monolayers of macrophages, previously exposed to interferon (1000 U/ml) for 16 hr at 37°C, were pulsed with various molar (M) concentrations of the cyclic nucleotide for 30 min at 37°C. Macrophage cultures were washed and MBL-2 leukemia target cells added. MBL-2 growth inhibition by treated macrophages was determined after 48 hr incubation.

activated macrophage cytotoxicity. There was no demonstrable effect of the dibutyryl cyclic nucleotides on resting macrophages in the absence of interferon.

Glucocorticoids have been shown to inhibit a number of macrophage functions. Werb *et al.*[8] reported that monocytes and macrophages contain saturable glucocorticoid-binding proteins with specificity of binding of cortisol, corticosterone, and related synthetic steroids such as dexamethasone and that they have dissociation constants for binding within physiological ranges. In the present report, corticosteroids suppressed the cytotoxicity of interferon-treated macrophages at what can be considered physiological concentrations. Although the mechanisms by which they act on inhibiting macrophage tumoricidal activity is unknown, their activity may be mediated by either stabilization of cell membranes or stimulation of production of cyclic AMP.[9]

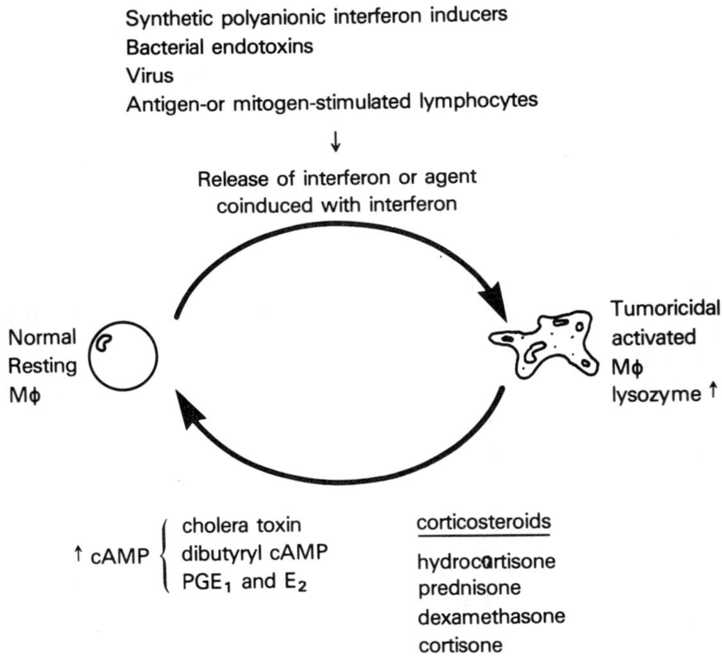

FIGURE 3. Pathway for reversible inhibition of nonspecifically activated macrophages.

Prostaglandins of the E-series have been previously reported to exert a number of inhibitory effects on macrophages besides cytotoxicity, including random locomotion,[10] lessened production of plasminogen activator,[11] and colony-stimulating factors for macrophage stem cells.[12]

The process of macrophage activation appears to be self-limiting, since it has been reported that activated macrophages release high levels of PGE_2.[13] Our present results indicate that PGE_1 and PGE_2, but not $PGF_{2}\alpha$, abrogate the ability of interferon to activate macrophages to their tumoricidal capacity. Such prostaglandins could act in a negative feedback inhibition to limit cell activities. This is illustrated in FIGURE 3. The tumoricidal activity of macrophages can be stimulated by several agents both by *in vitro* and *in vivo* conditions. The tumoricidal activity of the macrophage can be abrogated by inhibitory levels of prostaglandin (PGE_1 or PGE_2).

Preliminary evidence suggests that the ability of PGE's to inhibit macrophage cytotoxic function is related to elevated levels of intracellular cyclic 3′:5′-adenosine monophosphate. In addition, cells transformed by viruses or chemicals *in vitro* have been shown to produce severalfold more prostaglandins than do their normal counterparts.[14] These tumor cell products could subvert local macrophages and allow the tumor to progress in the presence of these potentially tumoricidal cells.

A more comprehensive knowledge of the stimuli and conditions under which the cytotoxic activity of macrophages is maintained *in vivo* may clarify the role of the activated macrophage in immunity. In the past, much emphasis has been placed on factors that enhance the functional activity of the macrophage system. It appears that there are opposing factors that may subvert the functional activity of the activated macrophage.

With the experience that macrophages are activated to a tumoricidal stage after exposure to interferon, or an interferon inducer such as pyran copolymer,[15] we attempted to assess the activity of these two agents in an *in vivo* tumor system. The schema of the assay is shown in FIGURE 4. In brief, C57BL/6 adult male mice were inoculated intraperitoneally with 1×10^6 MBL-2 leukemia cells. The following day animals were separated into control and treated groups (see TABLE 4). Treatment with bovine serum albumin, interferon or pyran copolymer was intraperitoneal and administered for 5 consecutive days beginning one day following tumor inoculation. On the sixth day, 5 mice from each group were sacrificed for peritoneal exudate and 10 mice were held for survival time observations. The peritoneal exudate from each experimental group was pooled, and macrophages separated by adherence on tissue culture plates and the non-adherent MBL-2 tumor cells in the supernatant collected. The supernatant was used for the visual counting of dead vs. live MBL-2 leukemic cells with a hemocytometer. The adherent macrophages were washed in RPMI-1640

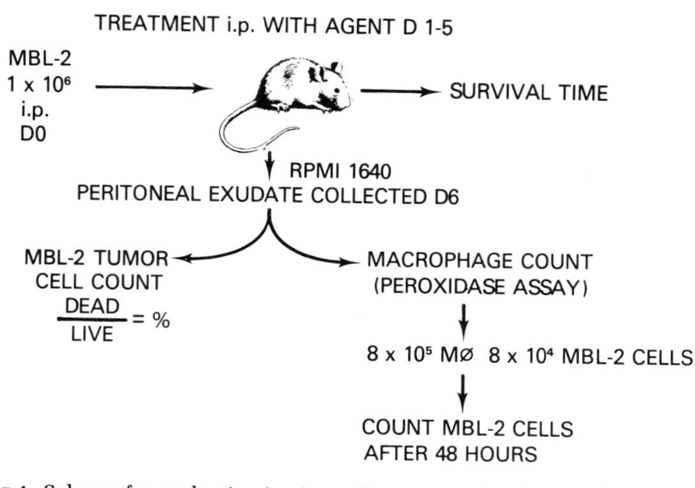

FIGURE 4. Scheme for evaluating *in vivo* antitumor activity of macrophage activators.

TABLE 4

IN VIVO RESPONSE OF MBL-2 TUMOR TO INTERFERON AND PYRAN COPOLYMER

MBL-2 1×10^6	BSA 0.5 mg	IF 1×10^5U	Pyran 0.2 mg	*In Vitro* Evaluation*: Dead Tumor Cells (%)	*In Vitro* Evaluation*: MØ Tumor Cell Death (%)	*In Vivo* Evaluation†: MST (days)	*In Vivo* Evaluation†: S/T (%)
DO				12		18	0
DO	D1–5			15	25	23	0
DO		D1–5		56	30	38	30
DO			D1–5	48	80	48	40

*C57 B1/6 mice sacrificed on day 6 for *in vitro* evaluation of tumor cells and macrophage tumoricidal activity.

†MST = median survival time; S/T survivors/total after 60 days of observation.

medium and approximately 8×10^5 macrophages were seeded into 16-mm wells on tissue culture Cluster plates. The macrophages were overlaid with 8×10^4 MBL-2 leukemia cells contained in RPMI-FCS. All cultures were incubated at 37°C in an atmosphere of 5% CO_2 in air, and viable leukemia cells were counted after 48 hr with a hemocytometer. Results of a typical study employing this assay are shown in TABLE 4.

The number of dead tumor cells in the peritoneal ascites fluid was markedly higher in the animals treated with interferon (56%) or pyran copolymer (48%). Was death of leukemic cells due to a tumoricidal effect of interferon, or interferon induced by pyran *per se*, or the result of *in vivo* macrophage-activated tumoricidal activity? Macrophages collected from the treated mice and separated from the peritoneal ascitic fluid from tumor cells and again incubated with MBL-2 target cells resulted in significant tumoricidal activity. The results indicate that macrophages from pyran-treated mice were capable of an 80% tumoricidal effect. In contrast, macrophages from animals treated with either bovine serum albumin or interferon exerted only a 25 and 30% tumoricidal effect, respectively. The increase in median survival time (MST) and percent survival, however indicate that interferon and pyran were both significantly effective in retarding tumor growth. The implications of this study are that: (1) macrophages, activated *in vivo* by interferon and pyran copolymer, were in part, responsible for tumor killing; (2) macrophages from pyran-treated mice exerted a stronger tumoricidal effect on tumor cells as reflected by their higher tumoricidal activity when tested *in vitro* and the resultant longer survival period of treated mice; (3) the resultant extension in survival time is due to the amount of tumor cell killing that occurred *in vivo* as the result of the treatment, and; (4) pyran copolymer is exerting an additional tumoricidal effect which may be unrelated to its capacity to induce interferon.

DISCUSSION

Since macrophage-mediated tumor destruction results predominantly from a nonphagocytic contact-mediated event, successful therapy is dependent on achieving adequate cell density at the tumor site. An example of this was shown in the last experiments which described the role of the macrophage in killing MBL-2 tumor cells *in vivo* in the peritoneal cavity where both tumor cells and macrophages were present. However, tumors themselves may produce soluble factors that interfere with effective macrophage mobilization.[16] Examples of this were seen when, the prostaglandins E_1 and E_2 or the corticosteroids were present at the same time as interferon, the macrophage-activated tumoricidal activity was markedly suppressed.

Many of the current efforts at immunotherapy of neoplasia employ nonspecific agents such as BCG, *Corynebacterium parvum*, glucan, and more recently interferon, which in part presumably acts by induction of nonspecifically tumoricidal macrophages. The greatest clinical success has been achieved when these adjuvants were injected directly into, or near, the tumor lesion, allowing for both mobilization of macrophages to the tumor site and subsequent activation in intimate contact with tumor. Similarly, Hibbs[17] has shown that the presence of cytotoxic activated macrophages in the tissue tends to be a local phenomenon, confined to the anatomical compartment(s) that contain high levels of inducing antigen. The continuing presence of activated macrophages requires that the specific agent, e.g., BCG or toxoplasms, which induced the production of cytotoxic macrophages remains in the tissue and provides a continuing stimulus for elaboration of a chemical signal that maintains macrophage activation. This may be the case for the better response noted for pyran (TABLE 4). Interferon has a very short half-life *in vivo* where, in contrast, pyran copolymer is present in diminishing quantities for a longer period of time,[18] thus serving as a continuing stimulus for macrophage activation.

There appears to be a strong need for understanding the immunopharmacology of nonspecific macrophage stimulants, such as interferon and interferon inducers, to improve on the clinical effects conferred by empirical therapy of this type.

This is especially true in view of the conflicting stimuli that abrogate the ability of agents to induce tumoricidal macrophages, e.g., prostaglandins, corticosteroids and other agents which increase cellular levels of cyclic AMP. Sufficient quantities of these opposing factors in the microenvironment of the tumor may severely compromise adjuvant-induced host resistance against neoplasms. Development of capabilities to control local production of agents that negate macrophage chemotaxis and/or functional activity may allow for improved immunotherapy of cancer.

REFERENCES

1. SCHULTZ, R. M., & M. A. CHIRIGOS. 1978. Similarities among factors that render macrophages tumoricidal in lymphokine and interferon preparations. Cancer Res. **38:** 1003–1007.
2. SCHULTZ, R. M., J. D. PAPAMATHEAKIS & M. A. CHIRIGOS. 1978. Correlation between antitumor activity and macrophage activation by polyanions. *In* Immune Modulation and Control of Neoplasia by Adjuvant Therapy. M. A. Chirigos, Ed. Vol. **7:** 459–469. Raven Press. New York.
3. SCHULTZ, R. M., N. A. PAVALIDIS, W. A. STYLOS & M. A. CHIRIGOS. 1978. Regulation of macrophage tumoricidal function: A role for prostaglandins of the E series. Science **202:** 320–321.
4. CHIRIGOS, M. A. & R. M. SCHULTZ. 1979. Animal models in cancer research which could be useful in studies of the effect of alcohol on cellular immunity. Cancer Res. **39:** 2894–2898.

5. SYKES, J. A. & I. S. MADDOX. 1972. Prostaglandin production by experimental tumors and effects of anti-inflammatory compounds. Nature (New Biol.) **237:** 59–63.
6. ECCLES, S. A. & P. ALEXANDER. 1974. Macrophage content of tumours in relation to metastatic spread and host immune reaction. Nature **250:** 667–673.
7. HIBBS, J. B. 1976. The macrophage as a tumoricidal effector cell: A review of *in vivo* and *in vitro* studies on the mechanism of the activated macrophage nonspecific cytotoxic reaction. *In* The Macrophage in Neoplasia. M. A. Fink, Ed.: 83. Academic Press. New York.
8. WERB, A., R. FOLEY & A. MUNICH. 1978. Interaction of glucocorticoids with macrophages. Identification of glucocorticoid receptors in monocytes and macrophages. J. Exp. Med. **147:** 1684–1691.
9. LOGSDON, P. J., E. MIDDETON & R. J. COFFEY. 1972. Stimulation of leucocyte adenylcyclase by hydrocortisone and isoproterenol in asthmatic and non-asthmatic subjects. J. Allergy Clin. Immunol. **50:** 45–51.
10. GALLIN, J. E., J. A. SANDLER, R. I. CEYMAN, V. C. MANGANIELLO & M. VAUGHAN. 1978. Agents that increase cyclic AMP inhibits accumulation of cGMP and depress human monocyte locomotion. J. Immunol. **120:** 492–496.
11. VASSALI, J., J. HAMILTON & E. REICH. 1976. Macrophage plasminogen activator: Modulation of enzyme production by anti-inflammatory steroids, mitotic inhibitors and cyclic nucleotides. Cell **8:** 271–281.
12. KIRKLAND, J. E., J. W. HADDEN & M. A. S. MOORE. 1977. Role of cyclic nucleotides in the proliferation of committed granulocytemacrophage proginator cells. Cancer Res. **37:** 4534–4538.
13. BRAY, M. A., D. GORDON & J. MORLEY. 1974. Role of prostaglandins in reactions of cellular immunity. Br. J. Pharmacol. **52:** 453–458.
14. HONG, S. L., C. M. WHELESS & L. LEVINE. 1977. Elevated prostaglandins synthetase activity in methylcholanthrene-transformed mouse BALB/3T3. Prostaglandins **13:** 271–279.
15. SCHULTZ. R. M., J. D. PAPAMATHEAKIS & M. A. CHIRIGOS. 1977. Direct activation *in vitro* of mouse peritoneal macrophages by pyran copolymer (NSC 46015). Cell Immunol. **29:** 403–409.
16. PIKE, M. C. & R. SNYDERMAN. 1976. Depression of macrophage function by a factor produced by neoplasms: A mechanism for abrogation of immune surveillance. J. Immunol. **107:** 1243–1249.
17. HIBBS, J. B., L. H. LAMBERT & J. S. REMINGTON. 1972. Control of carcinogenesis: A possible role for the activated macrophage. Science **177:** 998–1000.
18. PAPAMATHEAKIS, J. D., R. M. SCHULTZ, M. A. CHIRIGOS & J. G. MASSICOT. 1978. Cell and tissue distribution of ^{14}C-labeled pyran copolymer. Cancer Treat. Rep. **62:** 1845–1851.

CELLULAR INTERACTIONS IN THE AUGMENTATION OF HUMAN NK ACTIVITY BY INTERFERON

Eero Saksela,*† and Tuomo Timonen

Department of Pathology
University of Helsinki
00290 Helsinki 29 Finland

Kari Cantell

Central Public Health Laboratory
00280 Helsinki 28 Finland

Human natural killer cells (NK cells) can be greatly enriched by adsorption-elution procedures utilizing target-cell-coated plastic beads as adsorbants.[1] Among the eluted cells large granular lymphocytes (LGL) are present as a majority and by contact analyses on susceptible NK targets such as K-562 it can be demonstrated that the level of cytotoxicity obtained is directly proportional to the number of LGL making contact with the targets.[2] This and other evidence has, therefore, allowed us to conclude that cells with LGL morphology are responsible for the human NK activity and this cell type has been characterized in detail (for review see Saksela *et al.*[3]).

Interferon (IF) is known to augment the NK activity of human as well as various animal lymphoid cells both *in vivo* and *in vitro*.[4–6] On the other hand, Trinchieri and Santoli[7] have shown that contact of lymphoid effector cells with suitable, mainly tumor target cells results in the production of interferon by the lymphoid cells. At the same time the NK activity of the lymphoid effector cell population is enhanced. In the present communication we have investigated the cellular interrelationships in these phenomena using the cell fractionation procedures outlined above.

Materials and Methods

Effector Cells

Mononuclear cells were isolated from buffy coats derived from healthy donors' blood by the Ficoll-Isopaque method of Bøyum.[8] Surface-adherent cells were depleted by the incubation of Ficoll-Isopaque purified mononuclear cells in glass bottles and nylon-wool columns (Julius *et al.*[9]). Nylon wool adherent cells were recovered with a gentle pressing of the column.

Target Cells

K 562, the erythroleukemic cell line (Andersson *et al.*[10]) was grown in stationary suspension cultures and subcultured twice a week. HeLa, the cell line

*Supported by National Institutes of Health-National Cancer Institute Grant No. 1 RO 1 CA 23809-01 and by the Sigrid Juselius Foundation.

†*Address for correspondence:* Eero Saksela, MD, Department of Pathology, University of Helsinki, Haartmaninkatu 3, 00290 Helsinki 29, Finland.

0077–8923/80/0350–0102 $01.75/0 © 1980, NYAS

derived from a carcinoma of uterine cervix, and fetal lung fibroblasts were cultured in Degalan beads as previously described (Timonen and Saksela[11]). Both were subcultured once a week. The growth medium used was Ham's F 10 (Microbiological Associates, Walkersville, MD) supplemented with 10% fetal bovine serum (Microbiological Associates), 0.29 mg/ml L-glutamine (Oriola, Mankkaa, Finland) and antibiotics. This medium was also used in the cytotoxicity experiments.

Anti-interferon Antiserum

The antiserum against human leukocyte IF prepared in sheep as described earlier (Mogensen et al.[12]) contained 450,000 neutralizing units per ml.

Human Leukocyte Interferon

The human leukocyte IF was produced and partially purified as previously described (Cantell and Hirvonen[13]; Cantell et al.[14]).

Interferon Assay

The IF activity in coculture supernatants was assayed by the reduction of vesicular stomatitis virus plaques on human amnion cells (U), and expressed in terms of the unit assigned to the international research standard 69/19 (Mogensen and Cantell[15]).

Cytotoxicity Assay

Chromium ^{51}-release assays were used as previously described.[11] HeLa and fetal fibroblast targets were cultured on beads. E:T ratios used were 15:1 (for fetal fibroblasts) and 25:1 (for K 562 and HeLa), and exposure time was 18 hours. Percent release of radioactivity (PRR) was calculated from the following formula for each centrifuged triplicate tube: PRR = SN × 2/BT + SN × 100, in which SN = counts from a tube with half of supernatant from original triplicate tube, BT = counts from the tube with half of the supernatant and the remaining target cells (the original triplicate tube). Percent cytoxicity was calculated from the following formula: Cx% = (T − S)/(M − S) × 100, in which T = average PRR in the tubes with effector cells, S = average PRR in the tubes with medium only (spontaneous release), M = average PRR in the tubes with 10% Triton X-100 (maximal release).

Adsorption and Elution of Effector Cells from Target Cells

To enrich natural killer cells, Ficoll-Isopaque-purified blood mononuclear cells depleted of surface-adherent cells were allowed to attack either fetal fibroblasts or HeLa cells grown on Degalan beads, or K 562 in suspension. The formed attacker-target cell aggregates were fractionated in one-step gradients, and the attacker cells eluted according to the methods described earlier.[3]

Depletion of Natural Killer Cells by Incubation with Medium Containing Na-Butyrate

Ficoll-Isopaque-purified, surface-adherent-cell-depleted blood mononuclear cells were incubated overnight in Ham's F 10 medium containing 4mM of sodium butyrate. This treatment is known to selectively deplete the large granular lymphocytes (LGL) responsible for NK activity (Timonen and Saksela, manuscript in preparation).

Percoll Gradient Fractionation

Discontinuous Percoll (Pharmacia Ltd., Uppsala, Sweden) gradients were prepared in Ham's F10 medium with 10% FCS. The gradients ranged from 37.5–47.5% (vol/vol) with 2.5% intervals. 150–200 × 10^6 cells in 5–10 ml of the same medium were layered on top of the gradient and spun at 360 × g for 45 min. Visible bands formed at the interphases and were carefully collected in 5 fractions, washed twice in medium, and used (Timonen and Saksela[19]).

Giemsa Staining

Cytocentrifuged slides were air-dried, fixed for 10 min in methanol, and stained for 3 min in 10% aqueous Giemsa.

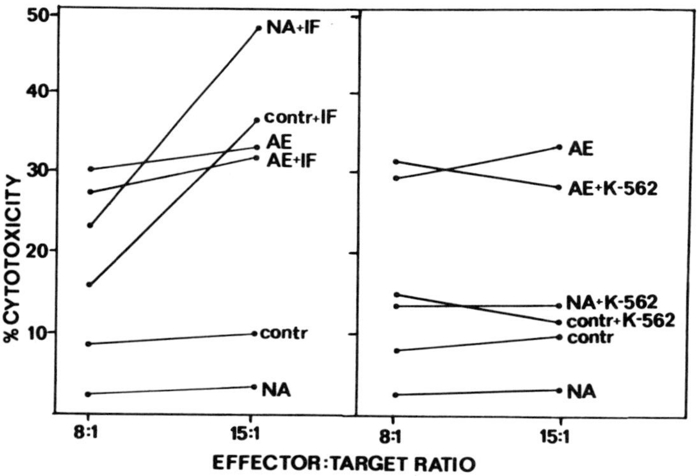

FIGURE 1. *Left-hand panel*: The effect of partially purified interferon (IF) on the natural killer activity of the various fractions obtained by adsorption-elution from fetal fibroblasts. NA = non-adherent cells. AE = adsorbed-eluted cells. Fractions were preincubated overnight with either 1:1000 final concentration of IF or medium only before tests for cytotoxicity against fetal fibroblasts in a 20-hr ^{51}Cr-release assay.

Right-hand panel: The same fractions as described above, but cocultured overnight with either K-562 cells at 15:1 lymphocyte:K-562 ratio or medium only before tests for cytotoxicity against fetal fibroblasts.

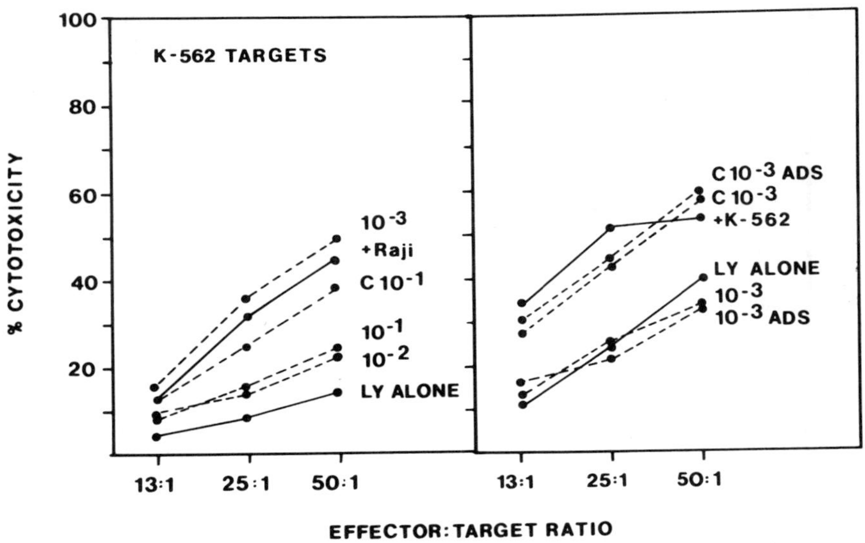

FIGURE 2. *Left-hand panel:* Effect of sheep anti-interferon antiserum on the augmenting effect of Raji cells measured against K-562 cells in 20-hr ^{51}Cr-release assay. LY alone = preincubation in medium only; + Raji = preincubation with Raji cells in 15:1 lymphocyte to augmentor ratio; 10^{-1} – 10^{-3} = serum dilutions present during the preincubation; C = control sheep serum.

Right-hand panel: Effect of preadsorbed (with packed suspensions of K-562 cells and lymphocytes used as effector cells) and nonadsorbed anti-interferon antiserum and control serum on the augmenting capacity of K-562 cells. LY alone = preincubation in medium only; K-562 = preincubation with K-562 cells in 30:1 lymphocyte to augmentor ratio; 10^{-3} = concentration of anti-interferon antiserum and control (C) serum in the lymphocyte-augmentor cell coculture; ADS = adsorbed.

RESULTS

Augmentation of NK Activity of Fractionated Cells

The cytotoxic activity of human NK cells can be augmented either through contact with tumor target cells or by addition of exogeneous interferon. We fractionated the effector cells using target-cell adsorption elution with fetal fibroblasts as adsorbants and investigated the response of such fractions to the above two modes of augmentation. As shown in FIGURE 1 the cytotoxic activity of the input cell population was augmented by both treatments. The cytotoxic activity of the fibroblast-nonadherent (NA) population was also greatly enhanced by the tumor cell contact or by interferon. However, both treatments failed to increase further the NK activity of the target-cell-adherent eluted cells containing the majority of "mature" NK cells of the LGL morphology. The findings indicated that fibroblast adsorption-elution had left behind an initially noncytotoxic population of cells rapidly augmentable to NK-activity by IF or by tumor cell contact. We termed such cells "pre-NK" cells. It is known that IF is released at the lymphocyte-tumor cell contact (see above). Anti-interferon antiserum added to the coincubation mixture of tumor cells and lymphocytes abolished the

NK augmentation induced by the tumor cells (FIGURE 2) corroborating previous suggestions that IF acts as a soluble mediator even under these conditions.

Nature of the Interferon-producing Cells

The source of the IF produced in lymphocyte tumor cell contact was then investigated. We analyzed first the effect of the various prepurification steps aimed at removing most of the macrophage-monocytes and the remaining polymorphonuclear cells. As seen in TABLE 1 removal of the glass or nylon-wool-adherent cells increased the IF production induced by an 18-hr contact with K-562 cells. Adherent cells recovered from the nylon-wool columns were

TABLE 1

EFFECT OF ADHERENT CELL DEPLETION ON THE DIFFERENTIALS, NK ACTIVITY, AND TARGET-CELL-INDUCED INTERFERON PRODUCTION IN VARIOUS FRACTIONS OF HUMAN PERIPHERAL BLOOD MONONUCLEAR CELLS

Experiment	Fraction*	Cx†	Differential Analysis‡ % LGL	Differential Analysis‡ % MON	IF IU/10^7 Cells§
238	FI	19	20	24	600
	FI + glass	29	26	3	600
	FI + NW	43	26	5	1100
	NW ADH	6	4	45	200
239	FI	7	22	19	>110
	FI + glass	33	28	15	600
	FI + NW	34	28	3	1100
	NW ADH	15	13	29	600
240	FI	14	19	22	1100
	FI + glass	36	25	3	>2000
	FI + NW	38	37	3	>2000
	NW ADH	23	9	47	350
241	FI	20	16	27	600
	FI + NW	21	32	2	>2000

*Abbreviations: FI = Ficoll-Isopaque-passed cells; NW = nylon-wool-passed cells; NW ADH = nylon-wool-adherent cells.

†NK activity against K 562, E:T ratio 25:1, exposure 20 hr.

‡LGL = large granular lymphocytes; MON = monocytes; the frequency of other lymphocytes complementary to % LGL + % MON.

§Interferon induced by K 562 cells in 1:5 ratio to lymphocytes for 18 hr. Supernatants tested as described in MATERIALS AND METHODS.

poor producers of interferon (TABLE 1). Further analysis of the IF-producing cells was carried out by fractionating the glass and nylon-wool-adherent (NA) cells by target-cell adsorption elution procedures using fibroblasts, K-562 or HeLa cells as adsorbants. The results are shown in TABLE 2. The highest titers of IF induced by contact with K-562 or HeLa cells were obtained when target-cell-adsorbed-eluted (AE) cells were used. The target-cell-nonadherent cells were the least effective IF producers. As seen in TABLE 2, lymphocytes of LGL morphology were also enriched in the AE fractions and depleted in the NA fractions, suggesting a relationship of LGL and IF production induced by the target cell contact.

TABLE 2

DIFFERENTIALS AND INTERFERON PRODUCTION OF VARIOUS FRACTIONS OBTAINED BY ADSORPTION AND ELUTION OF NK CELLS FROM FETAL FIBROBLASTS, K 562, AND HeLa CELLS

				Differential Analysis‡		
Experiment	Adsorbant	IF Inducer*	Fraction†	% LGL	% MON	IF IU/10^6 Cells
131	K 562	K 562	Input	21	1	50
			NA	13	1	72
			AE	76	0	153
141	K 562	K 562	Input	13	5	300
			NA	7	4	150
			AE	74	1	550
153	K 562	K 562	Input	14	3	200
			NA	8	3	>200
			AE	59	1	600
182	FF	K 562	Input	12	0	>20
			NA	14	0	35
			AE	33	0	200
191	FF	K 562	Input	nd	nd	nd
			NA	10	0	>200
			AE	37	0	600
196	FF	K 562	Input	28	1	>200
			NA	21	0	>200
			AE	57	1	200
198	HeLa	HeLa	Input	37	1	1000
			NA	41	1	300
			AE	61	1	1000

*See footnote § to TABLE 1.
†NA = target-cell non-adherent cells; AE = target-cell adsorbed eluted cells.
‡See footnote ‡ to TABLE 1.

TABLE 3

EFFECT OF SODIUM BUTYRATE ON NK ACTIVITY, DIFFERENTIAL ANALYSIS, AND INTERFERON PRODUCTION OF HUMAN PERIPHERAL BLOOD MONONUCLEAR CELLS

			Differential Analysis‡			
Experiment	Fraction*	Cx†	% MON	% LGL	IF IU/10 × 10^6 Cells	Yield§
236	Control	37	nd	nd	350	
	NA-butyr	24	nd	nd	>110	90
246	Control	69	7	44	600	
	Na-butyr	11	3	16	>200	79
247	Control (AE)	52	2	60	200	
	Na-butyr	19	3	5	>200	50
249	Control (AE)	73	1	41	nd	
	Na-butyr	1	1	6	nd	62

*AE = cells adsorbed and eluted from HeLa (247) or K 562 (249).
†See footnote † to TABLE 1.
‡See footnote ‡ to TABLE 1.
§Recovery of cells after Na-butyrate treatment as compared to control.

The relationship of LGL and IF production upon tumor cell contact was further analyzed by selective depletion of LGL from the effector cell populations. This was achieved by treatment with suitable concentrations of sodium butyrate, as will be reported in detail elsewhere (Timonen and Saksela, manuscript in preparation, 1979). The results of such experiments are shown in TABLE 3. The depletion of LGL from the effector cell populations resulted in loss of IF production at target cell contact, although the remaining cells of mainly medium sized and small lymphocyte morphology were shown to be viable and capable of other specialized responses such as PHA blast transformation and MLC (data not shown).

We have recently developed methods to fractionate Ficoll-Isopaque separated, glass- and nylon-wool-adherent cell-depleted human buffy coat lymphocyte populations in Percoll gradients to achieve an efficient and rapid purification of LGL. As shown in FIGURE 3, practically all of the NK activity resided in fractions enriched to up to 70–95% purity of LGL. These fractions were also most efficient in the production of IF upon contact with K-562 erythroleukemia cells,

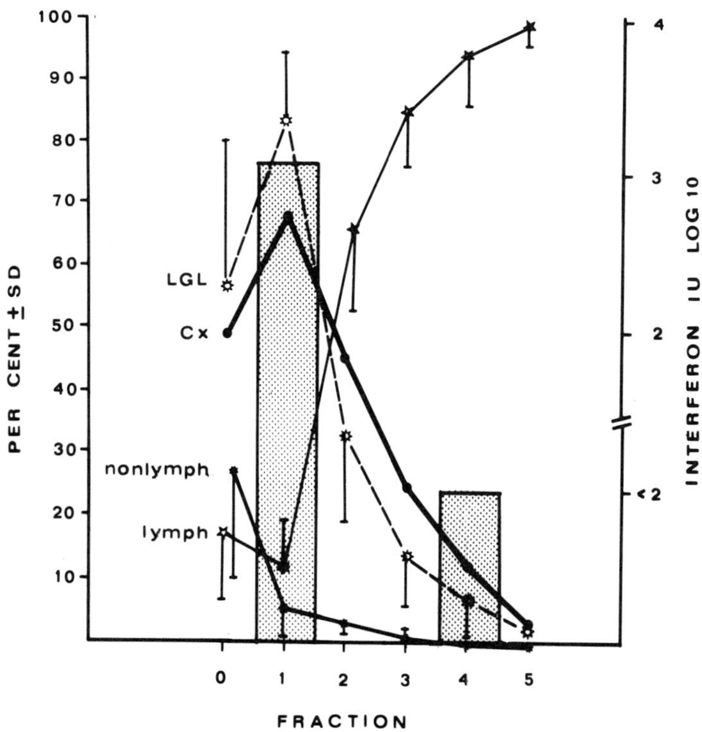

FIGURE 3. Percoll fractionation of Ficoll-Isopaque, glass and nylon-wool-passed human buffy coat cells. The NK activity measured on ^{51}Cr-labeled K-562 cells (E:T ration 25:1, 18 hr-assay), and differentials of the cell types indicated are given for each fraction. Columns represent international units of interferon obtained by 18-hr coculture with K-562 cells (E:T ratio 5:1) calculated per 10^7 lymphocytes of the fractions indicated.

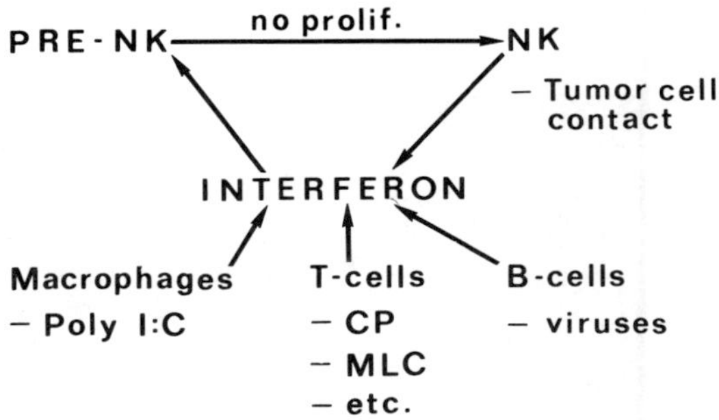

FIGURE 4. A schematic illustration of pathways involved in the regulation of human NK cell activity.

whereas no detectable IF was obtained from the other, mainly small and medium sized lymphocytic fractions.

Anti-Interferon Immunofluorescence Studies

In these experiments we induced IF synthesis by K-562 contact and after various periods of coculture let the cells adhere on poly-lysine-coated microscopic slides. The cells were fixed with 2.5% paraformaldehyde, reacted with a potent sheep anti-IF antiserum at various concentrations, and stained with fluorescein-coupled anti-sheep antiserum. The cells in contact with K-562 cells (mainly LGL as shown previously) were analyzed in ultraviolet microscopy. A proportion of the cells maximally ranging from 30 to 50% were brightly fluorescent after 6 hr, and simultaneous phase-contrast microscopy revealed the characteristic cytoplasmic granules (FIGURE 4). Fluorescence was detected in down to 1:2000 dilutions of the anti-IF antiserum, suggesting that possible contaminating specificities in the serum were not responsible for the fluorescence, and the reaction could be inhibited by the most purified interferon preparations available to us (4×10^6 IU interferon per mg protein). The results thus suggested a direct visualization of induced interferon within the LGL cytoplasm.[20]

DISCUSSION

These results show a clear association of the tumor-cell-induced IF production of human lymphocytes and the presence of large granular lymphocytes in the effector cell population. Cells of the monocyte-macrophage series did not produce significant amounts of IF in response to tumor cell contact and neither did the medium sized and small lymphocytes play a measurable role in such a response. We have already previously shown that the LGL are the effector cells of human NK activity.[3] Direct immunofluorescence studies with potent anti-IF antiserum revealed bright cytoplasmic fluorescence of granular cells making contact with K-562 cells and we know from previous experiments[2] that the number of LGL but not of the other types of lymphoid cells is directly proportional to the level of NK cytotoxicity measured by chromium release. All available evidence thus suggests that in man the NK cells and cells producing IF upon contact with tumor cells are similar if not identical cells.

Although LGL seem to be the major producers of IF in response to tumor cell contact they do not produce detectable amounts of IF spontaneously or by Sendai

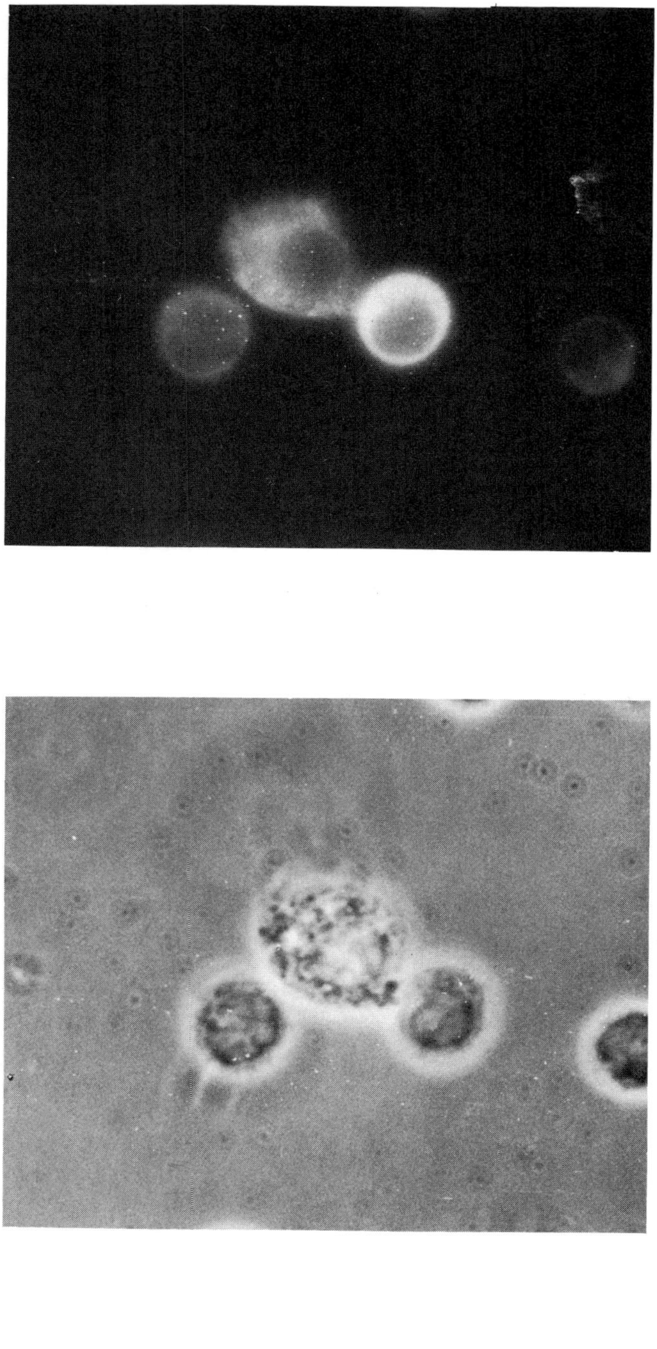

FIGURE 5. *Left:* Phase contrast photograph of lymphocytes in contact with K-562 erythroleukemia target cell. *Right:* Same field. Bright cytoplasmic fluorescence of a large granular lymphocyte in close contact with K-562 cell. Anti-interferon antiserum 1:2000 dilution after 4-hr lymphocyte target cell cocultvation.

virus infection. They are, however, obviously not the only blood cells capable of IF production. Non-T cells (Yamaguchi *et al.*[16]) probably B cells (K. Kumagai, personal communications) are known to be major producers of IF as a result of Sendai virus infection. T cells produce interferon when responding to mitogens and antigens (Epstein[17]), and monocyte-macrophages are potent producers of IF after treatment with polyinosinic:polycytidylic acid (Djeu *et al.*[18]). As the activation of NK cells by IF seems to be independent of the interferon source, whether exogeneous or endogeneous, leucocyte or fibroblast, type I or II, one may expect that regulation of the level of NK activity may occur in variety of conditions.

We have termed the initially cytotoxic circulating NK cells enriched by use of fetal fibroblast adsorbants, which by themselves do not induce interferon synthesis, "mature" NK-cells. Fetal fibroblast adsorption leaves behind a population of NK cells, also of LGL morphology, that can be recruited to full cytotoxic activity by IF or by contact with IF-inducing cells such as K-562. These cells have been termed "pre-NK cells." The present experiments indicate that at least the "mature"NK cells are capable of IF production, because fetal fibroblast adsorbed-eluted cells produced IF when stimulated with K-562 contact. It is not known whether "pre-NK" cells upon activation also gain this ability.

As shown above IF does not increase the cytotoxic activity of "mature" NK cells but exerts its action by recruiting "pre-NK cells" to active killer cells. On the other hand, "mature" NK cells are able to produce IF upon contact with tumor cells, which suggests an internal amplification mechanism of a positive feed-back type within the NK killer cell system. This has been schematically illustrated in FIGURE 5 together with some of the other pathways apparently implicated in the regulation of NK cell activity.

REFERENCES

1. TIMONEN, T. & E. SAKSELA. 1978. Cell Immunol. **40:** 69–78.
2. TIMONEN, T., E. SAKSELA, A. RANKI & P. HÄYRY. 1979. Cell Immunol. **48:**
3. SAKSELA, E., T. TIMONEN, A. RANKI & P. HÄYRY. 1979. Immunol. Rev. **44:** 71–123.
4. GIDLUND, M., A. ÖRN, H. WIGZELL, A. SENIK & I. GLESSER. 1978. Nature **273:** 759–761.
5. OHLER, J. R. & R. B. HERBERMAN. 1978. Int. J. Cancer **21:** 221–229.
6. EINHORN, S., H. BLOMGREN & H. STRANDER. 1978. Int. J. Cancer **22:** 405–412.
7. TRINCHIERI, G. & D. SANTOLI. 1978. J. Exp. Med. **147:** 1314–1333.
8. BÖYUM, A. 1968. Scand. J. Clin. Lab. Invest. **21,** Suppl. 97: 1–109.
9. JULIUS, M. H., E. SIMPSON & L. A. HERZENBERG. 1973. Eur. J. Immunol. **3:** 645–649.
10. ANDERSON, L. C., K. NILSSON & C. G. GAHMBERG. 1979. Int. J. Cancer **23:** 143–147.
11. TIMONEN, T. & E. SAKSELA. 1977. J. Immunol. Methods **18:** 123–132.
12. MOGENSEN, K. E., L. PYHÄLÄ & K. CANTELL. 1974. Acta Path. Microbiol. Scand. Sect. B **83:** 443–450.
13. CANTELL, K. & S. HIRVONEN. 1978. J. Gen. Virol. **39:** 541–543.
14. CANTELL, K., S. HIRVONEN, K. E. MOGENSEN & L. PYHÄLÄ. 1974. *In* The Production and Use of Interferon for Treatment and Prevention of Human Virus Infections. C. Waymouth, Ed. In Vitro Monograph **3:** 35–38. Tissue Culture Assoc. Rockville, MD.
15. MOGENSEN, K. E. & K. CANTELL. 1974. J. Gen. Virol. **22:** 95–103.
16. YAMAGUCHI, T., K. HANDA, Y. SHIMIZU, T. ABO & K. KUMAGAI. 1977. J. Immunol. **118:** 1931.
17. EPSTEIN, L. M. 1977. *In* Interferons and Their Actions. W. E. Stewart II, Ed.: 91–132. CRC Press. Cleveland, OH.
18. DJEU, J. Y., J. A. HEINBAUGH, H. T. HOLDEN & R. B. HERBERMAN. 1979. J. Immunol. **122:** 182.
19. TIMONEN, T. & E. SAKSELA. 1980. J. Immunol. Method. In press.
20. TIMONEN, T., I. VIRTANEN, K. CANTELL, & E. SAKSELA. 1980. Eur. J. Immunol. In press.

EFFECTS OF INTERFERON ON HUMAN LYMPHOID CELLS AND THEIR FUNCTION*

I. Heron, M. Hokland, P. Hokland, and K. Berg

Institute of Medical Microbiology
University of Aarhus
DK-8000 Aarhus C, Denmark

INTRODUCTION

It was already shown some years ago in mice that interferon exerts nonantiviral effects on lymphoid cells *in vitro* as well as *in vivo*. In parallel with progress in procedures to purify human interferon (IF), and with the acceleration of clinical use of human interferon, growing interest in the various biological effects exerted by the compound is becoming apparent. The influence on cells of the lymphoid apparatus in man will in this context stand as a subject of major importance and the present paper will deal with this. We have made observations in three different experimental systems. One includes methods to quantitate the amounts of major histocompatibility antigen (MHC) expressed on the membrane of lymphocytes and monocytes, another the assessment of natural killer cell (NK) function, and the third is a system where human lymphocytes become stimulated during mixed lymphocyte reactions (MLR) to develop alloaggressive cytolytic effector T cells that are assessed in a cell-mediated lympholysis assay (CML). In the two former systems different species of completely pure human leukocyte interferons have been assessed.

Complete purification of leukocyte interferon was accomplished as described in previous papers.[1,2] Partially purified leukocyte interferon (PIF) with a specific activity of 1×10^6 IFU/mg was a generous gift from Dr. K. Osther, Copenhagen. This material was used for further purification. FIGURE 1 shows the stained protein bands with an input of 1×10^6 international interferon units (IFU) on the SDS gels.

The upper curve of the FIGURE gives the antiviral (a-v) activity recovered from gel slices; it is apparent that the a-v activity appears in two major molecular species, and three additional minor species are disclosed by the analysis.

EFFECT OF INTERFERON ON MHC ANTIGEN EXPRESSION

Healthy nonrelated volunteers served as lymphocyte donors for the experiments. Lymphocytes were isolated from heparinized venous blood by centrifugation on Ficoll-Isopaque.[3] Mononuclear cells were washed twice, counted, and cultured in medium (RPMI 1640, GIBCO) containing 15% normal pooled heat-inactivated human serum in 10 ml test tubes at a concentration of 3×10^6 cells per ml. IF was added in microliter quantities to the suspensions. Cultures were incubated at 37°C in a humidified atmosphere of 5% CO_2/95% air. Thymidine incorporation was measured in selected cultures by the addition of 0.02 μCi of [^{14}C]thymidine to 0.2 ml of cell suspension in microtiter plates, which were

*This work was supported by grants from the Danish Medical Research Council to I. Heron and P. Hokland and from the Danish Cancer Society to M. Hokland and K. Berg.

0077-8923/80/0350-0112 $01.75/0 © 1980, NYAS

harvested and assayed for radioactivity 12–16 hr later, according to standard procedures.

Cells were washed two or three times in medium containing 5% fetal calf serum and 15 mM Na azide and then were incubated with 1:25 diluted fluorescein isothiocyanate (FITC)-labeled specific rabbit anti-human β_2-microglobulin (β_2-m) (Dakopatts, code F112, Dakopatts, Copenhagen) or with an indirect immunofluorescence technique to detect HLA and DR antigens. The first layer was monoclonal mouse hybridoma antibodies (kindly provided by Dr. Garotta, The Basel Inst. for Immunol). One of these reagents detects a common determinant on

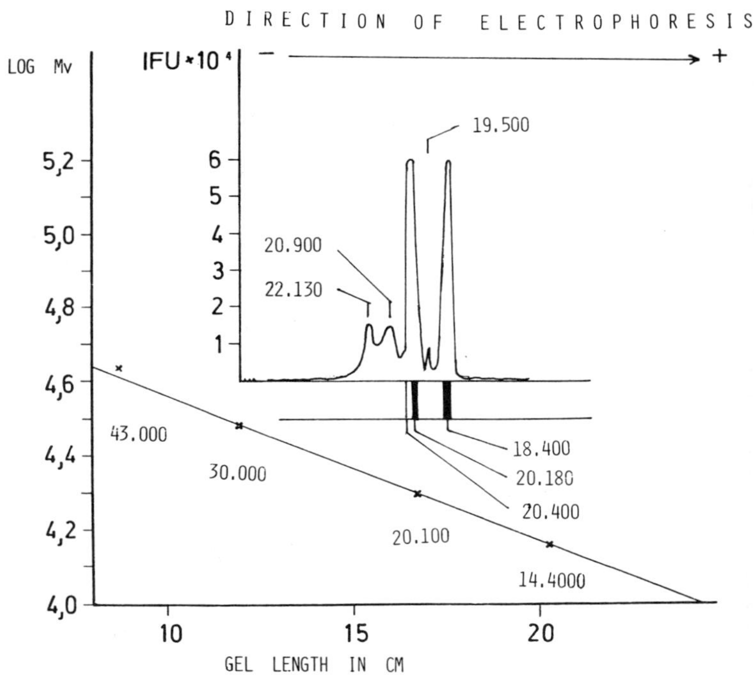

FIGURE 1. SDS-electrophoresis on acrylamide slab gels (SDS-PAGE) of pure human leukocyte interferon. The samples (30 μl) were examined in a 20-cm long exponential 12–18% acrylamide slab gel, 0.75 mm thick and 15 cm wide including a stacking gel of 5% acrylamide (10 cm high). After electrophoresis overnight (8–10°C, 10 mA constant current), one of the interferon-containing acrylamide-strips was cut off the gel and further subdivided into 1 mm pieces. Each piece was minced by means of a Teflon rod and eluted with 0.4 ml of 0.01% SDS at room temperature for 5 hours (rocking) and titrated on the same day. Total recovery of interferon activity from the eluted slices was 45%.

HLA molecules, and of the two anti-DR reagents one detects common DR determinants, and the other part of the DRW6 antigen. The fluorescent antibodies used to detect binding of monoclonal antibodies to the lymphocyte surface were a goat anti-mouse IgG (Bionetics code 8508-13).

Cells to be analyzed in the fluorescence-activated cell sorter (FACS) were washed three times and suspended in medium containing 5% fetal calf serum and 15 mM Na azide at a concentration of approximately 1×10^6 cells per ml. Cells (20,000–100,000) of each sample were analyzed at 4°C for green fluorescence, and a histogram showing the number of stained cells against the intensity of fluorescence was recorded. The scatter signals given by the passed cells were likewise recorded. Controls analyzed included nonstained cell suspensions to correct for background fluorescence and lymphocytes stained as if for detection of HLA antigens but without the first layer (cells labeled in this way gave essentially no fluorescence above "machine" background). The mean fluorescence intensity per cell was computed by using the formula $\Sigma i.c/\Sigma i$ in which i is the channel number and c is the number of cells appearing in the channel. When the same suspension of labeled cells was assessed twice, less than a 2% difference in the computed mean fluorescence intensity was found.

Cells were kept in culture in normal human serum under nonstimulatory conditions. Identical samples in the presence or absence of interferon were compared. Cell survival before labeling with antibodies was identical, and [^{14}C]thymidine uptake during culture was negligible. After incubation at 37°C overnight and labeling with anti-β_2m antibodies, scatter signals and fluorescence intensity of the cultured cells were as shown in FIGURE 2. Scatter profiles exhibited by the treated and nontreated cells were identical, but the IF-pretreated cells gave a positively skewed fluorescence intensity curve compared with the non-IF-treated cells. Such changes in fluorescence intensity curves of IF-treated cells were observed in every individual experiment, including studies with cells from 12 donors. The curve shift could be registered by a change in the position of the peak of the fluorescent cell intensity as well as by an increase in the computed mean intensity per cell. The relative increase in mean fluorescence intensity with anti-β_2-m and anti-HLA antibodies and nonseparated blood lymphocytes subjected to a standard dose (500 IF units/ml) for 16 hr varied from 21 to 48%, depending on the donor.

Lymphocytes were also tested in a number of experiments to determine the quantity of membrane-bound Ig. The IF-pretreated cells expressed more β_2-m, but the surface Ig profile was no different from that of the untreated controls. Similarly, the antigens on the lymphocyte surface, which could be determined by a rabbit anti-human T-lymphocyte antiserum, did not change quantitatively subsequent to IF treatment.

Absorption experiments performed previously,[4] and later confirmed by others,[5,6] have supported the conclusions of enhanced HLA antigen expression.

The selective increase in β_2-m-associated MHC antigen expression was obtained when PIF was used.[4] Each of the two pure major IF species as well as two minor species (FIGURE 1) were assayed in doses around 100 IFU per ml culture medium. *The effect was found using these pure molecular species,* whereas eluates from gel slices outside the regions where a-v activity was

FIGURE 2. Photographs from the screen of the FACS. The lower curves give results from control-incubated cells and the upper set from IF-treated cells. The left curves are the recorded light scatter signals. The abscissa represents size (increasing from left to right) and the ordinate shows number of particles or cells. Viable lymphocytes are seen as the main peak roughly in the center of the scatter diagram. The right curves are the recorded fluorescent signals. The ordinate gives number of cells and the abscissa the relative fluorescent intensity increasing from left to right. It will be seen when the upper and lower profiles are compared that the scatter signals are identical whereas the fluorescence curve given by the IF-treated cells is displaced to the right.

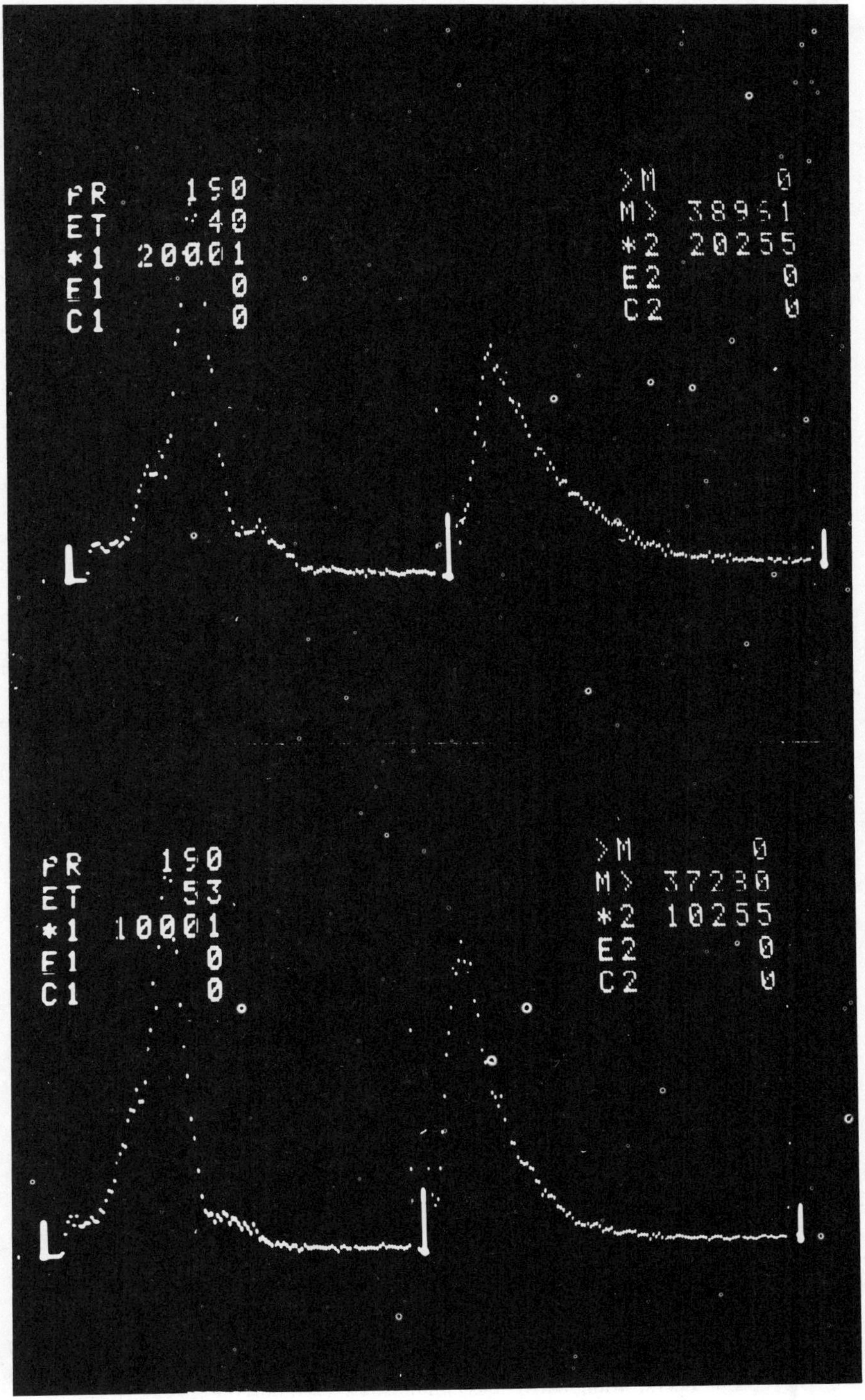
FR 190
ET 40
*1 20001
E1 0
C1 0
>M 0
M> 38961
*2 20255
E2 0
C2 0
FR 190
ET 53
*1 10001
E1 0
C1 0
>M 0
M> 37280
*2 10255
E2 0
C2 0

recorded had no effect. It has thus been proved that the effect of selective enhancement of MHC antigen expression on lymphoid cells is an inherent feature of the IF molecules.

DETERMINATION OF MHC PRODUCTS BY RADIOBINDING

Lymphocytes in numbers varying within experiments from 2 to 15 × 10^5 were incubated with the monoclonal antibodies as described above, and this was done using different dilutions. Following three washes, around 300,000 counts per minute of ^{125}I-labeled $F(ab)_2$ rabbit anti-mouse Ig reagent (kindly provided by Drs. Garotta and Trucco, The Basel Institute) was added to the tubes. Following incubation in the cold and 3 washing cycles, the pelleted lymphocytes were assessed for radioactivity in a gamma counter. A typical example is shown in FIGURE 3.

Comparison of the binding curves of IF-treated and nontreated cells show a marked difference when HLA or β_2-m determinants are assessed, whereas only slightly higher binding is observed when antibody against DR determinants are used. This minor difference, however, was reproduced several times employing cells from different donors and was seen with both of the monoclonal anti-DR reagents. Removal of phagocytic and adherent cells prior to the assay reduced the difference between IF-treated and control cells further.

The FACS was helpful in solving the question whether the increase in DR antigen content was solely due to monocyte DR antigens. From the light scatter signals thresholds can be applied and cells of different sizes can thus be assessed separately for fluorescent antibody binding. Blood monocytes appear mainly in a fraction of larger cells that can be seen on the scatter curve as a small peak to the right of the main lymphocyte peak[7] as will also be obvious in FIGURE 2. The small lymphocyte fraction assessed separately for fluorescence showed the following:

1. When anti HLA or anti β_2-m was used, the "normal" increase in fluorescence intensity was found on IF-treated cells.
2. When anti-DR antibodies were used only minute increase was observed.

The monocyte-rich function (>70% phagocytic) assessed separately showed

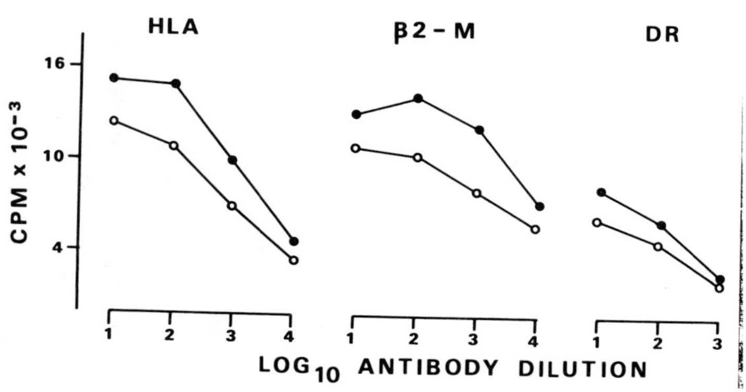

FIGURE 3. Binding of monoclonal mouse hybridoma antibodies against MHC products of human lymphoid cells assessed by uptake of ^{125}I-labeled anti-mouse antibodies. The open symbols represent control-incubated cells and the closed symbols the IF-treated cells.

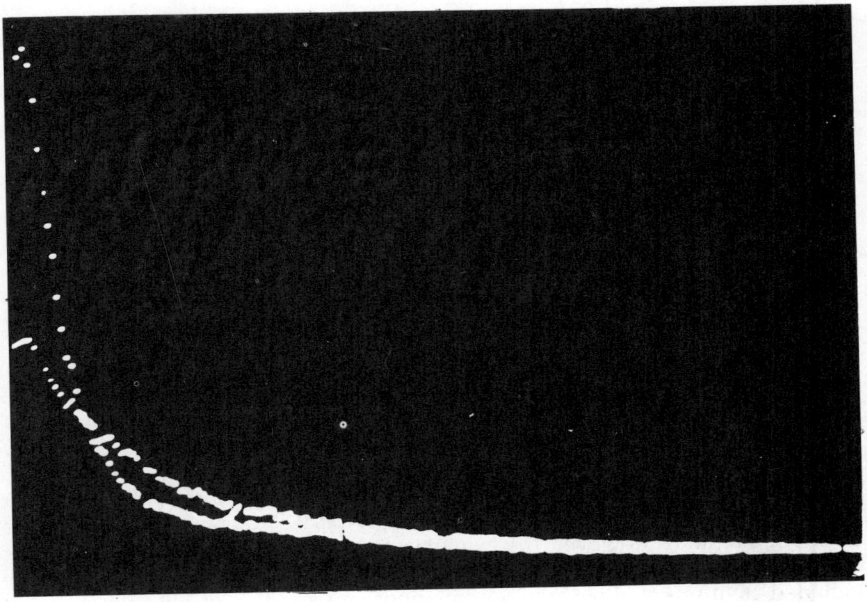

FIGURE 4. Fluorescence signals recorded when the monocyte-rich cell fraction was assessed separately for fluorescence intensity on the FACS. Cells were labeled with anti-DR antibodies. The signals recorded by IF-treated and control cells have been superimposed. The IF-treated cells are monitored in the curve showed to the right compared with control cells.

that IF-treated suspensions gave a clear increase in anti β_2-m as well as in anti-DR antibody binding (FIGURE 4).

The latter finding was reproduced using monocytes purified initially before culture by means of adherence to plastic surfaces and assayed in the absence of nonadherent cells.

The possible importance of this observation comes from the well known effect of macrophages presenting antigen in conjunction with I-region products to lymphocytes. We can hypothesize that the macrophage presentation of antigens that induce IF *in vivo* might be changed quantitatively as a result of increased amounts of surface I-region product.

EFFECT OF PURE LEUKOCYTE INTERFERON ON NATURAL KILLER CELL (NK) FUNCTION

Unsensitized human lymphocytes from normal donors are spontaneously cytotoxic *in vitro* for certain target cells.[8] This spontaneous cytotoxicity is enhanced by IF *in vitro* as shown by Trinchieri *et al.*[9] and by ourselves.[10] When IF was injected in patients, Einhorn *et al.*[11] showed that similar activation of NK cells apparently took place *in vivo*, since increase in NK was observed when lymphocytes were taken 12 hours after injection of IF and assessed for cytotoxicity in the absence of exogenous IF.

Although Heron *et al.*[10] and Zarling *et al.*[12] determined that highly purified preparations of leukocyte and fibroblast IF, respectively, were active in augmenting NK activity *in vitro*, formal proof that the activity is due to the pure IF molecules *per se* has not been presented previously.

FIGURE 5 shows a comparison between the four pure molecular IF species and PIF assessed in NK, where normal blood lymphocytes served as effector cells against K562 target cells. IF was added during the 5-hour incubation period in some experiments, and lymphocytes alone had been pretreated overnight with IF at 37°C in others before addition of target cells. Doses of 100 IFU per ml were equally effective in either way, and as shown in FIGURE 5 all four species and PIF were found to augment NK function to the same extent.

EFFECTS OF INTERFERON ON T-CELL RESPONSES *IN VITRO*

Blomgren *et al.*[13] reported that PIF added to human lymphocytes stimulated with PHA and Con A caused some degree of inhibition of DNA synthesis. Similarly, mixed lymphocyte culture reactions (MLR) were inhibitable by IF added to cultures. This effect is generally considered to reflect the "anti-cellular" properties of IF exerted on lymphocytes. Heron *et al.*[14] found (and it was later confirmed by Zarling *et al.*[15]) that addition of IF to MLR decreased the thymidine uptake moderately; however, the cytotoxic response of T-cells to the allogeneic cells generated during the MLR was increased. In 18 experiments,[16] which included 10 different allogeneic combinations and addition of 500 IFU per ml of culture medium, the average inhibition of thymidine uptake was 22% and the increase in lytic units was on average 121%. The effects were clearly dose-dependent and as shown in FIGURE 6, the optimal enhancement of cell-mediated lympholysis (CML) potential was observed with 500 IFU added per ml to the MLR. Higher doses not only depressed thymidine uptake further but also caused

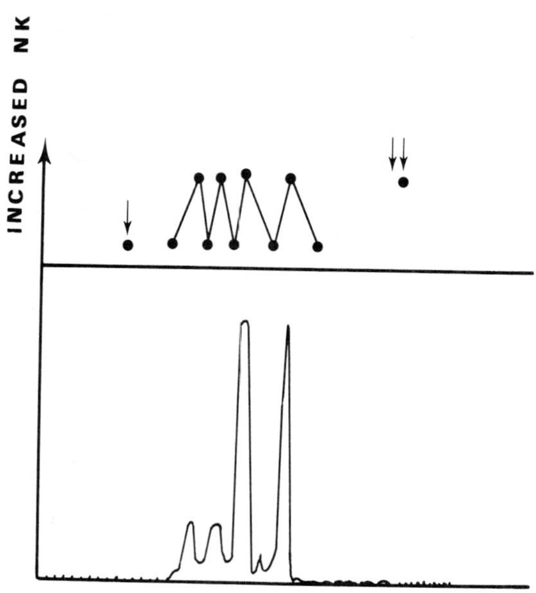

FIGURE 5. Pure molecular leukocyte IF species from gel cuts were assessed for NK enhancing activity. Fractions that have a-v activity as shown in the lower curve gave increased NK, whereas "base-line" fractions did not. One arrow indicates only saline added as negative control and two arrows indicate PIF used as positive control. Around 100 IFU a-v units of each IF preparation were added per ml.

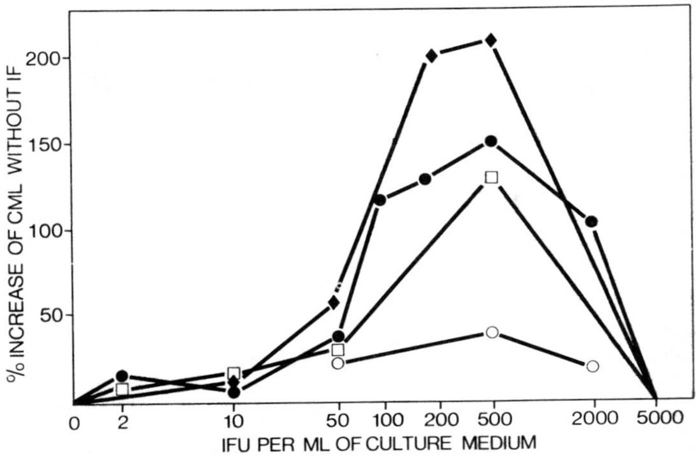

FIGURE 6. IF dose-response curves from four experiments where CML-enhancing effects of different PIF concentrations have been assessed.

inhibition of killer cell generation. The effect of IF on killer T-cell generation was further analyzed in a recent paper.[16] Leukocyte IF purified to a specific activity of 2×10^8 IFU/mg protein showed an effect similar to PIF. The experiments have, however, not yet been done using the pure material.

Various attempts to analyze the interactions induced by IF and leading to increased generation of cytolytic alloreactive T cells have been performed.[16] The possibilities that the effect is due to enhanced HLA antigen expression on the lymphocytes or to activation of NK cells have been excluded. Likewise, it was found to be unlikely that the effect was due to proliferating responder B cells or suppressor cells. The suppressor possibility was assessed in experiments where T-cell mitogens had been used to induce suppressor cells. It has not been possible to exclude the possibility that suppressor-cell populations normally generated during MLR become selectively inhibited by IF. Immunoselection was found to take place differently in IF-containing MLR as compared to control MLR, in a way giving selective support to killer precursor cells.

DISCUSSION

The possible immunomodulatory effects of IF *in vivo* still remain hypothetical. Nevertheless we are tempted to suggest that the *in vitro* effects of MHC enhancement and increased T-killer cell generation might play their roles *in vivo* during the host response against viral infection. Most viruses are good IF inducers, and from immunodeficiency syndromes in man it is known that T cells are particularly important for the immunological defense against viral disease. It is known that T cells initially recognize antigen in the context of I-region products and IF-induced increase in these on macrophages might assist in the recognition. In the second phase, killer T cells might receive preferential support due to IF and this might be further augmented by fever, as shown *in vitro*.[17] The killer T cells recognize virus antigen on infected target cells in conjunction with

MHC (H-2K-D, HLA-AB) products and IF-induced increase of these products in this stage might ease the recognition process.

Acknowledgments

We wish to thank Mrs. I. Sørensen and Mr. K. Vestergård for excellent technical assistance.

References

1. Berg, K., I. Heron & R. Hamilton. 1978. Purification of human interferons by antibody affinity chromatography using highly absorbed anti-interferon. Scand. J. Immunol. **8:** 429–439.
2. Berg, K. & I. Heron. 1980. The complete purification of human leukocyte interferon. Scand. J. Immunol. **11:** 489–502.
3. Bøyum, A. 1968. Separation of leukocytes from blood and bone marrow. Scand. J. Clin. Lab. Invest. **21,** Suppl. 97: 69.
4. Heron, I., M. Hokland & K. Berg. 1978. Enhanced expression of β_2 microglobulin and HLA on human lymphoid cells by interferon. Proc. Nat. Acad. Sci. USA **75:** 6215–6262.
5. Attallah, A. M. & D. M. Strong. 1979. Differential effects of interferon on the MHC expression of human lymphocytes. Int. Arch. Allergy Appl. Immunol. **60:** 101–105.
6. Fellous, M., M. Kamoun, I. Gresser & R. Bono. 1979. Enhanced expression of HLA and β_2-microglobulin on interferon-treated human lymphoid cells. Eur. J. Immunol. **9:** 446–449.
7. Cochrum, K., D. Hanes, G. Fagan, J. Van Speybroeck & F. K. Stur-Aevant. 1978. A simple and rapid method for the isolation of human monocytes. Transplant. Proc. **10:** 867–870.
8. Takasugi, M., M. R. Mickey & P. I. Terasaki. 1973. Reactivity of lymphocytes from normal persons on cultured tumor cells. Cancer Res. **33:** 2898–2905.
9. Trinchieri, G., D. Santoli & H. Koprowski. 1978. Spontaenous cell-mediated cytoxicity in humans. Role of interferon and immunoglobulins. J. Immunol. **120:** 1849–1855.
10. Heron, I., M. Hokland, A. M. Larsen & K. Berg. 1979. The effect of interferon on lymphocyte-mediated effector cell functions: Selective enhancement of natural killer cells. Cell. Immunol. **42:** 183–187.
11. Einhorn, S., H. Blomgren & H. Strander. 1978. Interferon and spontaneous cytotoxicity in man II. Acta Med. Scand. **204:** 477–483.
12. Zarling, J. M., L. Eskra, E. C. Borden, J. Horoszewicz & W. A. Carter. 1979. Activation of human natural killer cells cytotoxic for human leukemia cells by purified interferon. J. Immunol. **123:** 63–70.
13. Blomgren, H., H. Strander & K. Cantell. 1974. Effect of human leukocyte interferon on the response of lymphocytes to mitogenic stimuli in vitro. Scand. J. Immunol. **3:** 697–705.
14. Heron, I., K. Berg & K. Cantell. 1976. Regulatory effect of interferon on T cells in vitro. J. Immunol. **117:** 1371–1373.
15. Zarling, J. M., J. Sosman, L. Eskra, E. C. Borden, J. Horoszewicz & W. A. Carter. 1978. Enhancement of T cell cytotoxic responses by purified human fibroblast interferon. J. Immunol. **121:** 2002–2004.
16. Heron, I. & K. Berg. 1979. Human leucocyte interferon: Analysis of effect on MLC and effector cell generation. Scand. J. Immunol. **9:** 517–526.
17. Heron, I. & K. Berg. 1978. The actions of interferon are potentiated at elevated temperature. Nature **274:** 508–510.

DUAL MECHANISM OF INTERFERON AUGMENTATION OF NATURAL KILLER CYTOTOXICITY (NKCC)*

Stephan Targan†

Immunology and Gastroenterology Section
Medical and Research Services
Veterans Administration, Wadsworth Medical Center
Los Angeles, California 90073

Department of Medicine
UCLA School of Medicine
Los Angeles, California 90024

Fred Dorey

Department of Biomathematics
UCLA Center for the Health Sciences
Los Angeles, California 90024

INTRODUCTION

The human natural killer (NK) cell is capable of lysing tumor-related and virally infected target cells *in vitro*, without known prior *in vivo* sensitization.[1-4] In addition, several parameters such as fetal calf serum, mixed lymphocyte culture with B-cell lines, and mitogens can induce this activity over long time periods. In fact, some can induce active NK-like cells from lymphocyte populations that have been depleted of this activity.[2,5,6] On the other hand, rapid augmentation of NK lysis can be produced with interferon (IF).[2,3,7]

The actual significance of this latter NK activation in the role of this class of cytotoxic cell in host defenses against tumor transformation and viral infections is not known. However, recent studies suggest that the IF-mediated process might be important in increased protection against endogenous tumors and exogenous virus infection.[8-10] Thus, a clear understanding of the mechanism of this activation is an important consideration.

To date, the cytotoxic augmentation of NK cellular cytotoxicity has been documented using a ^{51}Cr-release assay.[7-9] Because of this assay's technical limitations, the questions of whether the IF augmentation is related to (1) increased numbers of effector cells; (2) actual activation of individual effector cells; or (3) a combination of both, could not be properly addressed. Recently, using a single cell assay where NK killing is directly visualized by the reading of trypan blue dye uptake at various time points by NK cell-target cell conjugates

*This work was supported in part by Wadsworth Veterans Administration Hospital Research Funds and in part by USPHS Grant CA-12800-08, "Immune Functions and Cancer."

†Address all reprint requests and correspondence to: Stephan R. Targan, M.D., Department of Medicine, Division of Gastroenterology, UCLA Center for the Health Sciences, Los Angeles, California 90024.

0077-8923/80/0350-0121 $01.75/0 © 1980, NYAS

plated in agarose gel, we have demonstrated that the frequency of active NK cells in normal peripheral blood lymphocyte populations is 2 to 4%.[11] In addition, we have shown the advantage of this assay over the standard ^{51}Cr-release assay in assessing the first order kinetics of spontaneous killer (NK) killing at the single cell level.[12] It is with this single cell assay where no recycling of effector cells can occur and killing can immediately and directly be visualized that the above questions concerning killer cellular cytotoxic augmentation can best be answered. The present report assesses the *in vitro* mechanism of IF activation of NKCC at the single cell level.

Materials and Methods

Lymphocytes

Peripheral Blood Lymphocytes

Fresh blood lymphocytes were obtained from normal volunteers after serial Ficoll-Hypaque centrifugation and iron carbonyl treatment removing macrophages and monocytes.[5]

Single Cell Assay

A modification of the single cell cytotoxic assay in agarose of Grimm and Bonavida[13] was employed using the NK-sensitive target cell K562. Test plates were prepared by melting 10 ml of agarose (1.0% in RPMI-1640 with HEPES buffer) in boiling water and then placing into a water bath at 42°C before mixing with the cells. Effector and target conjugates were formed by mixing equal volumes of lymphocytes and target cells in a total volume of 1 ml of RPMI-1640 with 10% fetal calf serum in V-shape 15 ml centrifuge tubes (Corning 25310). The cells were kept in a 37°C water bath for 5 minutes and spun at 1000 rpm for 5 minutes. All but 0.5 ml of media was aspirated and the cells were resuspended by using a Pasteur pipette and gently mixing the pellet ten times in the pipette. The melted agarose (at 42°C) was cooled by mixing in a 5 ml pipette four times and then 2 to 4 ml rapidly added and mixed to the suspended cells and conjugates. Before the agarose solidified 0.3 to 0.5 ml aliquots were rapidly added into the petri dishes (Corning 35 × 100 mm tissue culture 25000). No more than 2.5×10^5 of each cell was layered in each agarose test plate. Control dishes with target cells alone were prepared in a similar manner. After the agarose solidified, 1 ml of media was gently layered on top to avoid dehydration during incubation. Dishes were incubated at 37°C in a 5% CO_2 atmosphere. At appropriate time points (0, ½, 3 hr) (see RESULTS) test and control plates were removed from the incubator and the media aspirated (0 time actually represents approximately 5 to 10 min of reaction because of the 5 min of incubation required for maximum target binding). We then added 1.5 ml of trypan blue for 5 min, rinsed the plates, and added 2 ml of media and let them stand for 5 min. Coded dishes were counted at a later time after aspirating and adding 1 ml of 0.5% formaldehyde solution.

The percentage of conjugates was determined by counting the number of lymphocytes bound to targets in 100 counted lymphocytes. Cytotoxicity was determined by counting the number of dead target cells in 60 to 100 conjugates. The background spontaneous death is determined by counting the number of dead target cells in control dishes at appropriate time points. The percentage of bound cells that are cytotoxic at each time point is calculated by: (percentage of dead targets in conjugates) − (fraction of spontaneous dead targets × the percentage of dead targets in conjugates). Furthermore, the percentage of active killer cells for a given lymphocyte population at a given time is calculated by: (the percent bound cells that are cytotoxic at 3 hr) × (percentage of total lymphocytes bound to K562).

Effector Cell Activation

Interferon

Human leukocyte interferon (National Institutes of Allergy and Infectious Disease, United States Department of Health, Education and Welfare, Public Health Services, National Institutes of Health, Catalog No. G-023-901-527) at a final dilution of 1:2000 (10 units) was cultured with 2.5×10^6 cells/ml in RPMI-1640 plus 10% autologous serum. The cultures were incubated for 1 hr at 37°C in a 5% CO_2 atmosphere. These conditions for IF activation had been predefined using a ^{51}Cr-release assay to assess the minimal concentration and time for cytotoxic activation. These were used in order to look at any cytotoxic changes that might be produced by low levels of interferon. The cells were washed ×3 with PBS-A and counted for viability using the trypan blue dye exclusion.

Statistical Methods

The data were analyzed using a paired t-test at each time point as well as using a mixed model analysis of variance technique.[14]

Results

Table 1 shows results from seven experiments using the single cell assay for analysis before and after 1 hr of IF incubation. The time points 0, 30′, and 3 hr were based on previous results[11] that demonstrated the importance of measuring both early time points to define possible alteration in kinetics of NK lysis and the 3-hr point to evaluate maximum killing of nonactivated NK cells. There was no significant difference in percentage of lymphocytes that bound to the K562 target cells before or after interferon (8.9 ± 1.1 vs. 9.9 ± .7) (based on the paired sample t-test). In all experiments, there was a greater number of cells which had presumably been target bound that became active killers after interferon. In addition, while control NK cells did not reach maximum killing until 3 hr, the time point where nonaugmented NK lytic events are essentially complete, activated NK killing peaked by 30 min.

Figure 1 demonstrates these points graphically using combined data from the seven experiments. Results are expressed using both percentage of conjugates that are active NK cells and the total number of active NK cells in each

TABLE 1

FREQUENCY AND KINETICS OF NKCC BEFORE AND AFTER INCUBATION WITH INTERFERON

		Control			Interferon		
Subject	Time of Incubation (Hr)	% Lymphocytes Forming Conjugates	% Lymphocyte-Target Conjugates with Dead Targets	% Total Lymphocytes That Have Lysed Targets	% Lymphocytes Forming Conjugates	% Lymphocyte-Target Conjugates with Dead Targets	% Total Lymphocytes That Have Lysed Targets
1	0	13	4	.52	12	4	.48
	.5		9	1.17		38	4.56
	3		25	3.25		40	4.80
2	0	6	0	0	7	0	0
	.5		7	.42		24	1.68
	3		15	.90		24	1.68
3	0	9	0	0	10	18	1.80
	.5		5	.45		26	2.60
	3		15	1.35		23	2.30
4	0	7	0	0	9	25	2.25
	.5		7	.49		26	2.34
	3		18	1.26		21	1.89
5	0	11	0	0	12	0	0
	.5		9	.97		59	7.00
	3		26	2.86		60	7.20
6	0	9	0	0	9	0	0
	.5		5	.45		41	3.69
	3		26	2.28		40	3.60
7	0	9	3	.27	10	23	2.30
	.5		10	.90		25	2.50
	3		15	1.35		25	2.50
		8.9 ± 1.1			9.9 ± .7		

lymphocyte population at each of the three timepoints measured. Looking at the 3-hr timepoint, 20 ± 2% of the control target-bound lymphocytes and 1.77 ± .33% of the total control lymphocytes were active NK cells. After incubation with IF for 1 hr, these values were increased to 34 ± 5% and 3.5 ± 0.7%, respectively ($p < .01$). Since there was no significant increase in number of cells binding the K562 target it appears as though the majority of these new killer cells came from prior target bound yet inactive lymphocytes. Moreover, looking at the 0, ½, and 3-hr timepoints, to measure kinetics of lysis, control lymphocytes did not reach maximum killing until 3 hr of the assay, and only 37.5% of the potentially killing nonaugmented NK lymphocytes had killed after 30 min of reaction. In contrast, after IF, 100% of the activated NK cells had killed by 30 min, indicating marked

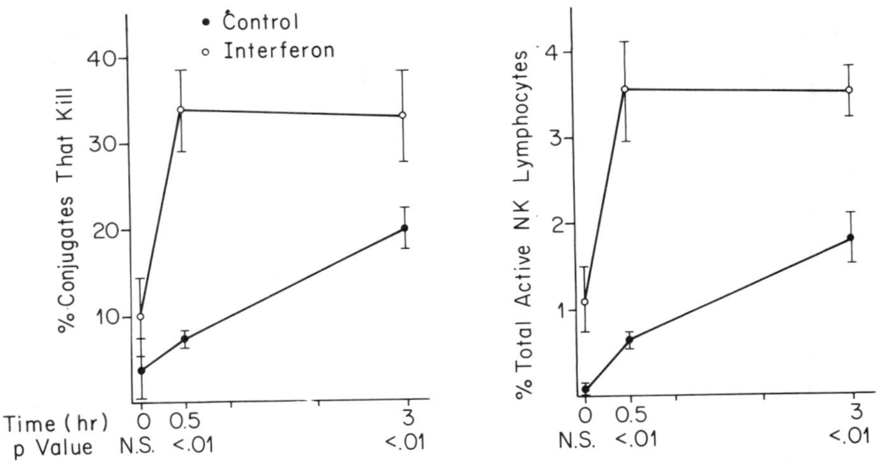

FIGURE 1. A comparison of killing of K562 targets at 0, ½, and 3 hr of a single cell assay before and after 1 hr incubation with 10 units/ml of interferon. Data represent results of seven experiments expressed in two ways. The left graph shows data as the number of effector/target conjugates which have dead targets at 0 (5 minutes), ½ hour and 3 hr. The right graph shows data as number of total active NK lymphocytes at the same time points (= % lymphocytes forming conjugates × % of conjugates with dead target cells). ●-●-Control; O-O-Interferon.

alteration of the usual first order of kinetics of lysis.[12] Because all post-IF and NK lytic events had been completed by 10 min, analysis of the specific kinetic pattern for this population over such a short time span was not possible.

These results were also confirmed using a mixed analysis of variance procedure with control of IF-treated lymphocytes as one fixed factor, time as another fixed factor, and each individual a random factor. As also indicated by the graphs in FIGURE 1, this analysis showed that incubation with IF resulted in a highly significant increase ($p < .01$) in percent killing during the 3-hr time period. Also there was a significant increase with time ($p < .01$) as well as a significant control-IF time interaction ($p < .05$). Thus, the killing curves over time differ significantly for the two groups. Of further interest is the fact that the variance component for individuals was not significant at the 5% level. This suggests a similarity in kinetics response of NK cells from different individuals, a result observed in earlier work with kinetics of nonaugmented NK cells.

Discussion

Ever since the human NK cell has been discovered, there had been much speculation as to how and where the endogenous arming and activation of this class of cytotoxic cell occurs. The cell has been most accurately defined functionally by the ability to lyse sensitive target cells;[1,3,15,16] however, the active NK cell appears to be Fc receptor positive and possibly of T-cell lineage.[7] Recent observations have shown that NK activity can be augmented by various *in vitro* modalities.[3,5,8,10,17,18] These stimuli appear to be divided into those that can augment NK activity within minutes to 24 hr of culture (interferon, poly IC, viruses) and those that require 48 to 72 hr of incubation before appearance of this augmentation (B-cell lines, pokeweed mitogen, and fetal calf serum).[3,5,7-9,18] In addition, the latter stimuli can induce NK-like cells from cell populations originally depleted of this NK activity.[18] This variable length of exposure required for each of this class of agents to augment NK activity suggests that there may be multiple stages of differentiation and responsiveness of NK cells.

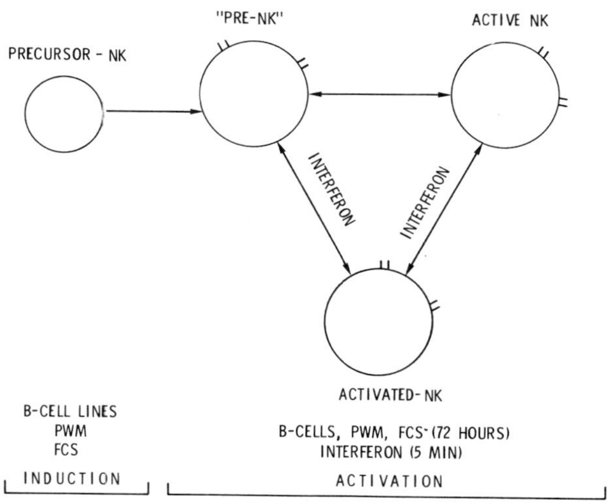

FIGURE 2. A conceptualization of the possible mode of NK modulation. The precursor NK is an Fc-negative cell which requires 48 to 72 hr of induction to be transformed into a potential pre-NK and then an activated NK cell. This process can be accomplished *in vitro* by mitogens, mixed lymphocyte cultures (MLC) or fetal calf serum, but at present it has not been seen with inteferon. The pre-NK cell has NK receptors and can bind to target cells but to kill needs to be activated by the various modalities shown in the figure. This process can occur within 5 min and is rapidly a reversible phenomenon. In addition, interferon will activate already active NK cells to become activated NK cells (see text). -NK-receptor.

FIGURE 2 is a conceptualization of the proposed mechanism of NK augmentation concentrating on the rapidly activating stage. However, it also illustrates the idea of the precursor-NK-cell which requires some differentiation over time to acquire NK receptors in order to bind to targets and more time to be programmed to become an active NK cell.[5,18] The data in this study only investigate the mechanism of rapid activation of all potentially responding NK cells.

One aspect of this mechanism seems to relate to recruitment of a new cell population. Using a single cell assay we have recently shown that the direct measurement of the frequency of active NK cells is possible. In doing this analysis, besides active NK cells, we found one or more subpopulations of freshly isolated peripheral blood lymphocytes that can bind sensitive NK targets but do not produce lysis.[11] The nature of these cells and whether they are potential NK killers has previously been suggested but not directly demonstrated.[3,7,11] In the present study, using the rapidly activating stimuli IF to augment NK activity, we have clearly demonstrated that a small percentage of these inactive target-bound lymphocytes can be rapidly programmed to kill. We interpret this to mean that a subset of "pre-NK" cells exist in peripheral blood lymphocytes which have NK receptors and can bind targets but remain inactive until they interact with appropriate stimuli such as interferon that initiates their killer potential (FIGURE 2). These findings are consistent with the speculation of others that such a population of cell might exist and be activated by IF or viruses.[3,7] The questions of the characteristics of these cells, what other stimuli activate these cells, and whether they can be driven to become active rather than activated NK cells (FIGURE 2), is presently being investigated. In addition, these newly activated cells may have a role in the altered killing potential or specificity of NK cells for fresh tumor cells after interferon incubation recently demonstrated by Zarling *et al.*[8]

The second aspect of NK augmentation relates to alteration in kinetics of lysis. In addition to being able to directly visualize frequency of active NK cells, the single cell assay is a sensitive technique to assess kinetics of lysis of cytotoxic lymphocyte populations. Recently, we have demonstrated at the single cell level first order kinetics of NK lysis over a three hour time span.[12] In the present study we have shown that these kinetics of active NK and the new pre-NK cell lysis are significantly altered after IF incubation, and, in fact, the entire NK population (now termed "activated NK-cells," FIGURE 2) has completed all lytic events by as early as 10 minutes. In fact all lytic events are completed so quickly that statistical kinetic analysis over this time span cannot be accurately assessed.

Using this single cell assay, the rates of effector cell recycling are not measured and these data represent alterations only at the single effector cell-target cell level. The first order kinetics of lysis of nonaugmented active NK cells suggests that a single factor is the limiting step in the lytic process.[12] In order to account for this tremendous lytic activation after IF, this rate-limiting factor must be either highly potentiated or additional factors which override this step are recruited by IF exposure. The molecular basis for this kinetic alteration in NK lysis, an event which is rapidly reversible[19] is presently being investigated.

Based on data from this study, FIGURE 2 represents an attempt to put both aspects of the rapid interferon NK augmentation process into a single concept. Hence, IF rapidly activates "pre-NK" cells, which have NK receptors and can bind to targets but are inactive killers, to become "activated NK" cells. Thus, there is a reserve of potential killer cells rapidly available to be activated when approrpriately stimulated. In addition, IF can stimulate already "active NK" cells to become "activated NK" cells which now kill sensitive targets much more rapidly. Since both of these processes are rapidly reversible[19] *in vitro*, there is a suggestion that this may be an important and tightly controlled *in vivo* system which can be turned on to respond to exogenous or endogenous stimuli such as viral infections or stress, and off once they are no longer present. Investigations into the possibility of such an *in vivo* control system are presently being performed.

In summary, using a single cell assay to measure differences in frequency and kinetics of lysis of IF-activated NK cells, we have demonstrated that this augmentation in cytotoxicity is due to both recruitment of new effector cells and an activation of both new and already active NK cells. The true *in vivo* significance of this activation mechanism to host tumor or viral defense remains to be shown.

Acknowledgments

The authors wish to acknowledge and thank Ms. Deborah Brown for her technical assistance and Ms. Linda Renée for her preparation of this manuscript.

References

1. Pross, H. F. & M. G. Baines. 1977. Spontaneous human lymphocyte-mediated cytotoxicity against tumor target cells. VI. A brief review. Cancer Immunol. Immunotherap. **3:** 75.
2. Trinchieri, G., D. Santoli, R. R. Dee & B. B. Knowles. 1978. Anti-viral activity induced by culturing lymphocytes with tumor-derived or virus-transformed cells. Identification of the anti-viral activity as interferon and characterization of the human lymphocyte subpopulation. J. Exp. Med. **147:** 1299.
3. Santoli, D. & H. Kaprowski. 1979. Mechanisms of activation of human killer cells against tumor and virus infected cells. Immunological Rev. **44:** 125.
4. Ono, A., D. B. Amos & H. S. Koren. 1977. Selective cellular natural killing against human leukaemic T cells and thymus. Nature (Lond.) **266:** 546.
5. Jondal, M. & S. Targan. 1978. In vitro induction of cytotoxic effector cells with spontaneous killer cell specificity. J. Exp. Med. **147:** 1621.
6. Targan. S. & M. Jondal. 1979. Lack of Fc receptor expression of cytotoxic effector cells with spontaneous killer (SK) cell specificity induced by stimulation with B cell lines. J. Clin. Lab. Immunol. **1:** 343.
7. Herberman, R., H. Djeu, D. Kay, J. R. Ortaldo, C. Ricardi, G. D. Bonnard, H. T. Holden, R. Fagnani, A. Santoni, and P. Puccetti. 1979. Natural killer cells: Characteristics and regulation of activity. Immunological Rev. **44:** 43.
8. Zarling, J. M., L. Eskra, E. C. Borden, J. Horoszcwicx & W. A. Cantar. 1979. Activation of human natural killer cells cytotoxic for human leukemia cells by purified interferon. J. Immunol. **123:** 63.
9. Ault, K. A. & H. L. Weiner. 1979. Natural killing of measles—infected by human lymphocytes. J. Immunol. **122:** 2611.
10. Kasai, M., J. C. Leclerc, L. McVay-Boudreau, F. W. Sheni & H. Cantor. 1979. Direct evidence that natural killer cells in nonimmune spleen cell populations prevent tumor growth in vivo. J. Exp. Med. **149:** 1260.
11. Targan, S., E. Grimm & B. Bonavida. 1979. Direct measurement of active spontaneous killer (SK) cells by a single cytotoxic cell assay. J. Clin. Lab. Immunol. In press.
12. Targan, S., F. Dorey, E. Grimm & B. Bonavida. 1979. First order kinetics of human spontaneous killer cellular cytotoxicity (SKCC). Comparison of a single cell cytotoxic assay with the standard ^{51}Cr release assay. Submitted.
13. Grimm, E. & B. Bonavida. 1979. Target cell lysis at the single cell-level. I. Determination of CTL frequency and relative lytic efficiency of individual effector cell populations. J. Immunol. In press.
14. Snedecor, G. W. & W. G. Cochran, Ed. 1967. Statistical Methods, 6th Edition. State University Press, Ames, IA.
15. Jondal, M., C. Spina & S. Targan. 1978. Human spontaneous killer cells selective for tumor-derived target cells. Nature (Lond.) **272:** 62.

16. BONNARD, G. D. & H. W. WEST. 1978. Cell mediated cytotoxicity in humans. A critical review of experimental models and clinically oriented studies. *In* Immunodiagnosis of Cancer. R. B. Herberman, and K. R. McIntire, Eds. Marcel Dekker Publishers. New York.
17. TARGAN, S. R. & R. P. GALE. 1979. Bone marrow modulation of spontaneous killer cellular cytotoxicity (SKCC) induction. J. Clin. Lab. Immunol. In press.
18. SEELEY, J. K. & S. H. GOLUB. 1978. Studies on cytotoxicity generated in human mixed lymphocyte cultures. I. Time course and target spectrum of several distinct concomitant cytotoxic activities. J. Immunol. **120:** 1415.
19. SILVA, A., B. BONAVIDA & S. TARGAN. 1979. The in vitro interferon NK activation system: Time, concentration and rapid reversibility of interferon augmentation. J. Immunol. In press.

IMMUNE INTERFERON: SOME PROPERTIES AND FUNCTIONS

Samuel Baron, J. Edwin Blalock, Ferdinando Dianzani, W. Robert Fleischmann, Jr., Jerzy A. Georgiades, Howard M. Johnson, and G. John Stanton

Department of Microbiology
University of Texas Medical Branch
Galveston, Texas 77550

Immune interferon (type II) is produced with other lymphokines by T lymphocytes stimulated by mitogens or by antigens to which they are sensitized.[1-4] It may function as an antiviral, antitumor, and immunoregulatory agent. Relatively large amounts of both mouse and human immune interferons (IF) are produced in leukocyte cultures stimulated with the T-lymphocyte mitogen, staphylococcus enterotoxin A.[5] Ten-thousandfold purification of human immune IF has been achieved using a series of procedures.[6] Antibody to mouse immune IF distinguishes it from virus-induced and lipopolysaccharide-induced interferons.[7] Unlike virus-induced interferons, immune IF preparations activate cells slowly[8] because the immune may induce an intermediary cellular protein which then induces the antiviral protein.[9] It exhibits highly potent antitumor cell activity even when partially purified.[10] The production and action of immune IF compared to other IFs, is under study in our laboratories and our results to date are presented here. A description of broadly active antiviral substance that is spontaneously produced by most cells in culture is also presented so it may be distinguished from IF.

ENZYMATIC INDUCTION OF INTERFERON PRODUCTION BY GALACTOSE OXIDASE TREATMENT OF HUMAN LYMPHOID CELLS

Because lymphocyte activation has been obtained after oxidation of membrane-bound galactose residues by galactose oxidase,[11-14] we initiated studies to investigate whether this enzyme, whose mechanism of action is known, is also capable of IF induction.[15] The results of a representative dose-response experiment are shown in FIGURE 1 in which IF production (FIGURE 1A) and DNA synthesis (FIGURE 1B) are presented for each dose of galactose oxidase. It may be seen that every dose of the enzyme applied induced both IF production and DNA synthesis. These two parameters show remarkable correlation, both reaching the maximum response at the level of 5 units of galactose oxidase. However, the IF response, which appeared exceptionally high in cultures treated with 5 to 20 units of galactose oxidase, was already maximal at 24 hr whereas DNA synthesis developed later, between 24 and 48 hr, and reached the maximum level at 72 hr. Both IF synthesis and [^{3}H]thymidine incorporation were completely prevented in cultures pretreated with actinomycin D. Pretreatment with β-galactosidase or with neuraminidase followed by β-galactosidase strongly reduced the response (up to 99%). Additionally, IF production did not occur in cells treated with heat-inactivated galactose oxidase (60° C for 30 min).

0077-8923/80/0350-0130 $01.75/0 © 1980, NYAS

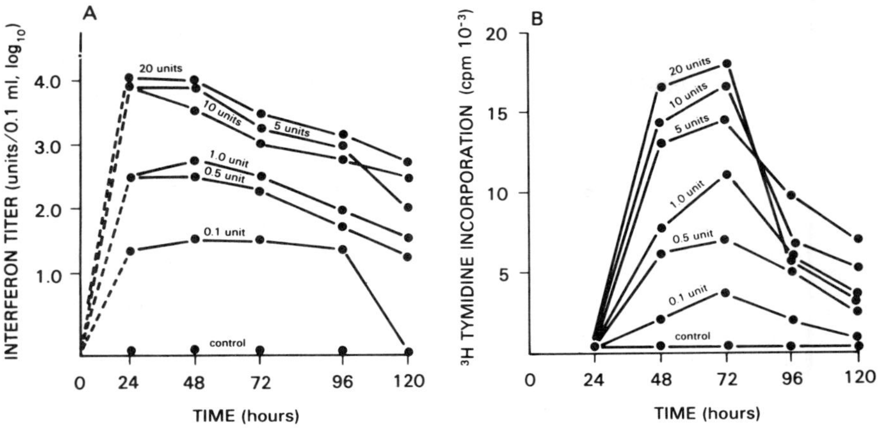

FIGURE 1. IF production (A) and activation of DNA synthesis (B) in lymphocyte cultures at different times after induction with various concentrations of galactose oxidase.

Kinetics of Interferon Production After Galactose Oxidase Treatment

To determine the kinetics of IF production more accurately, we treated lymphocyte cultures with galactose oxidase (5 and 20 units/ml) and harvested samples for IF titration after 3, 6, 11, 24, and 48 hr. The results of a representative experiment are shown in FIGURE 2. It may be seen that very low levels of IF were already detectable at 3 hr post-treatment; the levels increased substantially between 3 and 11 hr and reached the maximum titer between 11 and 24 hr. Lymphocyte cultures from six different donors showed slightly different

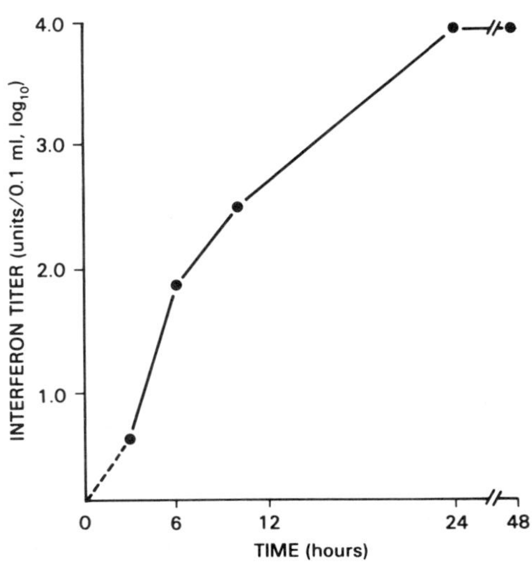

FIGURE 2. Kinetics of IF production in lymphocyte cultures treated with galactose oxidase (20 U/ml).

responses (not exceeding 30% of the response shown) only during the first 6 hr, whereas the later samples showed nearly identical responses. No significant differences were observed between cultures induced with 5 units of galactose oxidase and those induced with 20 units.

Characterization of Galactose Oxidase-induced Interferon

The properties of representative samples of galactose oxidase-induced IF were studied in comparison with samples of previously identified human leukocyte and immune IF. Galactose oxidase-induced IF shares with immune IF all the properties tested (unstable at pH 3, slow kinetics of cell activation, and not neutralized by antiserum to fibroblast or leukocyte IF) and it may therefore be temporarily identified as immune IF.

Immune-type Interferon-induced Transfer of Viral Resistance

We have recently demonstrated that cells made resistant to virus infection by treatment with their homologous virus-type IF can transfer viral resistance to cells of a heterologous species insensitive to that IF.[16–18] This transfer process is thought to represent a means of cell to cell communication that is mediated by a secondary messenger molecule(s) that transmits the IF signal from the cell membrane to the nucleus.[19]

The experimental plan was to determine whether immune-type IF-treated mouse L cells could transfer their antiviral resistance to cocultivated human WISH cells. Also, if transfer occurred, what was its quantitative relationship to the transfer caused by virus-type IF? Mouse L cells were cultured with human WISH cells in the presence or absence of serial dilutions of mouse immune or virus-type IF. Controls consisted of an equivalent total number of either cell species alone in the presence or absence of mouse immune or virus-type IF.

Figure 3 shows that whereas human WISH cells alone are not sensitive to the action of mouse immune-type IF, cocultivation of these cells in the presence of immune-type IF and sensitive mouse L cells resulted in a marked inhibition of the expected virus yield from the IF-insensitive human cells. Control cell mixtures in the absence of IF yielded the expected amount of virus as compared with the virus yield from either cell type alone. These data indicated that the presence of immune-type IF with its homologous cell can induce antiviral activity in heterologous cells. The controls show that inhibition of virus yield does not result from cocultivation of human and mouse cells but results from the presence of the mouse immune-type interferon preparation with the cocultivated cells.

The dose response (Figure 3) shows that transfer of viral resistance requires about 3 units IF/ml and that the maximum transfer of resistance can be demonstrated with between 10 and 30 units/ml of mouse immune-type IF. These data show that whereas transfer of viral resistance to human cells requires more IF than that required for development of resistance in mouse cells, the process is still fairly efficient in terms of the concentrations of immune-type IF required. Also shown in Figure 3 is that immune-type IF is about 3 to 10 times more efficient on a per unit basis than is virus-type IF at causing the transfer of viral resistance. The more efficient transfer by immune- relative to virus-type IF has been observed in repeated experiments.

Kinetics of Mouse Immune-type Interferon Action on Mixed Cultures of L and WISH Cells

Experiments were conducted to determine the time of treatment required for mixed cultures to manifest transferred resistance. FIGURE 4 shows that L cells

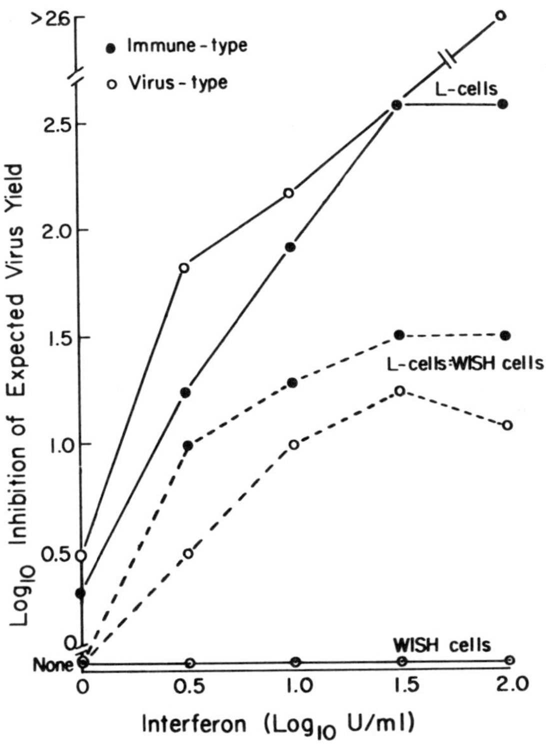

FIGURE 3. Dose responses of mouse immune- and virus-type interferon-induced transfer of viral resistance.

required 4 hr of treatment with 100 units/ml of immune-type IF to develop detectable antiviral activity, whereas transferred resistance required about 6 hr. The progressive development of resistance in L cells precedes by 2 hr the development of resistance in the heterologous cells. This suggests that the mouse immune-type IF initiated an antiviral process in the L cells that is subsequently transferred to the human WISH cells. Interestingly, L cells respond more rapidly (after 1 to 2 hr) to virus-type than immune-type IF, yet transferred resistance is similarly delayed with both IFs (data not shown). This suggests that the transfer

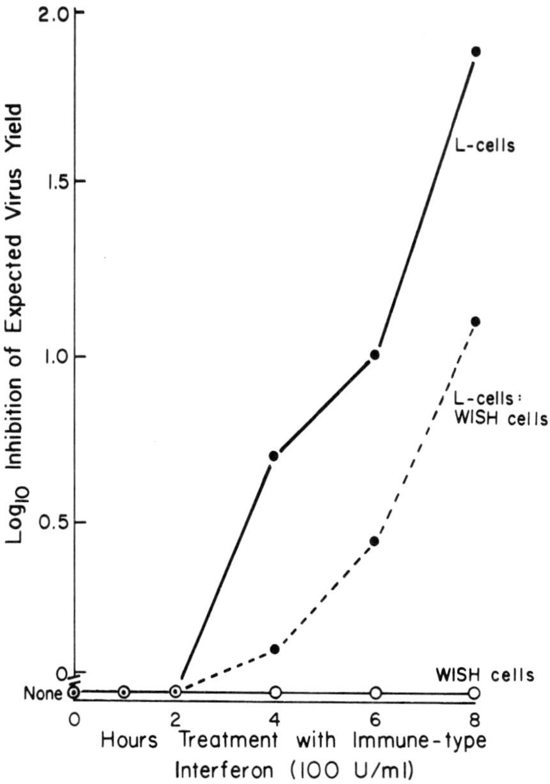

FIGURE 4. Kinetics of mouse immune-type interferon action on mixed cultures of mouse L and human WISH cells.

process and its expression in WISH cells may be very similar with both IF types whereas the initial events by which the two IFs activate L cells may be different.

Human Leukocyte Transfer of Viral Resistance to Heterologous Cells

Cocultivation of nonsensitized human leukocytes with xenogeneic cells leads to the production of human leukocyte IF.[20,21] These findings raise the interesting possibility that cells of the immune system, including mobile cells, might directly transfer IF-induced viral resistance to other cell types following exposure to endogenously produced leukocyte IF. When this possibility was tested it was found that human leukocytes could respond to foreign cells by producing leukocyte IF and then transfer their antiviral activity to the foreign mouse L cells which induced the IF.[22] The studies newly suggest an efficient host defense mechanism against virus infections that may be operating *in vivo*. The system would be activated by IF. Once activated by "foreign" or infected cells, migrating leukocytes could transfer resistance to other tissues, including lymph nodes, spleen, liver, nerves, and other target tissues. Unlike cytotoxic cells, cells capable of transferring resistance could rapidly help protect uninfected and recently infected cells without destroying them.

Interferon-induced Suppressor Factor: Possible Mechanism of Regulation of Normal and Tumor Cells

Suppression of the *in vitro* plaque-forming cell (PFC) response to sheep red blood cells by mouse fibroblast IF was shown to occur via the induction of suppressor cell activity in spleen cells.[23,24] Initially dose-response studies indicated that IF-treated 2×10^5 suppressor cells in the presence of 1.5×10^7 untreated spleen cells resulted in significant suppression of the PFC response. The high ratio (approximately 100:1) of untreated cells to IF-treated suppressor cells that resulted in suppression of the PFC response suggested that direct cell-cell contact of the effector (suppressor) and responder (untreated) cell was not required. Further, this suggested that a mediator derived from the suppressor cell population probably was responsible for the suppression. Direct evidence for such a mediator was obtained by incubating high concentrations of IF-treated cells for 2 hr at 37°C and adding the supernatants to untreated cultures (TABLE 1). The PFC response was suppressed over 95% and the suppression was not affected by prior incubation of suppressor supernatants with antibody to IF. The suppressor factor may be a macromolecule, since it did not pass through an Amicon filter with a molecular weight cut-off of 10,000, and in fact was concentrated under these conditions. Thus IF-induced suppressor cells, produced a suppressor factor that was capable of suppressing the *in vitro* PFC response.

It was of interest to ascertain whether the suppressor factor possessed

TABLE 1

Immunosuppressive Effect of Supernatants from Interferon-treated Spleen Cells*

Supernatants (1:10 final dil.) Suppressor Cells	Control Cells	Treatment	Anti-SRBC PFC/culture ± SD	% Inhibition
+	−	Anti-interferon	170 ± 113	98
+	−	NRS	150 ± 212	97
+	−	None	60 ± 57	99
−	+	Anti-interferon	10200 ± 792	4
−	+	NRS	6320 ± 4130	−41
−	+	None	5140 ± 990	30
−	+	Anti-interferon	10680 ± 3564	—
−	−	NRS	4480 ± 792	—
−	−	None	7380 ± 537	—

*Suppressor cells were obtained from the same population as those used in TABLE 2. Supernatants were obtained by incubating the cells at 1×10^8/ml at 37°C for 2 hr. After removal of the cells by centrifugation, the supernatants were incubated with anti-interferon serum, normal rabbit serum (NRS), or culture media as described for the cells in TABLE 2 prior to addition to syngeneic cultures.

antiviral activity. Undiluted suppressor factor preparation contained antiviral activity equivalent to 10 to 30 units of IF/ml which could be residual after washing. All of this antiviral activity was neutralized by antibody to interferon which failed to neutralize the suppressor activity (TABLE 2). IF-induced suppressor factor, then, was active in suppression of the PFC response, but lacked antiviral properties.

Titration of the factor showed a linear relationship between inhibition of PFC response versus suppressor factor dilution (data not shown). Induction of suppressor factor by IF was completely blocked if the IF was first neutralized by specific antibody prior to addition to spleen cell cultures. This is evidence that interferon was the inducer of the suppressor factor.

POTENTIATION OF ANTIVIRAL ACTIVITY BY MIXED PREPARATIONS OF IMMUNE AND FIBROBLAST INTERFERON

Possible synergistic interactions of immune and fibroblast interferons were studied by contrasting the separate protective abilities of immune and fibroblast interferons with the combined protective ability of mixed preparations of immune and fibroblast IFs.[25] L-cell monolayers were treated with IF samples for 12 hr and then challenged with mengovirus at a multiplicity of 10 PFU/cell. Progeny virus yields were harvested at 24 hr post-infection to allow completion of a one-step virus growth cycle. The virus yields were determined by plaque assay. Protection of IF-treated monolayers was determined by dividing the virus yield of untreated monolayers by the virus yield of IF-treated monolayers to obtain a fold inhibition value. Results of a representative experiment are presented in TABLE 3. Both immune IF and fibroblast IF provided protection against virus yield when employed separately. Three units of immune IF reduced virus yield by approximately 3-fold while 26 units of fibroblast IF reduced virus

TABLE 2

ANTIVIRAL ACTIVITY OF INTERFERON-INDUCED SUPPRESSOR FACTOR

Supernatant	Treatment	Interferon or Antiviral Activity (units/ml)
Suppressor factor*	None	30
	Anti-interferon†	<3
Control suppressor factor‡	None	<3
Interferon recovered after suppressor cell induction§	None	1000
Interferon used to induce suppressor cells¶	None	1000

*Suppressor factor obtained from cells treated with 1000 units of interferon/ml, washed, resuspended to 1×10^8 cells/ml, and incubated at 37°C for 2 hr.

†Equal volumes of suppressor factor (undiluted) and antibody to inteferon (1:20 dilution) were incubated together for 1 hr at room temperature prior to titration for antiviral activity.

‡Control suppressor factor obtained from cells incubated in culture media, washed, resuspended to 1×10^8 cells/ml, and incubated at 37°C for 2 hr.

§Residual interferon concentration after treatment of cells for suppressor cell induction.

¶Interferon concentration used to induce suppressor cells.

TABLE 3

POTENTIATION OF INTERFERON ACTIVITY BY MIXED PREPARATIONS OF IMMUNE INTERFERON AND FIBROBLAST INTERFERON*

IF Sample	Virus Yield PFU/ml ± S.D.	Fold Inhibition	IF Titer (units/ml) Actual†	Expected‡	Fold Potentiation§
No IF	$1.0 \times 10^9 \pm 0.1$				
IIF	$3.8 \times 10^8 \pm 0.4$	2.6	3		
FIF	$2.3 \times 10^7 \pm 0.1$	43	26		
IIF + FIF	$1.4 \times 10^6 \pm 0.03$	714	320	29	11

*Mouse L-cell monolayers were treated for 12 hr with growth medium (No IF), immune interferon (IIF), fibroblast interferon (FIF), and immune interferon and fibroblast interferon in combination (IIF + FIF). The monolayers were challenged with mengovirus at a multiplicity of infection of 10 PFU/cell and virus yields were harvested 24 hr later.

†Actual interferon titers were determined by comparison of virus yield with a standard yield reduction curve of interferon activity determined concurrently.

‡Expected interferon titer was determined by adding the actual titers of the interferons present in the mixed interferon preparation.

§The potentiation factor was determined by dividing the actual interferon titer by the expected.

yield by 43-fold. More important, the level of protection observed when immune and fibroblast IFs were added in combination was 714-fold, much greater than predicted on the basis of their separate protective abilities. The virus yields were compared to a standard curve of virus yields generated concurrently for known amounts of fibroblast IF in order to convert the observed virus yield into units of actual IF activity. The virus yields by monolayers treated with a combined total of 29 units of mixed IFs (3 units of immune IF plus 26 units of fibroblast IF) were at a level expected for monolayers treated with more than 300 units of IF. Thus, an 11-fold potentiation of IF activity occurred. More than a dozen separate immune IF preparations have been examined and shown to have potentiating abilities of from 5- to 20-fold. No potentiating activity has been observed when fibroblast IF was mixed with supernatant fractions from unstimulated spleen cells.

The potentiating effect is a nonadditive, synergistic effect that may not even be simply multiplicative. For a multiplicative effect, the anticipated level of virus yields by monolayers treated with mixed IF for the experiment shown in TABLE 3, would have been less than 120-fold (2.6-fold × 43-fold). The actual yield was reduced by 714-fold, 6-fold lower than would be predicted by a simple multiplicative effect.

PRODUCTION AND FUNCTION OF THE INHIBITOR OF INTERFERON ACTION FOUND IN MOUSE LYMPHOKINE PREPARATIONS

An inhibitor of IF action was obtained by stimulating dissociated mouse spleen cells with the T-cell mitogen, staphylococcal enterotoxin A (SEA) for at least 3 days.[26] Immune IF was also produced under these conditions. The inhibitor was first detected because it lowered the protective capacity of these immune IF preparations relative to fibroblast IF preparations. The inhibitor was separable from immune IF by gel filtration chromatography and was partially purified by two-step BSA-Affi-Gel and gel filtration chromatography.

Kinetics of Inhibitor Production

Since the inhibitor of IF was also induced by mitogen stimulation, the kinetics of inhibitor production were examined to determine whether IF production and inhibitor production might be related.[27] First, however, it was necessary to devise

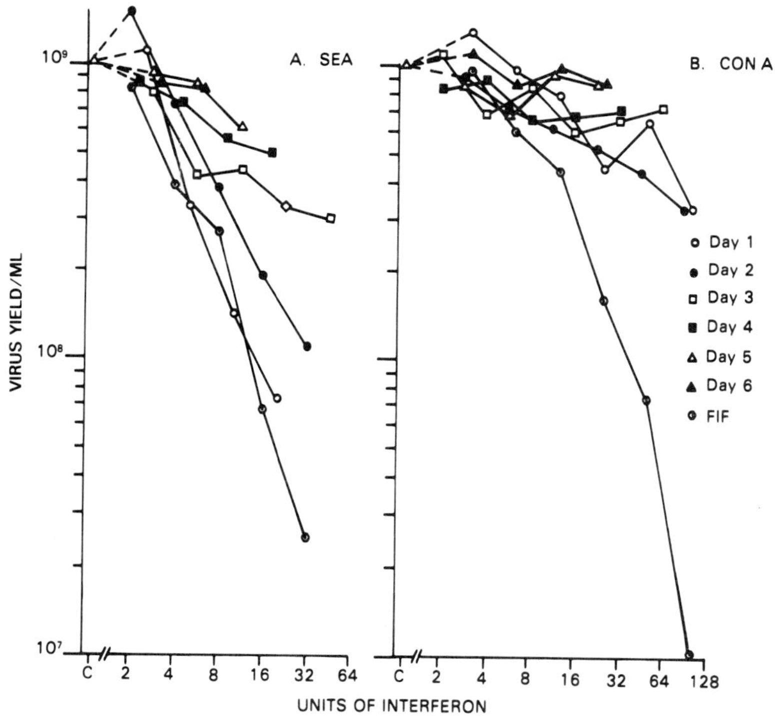

FIGURE 5. Kinetics of production of inhibitor. C57BL/6 mouse spleen cells in culture were stimulated with a final concentration of 0.02 μg/ml of SEA or 2 μg/ml of Con A. Supernatant fluids were harvested at the indicated times after mitogen stimulation and assayed for interferon activity by plaque reduction assay. The yield reduction protective capability of serial dilutions of each sample were determined and plotted against the interferon titer of the sample. Inhibitor was detected by the decrease yield reduction capability of the immune interferon samples. The shallower the slope of the yield reduction curve for a given sample, the greater the concentration of inhibitor in that sample.

methods of separately assaying each activity, since both immune IF and inhibitors were present in the same lymphokine preparations. Immune IF was conveniently titered by plaque reduction assay. The amount of IF present could be accurately quantitated for all preparations except those with very high inhibitor levels because the plaque reduction assay is a limit dilution assay in which the inhibitor is diluted out. The presence of inhibitor was detected in one-step yield reduction assays. The low dilution of IF in this assay permits the expression of the inhibitory activity as a reduction, relative to fibroblast IF alone, in the protective capacity of the lymphokine preparations.

The kinetics of inhibitor production after stimulation with SEA and with concanavalin A (Con A) are shown in FIGURE 5. The protective capacities of the immune and fibroblast IF preparations were measured as the virus yield per plaque reduction unit of IF. The shallower the slope of the immune IF protective capacity curves, compared to the fibroblast IF standard, the greater the amount of inhibitor in the immune IF preparation. As shown in panel A for SEA-stimulated spleen cells, the supernatant fluids from cells stimulated for 1 day had the same protective slope as fibroblast IF. By the third day of SEA stimulation a substantial amount of inhibitor had been produced and its concentration appeared to increase thereafter. In contrast to the delayed production of detectable levels of inhibitor observed with SEA stimulation, Con A stimulation caused the production of inhibitor within the first 24 hr (Panel B). The results observed for phytohemagglutinin (PHA) stimulation (not shown) were not so clear-cut since the maximum amount of immune IF induced by PHA was less than 30 units. However, the kinetics of inhibitor production appeared to be intermediate between those seen for SEA and Con A stimulation.

Partial Purification of Inhibitor

Immune IF preparations containing inhibitor activity were used to prepare a partially purified inhibitor preparation. The spleen cell supernatants were subjected to differential precipitation with ammonium sulfate. The precipitates obtained when the ammonium sulfate saturation levels were raised from 55 to 80% saturation were resuspended, dialyzed, and sequentially chromatographed on a BAS-Affi-Gel column followed by an Ultrogen AcA 54 column. Inhibitor activity was detected by mixing column fractions with fibroblast IF and assaying for decreased antiviral activity in a one-step virus yield reduction assay.

As shown in FIGURE 6, inhibitor activity could be detected in Ultrogel fractions 42–72. The inhibitor migrated with molecules having a molecular weight in the range of 8000 to 10,000.

A NON-INTERFERON, BROADLY ACTIVE ANTIVIRAL SUBSTANCE(S) SPONTANEOUSLY PRODUCED BY MOST CELLS

We detected a soluble viral inhibitor which appeared spontaneously in supernatant fluids form cell cultures. In these early experiments, a unit of inhibitor activity was defined as the highest dilution of the preparation that inhibited the specified virus yield by threefold (0.5 $\log_{10}$) when the virus was propagated in the continuous presence of the inhibitor. Decreased virus yield due to the inhibitor was usually accompanied by proportional protection of the cells against cytopathic effects. In subsequent experiments, a virus plaque reduction assay was employed. Inhibitor activity was assayed by mixing serial twofold dilutions of each sample with one-fifth volume of vaccinia virus (or the specified virus) and then plating 0.1 ml of the mixture on mouse L cells in a virus

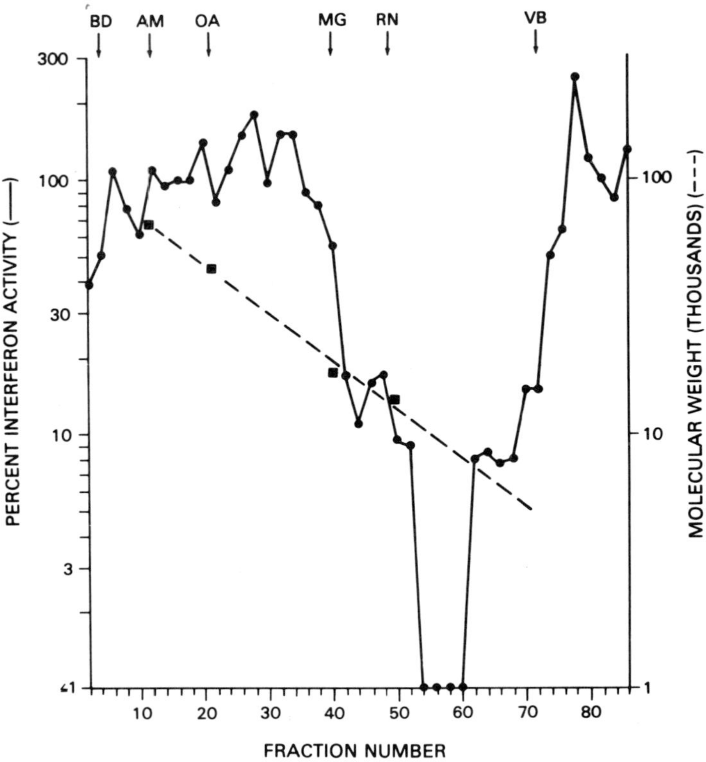

FIGURE 6. Ultrogel AcA 54 profile of BSA-Affil-Gel purified inhibitor activity. Inhibitor containing fractions from a BSA-Affi-Gel column were passed through a 2.5 cm ×82.5 cm. Ultrogel AcA 54 gel filtration column. Equal volumes of fraction sample were mixed either with growth medium or with fibroblast interferon (final concentration: 25 units fibroblast interferon per ml) and were tested for their protective capabilities in one-step yield reduction assays. Fractions containing inhibitor can be detected by their decreased capability to reduce the activity of added interferon. Arrows indicate the elution position of the protein standards used for calibration of the column (BD: blue dextran, >70,000 daltons; AM: albumin monomer, 67,000 daltons; OA: ovalbumin, 45,000 daltons; MG: myoglobin, 17,500 daltons; RN: ribonuclease A, 13,700 daltons; VB: vitamin B12, <5,000 daltons). (From Fleischmann *et al. Infect. Immun.* In press.)

plaque assay. The plaque inhibitory endpoint was defined as the highest dilution of the sample that inhibited 50% of the virus plaques.

The virus plaque inhibition titer in different culture fluids assayed on a variety of cells with different viruses is shown in TABLE 4. Several points are notable: the highest production of inhibitor was from mouse embryo, human HEP-2, and human lung cell cultures; the inhibitor was active against a variety of viruses in different cell cultures from unrelated animals, which is unlike IF; mouse L cells infected with vaccinia virus were most sensitive to its action; and poliovirus type 1 in HEP-2 cells showed intermediate sensitivity while several viruses showed lower sensitivity. In the yield reduction assay the degree of protection against vesicular stomatitis virus by the inhibitor was much greater than in a plaque reduction assay. An example of the yield inhibition of vesicular stomatitis virus (VSV) by various plaque reduction units of this cell-produced viral inhibitor (CVI) after infection with a low multiplicity of virus, is shown in FIGURE 7. Notworthy is the strong inhibition of virus yield from human WISH cells by low doses of CVI even though VSV is of low sensitivity to CVI in the plaque reduction assay. Thus, 2.5 units of CVI reduced the virus yield by a factor of approximately 100, and 5 units reduced it by a factor of 500 to 6000, thereby demonstrating a steep slope which may be advantageous during natural resistance to viruses and during attempts at therapy. A similarly steep slope occurred with sindbis virus.

Kinetics of appearance in culture fluids is shown in FIGURE 8. As may be seen, high titers of the inhibitor were released into culture fluids within a few hours. The rapid appearance of the inhibitor in culture fluids permitted the use of selective metabolic inhibitors in pilot studies to help determine the pathways of synthesis. The 96% inhibition of cellular RNA synthesis by 5 μg/ml of actinomy-

TABLE 4

INHIBITOR TITER* IN FLUIDS FROM MONOLAYER CELL CULTURES AGAINST VARIOUS VIRUSES IN DIFFERENT CELL TYPES

Cell Producer of Inhibitor	Treated Cells	Challenge Virus	Virus Dose (PFU)	Titer of Inhibitor
Mouse embryo	L	Vaccinia	10	1024
		VSV	10	2
		Sindbis	30	<2
	WISH	Vaccinia	10	32
		VSV	100	6
		Polio 1	30	4
	HEP-2	Vaccinia	10	5
		HSV 1	30	2
		HSV 2	10	2
		Polio 1	100	64
	Mouse Embryo	Vaccinia	10	6
	Hela	Polio 1	100	2
Mouse L	WISH	VSV	100	3
		VSV	100	<2
Human HEP-2	WISH	Polio	100	8
		VSV	100	12
	HEP-2	HSV-1	100	2
		Vaccinia	100	12
		Polio 1	100	32
	L	Vaccinia	10	16
		VSV	10	2
	Hela	Vaccinia	100	2
	ME	Vaccinia	10	64
Human WISH	WISH	VSV	100	3
Human lung	L	Vaccinia	50	96
Human skin-muscle	L	Vaccinia	50	16
Human thyroid	L	Vaccinia	50	8

*The plaque reduction assay with listed viruses was used to titer inhibitor (see text).

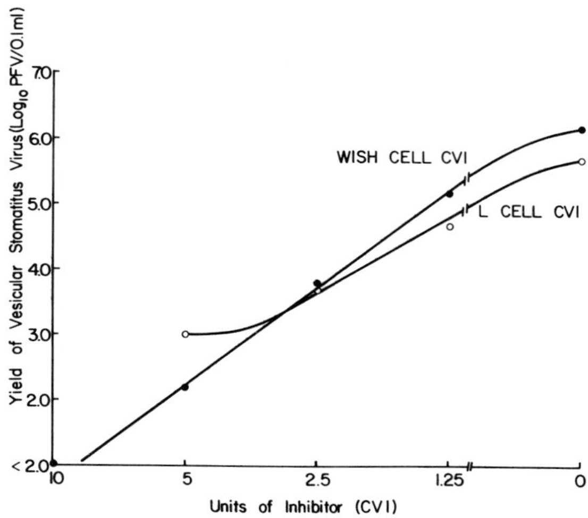

FIGURE 7. Inhibition of the yield of vesicular stomatitis virus by various doses of inhibitor. One thousand plaque-forming units of virus were mixed with inhibitors produced by human WISH or mouse L cells and then plated on human WISH cells. Culture fluids were collected after a 24-hr incubation at 37°C and assayed for infectious plaque-forming units (PFU) on WISH cells.

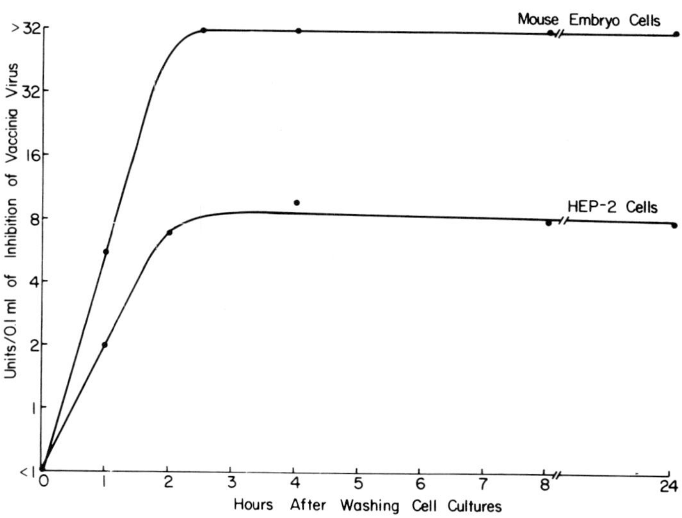

FIGURE 8. Kinetics of appearance of cell-produced viral inhibitor (CVI) in supernatant fluids from human HEP-2 and mouse embryo cell cultures. Monolayer cultures were washed, refed with Eagle's medium containing 2% fetal bovine serum and antibiotics, incubated and the fluid sampled at the times indicated for assay of CVI.

cin D decreased production of CVI at 4 hr by >90%, indicating that the inhibitor is newly synthesized by cells and that its formation may require RNA and protein synthesis. The 95% inhibition of protein synthesis by 10μg/ml of cycloheximide also inhibited its formation at 4 hr to the same degree, thereby suggesting the requirement for protein synthesis. Actinomycin D and cycloheximide controls indicated that residual metabolic inhibitors in the virus inhibitor assay were diluted well beyond concentration which would affect the assay. Taken together, the production of the inhibitor by normal cells and the apparent requirement for cellular protein synthesis indicate that it is a cell-produced viral inhibitor (CVI).

CVI's relationship to previously described inhibitors[28,29] requires study. At this early stage CVI appears to be distinct not only from IF (TABLE 5) but also from many previously described viral inhibitors of animal origin[30,31] because of CVI's unusually broad antiviral activity and absence of lipid in its active structure (data not presented). CVI is probably not composed of cellular receptors for virus, since mouse cells that do not have receptors for poliovirus[32] produce CVI which

TABLE 5

PROPERTIES OF CVI AND INTERFERON

Property	CVI	Interferon
Broadly active against viruses	+	+
Protein structure required for activity	+	+
Cell species specificity	0	+
Induces cell-bound (intracellular) antiviral activity	0	+
Inhibits virus attachment	+	0
Produced by VERO cells	+	+
Inhibits herpes simplex and vaccinia viruses	+	±
Spontaneously produced	+	0

is active against poliovirus (TABLE 4). Further study of CVI in comparison with some of the previously detected inhibitors from cell culture[28] and milk[29] will be required to test the possibility of a relationship. Important characteristics for comparison will be antigenic specificity, chemical structures, and mode of action. Purification studies of CVI will also be necessary to determine whether it is one substance or several.

REFERENCES

1. WHEELOCK, E. F. 1965. Science **149:** 310.
2. GREEN, J. A., S. R. COOPERBAND & S. KIBRICK. 1969. Science **164:** 1415.
3. SALVIN, S. B., J. S. YOUNGNER & W. H. LEDERER. 1973. Infect. Immun. **7:** 68.
4. YOUNGNER, J. S. & S. B. SALVIN. 1973. J. Immunol. **111:** 1914.
5. JOHNSON, H. M., G. J. STANTON & S. BARON. 1977. Proc. Soc. Exp. Biol. Med. **154:** 138.
6. GEORGIADES, J. A., M. L. LANGFORD, G. J. STANTON & H. M. JOHNSON. 1979. IRCS Medical Science: Biochemistry; Biomedical Technology; Cell and Membrane Biology; Immunology and Allergy; Microbiology, Parasitology and Infectious Diseases. **7:** 559.
7. OSBORNE, L., J. A. GEORGIADES & H. M. JOHNSON. 1980. Infect. Immun. In press.
8. DIANZANI, F., L. SALTER, W. R. FLEISCHMANN & M. ZUCCA. 1978. Proc. Soc. Exp. Biol. Med. **159:** 94.

9. DIANZANI, F., M. ZUCCA, A. SCUPHAM & J. A. GEORGIADES. 1980. Nature. **283**:400.
10. BLALOCK, J. E., J. A. GEORGIADES, M. P. LANGFORD & H. M. JOHNSON. 1980. Cellular Immunol. **49**:390.
11. BINIAMINOV, M., B. RAMOT, E. ROSENTHAL & A. NOVOGRODSKI. 1975. Clin. Exp. Immunol. **19**: 93.
12. DIXON, J. F., J. W. PARKER & R. L. O'BRIEN. 1976. J. Immunol. **116**: 575.
13. MONAHAN, T. M. & C. W. ABELL. 1978. Exp. Cell Res. **116**: 47.
14. NOVOGRODSKY, A. & E. KATCHALSKI. 1973., Proc. Nat. Acad. Sci. USA **70**: 1824.
15. DIANZANI, F., T. M. MONAHAN, A. SCUPHAM & M. ZUCCA. 1979. Infect. Immun. **26**: 879.
16. BLALOCK, J. E. & S. BARON. 1977. Nature. **269**: 422.
17. HUGHES, T. K., J. E. BLALOCK & S. BARON. 1978. Arch. Virol. **58**: 77.
18. BLALOCK, J. E. & G. J. STANTON. 1978. J. Gen. Virol. **41**: 325.
19. BLALOCK, J. E. & S. BARON. 1979. J. Gen. Virol. **42**:363.
20. TRINCHIERI, G., D. SANTOLI, R. R. DEE & B. B. KNOWLES. 1978. J. Exp. Med. **147**: 1299.
21. BLALOCK, J. E., M. P. LANGFORD, J. A. GEORGIADES & G. J. STANTON, 1979. Cell Immunol. **43**: 197.
22. STANTON, G. J., D. A. WEIGENT, M. P. LANGFORD, & J. E. BLALOCK. 1980. *In* Interferons, Properties and Clinical Uses. A. Kahn, N. O. Hill & G. Dorn, Eds. Wadley Institute of Molecular Medicine, Dallas, TX. In press.
23. JOHNSON, H. M. & J. E. BLALOCK. 1980. *In* Interferons, Properties and Clinical Uses. A. Kahn, N. O. Hill & G. Dorn, Eds. Wadley Institute of Molecular Medicine, Dallas, TX. In press.
24. JOHNSON, H. M. & J. E. BLALOCK. 1980. Infect. Immun. In press.
25. FLEISCHMANN, W. R., JR., J. A. GEORGIADES, L. C. OSBORNE & H. M. JOHNSON. 1979. Infect Immun. **26**: 248.
26. FLEISCHMANN, W. R., JR., J. A. GEORGIADES, L. C. OSBORNE & H. M. JOHNSON. 1979. Infect. Immun. **26**: 949.
27. FLEISCHMANN, W. R., JR., E. J. LEFKOWITZ, J. A. GEORGIADES & H. M. JOHNSON. 1980. *In* Interferons, Properties and Clinical Uses. A. Kahn, N. O. Hill & G. Dorn, Eds. Wadley Institute of Molecular Medicine. Dallas, TX. In press.
28. BUCKLER, C. E. & S. BARON. 1966. J. Bacteriol **91**: 231.
29. MATTHEWS, T. H. J., M. K. LAWRENCE & D. A. J. TYRRELL. 1976. Lancet. 1387.
30. SMORODINTSOV, A. A. 1960. Advances in Virus Research. **7**: 327.
31. WASSERMAN, F. E. 1968. Methods Virol. **4**: 53.
32. HOLLAND, J. J. & L. C. MCLAREN. 1959. J. Exp. Med. **109**: 487.

PROPERTIES OF MOUSE IMMUNE T-INTERFERON (TYPE II)

Ernesto Falcoff, Juana Wietzerbin, Simon Stefanos, Miguel Lucero, Claude Billardon, and Liliane Catinot

Section de Biologie
Institut Curie
75231 Paris, Cédex 05, France

Françoise Besançon and Helmut Ankel

Department of Biochemistry
Medical College of Wisconsin
Milwaukee, Wisconsin 53226

I would like, if I may, to start my talk on T-interferon by attempting to justify the reason for this nomenclature.

We used the term "Immune Interferon" for the first time in 1972[1] to define the types of interferon (IF) exclusively produced in immunocompetent cells stimulated by specific antigens or by nonspecific stimulants like mitogens and lectins. The term "immune-interferon" is frequently used in the literature. The work done in this field by our group and other laboratories[2-5] has led to the conclusion that there are two different types of immune-interferons: firstly, those induced by stimulants dependent on B lymphocytes—acid-stable, antigenically related to viral IF—and secondly, IFs induced by T-lymphocyte stimulants; these are acid-unstable and antigenically distinct from viral IF (FIGURE 1).

We shall refer to these interferons as Type B and Type T, taking into account inducer selectivity exclusively.

Youngner introduced another very popular nomenclature for antigen-induced IF, which he defined as acid-unstable and antigenically distinct from viral IF: he called it Type II interferon.[3]

Immune and Type II interferon are often synonymous in the literature. However, according to the criteria we have just defined (antigenic properties and stability at acid pH) these terms cannot be used synonymously.

As a function of these two criteria we therefore consider that among immune interferons a distinction must be made between Type T, which is similar to Youngner's Type II, and Type B, which shares some of the characteristics of viral interferon. This is schematized in FIGURE 2. We do not claim here to suggest a final classification for immune-induced IFs, for I think it is still too early to achieve this. The present comments simply aim to avoid the confusion caused by the use of the term "immune-interferon" as a synonym for Type II interferon.

The T-interferon prototype used in our research over the past few years was prepared by PHA stimulation of mouse splenocytes, since, as you know, PHA stimulates T lymphocytes.

The method has been optimalized and at the present time we are able to prepare considerable quantities of this interferon. The crude preparation has a

*This work was supported by grants from the Institut National de la Santé et de la Recherche Médicale (78.4.082.1), Délégation Générale à la Recherche Scientifique et Technique (77.7.1375; 79.7.1037) and Centre National de la Recherche Scientifique.

0077-8923/80/0350-0145 $01.75/0 © 1980, NYAS

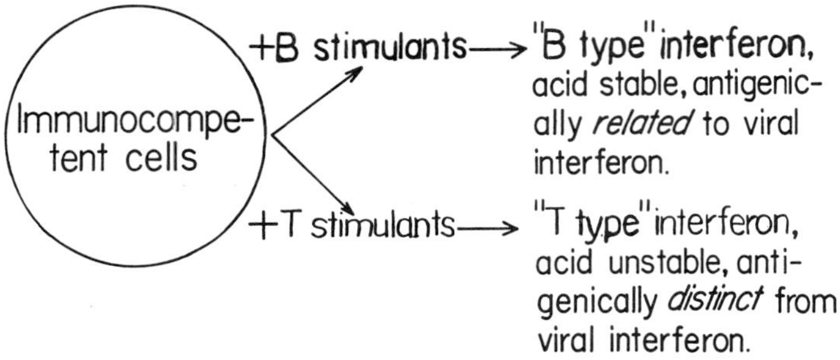

FIGURE 1. Induction of immune interferon.

titer of several thousand units per milliliter, with very slight specific activity of a few hundred units per milligram of protein.[6]

In order to define a method for purifying this interferon, we completed a preliminary study of its chromatographic properties, in cooperation with E. Sulkowski and J. O'Malley of the Roswell Park Memorial Institute, Buffalo, NY. The conclusions reached may be summarized as follows:[6]

T-interferon consists of heterogeneous populations of molecules that share some properties with viral IF: they are capable of interaction with matrices possessing hydrophobic and electrostatic properties, and they are irregularly glycosylated. In our work with Thang, of the Institut de Biologie Physicochimique in Paris, we also showed that like viral IF, T-interferon molecules have a polynucleotide recognition site.

These studies enabled us to work out a purification process comprising the following steps: fractionation of crude preparations with ammonium sulfate, dialysis, vacuum concentration, and Blue-Sepharose and Phenyl-Sepharose chromatography. This method allowed 1000-fold purification, with a titer of 10,000 units of interferon per milliliter and a specific activity of 1-2 $\times$ 10^5 units per milligram of protein.[6,8,9]

We prepared a serum against T-interferon by repeated inoculation of rabbits with a semi-purified preparation of this type of interferon.[8]

As shown in TABLE 1, the anti T-interferon serum is also capable of neutralizing Type II IF, but has no effect on viral interferon, indicating that antigen-induced IF and T-mitogen-induced IF are antigenically related.

In cooperation with Wolf H. Fridman from the Institut de Recherches sur le Cancer at Villejuif (France) and Miguel Lucero from our group, we studied the immunosuppressive properties of T-interferon, using the Mishell and Dutton test.[9]

Our results show that purified T-interferon with a specific activity of 1 to 2 $\times$ 10^5 units per milligram of protein inhibits *in vitro* antibody synthesis against

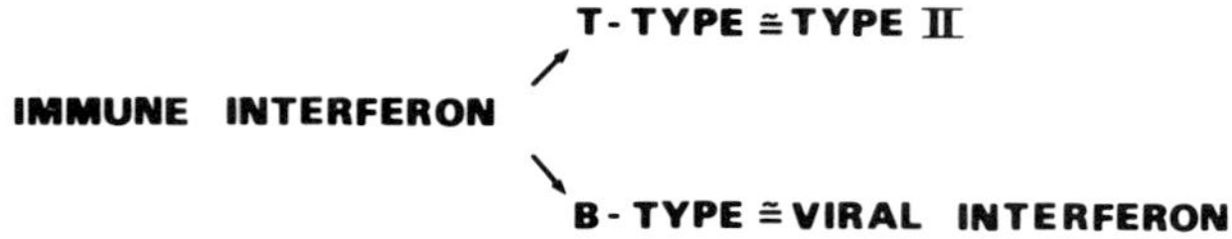

FIGURE 2.

TABLE 1

NEUTRALIZATION CAPACITY OF ANTI-T-INTERFERON SERUM

Interferons	Neutralization Titer (against 10 interferon units)	
	Antiviral Interferon Serum	Anti-PHA Interferon Serum
Viral interferon (NDV)	40,000	<20
Type T-interferon (PHA)	<20	2,000
Type II-interferon (BDG-PPD)	<20	3,600

sheep red blood cells. After fractionation on different chromatographic sorbents such as Con A-Sepharose and Blue-Sepharose, inhibitory activity could not be dissociated from antiviral activity. The kinetics of the action of T-interferon on antibody synthesis show that it interferes with the early events in lymphocyte activation.

Inhibition was at its maximum when T-interferon was added either 6 hours before the antigen or together with it, but a significant effect was still obtained when T-interferon was added 24 or 48 hours after the antigens. These kinetics were similar to those obtained with viral interferon.

Pretreatment of T-interferon for 24 hours at pH 2 destroyed both the antiviral and immunosuppressive activities.

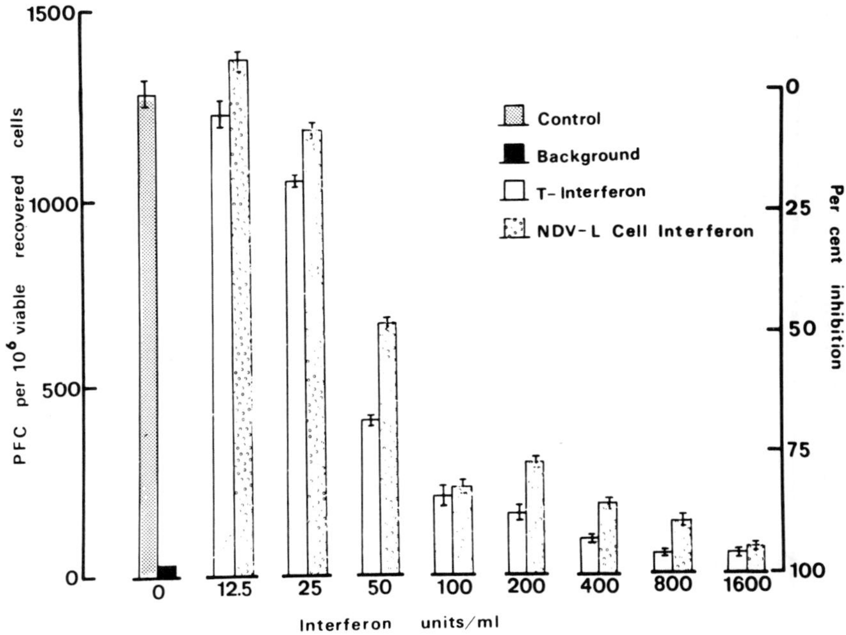

FIGURE 3. Dose effect of viral and T-interferon on the number of anti-SRBC plaque-forming cells.

FIGURE 3 shows the comparative effects of doses of T and viral IF on PFC inhibition. Graded doses of 12 to 1600 units of purified T or of viral interferon were added at the same time as antigen to spleen cells stimulated by SRBC, and the inhibitory effect on direct PFC generation was measured at Day 5. As shown in FIGURE 3, inhibition increased as a function of the dose of IF added, and no significant differences were observed when the same dose of T or viral IF was added to the culture.

Viral and T-interferon were also compared with respect to another biological property—the spontaneous cytotoxicity of natural killer (NK) cells.

Several laboratories recently demonstrated that cytotoxicity of these cells against different lines of tumor cells increases after treatment with viral interferon.[10-12]

In collaboration with Anna Senik of the Institut de Recherche sur le Cancer at Villejuif in France, we studied murine NK cell activation after treatment with different doses of T or viral interferon.[13] The Yac 1 cell line was used as target. Spleen cells from BALB/c were treated with IF for 3 hours and mixed with target cells at the ratio of 100:1, and specific ^{51}Cr release was determined 4 hours later (FIGURE 4). From this and other experiments of the same type we concluded that under our experimental conditions, nonsignificant differences can be observed in the capacity of the NK system to be activated by viral or T-interferon.

During the past few years there has been considerable progress in our knowledge of the molecular mechanism governing the antiviral action of virus-induced interferons. As regards T-interferons, on the other hand, nothing was known about this mechanism.

We report below the research undertaken on this question in cooperation with Dr. A. Hovanessian of the Pasteur Institute and Catherine Vaquero and Odile Aujean of our group.[14]

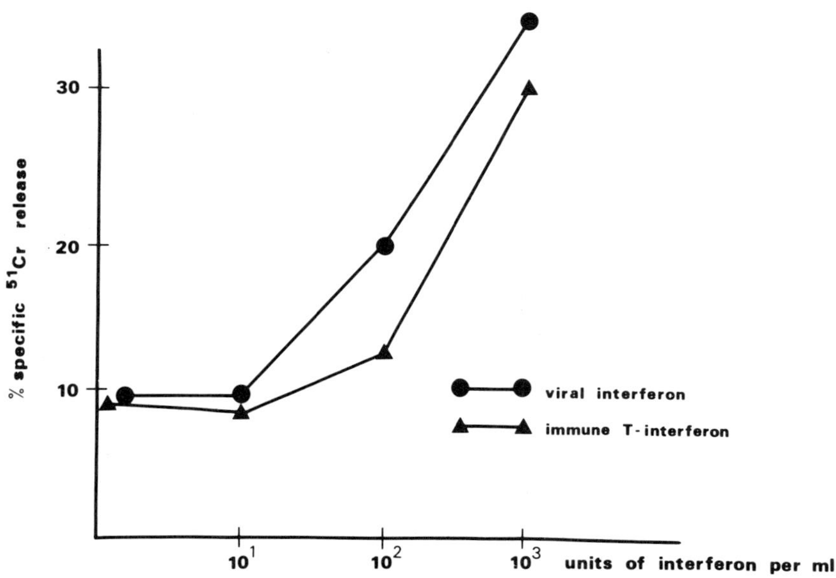

FIGURE 4. Mouse NK cell activation by viral and T-interferon.

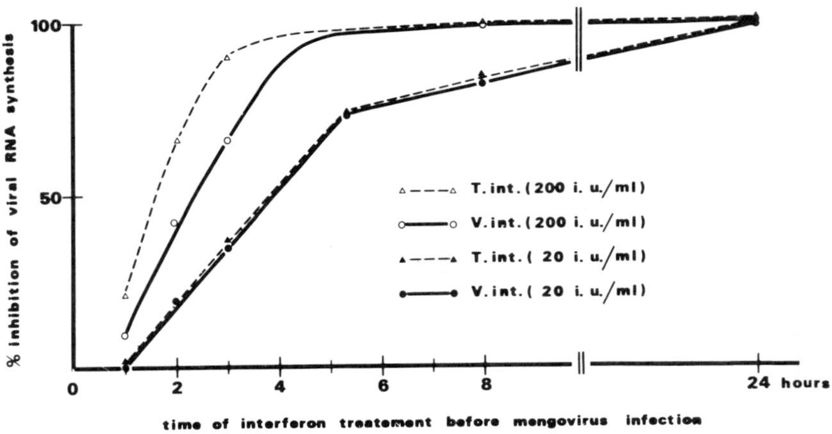

FIGURE 5. Development of antiviral activity in L-cells treated for various periods of time with either T-type or viral-type interferon.

During the first phase of this work, we compared the kinetics of the two interferons as regards the establishment of the antiviral state.

To increase the accuracy of the antiviral state measurements, particularly those made early after infection, we measured the inhibition of mengovirus RNA synthesis. The results are given in FIGURE 5. The procedure was as follows:

L-cells were treated for periods of one to 24 hours with either 20 or 200 units of viral or T-interferon. After that, cells were infected with Mengo-virus in the presence of actinomycin. Tritiated uridine was added during the last 30 minutes of infection. Inhibition of viral multiplication was expressed as the percentage of tritiated uridine incorporation measured in the control cells. The kinetics for the development of the antiviral state were found to be almost the same for viral and T-interferon, whether cells were treated with 20 or 200 IF units.

FIGURE 6 shows the phosphorylation of 67 K protein (Channels 1 to 3) and the phosphorylation of an exogenous substrate: calf thymus histones (Channels 4 to 6). Protein kinase activity from nontreated control cells (1 and 4) and from cells treated with viral-interferon (2 and 5) or with T-interferon (3 and 6) was purified on columns of poly (I).poly (C)-Sepharose before assay.

The phosphorylated proteins were analyzed on polyacrylamide slab gels containing SDS. An autoradiograph of a stained, dried gel is shown. The numbers on the left give the molecular weights of protein markers in thousands. The respective positions of the 67 K protein (arrow) and histones (H) are indicated to the right of the gel. Phosphorylation levels for the 67 K protein and the histones in extracts from control cells varied from one preparation to another. However, the enhanced level of kinase activity after treatment with IF was strikingly similar in extracts from cells treated with viral or T-interferon preparations.

FIGURE 7 shows the kinetics of protein synthesis in a Mengo-RNA programmed cell-free system from rabbit reticulocytes, in the absence and presence of 2′-5′ A synthesized by enzyme fractions from nontreated control cells, and from cells treated with either viral-induced or T-interferon. The 2′-5′ A was assayed at a final 10^3-fold dilution. The ordinate gives the ^{14}C-labeled amino

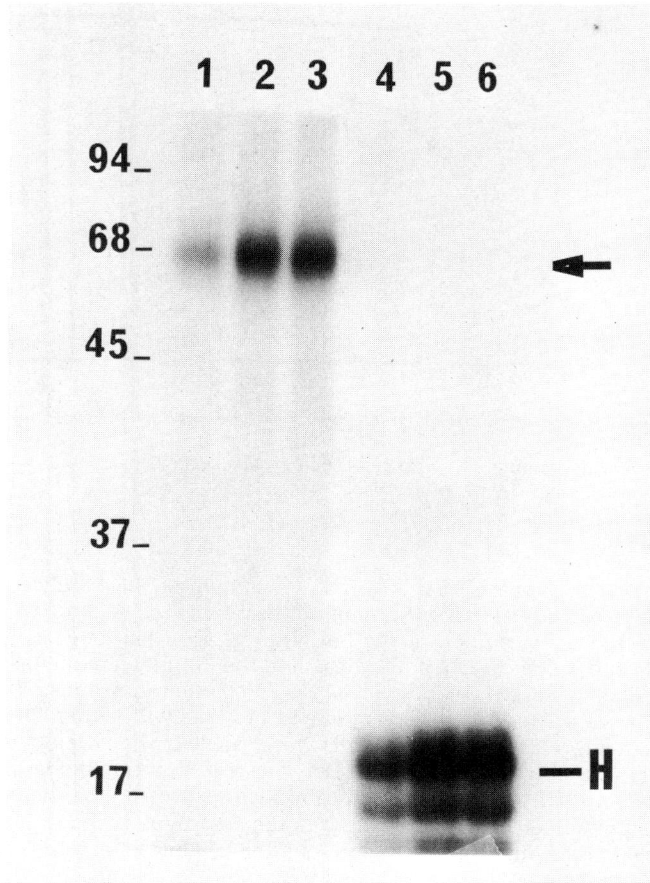

FIGURE 6. Protein kinase activity from cells not treated or treated with viral and T-interferons.

acid incorporation per 10 μl sample. As shown in FIGURE 7, the same level of inhibition was obtained with both interferons.

The inhibitor generated by incubation of enzyme fractions from T-interferon-treated cells was heat stable and showed the same spectrum of resistance and sensitivity to alkali, micrococcal nuclease, snake venom phosphodiesterase and bacterial alkaline phosphatase as the corresponding material synthesized with extracts from viral interferon-treated cells or rabbit reticulocytes.

These results confirmed that the inhibitor synthesized was the 2′-5′-linked oligoadenylic acid triphosphate.

In collaboration with Helmut Ankel and Françoise Besançon from the Medical College of Wisconsin, we studied the interaction of gangliosides with T-interferon.[15] Previous investigations by these authors suggested that viral interferon interacts with carbohydrate-containing cell membrane constituents.[16,17] Its antiviral action is blocked after preincubation with gangliosides. Gangliosides, covalently attached to Sepharose, avidly bind viral IF, and this binding is reversed in the presence on *N*-acetyl-neuraminyl lactose, the trisaccharide common to many gangliosides. Although the biological activities of T-interferon resemble those of viral IF, T-interferon neither binds to these glycolipids nor is inhibited by them. This is shown in the experiment represented in FIGURE 8, in which 1,000 units of viral or T-interferon were loaded on a small column containing 0.2 ml of Sepharose gangliosides. The column was first eluted with buffer. Where indicated by the arrow, elution was continued with a solution of *N*-acetyl-neuraminyl lactose and the antiviral activity in each fraction was measured.

Ninety percent of the viral IF activity is retained by the columns and eluted with *N*-acetyl neuraminyl lactose, as shown in the left part of FIGURE 8. Under the same experimental conditions, T-interferon passes through the column (right part of figure).

In the experiment depicted in FIGURE 9, we compared the effect of bovine brain gangliosides on the antiviral activities of both viral and T-interferon. At ganglioside concentrations that completely inhibited the antiviral activity of viral interferon, T-interferon activity remained unchanged. In this experiment we also show that T-interferon remained insensitive to ganglioside inhibition even after passing through the affinity column, which rules out the possibility that a noninterferon contaminant with a high affinity for gangliosides had been removed by this procedure.

Furthermore, individual glycolipids that inhibited viral interferon had no effect when tested with T-interferon under identical conditions at concentrations up 100 μM. These included GM_3, GM_2, GM_1, GD_{1a}, GT_1 and GL_4.

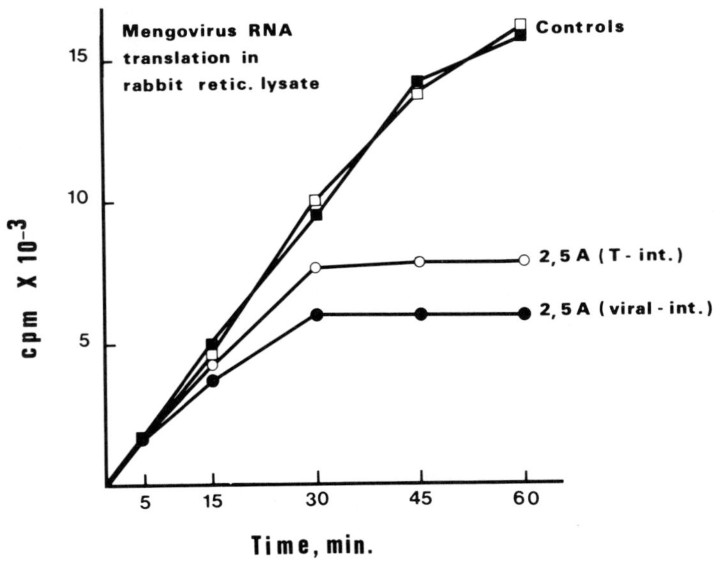

FIGURE 7. Synthesis of 2′, 5′ A with the synthetase bound to poly(I). poly(C)-Sepharose.

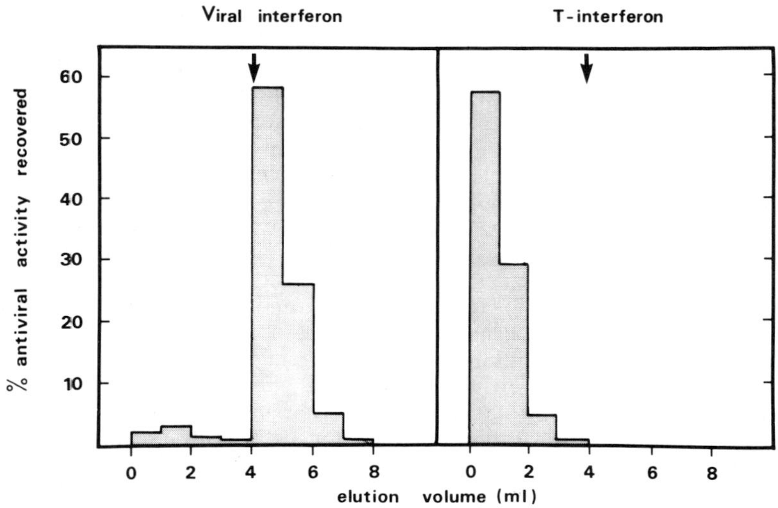

FIGURE 8. Binding of interferon to Sepharose-ganglioside columns.

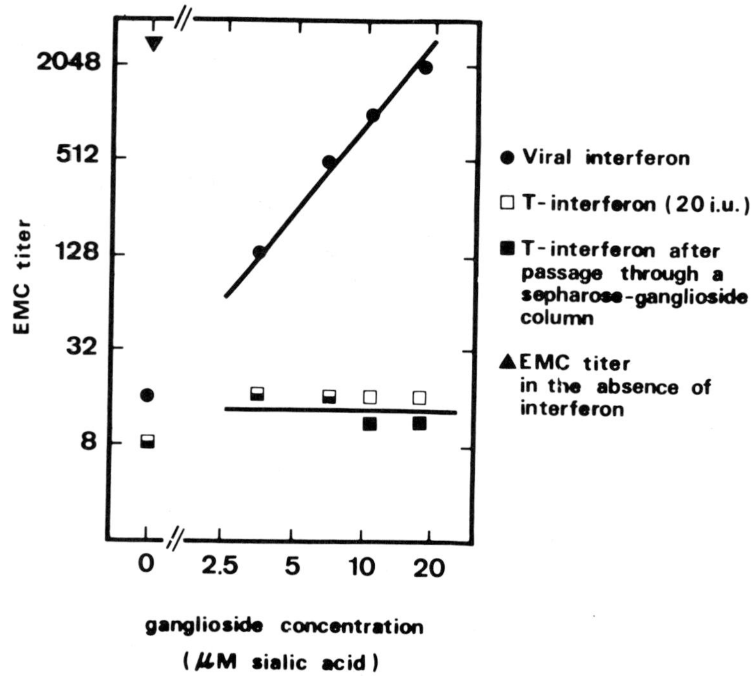

FIGURE 9. Comparison of the effects of bovine brain gangliosides on the antiviral activities of viral and T-interferon.

If the affinity of viral IF for gangliosides is linked to its functional interaction with mouse cells, then clearly T-interferons must interact with different components of these cells, as it does not bind to gangliosides. Consequently, if the sites on the membrane of the L-1210 R cells selected by Gresser[18] for their resistance to viral IF had altered or became inaccessible and no longer allowed productive interaction with viral IF, then T-interferon might still be active in these cells. The next experiment shows that this is indeed the case (FIGURE 10).

In this experiment, we compared the antigrowth effects of viral IF on L-1210 sensitive and resistant cells in the presence and absence of gangliosides. Cells were counted after 3 days of culture. L-1210 S cells were found to be equally sensitive to the antigrowth activities of both IFs. However, L-1210 R cells,

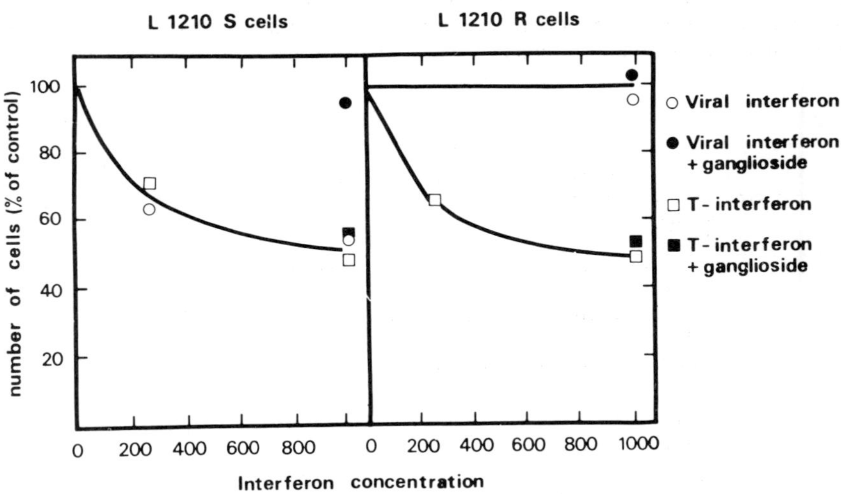

FIGURE 10. Comparison of the antigrowth activities of viral and T-interferon. Effect of gangliosides.

although insensitive to viral IF, were just as sensitive to T-interferon as L-1210 S cells. In addition, the antigrowth effect of T-interferon, like its antiviral effect, was found to be resistant to inhibition by gangliosides at concentrations that completely reversed the antigrowth effect of viral interferon.

The following conclusions may be drawn from the results obtained in collaboration with Ankel and Besançon:[15]

(1) neither the antiviral nor the antigrowth effects of T-interferon are inhibited by gangliosides, and T-interferon does not bind to them, and

(2) mouse leukemia L-1210 R cells selected for their resistance to viral interferon retain unchanged sensitivity to T-interferon.

It is not known whether viral or T-interferons, or parts of them, have to enter target cells in order to produce antiviral or antigrowth responses. The fact that viral interferon interacts with carbohydrate constituents of ganglioside molecules, and that the sensitivity to its antiviral effect of certain transformed mouse cells increases after uptake of exogenous gangliosides by the cell membrane[19] tempts us to speculate that the interaction of viral IF with cell membrane gangliosides is of functional significance. If this were the case, T-interferon, although it produces the same biological effects as viral IF, would clearly have a different mechanism of interaction with its target cells, since it does not bind to gangliosides and is active with cells selected for their resistance to viral interferon.

TABLE 2 shows the similarities and differences in the properties of viral and T-interferon.

The most significant feature of these properties is the difference between each IF's affinity for gangliosides. It is conceivable that there are two classes of interferon-binding sites on the cell membrane, each of them specific for productive interaction with one type of IF only. Thus, prolonged growth of L-1210 cells in the presence of viral IF could select those cells that have nonfunctional binding sites for viral IF but still carry unaltered binding sites for T-interferon. Alternatively, the uptake mechanisms for both interferons or their active fragments might be different, one involving gangliosides, and the other, a different type of glycolipid or none at all.

TABLE 2

PROPERTIES OF VIRAL AND T-INTERFERONS

Similar
Physico-chemical:
Hydrophobicity, Glycosilation, Polynucleotide binding site
Biological:
Antiviral action on L-cells (Kinetic, 2′-5′ A, Phosphorylation)
Activation of NK cells
Inhibition of antibody synthesis
Different
Acid stability
Antigenic structure
Affinity for gangliosides

Two aspects of our observations may have medical significance: Firstly, it is known that cancer patients often have elevated levels of circulating gangliosides, which may reflect increased concentrations of these glycolipids in the tissue surrounding the tumor.[20] Treatment of such patients with human fibroblast or leukocyte IF might therefore not be very effective, as these two IFs also bind to gangliosides. Consequently, the use of human T-interferon as an alternative treatment in cases where fibroblast or leukocyte IF fail to show the desired effects might have obvious advantages, providing that the human T-interferon is comparable to mouse T-interferon in its resistance to ganglioside inhibition. Secondly, the observations of Gresser *et al.*[18] concerning the selection of viral interferon-resistant leukemia cells might be relevant to interferon therapy of leukemia patients, whose organism might select resistant cells that would escape from the desired growth inhibition. Our data suggest that alternate administration of viral and T-interferon might be a useful approach in preventing such selection.

REFERENCES

1. FALCOFF, R. 1972. Some properties of virus and immune induced human lymphocyte interferon. J. Gen. Virol. **16:** 250–253.
2. WIETZERBIN, J., R. FALCOFF, L. CATINOT & E. FALCOFF. 1977. Affinity chromatographic analysis of murine interferons induced by viruses and by T and B cell stimulants. Ann. Immunol. (Inst. Pasteur) **128 C:** 699–708.
3. YOUNGNER, J. S. & S. B. SALVIN. 1973. Production and properties of migration inhibitory factor and interferon in the circulation in mice with delayed hypersensitivity. J. Immunol. **111:** 1914–1922.
4. JOHNSON, H. M. & S. BARON. 1976. The nature of the suppressive effect of interferon and interferon inducers on the "in vitro" immune response. Cell. Immunol. **25:** 106–115.
5. VALLE, M. J., G. W. JORDAN, S. HAAHR & T. C. MERIGAN. 1975. Characteristics of immune interferon produced by human lymphocyte cultures compared to other human interferons. J. Immunol. **115:** 230–233.
6. WIETZERBIN, J., S. STEFANOS, M. LUCERO, E. FALCOFF, J. O'MALLEY & E. SULKOWSKI. 1979. Physico-chemical characterization and partial purification of mouse immune interferon. J. Gen. Virol. **44:** 773–781.
7. WIETZERBIN, J., S. STEFANOS, M. LUCERO, E. FALCOFF, D. C. THANG & M. N. THANG. 1978. Presence of a polynucleotide binding site on murine interferon (T-type). Biochem. Biophys. Res. Commun. **85:** 480–489.
8. STEFANOS, S., L. CATNINOT, J. WIETZERBIN & E. FALCOFF. Production of antibodies directed against mouse T-interferon and their neutralization properties. J. Gen. Virol. In press.
9. LUCERO, M., J. WIETZERBIN, S. STEFANOS, C. BILLARDON, E. FALCOFF & H. W. FRIDMAN. 1979. Immunosuppressive properties of purified immune T-interferon. Cell. Immunol. In press.
10. TRINCHIERI, G., D. SANTOLI, R. R. DEE & B. B. KNOWLES. 1978. Anti-viral activity induced by culturing lymphocytes with tumor-derived or virus transformed cells. J. Exp. Med. **147:** 1299–1313.
11. GIDLUND, M., A. ORN, H. WIGZELL, A. SENIK & I. GRESSER. 1978. Enhanced NK cell activity in mice infected with interferon and interferon inducer. Nature **273:** 759–761.
12. HERBERMAN, R., J. Y. DJEU, J. R. ORTALDO, H. T. HOLDEN, W. H. WEST & G. D. BONNARD. 1978. Role of interferon in augmentation of Natural and cell-mediated cytotoxicity. Cancer Treatment Rep. **62:** 1893–1896.
13. SENIK, A., M. LUCERO, M. CASTAGNA, S. STEFANOS & E. FALCOFF. T-interferon (type II) enhances NK cell activity. Manuscript in preparation.
14. HOVANESSIAN, A., E. MEURS, O. AUJEAN, C. VAQUERO, S. STEFANOS & E. FALCOFF. Antiviral response and induction of specific proteins in cells treated with immune T (Type II) interferon analogous to that from viral interferon (Type I). Virology. In press.
15. BESANÇON, F., H. ANKEL, C. KRISHNAMURTI, S. STEFANOS & E. FALCOFF. Mouse type I and immune T-type (type II) interferons: Pronounced differences in affinity for gangliosides and in antiviral and in antigrowth effects on mouse leukemia L 1210 R cells. Proc. Nat. Acad. Sci. USA. In press.
16. BESANÇON, F. & H. ANKEL. 1974. Binding of interferon to gangliosides. Nature (London) **252:** 478–480.
17. BESANÇON, F., H. ANKEL & S. BASU. (1976). Specificity and reversibility of interferon gangliosides interaction. Nature (London) **259:** 576–578.

18. GRESSER, I., M. T. BANDU & D. BROUTY-BOYÉ. 1974. Interferon and cell division IX. Interferon resistant L 1210 cells: Characteristics and origin. J. Nat. Cancer Inst. **52:** 553–559.
19. VENGRIS, U. E., F. H. REYNOLDS, JR., M. D. HOLLEMBERG & P. M. PITHA. 1976. Interferon action: Role of membrane gangliosides. Virology **72:** 486–493.
20. KLOPPEL, T. M., T. W. KEENAN, M. J. FREEMAN & D. J. MORRÉ. 1977. Glycolipid-bound sialic acid in serum: Increased levels in mice and humans bearing mammary carcinomas. Proc. Nat. Acad. Sci. USA **74:** 3011–3013.

SPONTANEOUS PRODUCTION OF T (TYPE II) INTERFERON BY A MURINE RETICULUM-CELL SARCOMA*

N. M. Ponzio† and K. L. Fitzgerald‡

Departments of Microbiology-Immunology and Pathology and the Cancer Center Northwestern University Medical School Chicago, Illinois 60611

J. Vilček§ and G. J. Thorbecke¶

Departments of §Microbiology and ¶Pathology New York University School of Medicine New York, New York 10016

INTRODUCTION

SJL/J mice exhibit a high incidence (>90%) of spontaneous reticulum-cell sarcomas (RCS) with advancing age.[1,2] The majority of primary RCS are pleomorphic, composed of diverse cell types, including reticulum cells, histiocytes, plasma cells, eosinophils, lymphocytes, and giant cells.[3] In primary RCS that have been serially transplanted in SJL recipients, however, there is a progressive loss of differentiation, with the predominant cell type resembling a lymphoblast.

The transplantable RCS have several distinguishing characteristics that are listed in TABLE 1. Whereas RCS show progressive growth in the lymph nodes and spleens of normal SJL recipients, they grow poorly in X-irradiated SJL mice.[4,5] Their growth in SJL F_1 hybrid mice varies, depending on the non-SJL parent; however, there appear to be both H-2-associated and other negative influences.[6] Transplantable RCS do not express surface markers characteristic of T or B lymphocytes: they are Thy-1^- and Ig^-, nor do they bear receptors for C3 (ref. 7, and unpublished observations). These tumor cells do, however, express Ia antigens (Ia. 4) of the SJL haplotype[7] and it has recently been shown that they also possess F_c receptors and Lyb-2 determinants (Scheid & Thorbecke, unpublished observations).

RCS cells exhibit migration properties that are typical of B lymphocytes, localizing in follicles of the lymph node (LN) following systemic injection.[8] X-irradiated (X-RCS) or mitomycin C-treated RCS cells stimulate marked proliferation of syngeneic Ly-1^+ T lymphocytes.[9-11] Although this phenomenon has been studied for the most part by coculture of X-RCS cells and SJL lymphoid

*Supported in part by United States Public Health Service Grants CA22544, AI07057, AI12948 and CA14462.

†Recipient of Research Career Development Award (CA00612) from USPHS.

‡Submitted in partial fulfillment of the requirements for the Doctor of Philosophy degree from Northwestern University Graduate School. Supported in part by a fellowship from the Chicago Baseball Cancer Charities.

0077-8923/80/0350-0157 $01.75/0 © 1980, NYAS

cells *in vitro*, a similar proliferation of T cells has also been demonstrated *in vivo*.[12] Despite their capacity to induce this marked proliferative response, no cytotoxicity is evident in either primary MLC or repeatedly immunized SJL recipients.[12]

A more recently described property of RCS cells is their natural-killer (NK)-like activity[13-16] and their ability to induce NK activity in syngeneic host cells.[15-16] In view of recent publications[17-19] suggesting that interferon (IF) strongly enhances the killer activity of normal NK cells, it seemed possible that RCS cells either induced IF production in host cells or else produced IF themselves, thereby stimulating NK activity in the SJL strain, which normally has low NK activity.[20] The present studies were undertaken to investigate these possibilities.

TABLE 1

CHARACTERISTICS OF TRANSPLANTABLE RETICULUM-CELL SARCOMAS (RCS) OF SJL/J MICE

Growth:	
Normal SJL recipients: progressive growth	
X-irradiated SJL recipients: dose-dependent negative influence on growth	
SJL F_1 recipients: variable, dependent on non-SJL parent	
Surface Markers:	
Thy-1^-	Ia^+ (Ia.4)
Ig^-	F_c^+
$C3^-$	Lyb-2^+
gp $69/71^-$	
gs 30^-	
Homing Properties:	
Localize in follicles after i.v. injection	
Capacity to Stimulate Immunity in SJL Lymphoid Cells:	
Induce proliferation of syngeneic, Ly-1^+ T lymphocytes	
Fail to stimulate syngeneic cytotoxic T lymphocytes	
Effector Function:	
Possess natural killer cell cytotoxic function	

MATERIALS AND METHODS

Mice and Tumors

SJL/J mice were purchased from the Jackson Laboratories (Bar Harbor, ME). The transplantable RCS tumors of SJL mice used in these studies were derived from spontaneous RCS and were maintained as transplantable lines by serial intravenous (i.v.) passage in syngeneic recipients at regular intervals, as previously described.[5,7,9-11]

To obtain purified tumor cells, RCS cells were grown in (SJL × A.TH) F_1 hybrid recipients. Since the F_1 host cells express H-$2D^d$ determinants that are not shared by RCS tumor cells, host cells were deleted from tumor-enlarged lymphoid tissues by treatment with alloantisera (anti-H-$2D^d$) and C. This antiserum, prepared by repeated immunizations of A.SW mice with A.TH thymus, lymph node and spleen cells, was used in a two-step cytotoxic assay with preselected rabbit C to treat RCS tumors grown in (SJL × A.TH) F_1 recipients.

Transplantable RCS cells were adapted to *in vitro* culture conditions by a "ping-pong" method, alternating *in vivo* and *in vitro* growth of tumor cells. Freshly explanted RCS cells were cultured in medium RPMI-1640, supplemented with 10% fetal calf serum (FCS), 2mM L-glutamine, and 5×10^{-5}M 2-mercaptoethanol for 1 week. Cells surviving this initial culture period were injected into several SJL recipients. When tumor growth was apparent (approximately 1–2 weeks), RCS cells were again explanted *in vitro* (referred to as passage 2) for a longer period of time, followed again by reinjection into SJL recipients. With each *in vitro* passage, RCS cells survived for increasingly longer intervals, as judged by cell viability and number. The RCS cells used in these studies, referred to as precultured RCS, were taken from *in vitro* passages 7–9. The doubling time of these cells *in vitro* was approximately 24 hours. The precultured RCS cells displayed all the known properties of the *in vivo* transplantable line from which they were derived. These cells are Thy-1^-, Ig^- and Ia.4^+; they induce high proliferative responses in SJL T cells and they grow in normal, but not in X-irradiated SJL mice (Ponzio, manuscript in preparation).

Mixed Cell Cultures

RCS tumor cells, either alone or combined with normal SJL thymus, lymph node or spleen cells, were cultured at various ratios in upright 75 cm^2 plastic tissue culture flasks in 10 ml of medium RPMI-1640, supplemented with FCS, L-glutamine and 2-mercaptoethanol, as described above. In some instances, RCS cells were pretreated with anti-Thy 1.2 serum (1:60) and rabbit complement (C, 1:15) to delete T lymphocytes. When used in mixed cell cultures, RCS cells were γ-irradiated (10,000R) prior to culture. In some experiments, combined anti-Thy 1.2 and irradiation treatment of RCS cells was used.

Natural Killer (NK) Cell Cytotoxic Assay

NK activity of RCS effector cells was assessed in a ^{51}Cr-release assay using YAC-1 (A-strain Moloney virus-induced lymphoma) target cells, the details of which have been previously described.[13,16] Briefly, ^{51}Cr-labeled YAC cells were incubated at various ratios with effector cells in round-bottomed 96-well microplates for 16 hours. Supernatants were harvested with the Titertek Supernatant Collector (Flow Labs.) and counted in a Beckman Gamma 8000 counter. Cytotoxicity was calculated by the following formula:

$$\% \ ^{51}\text{Cr-release} = \frac{\text{(cpm of effector/target cell mixtures)} - \text{(cpm:spontaneous release)}}{\text{(cpm:maximum release)} - \text{(cpm:spontaneous release)}} \times 100$$

where spontaneous release reflects cpm in supernatants of ^{51}Cr-labeled target cells incubated alone (or with unlabeled targets to compensate for cell densities) and maximum release represents cpm of ^{51}Cr-labeled target cells incubated with the nonionic detergent NP-40.

Interferon Assay

A semi-micromethod was employed for IF assay, based on the inhibition of vesicular stomatitis virus in cultures of mouse L cells grown in 96-well plastic trays.[21] One unit corresponds to approximately one reference unit, based on the value of mouse IF (Type I) reference standard G-002-904-511. Rabbit antiserum to Type I mouse IF (derived from L cells induced with Newcastle disease virus) was provided by the Antiviral Substances Program, National Institute of Allergy and Infectious Diseases, Bethesda, MD. When diluted 1:100 this antiserum completely neutralized ≥500 units/ml of Type I mouse interferon. To determine whether an IF preparation was neutralized by antiserum to Type I mouse IF, the tested samples were diluted to the desired potency, mixed with a 1:100 final dilution of antiserum or control serum, incubated for 1 hr at 37°C and assayed for residual IF activity.

RESULTS

Detection of Interferon in Sera of RCS-Injected SJL Mice

Groups of SJL mice were injected i.v. with 10^7 viable RCS cells. At various intervals, mice were bled from the retro-orbital plexus and the serum obtained was stored at −70°C until assayed for IF activity. Preinjection sera also tested at the same time did not show detectable IF activity. The appearance of IF in the

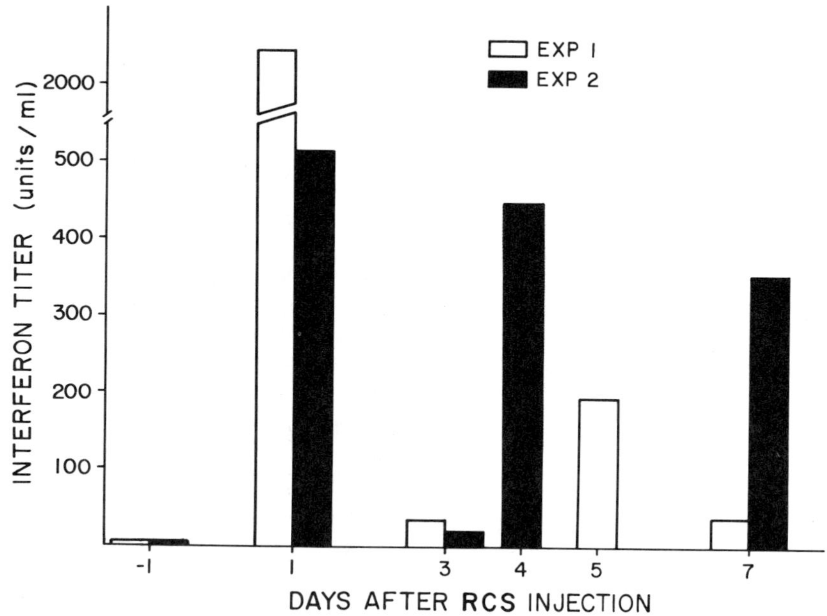

FIGURE 1. IF titers in sera taken from SJL mice various days after intravenous injection of 10^7 viable RCS cells. Two typical experiments are represented.

TABLE 2
PRODUCTION OF INTERFERON BY TRANSPLANTABLE RETICULUM-CELL SARCOMAS OF SJL/J MICE

RCS Cells		Interferon Titer*					
		Experiment 1		Experiment 2		Experiment 3	
Treatment	No. of Cells	24 hr	72 hr	24 hr	72 hr	24 hr	72 hr
Untreated	2×10^7	512	256	1024	256	192	192
	5×10^6	ND	ND	64	192	64	256
10,000R	2×10^7	64	256	ND	ND	ND	ND
Anti-Thy 1.2 + C	2×10^7	ND	ND	256	384	32	512
	5×10^6	ND	ND	64	192	4	96
Anti-Thy 1.2 + C + 10,000R	2×10^7	ND	ND	128	192	4	32
Anti-Ia^s + C†	2×10^7	ND	ND	ND	ND	<4	<4
	5×10^6	ND	ND	ND	ND	<4	<4

*Determined in supernatants taken from 24 or 72-hr cultures of freshly explanted RCS tumor cells.
†Anti-Ia^s serum: Specificity Ia.4 (A.TL × A.TFR5)F_1 anti A.TH.
ND = Not determined.

serum of RCS-injected SJL mice appeared to be biphasic in nature (FIGURE 1). Twenty-four hours after injection, serum IF titers were high. By 3 days, the serum IF titers were considerably lower. At time intervals beyond 3 days, however, there again was a significant rise in IF activity, with the titer in experiment 2 reaching levels that were similar to those obtained on day 1. On day 7 after injection, the serum IF levels differed between the two experiments. In experiment 1, titers were about as low as on day 3, whereas in experiment 2, significant levels of IF were still present. RCS growth (as judged by lymphoid organ weight/body weight ratios) was assessed in experiment 1 and showed progressive enlargement of lymph nodes and spleen over the 7-day test period (data not shown). This variability in IF levels on day 7 may be related to the fact that the mice are moribund 7 days after RCS injection. In order to analyze this potentially complex situation in more detail, the production of IF was studied *in vitro*.

Interferon Production in Supernatants of Freshly Explanted RCS Cells

Cells from grossly enlarged lymph nodes taken from SJL mice 7 days after i.v. injection of RCS cells were pretreated in various ways and placed in short-term culture. Supernatants taken 24 and 72 hours later were titrated for IF content (TABLE 2). High IF titers were present in supernatants from untreated cells at both times; the 24-hr yield was lower in cultures from 10,000 γ-irradiated RCS cells. Deletion of defined populations with specific antisera and C was used to determine whether RCS tumor cells themselves contributed to the IF detected in supernatants of freshly explanted RCS cells. Treatment of RCS cells with anti-Thy 1.2 + C tended to decrease the IF titers at 24 hours, but had no significant effect on titers seen at 72 hours. Although titers were lower, IF was still detected in supernatants from 2×10^7 RCS cells cultured after receiving both treatments. Cultures containing lower cell numbers of anti-Thy 1.2 + C treated and irradiated cells showed no detectable IF (data not shown). It was of interest that, after killing of the tumor cells with anti-Ia serum + C, IF was not detected in supernatants, even with high numbers of viable cells.

Another approach used to obtain purified RCS cells was by growing RCS cells in (SJL × A.TH) F_1 recipients and removing F_1 host cells with alloantisera directed against the non-SJL parental haplotype. To avoid possible problems of graft-versus-host reactions initiated by SJL T cells within the tumor cell preparations, RCS cells were treated with anti-Thy 1.2 serum and C prior to injection into F_1 recipients. When palpable tumors were apparent in RCS-injected (SJL × A.TH) F_1 mice, cell suspensions were prepared and host F_1 cells were deleted, using H-2D^d specific alloantiserum and C. Since the injected RCS cells expressed only the SJL haplotype (H-2^s) and are not susceptible to such alloantiserum pretreatment, a purified population of RCS tumor cells was obtained. To determine if any host F_1 cells remained after primary treatment with anti-H-2 serum, a second anti-H-2D^d treatment was also performed, which resulted in no further cytotoxicity above background levels.

Following pretreatment with anti-H-2D^d, anti-Ia^s (Ia.4) or normal mouse serum and C, the recovered cells were placed in culture tubes at two different densities. Individual tubes were harvested at various time intervals and the supernatant fluids were assayed for IF activity (TABLE 3). On the whole, anti-H-2D^d pretreated cells showed higher IF levels than NMS pretreated cells. In addition, following removal of host F_1 cells with alloantisera, the purified RCS cells showed a progressive increase in IF activity with increasing time in culture, whereas the IF titers of NMS pretreated cells were relatively constant over the 4-day interval.

RCS cells grown in (SJL × A.TH) F_1 recipients and pretreated with anti-Ia^s serum and C showed a different pattern of IF production *in vitro*. In this instance, RCS tumor cells, as well as Ia^+ F_1 host cells were deleted. Therefore, recovered cells would represent Ia^- F_1 host cells, presumably T cells, although this has not been tested. IF titers from anti-Ia^s pretreated RCS cells were lower, at all time intervals, than those from either NMS or anti-H-2D^d pretreated cells (TABLE 3). It is not clear whether this result, which differs somewhat from the results in TABLE 2, reflects the ability of host cells to produce IF or whether some tumor cells survive the treatment with anti-Ia serum + C, possibly due to variability in the quantitative expression of surface Ia determinants.

TABLE 3

DETECTION OF INTERFERON IN CULTURES OF RCS CELLS FOLLOWING REMOVAL OF F_1 HOST LYMPHOID CELLS*

Antiserum Pretreatment†	No. of RCS Cells Cultured	Interferon (units/ml) 24 hr	48 hr	72 hr	96 hr
NMS	2×10^6	128	192	512	192
	4×10^6	256	192	192	192
Anti-H-2D	2×10^6	128	256	384	512
	4×10^6	384	ND	384	768
Anti-Ia^s	4×10^6	24	128	128	64

*For these experiments RCS was grown in (SJL × A.TH)F_1 hosts, which are ssss × sssd in the H2 region.

†NMS: Normal mouse serum Anti-H-2D^d: A.SW anti-A.TH Anti-Ia^s: (A.TL × A.TFR5)F_1 anti-A.TH (Anti-Ia.4)

ND = Not determined.

TABLE 4

INTERFERON PRODUCTION BY RCS CELLS IN LONG-TERM CULTURE

RCS Passage No.	Weeks in Culture*	Culture Conditions for Supernatant Collection		IF Titer
		hr	Serum in Medium†	
7	1	24	10% FCS	768
	2	24	10% FCS	768
	3	24	10% FCS	192
9	8	48	2% FCS	1024
9	8	48	2% FCS	2048
9	8	24	1% NMS	1024
		48	1% NMS	1024

*After establishment of last *in vitro* culture (in 10% FCS).
†FCS, fetal calf serum; NMS, normal mouse serum.

Interferon Production in Supernatants of RCS Cells in Long-term Culture

These data suggested that Ia^+, Thy-1.2^- cells, possibly the RCS cells themselves, were producing IF, but a contribution by normal host cells was by no means excluded. RCS cells that had been cultured for more extended times were therefore also examined for IF production (TABLE 4). The RCS tumor cells of SJL/J mice have been notoriously difficult to grow in long-term culture. Although some cell lines derived from RCS have been obtained,[22,23] they display somewhat modified properties when compared to the *in vivo* transplantable RCS. The precultured RCS which are described here, cannot be regarded as established cell lines, but are relatively free of contaminating host T cells as judged by surface markers. In fact, >95% of these cells are killed by anti-Ia^s serum + C, and no killing above background is observed with anti-Thy-1.2 serum + C (data not shown). Furthermore, these cells were shown to grow as typical RCS in SJL mice within 1–2 weeks after transfer (Ponzio, manuscript in preparation).

These precultured RCS cells, grown in densities varying from approximately 3×10^6 to 3×10^7 cells per ml, produced high IF titers within 24 to 48 hours. This IF production occurred equally well in the presence of low concentrations of fetal calf serum or normal mouse serum (TABLE 4). The results, therefore, are consistent with the interpretation that RCS cells themselves are at least one source of the IF found in supernatants of cultured RCS.

Interferon Production by Cocultures of SJL Lymphoid Cells and X-RCS

As it has been shown that allogeneic mixed lymphocyte reactions (MLR) may cause IF synthesis in mouse lymphoid cells,[24] and as previous studies have indicated an overlap between MLR and RCS responsive SJL T cells,[10] it seemed likely that RCS could also induce IF production in host cells. Mixed cultures were therefore initiated between syngeneic normal thymus, lymph node or spleen cells and low numbers of irradiated RCS cells (X-RCS). Supernatant culture fluids were assayed for IF activity at 24 and 72 hours of culture (TABLE 5). In addition, cells harvested from these cultures at 72 hours were used as effector

TABLE 5

DETECTION OF INTERFERON AND NATURAL KILLER CELL ACTIVITY IN MIXED CULTURES OF X-RCS AND SJL/J LYMPHOID CELLS

Responder Cells (2 × 10⁷)	No. of X-RCS Stimulators*	Interferon (units/ml)		% ⁵¹CR Release from YAC Targets†	
		24 hr	72 hr	E/T = 50	25
Thymus	None	ND	<8	8.3	ND
	5×10^6	<8	16	25.3	21.6
	2×10^6	<8	<8	9.9	4.7
Lymph Node	None	<8	<8	4.1	2.6
	5×10^6	<8	96	58.3	53.9
	2×10^6	<8	16	46.8	32.5
Spleen	None	<8	16	27.1	19.1
	5×10^6	24	48	61.5	49.9
	2×10^6	12	16	55.9	31.5
None	5×10^6	<8	<8	5.3	ND
	2×10^6	<8	<8	4.7	ND

*Transplantable RCS received 10,000R (X-RCS) prior to culture.
†Effector cells taken from 72-hr cultures.
E/T = effector/target cell ratios.
ND = Not determined.

cells against ^{51}Cr-labeled YAC target cells to determine their capacity to express NK cytotoxic function (TABLE 5).

Supernatants from the mixed cell cultures collected at 72 hours contained significant amounts of IF, but at 24 hours they contained only low amounts of IF or were negative. Supernatants from responder cells cultured alone, with the exception of spleen cells at 72 hours, were negative for IF activity. No IF activity was detected in supernatants taken from cultures of X-RCS alone.

With respect to the NK activity of effector cells recovered from these cultures, there appeared to be a direct correlation between IF and NK activities. In mixed cultures, where IF was detected in culture supernatants, NK cytotoxicity was also evident. In mixed cultures where no IF was apparent (e.g. thymus × X-RCS at a 10:1 ratio) NK cytotoxicity was very low. Again, responder cells cultured alone showed low NK activity. The exception was spleen cells, which showed moderate levels of cytotoxic function. However, it should be noted that IF activity was also detected in the supernatant of these spleen cells cultured alone, and that when X-RCS stimulators were included with these splenic responders, both IF titers and NK cytotoxicity were significantly increased. X-RCS (10,000R) cells by themselves showed background levels of NK activity.

These results can be interpreted in two ways. Since the mixtures of RCS and normal lymphoid cells show a higher IF production, as well as NK activity, than either one population cultured separately, one of the cell types induces activity in the other. However, it is not immediately evident whether X-RCS induces the activity in the normal cells, or conversely, normal cells promote IF production by X-RCS. Further analysis of the surface markers of the NK cells and of the IF-producing cells, will be needed to settle this point, since differences in the expression of Ia determinants by host NK cells versus tumor NK cells have been found *in vivo*.[15,16]

Characterization of Interferon Type

Two major species of mouse IF can be clearly distinguished.[25-27] Type I IF is produced by most types of cells on induction with viruses and polynucleotides. Type II IF is made by some lymphoid cells on stimulation with specific antigens or mitogens. Type II IF is not neutralized by antiserum to Type I IF. Furthermore, Type II IF is inactivated at pH2, whereas Type I IF is stable. Greater thermal stability is another characteristic associated with Type II mouse IF.[25-27] It is not firmly established that Type I and II IF are produced by distinct cell populations. IF-containing supernatant fluids from cultures of RCS cells alone or from mixed cell cultures were examined (TABLE 6). Results on pH2 lability and resistance to neutralization by antiserum to Type I IF, both indicated that the bulk of IF produced *in vitro* in these experiments was always Type II. Stability at 56°C of the IF in culture supernatants was also greater than that of the reference Type I mouse IF examined (data not shown).

DISCUSSION

The present data show that the serum of RCS-bearing SJL/J mice contained high titers of IF. An attractive hypothesis to explain the biphasic appearance of IF in the sera would be that RCS cells first induced production of IF in host cells, causing the peak at 24 hours, whereas the second peak was caused by IF production by tumor cells themselves. This would compare with previous

TABLE 6

CHARACTERIZATION OF INTERFERON PRODUCED IN RCS TUMOR CELL CULTURES*

Culture Supernatant Derived from	Hours of Culture	Experiment No.	IF Titer After Treatment			
			Antiserum		Dialysis Against	
			Control	Mouse IF	pH 7	pH 2
Untreated RCS	24	1	32	24	ND	ND
	72	1	32	24	ND	ND
	24	2	512	512	1280	128
RCS (Anti-Thy 1.2)	24	2	256	512	ND	ND
	72	3	192	128	192	32
X.RCS (10,000R)	72	1	24	16	ND	ND
X.RCS (Anti-Thy 1.2 + 10,000R)	72	2	256	128	ND	ND
RCS p7 (precultured for 2 wk)	24	3	128	128	128	8
Lymph node + X.RCS (Anti-Thy 1.2 + 10,000R)	72	2	256	256	ND	ND
	72	3	96	96	128	2
Reference type I mouse IF	—	1	32	<2	ND	ND
	—	2	384	<2	512	640
	—	3	64	<2	64	64

*Derived from experiments shown in TABLES 2 and 4.
ND = Not determined.

observations regarding NK activity in RCS-injected mice, where host NK cells were induced, which were resistant to treatment with anti-Ia serum + C, followed by the appearance of tumor NK cells, which were susceptible to lysis by anti-Ia serum + C.[16] Upon further analysis, through study of IF production *in vitro*, it appeared that the tumor cells themselves were an important source of IF Type II. Relatively long-term cultures of the RCS cells showed the continued presence of IF in their culture supernatants, and this IF-producing cell appeared to be Ia-antigen bearing, like RCS. On the other hand, the production of Type II IF in mixed cell cultures was higher than in irradiated RCS or normal lymph node cells alone, suggesting that exposure to X-RCS induced lymph node cells to release IF or vice versa. More studies are needed to determine the cell(s) responsible for this IF production.

T cells are thought to be the major source of Type II IF[28-30]; however, the types of IF produced by B cells have not been completely characterized.[27] In a recent report,[31,32] the collaboration between $Ly-1^+$ cells and one or more other cells, including an Ia^+ cell, was found necessary for production of Type II IF by murine spleen cells in response to bacterial products. It was not determined which of these collaborating cells was actually synthesizing the IF. In the present studies, treatment with anti-Thy-1.2 and C did not abolish IF synthesis by RCS cells, whereas treatment with anti-Ia serum and C did. Thus, if a comparison can be made between these two studies, the RCS cells might represent the Ia^+ cell of the normal collaborating cell populations which had either already been activated *in vivo* to produce IF without further help from T cells, or else were producing IF spontaneously.

There are several reports of spontaneous production of human leukocyte (Type I) IF by lymphoblastoid cell lines derived from Burkitt's lymphoma.[30,33,34] As far as we know, this is the first demonstration of spontaneous IF production by mouse lymphoma cells. Type II IF has not yet been purified and thoroughly characterized because it is notoriously difficult to produce in large quantities. Without a good source of this IF it will be difficult to verify the claims that Type II IF is a more potent immunoregulator than Type I IF.[35] RCS cells should prove to be a useful source of mouse Type II IF. Our finding may stimulate the search for human lymphoma lines producing Type II IF.

It is of interest to note that a putative Ia^+ NK tumor cell was found here to produce Type II IF, while several reports in this symposium[36-38] suggest the normal Ia^- NK cell as a source for Type I IF. Further studies are needed to determine whether, like the normal NK cells, the Ia^+ NK cell described here is also activated by its own product.

References

1. MURPHY, E. D. 1963. Proc. Am. Assoc. Cancer Res. **4:** 46.
2. SEIGLER, R. & M. A. RICH. 1968. J. Nat. Cancer Inst. **41:** 125.
3. MURPHY, E. D. 1969. J. Nat. Cancer Inst. **42:** 797.
4. WANEBO, H., E. CARSWELL, L. J. OLD & E. A. BOYSE. 1969. Proc. Am. Assoc. Cancer Res. **10:** 97
5. LERMAN, S. P., E. A. CARSWELL, J. CHAPMAN & G. J. THORBECKE. 1976. Cell. Immunol. **23:** 53.
6. KATZ, I R., S. P. LERMAN, N. M. PONZIO, D. C. SHREFFLER & G. J. THORBECKE. 1980. J. Exp. Med. **151:** 347.
7. PONZIO N. M., C. S. DAVID, D. C. SHREFFLER & G. J. THORBECKE. 1977. J. Exp. Med. **146:** 132.

8. CARSWELL, E. A., S. P. LERMAN & G. J. THORBECKE. 1976. Cell. Immunol. **23:** 39.
9. LERMAN, S. P., J. M. CHAPMAN, E. A. CARSWELL & G. J. THORBECKE. 1974. Int. J. Cancer **14:** 808.
10. PONZIO, N. M., J. CHAPMAN-ALEXANDER & G. J. THORBECKE. 1978. Cell. Immunol. **41:** 157.
11. LERMAN, S. P., J. CHAPMAN-ALEXANDER, D. UMETSU & G. J. THORBECKE. 1977. Cell. Immunol. **43:** 209.
12. PONZIO, N. M., S. P. LERMAN, J. M. CHAPMAN & G. J. THORBECKE. 1977. Cell. Immunol. **32:** 10.
13. FITZGERALD, K. L. & N. M. PONZIO. 1979. Cell. Immunol. **43:** 185.
14. CHANG, K. S. S. 1977. *In* Adv. in Comp. Leuk. Res. P. Bentvelzen, J. Hilgers & D. S. Yohn, Eds. 327. Elsiever-North Holland. Amsterdam.
15. FITZGERALD, K. L. & N. M. PONZIO. 1979. Fed Proc. **38:** 1278 (Abstract).
16. FITZGERALD, K. L. & N. M. PONZIO. Submitted for publication.
17. TRINCHIERI, G. & D. SANTOLI. 1978. J. Exp. Med. **147:** 1314.
18. GIDLUND, D., A. ORN & H. WIGZELL. 1978. Nature **273:** 759.
19. OEHLER, J. R., L. R. LINDSAY, M. E. NUNN, H. T. HOLDEN & R. B. HERBERMAN. 1978. Int. J. Cancer **21:** 210.
20. HERBERMAN, R. B. & H. T. HOLDEN. 1977. *In* Advances Cancer Research, Vol 27. G. Klein & S. Weinhouse, Eds.: 305, Academic Press Inc. New York.
21. HAVELL, E. A. & J. VILČEK. 1972. J. Antimicrob. Ag. Chemother. **2:** 476.
22. FINKE, J. H., D. A. FYFE, B. C. DEL VILLANO, G. H. BUTLER & N. M. PONZIO. 1980. Transpl. Proc. **12:** 53.
23. BONAVIDA, B., J. ROMAN & E. HUTCHINSON. 1980. Transpl. Proc. **12:** 59.
24. GIFFORD, G. E., A. TIBOR & D. L. PEAVY. 1971. Infect. Immunity. **3:** 164.
25. YOUNGER, J. S. & S. B. SALVIN. 1973. J. Immunol. **111:** 1914.
26. OBORNE, L. C., J. A. GEORGIADES & H. M. JOHNSON. 1979. Infect. Immunity **23:** 80.
27. EPSTEIN, L. B. 1977. Texas Rep. Biol. Med. **35:** 42.
28. WIETZERBIN, J., S. STEFANOS, R. FALCOFF, M. LUCERNO, L. CATINOT & E. FALCOFF. 1978. Infect. Immunity **21:** 966.
29. EPSTEIN, L. B. & S. E. SALMON. 1974. J. Immunol. **112:** 1131.
30. HENLE, G. & W. HENLE. 1965. J. Bacteriol. **89:** 252.
31. SONNENFELD, G., A. D. MANDEL & T. C. MERIGAN. 1979. Immunology **36:** 883.
32. KIRCHNER, H., R. ZAWATSKY & V. SCHIRRMACHER. 1979. Eur. J. Immunol. **9:** 97.
33. DALTON, B. J. & K. PARKER. 1979. Infect. Immunity **23:** 244.
34. KLEIN, G. & J. VILČEK. 1980. J. Gen. Virol. **46:** 111.
35. SONNENFELD, G., A. MANDEL & T. C. MERIGAN. 1978. Cell. Immunol. **40:** 285.
36. MINATO, N., A. NEIGHBOUR, L. REID, B. R. BLOOM. 1980. Ann. N.Y. Acad. Sci. This volume.
37. PERUSSIA, B., D. SANTOLI & G. TRINCHIERI. 1980. Ann. N.Y. Acad. Sci. This volume.
38. SAKSELA, E., T. TIMONEN & K. CANTELL. 1980. Ann. N.Y. Acad. Sci. This volume.

PART IV. MECHANISMS OF CELL GROWTH INHIBITORY AND ANTITUMOR ACTION; GENETICS OF THE INTERFERON SYSTEM

MECHANISMS OF CELL GROWTH INHIBITORY AND ANTITUMOR ACTION; GENETICS OF THE INTERFERON SYSTEM

INTRODUCTORY REMARKS

Hans Strander

Radiumhemmet
Karolinska Hospital
104 01 Stockholm, Sweden

This section deals with two important topics: (1) the genetics of interferon production and action and, (2) the cell multiplication inhibitory effect exerted by interferons. For literature references, see Stewart.[9]

GENETICS OF INTERFERON PRODUCTION

Already in 1968 Guggenheim, Friedman and Rabson used heterokaryotic cells to study interferon production.[6] Later Chany and associates studied hybrids randomly losing chromosomes for one of the involved species to map the genetics of monkey interferon production.[2] The hybrid cell technique involving the sorting-out of chromosomes and making use of the species-specificity of the interferon produced by hybrid cells was used by Tan, Creagan and Ruddle in 1974 to demonstrate the importance of chromosomes 2 and 5 for human interferon production.[13] This work was followed up by experiments with aneuploid cells, and it was later suggested that interferon gene information resided in human chromosome 5 and probably in its long arm.[11] This concept has recently been challenged, and chromosome 9 considered to be important—as we shall learn in this section.

One of the draw-backs involved in these studies have been that in the human system only fibroblast interferon has been employed. Also the techniques employed are sometimes difficult to interpret because of epigenetic changes. The importance of studying *in vitro* the genetics of interferon production is obvious. It is not only important to learn more about the basic mechanisms of interferon production *per se*, but also such techniques could probably lead to the creation of high-producer cells by the correct mixing of chromosomes. These studies also have a direct bearing on gene manipulation techniques.

In vivo analysis has also been made of the genetics of interferon production. Strains of animals with high or low disease suspectibilities have been studied, and also mutants with different abilities to produce interferon have been employed in such studies. Experimental results obtained by involving the high or low suspectibility strains are rather difficult to interpret.[5] The mutant systems have been interesting, and such studies might throw some light on different aspects of the interferon-producing system.[3] Especially interesting is the aspect that different inducers *in vivo* might activate different loci in the animals.

GENETICS OF INTERFERON SENSITIVITY

Tan, Tischfield and Ruddle found, while working with human hybrid cells, that the human interferon-induced antiviral activity was linked to the indophenol oxidase-B gene.[15] This implied that the human chromosome 21 was involved in determining the action of interferon. Tan and associates also used aneuploid cells in studies on the same problem.[14] By using such techniques it could be shown that human chromosome 21 had an effect on the antiviral state. It was shown by Epstein and Epstein that the important gene was located on the distal portion of the long arm of chromosome 21.[4] Similar findings were made simultaneously by Tan and Greene.[12] It has been implied that chromosome 21 is of importance for the binding of interferon to cells in the human system.[16]

The importance of such studies both theoretically and clinically are obvious. These studies have led to the development of trisomic 21 cells, which are particularly sensitive to the action of interferon. Such cells have been used as test cells for interferon. It has been conclusively shown that chromosome 21-dependence in the human system applies to the antiviral action, to the binding of interferon, and to the cell multiplication inhibition effects exerted by interferons. Likewise, it has been shown that both type 1 and type 2 human interferons in their action are dependent on the long arm of chromosome 21 in human cells.

In addition, *in vivo* analysis has been made of the genetics of interferon sensitivity. As in the case of production strains of animals with high or low disease suspectibility have been used as have mutants with increased sensitivity to interferons. The problem with such studies is once again that epigenetic factors are strong and might make interpretation of the results difficult.

CELL-MULTIPLICATION-INHIBITION (CMI) BY INTERFERONS

In 1962 Paucker and coworkers showed that interferon preparations had an effect on the growth-rate of cells.[8] It has since been much debated whether this effect is due to the presence of the interferon *per se* or to some other component of the interferon preparations. The evidence is now overwhelming that interferon itself can exert such an action. It has been shown, (1) that purified interferons and interferoid are as active as they are in impure preparations, (2) that the ratio between the antiviral- and the CMI effect is independent of purity, (3) that the host-range of both effects is similar, (4) that cells resistant to the antiviral effects of interferon preparations are resistant also to the CMI effects, and (5) that cells which are more sensitive to the antiviral effect than other cells also are more sensitive to the CMI effect of interferon preparations. On the other hand, the CMI effects might be caused, at least partly, by other molecular mechanisms in the cells than the antiviral effects. In the human system CMI studies have led to the detection of extremely interferon-sensitive lymphoma cells.[1]

It is characteristic of CMI effects that they can occur both *in vitro* and *in vivo*, that they are reversible at least to some extent, and that they probably are caused by several operating mechanisms. Studies on the CMI effects are important not only for theoretical reasons but also because interferons have been shown to have an effect *in vivo*, also in humans, both against virus infections and tumor diseases.[7,10] Hence, they can conceivably have an important role to play in therapy since they might cause inhibition of tumor cell growth and also have an effect on growth of immunologically important cells. It is necessary now to determine whether therapeutic effects are mainly due to direct effects on virus-infected or tumor cells or whether interferon acts mainly indirectly through other, and then probably immune mechanisms. Probably both systems play a part in therapy.

I think we can look forward to an interesting session with impact both theoretically and clinically on the interferon field.

References

1. Adams, A., H. Strander & K. Cantell. 1975. Sensitivity of Epstein-Barr virus transformed human lymphoid cell lines to interferon. J. Gen. Virol. **28:** 207–214.
2. Cassingena, R., C. Chany, M. Vignal, H. Suarez, S. Estrada & P. Lazar. 1971. Use of monkey-mouse hybrid cells for the study of the cellular regulation of interferon production and action. Proc. Nat. Acad. Sci. USA **68:** 580–84.
3. De Maeyer, E. & J. De Maeyer-Guignard. 1969. A gene with quantitative effect on circulating interferon induction—further studies. Ann. N.Y. Acad. Sci. **173:** 228–236.
4. Epstein, L. B. & C. J. Epstein. 1976. Localization of the gene AVG for the antiviral expression of immune and classical interferon to the distal portion of the long arm of chromosome 21. J. Infect. Dis. **133:** A 56.
5. Gresser, J., M. G. Tovey, C. Maury & M. T. Bandu. 1976. Role of interferon in the pathogenesis of virus diseases in mice as demonstrated by the use of anti-interferon serum. II. Studies with herpes simplex, Moloney sarcoma, vesicular stomatitis, Newcastle disease and influenza viruses. J. Exp. Med. **144:** 1316–27.
6. Guggenheim, M. A., R. H. Friedman & A. S. Rabson. 1968. Interferon production by chick erythrocytes activated by cell fusion. Science **159:** 542–43.
7. Merigan, T. C., K. H. Rand, R. B. Pollard, P. S. Abdallah, G. W. Jordan & R. P. Fried. 1978. Human leukocyte interferon for the treatment of herpes zoster in patients with cancer. New Engl. J. Med. **18:** 981–987.
8. Paucker, K., K. Cantell & W. Henle. 1962. Quantitative studies on viral interference in suspended L-cells. III. Effect of interfering viruses and interferon on the growth rate of cells. Virology **17:** 324–334.
9. Stewart, W. E., II. 1979. The Interferon System. Springer-Verlag. Vienna New York.
10. Strander, H. 1977. Interferons: Anti-neoplastic drugs? Blut **35:** 277–288.
11. Tan, Y. H. 1977. Genetics of the human interferon system. *In* Interferons and Their Actions. W. E. Stewart. II, Ed.: 73–90. CRC Press, Inc. Cleveland, OH.
12. Tan, Y. H. & A. E. Greene. 1976. Subregional localization of the genes governing the human interferon-induced antiviral state in man. J. Gen. Virol. **32:** 153–57.
13. Tan, Y. H., R. P. Creagan & F. M. Ruddle. 1974. Assignment of the genes for the human interferon system to chromosomes 2 and 5. Cytogenet. Cell. Genet. **13:** 155–57.
14. Tan, Y. H., E. L. Schneider, J. Tischfield, C. J. Epstein & F. H. Ruddle. 1974. Human chromosome 21 dosage: Effect on the expression of the interferon induced antiviral state. Science **186:** 61–63.
15. Tan, Y. H., J. Tischfield & F. H. Ruddle. 1973. The linkage of genes for the human interferon-induced antiviral protein and indophenol oxidase-B traits to chromosome 6–21. J. Exp. Med. **137:** 317–330.
16. Wiranowska-Stewart, M. & W. E. Stewart II. 1977. The role of human chromosome 21 in sensitivity to interferons. J. Gen. Virol. **37:** 629–34.

ASSIGNMENT OF THE GENES FOR SENSITIVITY TO INTERFERON (*IfRec*) AND SOLUBLE SUPEROXIDE DISMUTASE (*SOD-1*) TO MOUSE CHROMOSOME 16*

Lois B. Epstein, David R. Cox, and Charles J. Epstein

Cancer Research Institute and the
Departments of Pediatrics and of Biochemistry
and Biophysics
University of California, San Francisco
San Francisco, California 94143

There is now abundant evidence that human chromosome 21 contains genetic material that controls the sensitivity of human cells to the antiviral effects of interferon.[1-5] This locus, termed *IfRec*, is believed to code for the interferon receptor,[6] and its localization on chromosome 21 has been further refined to the distal segment of the long arm.[7,8] The gene for soluble superoxide dismutase (*SOD–1*) (a ubiquitous enzyme that protects cells against the toxic effects of radiation-induced and oxygen-induced free radicals) is also present on this part of chromosome 21,[7,9] the same region that is responsible for the phenotype of Down's syndrome (DS) or trisomy 21.[10]

Given the location of *IfRec* on human chromosome 21 it was reasonable to expect that there would be functional differences in the response to interferon among cells containing different numbers of chromosome 21, and this has been proven to be true. Fibroblasts derived from patients with trisomy 21 are more responsive to exogenous interferon than are cells from normal individuals, whereas cells monosomic for chromosome 21 are less responsive.[2,5,7,11,12]

Thus it is possible to use sensitivity to human interferon to confirm the presence of chromosome 21 in human cells. The original mapping of *IfRec* (formerly designated *AVP*) to human chromosome 21 was carried out in human-mouse somatic cell hybrids in which sensitivity to human interferon could be correlated with the presence of this chromosome.[1] It is possible to use the same approach in hybrids of other types to identify the chromosome of another species which carries *IfRec* and may be partially homologous to human chromosome 21. Using this method we have found that *IfRec* and *SOD-1* are syntenic in the mouse, as they are in man, and that these genes map to chromosome 16.

Two approaches were used to map *IfRec* and *SOD-1* in the mouse. In the first, we prepared hamster × mouse somatic cell hybrids by fusing mouse peritoneal macrophages with an established hypoxanthine phosphoribosyltransferase (HPRT)-deficient Chinese hamster cell line.[13] Ten independent hybrid clones segregating mouse chromosomes were isolated in HAT medium and assayed for mouse *IfRec* and mouse *SOD-1*. The assay for mouse *IfRec*, which measured the ability of a cell line to be protected by mouse interferon against a viral challenge, was an adaptation of Armstrong's dye-binding assay for interferon.[14] Hamster × mouse hybrid cells or hamster parental cells were plated into

*This work was supported by Contract NO-1-HD-8-2858, Research Grant AI-12481, and Training Grant GM-07085 from the National Institutes of Health and a research grant from the National Foundation March of Dimes. C.J. Epstein is an investigator of the Howard Hughes Medical Institute.

microwell plates at a concentration of 2×10^4 cells/well and interferon was added 12 hours later. The cells were incubated at 37°C for 24 hours in the presence of interferon, the interferon was removed, and the cells were exposed to vesicular stomatitis virus (VSV). After one round of viral replication (approximately 20 hours), the cells were stained with crystal violet. Cells containing the mouse *IfRec* gene were protected by mouse interferon and were darkly stained by the dye. Cells without mouse *IfRec* were not protected by the mouse interferon and were lysed by the virus. Untreated cell controls were also prepared, as well as virus controls (cells exposed to virus, but no interferon).

As a result of limited species cross-reactivity, human interferon was found to protect hamster cells but not mouse cells. Therefore, because of the unavailability of high titered hamster interferon, we used human leukocyte interferon to assay for the integrity of the hamster interferon response system in each of the hybrid clones. While low concentrations of mouse interferon did not protect the hamster parental cells, high concentrations of mouse interferon did protect these hamster cells. Therefore, the assay for mouse *IfRec* in hybrid cells was done using interferon concentrations at which the hamster parental cells were protected by human, but not by mouse interferon. Mouse *SOD-1* was assayed in hamster × mouse hybrids by isoelectric focusing in polyacrylamide slab gels,[15,16] followed by staining for SOD-1 activity.[17]

When the 10 primary hamster-mouse hybrids were assayed for mouse *IfRec* and *SOD-1*, these genes demonstrated perfect synteny. Five hybrids retained both *IfRec* and *SOD-1*, while five hybrids retained neither of these mouse markers. To confirm this apparent linkage between *IfRec* and *SOD-1*, the 5 primary clones which retained both mouse markers were counterselected in 8-azaguanine and 25 secondary clones were isolated. Four of these secondary clones, each derived from an independent primary clone, lost *SOD-1*. Consistent with the proposed synteny between *IfRec* and *SOD-1*, each of these four secondary clones was also found to have lost mouse *IfRec*. When the remaining 21 secondary clones which retained mouse *SOD-1* were assayed for *IfRec*, these two loci were again found, with only one exception, to be concordant.

Chromosome analysis of four of the informative hybrid clones revealed that mouse chromosome 16 was the only mouse chromosome which segregated concordantly with *IfRec* and *SOD–1*. These two genes therefore, appear to map to mouse chromosome 16.

We used a second, somewhat different approach to confirm our assignment of mouse *IfRec* and *SOD–1* to mouse chromosome 16. A new set of hamster-mouse hybrids was prepared by fusing HPRT-deficient Chinese hamster cells with mouse peritoneal macrophages that were homozygous for a Robertsonian translocation involving chromosomes 16 and 17. In these hybrids, genes on mouse chromosomes 16 and 17 will be syntenic. If mouse *IfRec* and *SOD-1* map to mouse chromosome 16, then in these translocation hybrids, both markers should be syntenic with glyoxylase (GLO-1), a mouse enzyme which is coded for by chromosome 17. Twelve primary hamster-mouse translocation hybrids were isolated, and assayed for mouse *IfRec*, *SOD-1* and *GLO-1*.[18] Mouse *IfRec* and *SOD-1* again showed perfect synteny in these 12 translocation hybrids, as they did in the 10 original hybrids that did not contain the 16; 17 translocation chromosome. In contrast, while *IfRec* and *SOD-1* segregated concordantly with *GLO-1* in 11 of the 12 translocation hybrids clones, these two mouse markers were not syntenic with *GLO-1* in the original 10 hybrid clones. These results confirm the assignment of mouse *IfRec* and *SOD-1* to mouse chromosome 16.

In summary, we have used 12 hamster × mouse hybrids segregating a mouse 16; 17 Robertsonian translocation chromosome, in conjunction with 35 similar hybrids segregating normal mouse chromosomes, to show that *IfRec* and *SOD-1* are syntenic in the mouse, as they are in man, and to demonstrate that these loci map to mouse chromosome 16.[15] A region of mouse chromosome 16 therefore, appears to be homologous to that segment of human chromosome 21 which is responsible for the Down's, syndrome phenotype. We are presently breeding mouse embryos that are trisomic for chromosome 16, which will provide us for the first time with a mouse model for human trisomy 21. By studying these aneuploid embryos, we hope to gain a better understanding of the functional consequences of genetic imbalance of the loci now known to be on mouse chromosome 16, particularly as they relate to the interferon response system.

Acknowledgments

We thank Ms. Nancy McManus, Ms. Della Goldblatt, and Mr. Bruce Travis for excellent technical assistance. We thank Ms. Mary Joan Fredette for typing the manuscript.

References

1. Tan, Y. H., J. Tishchfield & F. H. Ruddle. 1973. J. Exp. Med. **137:** 317–330.
2. Chany, C., M. Vignal, P. Covillon, N. Van Cong, J. Boue & A. Boue. 1975. Proc. Nat. Acad. Sci. USA **72:** 3129–3133.
3. Creagan, R. P., Y. H. Tan, S. Chen & F. H. Ruddle. 1975. Fed. Proc. **34:** 2222–2226.
4. Morgan, M. J. & P. Faik. 1977. Brit. J. Cancer. **35:** 254.
5. Slate, D. L., L. Shulman, J. B. Lawrence, M. Revel & F. H. Ruddle. 1978. J. Virol. **25:** 319–325.
6. Revel, M, D. Bash & F. H. Ruddle. 1976. Nature **260:** 139–141.
7. Epstein, L. B. & C. J. Epstein. 1976. J. Infect. Dis. **133:** A56–A62.
8. Tan, Y. H. & A. E. Greene. 1976. J. Gen. Virol. **32:** 153–157.
9. Sinet, P. M., J. Couturier, B. Dutrillaux, M Poissonnier, U. Raoul, M. O. Rethore, D. Allard, J. Lejeune & H. Jerome. 1976. Exp. Cell Res. **97:** 47–55.
10. Hagemeijer, A. & E. M. E. Smit. 1977 Hum. Genet. **38:** 15–23.
11. Tan, Y. H., E. L. Schneider, J. Tischfield, C. J. Epstein & F. H. Ruddle. 1974. Science **185:** 61–63.
12. Wiranowska-Stewart M. & W. E. Stewart II. 1977. J. Gen. Virol. **37:** 629–634.
13. Davidson, R. L., K. A. O'Malley & T. B. Wheeler. 1976. Somatic Cell Genet. **2:** 271–280.
14. Armstrong, J. A. 1971. Appl. Microbiol. **21:** 723–725.
15. Cox, D.R., L. B. Epstein & C. J. Epstein. 1980. Proc. Nat. Acad. Sci. USA **77:** 2168–2172.
16. O'Farrell, P. H. 1975. J. Biol. Chem. **250:** 4007–4021.
17. Meera Kahn, P. 1971. Arch. Biochem. Biophys. **145:** 470–483.
18. Meera Kahn, P. & B. A. Doppert. 1976. Hum. Genet. **34:** 53–56.

SOMATIC CELL GENETIC ANALYSIS OF INTERFERON PRODUCTION AND RESPONSE*

Doris L. Slate† and Frank H. Ruddle

Department of Biology
Yale University
New Haven, Connecticut 06520

Somatic cell genetic techniques have permitted the analysis of gene arrangement in cultured mammalian cells. Hybrid cells produced by the fusion of cells from two different species generally lose chromosomes from one parental input preferentially. This segregation provides the basis for mapping genes to specific chromosomes for the species whose chromosomes are lost.[1] Synteny assignments can be made by correlating the presence of marker isozymes and the gene to be mapped. Identification of specific chromosomes retained in a hybrid through the use of differential staining and banding techniques is then used for the assignment of the gene to a particular chromosome.

The interferon system is amenable to somatic cell genetic analysis since species-specificity of interferon action allows the study of interferon production and response in interspecific heterokaryons and hybrids.[2] Both interferon synthesis and the attainment of the antiviral state after interferon treatment are inducible functions, requiring *de novo* RNA and protein systhesis. The genes governing these two functions are located on different chromosomes in the species that have been studied.[3]

Human/mouse and human/Chinese hamster hybrid cells, which usually segregate human chromosomes, have been used to map genes involved in the human interferon system. Sensitivity to human interferon is governed by human chromosome 21.[4,5] The exact nature of the chromosome 21-coded gene product responsible for conferring interferon sensitivity is unknown, but current models postulate that a cell surface receptor is involved in the species-specific interferon response.[6] Trisomy 21 cells are markedly more sensitive to human interferon than normal diploid fibroblasts, while monosomy 21 cells are less sensitive.[7]

Genes that govern the synthesis of human fibroblast interferon have been assigned to three human chromosomes (2, 5 and 9).[8–11] The roles played by each of these chromosomes are as yet unclear, but it is possible that multiple interferon structural loci exist.

In this report, we will discuss our recent work with somatic cell hybrids to further elucidate the genetic control behind interferon systhesis and response.

Mapping a Gene Governing Sensitivity to Mouse Interferon

In collaboration with Dr. P.-F. Lin, we have screened mouse/human somatic cell hybrids, which preferentially segregate mouse chromosomes, for their

*This work was supported by National Institutes of Health grant GM09966 and a grant from the American Cancer Society to F.H.R.

†*Current address:* Department of Biological Sciences, Stanford University, Stanford, California 94305.

0077-8923/80/0350-0174 $01.75/0 © 1980, NYAS

sensitivity to partially purified mouse interferon (Lin *et al.*, submitted for publication). A combination of isozyme analysis and interferon assays revealed that the murine genes for cytoplasmic superoxide dismutase and interferon sensitivity were syntenic. Karotype data from approximately 20 hybrid cell lines revealed that these genes are located on mouse chromosome 16.

The establishment of this linkage relationship is important since the genes for human cytoplasmic superoxide dismutase and interferon sensitivity also map to a single chromosome, human chromosome 21.[4,5] These two loci appear to be closely linked, and from an evolutionary standpoint, it might be expected that this synteny relationship may be preserved in other species.

In vivo studies on the genetics of interferon production have been done in mice by DeMaeyer and his colleagues,[12] and indicate that a number of genes are involved. The use of mouse/human hybrid lines segregating mouse chromosomes may permit chromosomal localization of these genes.

Antibodies to Human Chromosome 21-Coded Cell Surface Components That Block Human Interferon Action Show Differential Binding to Human Fibroblasts Differing in Chromosome 21 Dosage

Several reports have demonstrated that injecting human/mouse somatic cell hybrids into mice of the same strain as the murine parent of the hybrid results in the production of antibodies directed against cell surface determinants coded by the human chromosomes in the hybrids.[13,14] When human chromosome 21 is retained, the antibodies generated in this way can block the action of human interferon in human fibroblasts.[14,15] The blocking effect of such antiserum is more pronounced in monosomy 21 cells than in diploid fibroblasts, and decreases as the number of copies of this chromosome increases.[14] We are presently attempting to quantitate the binding of this antiserum to human chromosome 21 components on trisomy 21 fibroblasts (GM2504), diploid human cells (FS7) or monosomy 21 cells (TC265) using an indirect immunofluorescence assay and the fluorescence-activated cell sorter (FACS).

Spleens have been removed from mice that produce antibodies with interferon-blocking activity, and spleen cells fused to a myeloma cell line to give hybridomas (D'Eustachio, Slate and Ruddle, unpublished data). Antibodies produced by these hybridomas should prove useful in purifying and quantitating the putative human interferon receptor.

Role of Human Chromosomes 2, 5 and 9 in Human Interferon Production

The control of human interferon production appears to be a complex process. Not only are there at least three antigenic types of human interferon (designated fibroblast, leukocyte, and immune interferons), but the type produced by any given cell may differ depending on the inducer employed.[16] The time course of interferon messenger synthesis[17] and interferon release from cells[18] also varies with the inducer and cell type.

Studies with human/mouse and human/Chinese hamster hybrids by several investigators have produced human interferon gene assignments to chromosomes 2, 5 and 9. The first assignment was made by Tan, Creagan and Ruddle[8] who indicated that the presence of both human chromosomes 2 and 5 together was necessary for human interferon synthesis. Later studies indicated that there were at least two interferon loci, one on each of these chromosomes.[10] Most recently, Meager *et al.*[11] have reported that chromosome 9 bears a gene for human fibroblast interferon. They interpret their data to suggest that this chromosome 9 locus is the only gene for human fibroblast interferon.

Using chromosome-mediated gene transfer techniques,[19,20] C. Miller in our laboratory has generated a cell line (23/21-30B) which contains, in a mouse A9 background, a human translocation chromosome involving chromosomes 9 and X (see FIGURE 1). This translocation chromosome is the only human material cytologically detectable in the hybrid (Miller and Ruddle, unpublished data), and carries the selectable marker hypoxanthine phosphoribosyltransferase (HPRT) from the X chromosome and adenylate kinase (AK-1), a chromosome 9 marker.

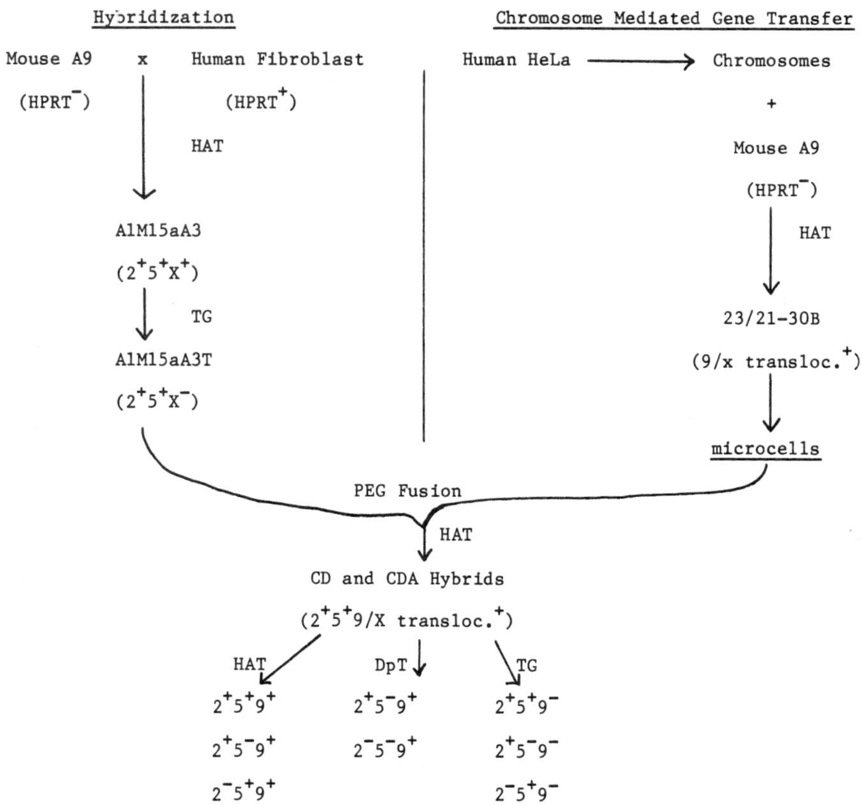

FIGURE 1. Generation of CD and CDA hybrids. The human/mouse hybrid cell line A1M15aA3T was fused with microcells from the chromosome-mediated gene transfer line 23/21-30B, which retained an X/9 translocation chromosome as the only detectable human genetic material. The resultant hybrids were subcloned in HAT or treated with diphtheria toxin (DpT) or thioguanine (TG), to give lines with various chromosome contributions.

This line was tested for human interferon production under poly(rI):poly(rC) superinduction and Newcastle disease virus-induction conditions,[10] and found to produce human fibroblast interferon, confirming the results of Meager *et al.*[11]

We then decided to test the effect of transferring the (X,9) translocation chromosome from 23/21-30B into a human/mouse hybrid that contained chromosomes 2 and 5 (but lacked 9), and could produce human interferon. We hoped to be able to analyze the effect of interferon gene dosage in the hybrid cells. This transfer was accomplished by generating microcells[21] from the 23/21-30B line and fusing them to the human/mouse hybrid AIM15a-A3T. FIGURE 1 illustrates the derivation of the parental cell lines and the generation of the 2^+5^+ $9/X^+$ hybrids. After selection in HAT medium,[22] hybrid clones were picked, expanded, and analyzed for the presence of human isozyme markers. Two separate microcell X hybrid cell fusions were performed; the hybrids generated were called CD and CDA lines, respectively.

AIM15aA3T, 23/21-30B and several CD and CDA clones were screened for human interferon production under superinduction and Newcastle disease virus-induction conditions. The results of these experiments suggested that each of the three previously implicated human chromosomes (2, 5 and 9) bears interferon genes. Elimination of either chromosome 5 (using diphtheria toxin selection) or the (X,9) translocation chromosome (using thioguanine selection) in CD or CDA clones reduces the amount of human interferon synthesized when compared with the parental 2^+5^+ $X/9^+$ lines. Eliminating chromosome 9 appears to have more of an effect on the decrease in human interferon production than eliminating chromosome 5 (Slate and Ruddle, unpublished data).

It has not been possible to determine if all three interferon loci are identical. Antigenically the interferon produced by cells with various combinations of chromosome 2, 5 and 9 complements is fibroblast type, but there may be differences in the interferon molecules encoded by the three chromosomes. Chany (personal communication) has found evidence in human/Chinese hamster hybrids for human fibroblast interferon structural genes on chromosomes 2, 5 and 9, but has failed to detect interferon production in a line with multiple copies of chromosome 9. This latter observation may be related to our findings regarding interferon production before and after loss of chromosome 9 in hybrids. Chromosome 9 may play a regulatory role in interferon synthesis or cell growth, in addition to its role in human interferon production.

Experiments designed to test the human interferon messenger RNA content of our hybrid cells are in progress. This work may provide information regarding the similarity of the interferon genes. The obvious question at this point involves why there should be multiple copies of an interferon structural gene. Perhaps the epigenetic state of a cell or the specific inducer triggering interferon synthesis affects the transcription of these genes differentially, Obviously, there is still much work to be done in clarifying the role of genetic factors in interferon synthesis.

ACKNOWLEDGMENTS

We wish to thank B. Barel, C. Colmenares, A. Cunningham, E. Nichols, and V. Salerno for excellent technical assistance, and M. Siniscalchi for typing the manuscript.

References

1. Ruddle, F. H. & R. P. Creagan. 1975. Parasexual approaches to the genetics of man. Ann. Rev. Genet. **9:** 407–486.
2. Slate, D. L. & F. H. Ruddle. 1979. Genetics of the interferon system. Pharmacol. Therap. **4:** 221–230.
3. Creagan, R. P., Y. H. Tan, S. Chen & F. H. Ruddle. 1975. Somatic cell genetic analysis of the interferon system. Fed. Proc. **34:** 2222–2226.
4. Tan, Y. H., J. A. Tischfield & F. H. Ruddle. 1973. The linkage of the genes for the human interferon induced antiviral protein and indophenol oxidase-B traits to chromosome G-21. J. Exp. Med. **137:** 317–330.
5. Chany, C., M. Vignal, P. Couillin, N. V. Cong, J. Boue & A. Boue. 1975. Chromosomal localization of human genes governing the interferon-induced antiviral state. Proc. Nat. Acad. Sci. USA **72:** 3129–3133.
6. Chany, C. 1976. Membrane-bound interferon specific cell receptor system: Role in the establishment and amplification of the antiviral state. Biomed. Express Paris **24:** 148–157.
7. Tan, Y. H., E. L. Schneider, J. Tischfield, C. J. Epstein & F. H. Ruddle. 1974. Human chromosome 21 dosage: Effect on the expression of the interferon induced antiviral state. Science **186:** 61–63.
8. Tan, Y. H., R. P. Creagan & F. H. Ruddle. 1974. The somatic cell genetics of human interferon: Assignment of human interferon loci to chromosomes 2 and 5. Proc. Nat. Acad. Sci. USA **71:** 2251–2255.
9. Morgan, M. J. & P. Faik. 1977. The expression of the interferon system in clones of Chinese hamster/human hybrid cells. Brit. J. Cancer **35:** 254.
10. Slate, D. L. & F. H. Ruddle. 1979. Fibroblast interferon in man is coded by two loci on separate chromosomes. Cell **16:** 171–180.
11. Meager, A., H. Graves, D. C. Burke & D. M. Swallow. 1979. Involvement of a gene on chromosome 9 in human fibroblast interferon production. Nature **280:** 493–495.
12. DeMaeyer, E., J. DeMaeyer-Guignard & D. W. Bailey. 1975. Effect of mouse genotype on interferon production I. Lines congenic at the *If-1* locus. Immunogenetics **1:** 438–443.
13. Dorman, B. P., N. Shimizu & F. H. Ruddle. 1978. Genetic analysis of the human cell surface: Antigenic marker for the human X chromosome in human-mouse hybrids. Proc. Nat. Acad. Sci. USA **75:** 2362–2367.
14. Revel, M., D. Bash & F. H. Ruddle. 1976. Antibodies to a cell surface component coded by human chromosome 21 inhibit action of interferon. Nature **260:** 139–141.
15. Slate, D. L. & F. H. Ruddle. 1978. Antibodies to chromosome 21 coded cell surface components can block response to human interferon. Cytogenet. Cell Genet. **22:** 265–269.
16. Havell, E. A., T. G. Hayes & J. Vilček. 1978. Synthesis of two distinct interferons by human fibroblasts. Virology **89:** 330–334.
17. Sehgal, P. B., B. Dobberstein & I. Tamm. 1977. Interferon messenger RNA content of human fibroblasts during induction, shutoff, and superinduction of interferon production. Proc. Nat. Acad. Sci. USA **74:** 3409–3413.
18. Mozes, L. W. & J. Vilček. 1975. Distinguishing characteristics of interferon induction with poly(I):poly(C) and Newcastle disease virus in human cells. Virol. **65:**100–111.
19. Miller, C. L. & F. H. Ruddle. 1978. Co-transfer of human X-linked markers into murine somatic cells via isolated metaphase chromosomes. Proc. Nat. Acad. Sci. USA **75:** 3346–3350.
20. Klobutcher L. A. & F. H. Ruddle. 1979. Phenotype stabilization and integration of transferred material in chromosome-mediated gene transfer. Nature **280:** 657–660.
21. Fournier, R. E. K. & F. H. Ruddle. 1977. Microcell-mediated transfer of murine chromosomes into mouse, Chinese hamster, and human somatic cells. Proc. Nat. Acad. Sci. USA **74:** 319–323.
22. Littlefield, J. W. 1964. Selection of hybrids from matings of fibroblasts in vitro and their presumed recombinants. Science **145:** 709–710.

GENETIC CONTROL OF INTERFERON FORMATION

Derek C. Burke and Anthony Meager

Department of Biological Sciences
University of Warwick
Coventry, CV4 7AL, West Midlands, England

Introduction

Somatic cell hybrids offer an attractive system for the study of the control of the interferon system, for the different types of interferons (mouse, human, *etc.*) produced by the hybrid can be distinguished by the interferon assay, and therefore the effect of various treatments upon the synthesis of the different interferons can also be distinguished. We have used mainly mouse-human hybrids, but also Chinese hamster-human hybrids, to investigate the control processes.

Such hybrids also offer the opportunity to discover which chromosome carries the interferon gene, and we have used the hybrids to assign the gene for human fibroblast interferon to chromosome 9. There are several reasons why such an assignment is important. First, it provides further characterization of the interferon system and makes it possible to determine whether the interferon gene is restricted to a single chromosome, or whether a number of interferon genes are distributed over several chromosomes. Second, it should throw some light on the mechanism responsible for producing two different types of human interferon (called fibroblast and leukocyte) by human fibroblast and leukocyte cells, respectively, and specifically may indicate whether these two interferons are products of two genes on different chromosomes or are produced by post-transcriptional modification of a single gene product. Third, it will be possible to determine whether the interferon system is controlled by genes on other chromosomes. Finally, such hybrids will be interesting systems to investigate when a cloned interferon gene becomes available.

Analysis of mouse-human hybrids has to date provided evidence for assignment of the human fibroblast interferon gene to human chromosomes 2 or 5 or to human chromosomes 2 and 5.[1-3,19] Such involvement of two chromosomes is puzzling, and because of this, and because also some of the hybrids used produced only low titers of interferon, we decided to reinvestigate the problem. Our initial aim therefore was to investigate a series of mouse-human hybrids in order to clarify the role of human chromosomes 2 and 5, as an essential prelude to a study of the control of human interferon production in hybrid cells.

Production of Interferon by Mouse-Human Hybrids

We have tested 42 primary mouse-human hybrids (4 with a human lymphocyte parent and 38 with a human fibroblast parent) for human interferon production after treatment with NDV strain F. All of the hybrids produced mouse interferon and eight produced human interferon (Table 1). The human interferon was trypsin-sensitive and pH 2-insensitive, and specifically primed interferon production in human cells. The eight producers could be divided into two classes (1) high producers—producing more than 200 units/ml/10^6 cells and (2)

0077-8923/80/0350-0179 $01.75/0

TABLE 1

PRODUCTION OF HUMAN INTERFERON BY MOUSE-HUMAN HYBRIDS

Hybrid	Interferon Yield (units/ml/10^6 cells) First Tested	Higher Passage Levels
CTP34	830*	70
HL15	670	100
HL53	250	45
CTP41	2†	ND
HL20	16	<4
HL35	4	2–3
HL42	9	5–10
HL57	12	<4

*At passage number 17.

†At passage number 13; all others at passage numbers 3–5.

low producers—producing less than 20 units/ml/10^6 cells. The human parental cell of the HL series produced 800 units/ml/10^6 cells. Both classes progressively lost the ability to produce human interferon on continued passage; because of this tendency to produce less interferon and because we could not be sure that the interferon production by the low producers was not due to a subpopulation of high-producer cells with a different karyotype, the low producers were not investigated any further.

CHARACTERIZATION OF HUMAN INTERFERON MADE BY MOUSE-HUMAN HYBRIDS

Since human cells can produce either leukocyte or fibroblast interferon, and since our hybrids were derived from both lymphocyte (CTP34) and fibroblast human parents (the HL series), it was important to determine whether only one or both types of human interferon were produced. Neutralization with antibody to leukocyte interferon or with antibody to fibroblast interferon showed that the product was predominantly the fibroblast type.[5] This was confirmed by titration of the interferon on cat lung cells, which are much more sensitive to human leukocyte interferon than to human fibroblast interferon.[6] This test showed that less than 3% of the human interferon activity was due to leukocyte interferon.[5] More recently we have shown that by using a line of bovine cells called EBTr (obtained from Dr. J. Vilček of New York University) that the product is exclusively of the fibroblast type, i.e. it produces no leukocyte interferon, whereas the human fibroblast parent cells produce interferon containing up to 20% leukocyte interferon,[18] a finding we have confirmed.

KAROTYPE AND ISOENZYME ANALYSIS OF THE MOUSE-HUMAN HYBRIDS

In collaboration with Dr. D. M. Swallow, of the MRC Human Biochemical Genetics Unit and Dr. J. R. Walker of this department, we karyotyped 11 primary hybrids, including all of the interferon-producing clones. The results, summarized in TABLE 2, showed that the three high-producer clones had many human chromosomes in common, including chromosomes 2 and 5, and also that chromosome 9 was present in all three hybrids but absent in all the low and nonproducers.

Sensitivity of the Mouse-Human Hybrids to Diptheria Toxin

Sensitivity to diptheria toxin requires the presence of human chromosome 5, and since this is one of the chromosomes that have been suggested as essential for human interferon production,[1-3] we expected to find a correlation between diptheria toxin sensitivity and human interferon production. However, this was not so,[5] although diptheria toxin sensitivity did correlate well with the presence of human chromosome 5, as shown by isoenzyme analysis by Dr. D. M. Swallow. This suggested either that chromosome 5 was not required or that a second chromosome, in addition to chromosome 5, was required.

Further information was sought by isolation of a series of diptheria toxin-resistant subclones of CTP34. Isoenzyme analysis by Dr. D. M. Swallow and karyotype analysis in this laboratory showed that none of the subclones contained chromosome 5, but that 7 out of 11 subclones still produced human interferon. This showed that chromosome 5 was not required in these hybrids. However, all the nonproducer subclones had lost chromosome 9 (Table 3), and when a series of randomly selected subclones derived from the high producers were analyzed, the only chromosome lost by low- or nonproducer subclones which was common to all three subclones was chromosome 9 (Table 3).

Chinese Hamster-Human Hybrids and Their Subclones

At this point, the evidence for human chromosome 9 had become rather strong, but we still had no evidence for, or against, human chromosome 2, which was present in all our producer clones and their subclones (Tables 3 and 4).

Table 2

Human Chromosomes of Primary Mouse-Human Hybrids

	Human Chromosomes Present																						
High Producers																							
CTP34		2		4	5	6	7		9			12		14	15	16	(17)*	18		20			X
HL15	1	2			5	6	7		9		11	12		14	15	16	(17)	18	19	20	21		X
HL53	1	2			5	6	7		9	10	11	12			15	16	17	18	19	20		22	X
Low Producers																							
CTP41		2				6	7							14	15	16		18		20			X
HL20		(2)				(6)																	
HL35	1	2			(5)						11	12	13	14	15	16		18			21	22	
HL42	1				5	(6)	(7)		†		11	12		14	15	16	17	18	19	20	21		X
HL57		(2)										12			15	16			(19)	20			
Nonproducers																							
DUR4			3		5					10	11	12	13	14			17	18			21	22	X
HORP9				4						10	11	12		14					19		21	22	X
HORP14		2					(7)			10	11			14							21		X
HL22					(5)	6					11			14		16	17	18		(20)			
HL44											11		13		15	16	17						X

*( ) indicates a ± result.
†AKl + ; AK3 −.

TABLE 3

HUMAN CHROMOSOMES LOST FROM MOUSE-HUMAN HYBRIDS ON SUBCLONING AND HUMAN INTERFERON YIELDS

Hybrid	Subclone	Human Interferon Yield (units/ml/10^6 cells)	Human Chromosomes Lost
CTP34		830	—
CTP34	DTR1	445	5
CTP34	DTR2	740	5 15 18 2022
CTP34	DTR3	106	5
CTP34	DTR4	21	5 6 (9)* 15 (X)
CTP34	DTR5	0	5 (6) 9 15 16 X
CTP34	DTR6	168	5 15
CTP34	DTR7	0	5 9
CTP34	DTR8	0	5 9
CTP34	DTR9	740	5 15 18
CTP34	DTR10	256	5 15 (18)
CTP34	SC4	0	2 9 15 18
HL15	SC9	190	(7)
HL15	SC14	9	1 9 (15) 20
HL53	SC3a	45	(10)
HL53	SC3b	0	1 (5) 7 9 (10) 17 18 2022

*( ) indicates a ± result.

However, use of a karyotyped Chinese hamster-human hybrid, 46.6.1, which was provided by Dr. A. Westerveld, of the Department of Cell Biology and Genetics, Erasmus University, Rotterdam, gave further evidence. This hybrid contained human chromosomes 5 and 9 among others, but lacked chromosome 2. Since it produced human fibroblast interferon,[5] chromosome 2 could not be essential. Chinese hamster interferon was also produced by the hybrid, although the parental Chinese hamster line was a poor producer. Analysis of eight subclones of this hybrid showed that only one, SC1, produced no human interferon and this had lost chromosome 9 but not chromosome 5 (TABLE 4). Another subclone, SC7, had only weak markers for chromosome 9 and produced the least human interferon of the seven producers.

Two other Chinese hamster-human hybrids (CL13 and CL23) obtained from Dr. R. Buckland of the University of Glasgow and known to be very similar in their chromosome composition were also tested. Only CL13 produced human fibroblast interferon, while isoenzyme analysis showed that CL23 differed from CL13 only in that it had lost the markers AK_3 and $ACON_S$ for the short-arm of chromosome 9 (TABLE 4). One of our low-producer hybrids, HL42, also contained only a portion of human chromosome 9, being positive for AK_1 and negative for AK_3 (TABLE 2). This considerably strengthened the evidence for chromosome 9 and suggested that the interferon gene was, like the marker AK_3, on the short arm of that chromosome.

USE OF AN X:9 TRANSLOCATION

Confirmation of the assignment to chromosome 9 was obtained by use of an X:9 translocation (q12; p24) in which all but the P-terminal portion of chromosome 9 is translocated onto the long arm of chromosome X. The X chromosome, and hence the translocated 9 chromosome, can be selected for by cultivation in HAT medium and against by cultivation with 8 aza-guanine in the medium. Hybrids were therefore made between GM705, a human fibroblast with this X:9 translocation, and the mouse lines L-A_9 or PG19. Hybrid GLA, a hybrid obtained from GM705 and L-A_9 was an interferon producer and contained human chromosomes 2, 5, and 9 (as the X:9 translocation) among others (TABLE 5). The diptheria toxin-resistant subclone GLB was also a human interferon producer but had lost chromosome 5, whereas the subclone GLC, obtained by treatment with 8 aza-guanine, had lost the capacity to make human interferon and the X:9 chromosome. Two hybrids, GP2 and GP3, obtained by fusion of GM705 and PG19, were interferon producers and both contained human chromosome 9 (as the X:9 translocation) while neither contained human chromosome 5. In addition, GP2 had no human chromosome 2. Treatment of GP2 with 8 aza-guanine also gave a subline that had lost the capacity to make human interferon. We concluded that the results obtained with these hybrids confirmed the assignment to chromosome 9.

Since the X:9 human chromosome is required for these hybrids to grow in HAT medium, we continuously passaged one of the hybrids for 42 passages, over a period of 6 months, first, to see if the capacity to produce human interferon remained unchanged and second, to see if, by continued shedding of human chromosomes, a hybrid could be obtained which contained few, and preferably only one, human chromosome. When GP2 was passaged in this way, there was little effect on the human interferon yield (TABLE 6). Under the same conditions the high yielding hybrid, CTP34, lost its capacity to produce human interferon, presumably because of human chromosome loss. GP2 lost few, if any, of its human chromosome complement over this period. However, recently we have

TABLE 4
HUMAN CHROMOSOMES 5 AND 9 IN SUBCLONES OF A CHINESE HAMSTER-HUMAN HYBRID AND ITS SUBCLONES AND HUMAN INTERFERON YIELD*

Hybrid	Subclone	Human Interferon Yield (units/ml/10^6 cells)	Chromosomes Present*
46.6.1		135	
46.6.1	SC1	0	5+ , 9−
46.6.1	SC2	84	5+ , 9+
46.6.1	SC3	230	5+ , 9+
46.6.1	SC5	420	5+ , 9+
46.6.1	SC7	37	5+ , 9 wk
46.6.1	SC8	375	5+ , 9+
46.6.1	SC9	167	5+ , 9+
46.6.1	SC10	71	5+ , 9+
CL13		140	5+ 9 AK_1 + AK_3 + $ACON_S$ +
CL23		0	5+ AK_1 + AK_3 − $ACON_S$ −

**Abbreviations:* AK_1, adenylate kinase-1; AK_3, adenylate kinase-3; $ACON_S$, soluble aconitase; wk, weak.

TABLE 5

HUMAN CHROMOSOME COMPOSITION AND HUMAN INTERFERON YIELDS IN HYBRIDS WITH AN X:9 TRANSLOCATION

Hybrid	Human Interferon Yield (units/ml/ 10^6 cells)	Human Chromosomes Present*																					
Hybrids between L-A_9 and GM705																							
GLA	125		2	3	5	6	7	8	(9)†		11	12		14	15	16		18	19	20	21	X	X:9
GLB	125		(2)	3		6	7	8			11	12		14	15	16		18	19	20	21	X	X:9
GLC	0		(2)	3		6	7	8			11			14	15	16		18	19	20	21		
Hybrids between PG19 and GM705																							
GP2	890	1		NT		6	NT	NT	9 ‡	(10)	(11)	12	13	14		16	17	18	19	20	21		X:9
GP3	450		2	NT		6	NT	NT	9 ‡	NT	11	12	NT	14	NT	16	17	18	19	20	NT	NT	X:9

*The GL series were characterized by isoenzyme analysis and karyotyping; the GP series by isoenzyme analysis only.

†Detected by karyotyping in about 5% of the cells.

‡Since isoenzyme analysis only was used, we cannot distinguish a free chromosome 9 from an X:9 translocation.

NT = not tested.

received, from Dr. T. Mohandas of the University of California, Torrance, a Chinese hamster-human lymphocyte hybrid that contained a human X:9 (q 13; q 34) as the only human chromosome present. This hybrid produces human interferon when induced with NDV-F, showing that human chromosome 9 is both necessary and sufficient for production of human fibroblast interferon.

THE USE OF THE HYBRIDS TO STUDY CONTROL OF THE INTERFERON SYSTEM

Since fibroblast interferon is a glycoprotein, the products of other genes, in addition to the structural gene, must be required for the secondary modification of the human fibroblast polypeptide. Several lines of evidence show this to be so. First, mouse-human hybrids, which are adherant cells in culture, produce only human fibroblast interferon, irrespective of whether the human parent was of fibroblast or lymphoid origin. Second, although all the hybrids respond to viral induction, the inducibility of hybrids by poly rI. poly rC depends on whether the mouse parent is inducible in the first place. For example, the hybrid CTP34 derived from the mouse PG19 cell line, which is inducible with poly rI. poly rC, and a human lymphoid cell that is almost certainly uninducible with poly rI. poly rC is, like the mouse parent, inducible with poly rI. poly rC. The hybrid HL15 derived from the mouse cell line L-A_9, which is not inducible with poly rI. poly rC, and the human fibroblast HEF cell stain, which is inducible with poly rI. poly rC, is not inducible (TABLE 7). Thus, although the human parent is inducible, the hybrid with L-A_9 is not, showing the mouse phenotype to be dominant.[7]

A similar effect was found with the superinduction effect, in which interferon yields can be increased by appropriate treatment of cells induced with poly rI. poly rC with metabolic inhibitors.[8-12] The superinduction procedure greatly increased the yield of interferon from human fibroblasts (HEF) and the PG19 mouse line, but L-A_9 cells still produce no interferon. The hybrid CTP34, derived

TABLE 6

EFFECT OF CONTINUED PASSAGE OF TWO MOUSE-HUMAN HYBRIDS ON INTERFERON PRODUCTION

		Interferon Yield (log_{10} units/ml/10^6 cells)	
Hybrid	Passage No.	Human Interferon	Mouse Interferon
GP2 (X:9)	3	3.0	>5.0
	6	2.7	NT
	7	2.8	4.25
	10	1.9	NT
	19	1.9	NT
	22	2.35	3.55
	28	2.3	3.4
	34	2.15	4.0
	42	2.3	NT
CTP34	17	2.9	4.6
	22	2.45	3.6
	24	2.15	3.9
	30	1.05	>5.0
	38	<0.6	NT

NT = not tested.

from PG19, was superinducible whereas the hybrid HL15, derived from L-A_9 was not, despite the fact that its human parent was also superinducible (TABLE 7). Again the mouse phenotype was dominant.[7] A similar effect was shown by primed cells where pretreatment of cells with low doses of interferon increases the yield of interferon when the cells are subsequently induced.[13-16] Here again the mouse phenotype was dominant (data not shown).

Finally, we have shown that interferon synthesis in human and mouse cells is differentially inhibited by 2-deoxy-D-galactose (2dGal). In mouse L-A_9 cells interferon production is inhibited at low concentrations of 2dGal (0.5 mM) whereas much higher concentration (>10 mM) are required to inhibit human interferon synthesis in human fibroblasts. However, in the mouse-human

TABLE 7

INDUCTION AND SUPERINDUCTION OF MOUSE-HUMAN HYBRIDS AND THEIR PARENTS

	Interferon Yield in Response to poly rI. poly rC* (units/ml/10^6 cells)			
	Human Interferon		Mouse Interferon	
Cell	Induction	Superinduction	Induction	Superinduction
Parental cells				
Mouse PG19			130	5100
L-A_9			0	0
Human HEF	200–400	2400–10000		
Hybrid formed from human T lymphocyte and PG19				
CTP34	2–6	250–320	10–70	4000–10000
Hybrid formed from human fibroblast and L-A_9				
HL15	0	0	0	0

*100 μg/ml.

hybrids HL15, GP2 and GP2 SC8, synthesis of both mouse and human interferons is inhibited by low concentrations of 2 dGal.[17] Thus, we conclude that once the human interferon gene has been incorporated into the hybrid cell, human interferon is subject to control and modification by products of the mouse genome.

Conclusion

The gene for human fibroblast interferon is on chromosome 9. We do not know whether there is another gene for human leukocyte interferon on this or another chromosome, or whether the distinct mRNAs for fibroblast and leukocyte interferon are produced by different processing pathways from a single gene product. However, the formation of fibroblast interferon by adherant cell hybrids, whether the human parent is leukocyte or fibroblast, suggests that this control may be post-transcriptional. Modulation of the interferon yield by either superinduction or priming in the mouse-human hybrids is characteristic of the mouse parent, although the exact mechanism of either effect is unknown. Finally glycosylation of the completed polypeptide is, as expected, characteristic of the mouse parent.

Acknowledgments

We are indebted to Mrs. H. E. Graves for excellent technical assistance and to the Medical Research Council for program grant support.

References

1. Tan, Y. H., R. P. Creagan & F. H. Ruddle. 1974. The somatic cell genetics of human interferon: Assignment of human interferon loci to chromosomes 2 and 5. Proc. Nat. Acad. Sci. USA **71:** 2251–2255.
2. Morgan, M. J. & P. Faik. 1977. The expression of the interferon system in clones of Chinese hamster-human hybrid cells. Brit. J. Cancer **35:** 254.
3. Tan, Y. H. 1977. Genetics of the human interferon system. *In* Interferons and their Actions. W. E. Stewart II, Ed.: 73–90. CRC Press. Cleveland, OH.
4. Knight, E., Jun. 1976. Interferon: Purification and initial characterization from human diploid cells. Proc. Nat. Acad. Sci. USA **73:** 520–523.
5. Meager, A., H. E. Graves, J. R. Walker, D. C. Burke, D. M. Swallow & A. Westerveld. 1979. Somatic cell genetics of human interferon production in human-rodent cell hybrids. J. Gen. Virol. **45:** 309–321.
6. Desmyter, J. & W. E. Stewart II. 1976. Molecular modification of interferon: Attainment of human interferon in a conformation active on cat cells but inactive on human cells. Virology **70:** 451–458.
7. Graves, H. E. & A. Meager. 1980. Superinduction and priming of interferons in human-mouse hybrids. J. Gen. Virol. **47:** 489–495.
8. Vilček, J. 1970. Metabolic determinants of the induction of interferon by a synthetic double-stranded polynucleotide in rabbit kidney cells. Ann N.Y. Acad. Sci. **173:** 390–403.
9. Tan, Y. H., J. A. Armstrong, Y. H. Ke & M. Ho. 1970. The regulation of cellular interferon synthesis: Enhancement by antimetabolites. Proc. Nat. Acad. Sci. USA **67:** 464–471.

10. HAVELL, E. A. & J. VILČEK. 1972. Production of high titred interferon in cultures of human diploid cells. Antimicrob. Ag. Chemo. **2:** 476–484.
11. BILLIAU, A., M. JONIAU & P. DESOMER. 1972. Production of crude human interferon with high specific activity. Proc. Soc. Exp. Biol. Med. **140:** 485–491.
12. TAN, Y. H. & W. BERTHOLD. 1977. A mechanism for the induction and regulation of human fibroblastoid interferon genetic expression. J. Gen. Virol **34:** 401–411.
13. ISAACS, A. & D. C. BURKE. 1958. Mode of action of interferon. Nature **182:** 1073–1074.
14. FRIEDMAN, R. M. 1966. Effect of interferon treatment on interferon production. J. Immunol. **96:** 872-877.
15. LEVY, H. B., C. E. BUCKLER & S. BARON. 1966. Effect of interferon on early interferon production. Science **152:** 1274–1276.
16. STEWART, W. E. II, L. B. GOSSER & R. Z. LOCKART, Jun. 1971. Priming: A non-antiviral function of interferon. J. Virol. **7:** 792–801.
17. MASON, T. & A. MEAGER. In preparation.
18. HAVELL, E. A., T. G. HAYES & J. VILČEK. 1978. Synthesis of two distinct interferons by human fibroblasts. Virology **89:** 330–334.
19. SLATE, D. L. & F. H. RUDDLE. 1979. Fibroblast interferon is coded by two loci on separate chromosomes. Cell **16:** 171–180.

THE CELL GROWTH INHIBITORY AND ANTIVIRAL EFFECTS OF INTERFERON IN CLONED TRANSFORMED MOUSE CELLS

L. Borecký, Valéria Hajnická, N. Fuchsberger, P. Kontsek, V. Lackovič, and G. Russ

Institute of Virology
Slovak Academy of Sciences
Bratislava, Czechoslovakia

J. Čapková

Institute of Molecular Genetics
Czechoslovak Academy of Sciences
Prague, Czechoslovakia

A growing number of papers indicate that we are witnessing a change in the conception of interferon (IF) from that of an autonomous nonimmunological antiviral factor to a hormone- and/or lymphokine-like cell-regulatory substance.[1] The slow progress in exploitation of IF in the therapy of viral diseases and the variety of its effects in normal and tumorous, homologous and heterologous, animal and bacterial cells lend support to the changing view.[2] However, the basic objections to polarization of these concepts, such as nonhomogeneity of the IF preparations and cells used as models have not been, as yet, eliminated completely and further studies are needed to gain a deeper insight into the mechanism of IF action. This paper summarizes the results of our studies, which have focused on the two best characterized effects of IF in the cell: the antiviral (AV) and the cell-growth inhibitory (CGI) activities.

Material and Methods

Viruses

Newcastle disease virus (NDV), Hertfordshire strain, was used for IF induction. The virus was maintained by repeated passage in the allantoic cavities of 9-day-old chick embryos. Unless otherwise stated, encephalomyocarditis (EMC) virus was used for cell challenge in AV tests. It was grown in monolayers of LB2 cells (a subline of L-929 mouse fibroblasts). The Harvey strain of mouse sarcoma virus (MSV) was obtained from the Institute of Experimental Oncology, Slovak Academy of Sciences, Bratislava. Stock suspension of the virus contained about 10^7 $TCID_{50}$ per ml of virus. Simian virus 40 (SV40) was obtained from the Institute of Sera and Vaccines (Prague). The virus was replicated in African green monkey kidney cells. Its titer was about 10^7 $TCID_{50}$ per ml.

Cells

Two sublines of the L-929 mouse cell line were employed. The LB2 cells, maintained in the Institute of Virology, Bratislava, were used for IF titration. The LG cells, which originated in the Imperial Cancer Research Fund Laboratories

0077-8923/80/0350-0188 $01.75/0 © 1980, NYAS

(London), were used for IF production. The CSV-21 cells are a subline of the LB2 cells.[3] Primary mouse embryonic fibroblasts (MEF) used in viral and chemical transformation were prepared from inbred C3H mouse embryos on day 17–19 of gestation. The cells were grown in Eagle's basal medium (BEM) supplemented with either 5% or 20% heated calf serum and antibiotics. In tests with human interferon, human amniotic U-cells, cervical carcinoma HeLa cells, and the BHK-21 line of hamster cells were used.[4]

Viral Transformation of Primary Mouse Embryonic Cells

Mouse embryonic fibroblasts in the second passage, two days after seeding and before a monolayer was formed, were used for transformation. The cultivation medium supplemented with 20% heated calf serum was changed for serum-free medium containing approximately 10^7 $TCID_{50}$ of SV40 or MSV. After 4 hr of absorption, the cells were washed and the complete cultivation medium was added. Foci of transformed cells appeared 4 to 6 weeks after seeding of cells. The cells in the first passage after foci were noticed were designated as the "first" passage of MEF-SV40 or MEF-MSV line, respectively.

Chemical Transformation of Primary Embryonic Cells

One part of C3H mouse embryonic fibroblasts cultures in the second passage was treated with 0.1 μg per ml of 20-methylcholanthrene (MCH). The carcinogen-treated cultures were exposed to carcinogen for 72 hours. The medium with the carcinogen was changed daily. BEM supplemented with 20% heated calf serum was used for the rest of the cultivation period. Foci of transformed cells appeared after 3 to 4 weeks of cultivation. The first subcultures of these cells were designated as the "first" passage of MEF-MCH.

The Growth of Cells in Soft Agar

The method of MacPherson and Mantagnier[5] was slightly modified. The bottom of Petri dishes 10 cm in diameter was covered with 10 ml of 0.5% agar medium supplemented with 20% heated calf serum. The upper layer was formed with 2 ml of 0.3% agar medium containing 2000 to 5000 cells per dish.

Isolation of Cell-clones

For cloning, the ability of cells to grow in semisolid agar was utilized. Two to five thousand cells were added to the 0.5% agar medium in a Petri dish. After 12 to 15 days, the colonies were picked up with a Pasteur pipette under microscopic control and transferred into tubes containing BEM supplemented with 20% heated calf serum. This subculture was considered the "first" passage of a clone.

Interaction of Cells with Lectins

For testing agglutinability of cells with Concanavalin A (Con A), each tested cell suspension in 0.2 volume (10^6 cells per ml) was mixed with an equal volume of the indicated concentration of Con A (Sigma Chem. Co., USA). After 1 hr of incubation at room temperature, the agglutination was registered.

For measuring the binding of lectin to cell surface, ^{125}I-labeled soybean lectin (Pharmacia, Sweden) was used according to the method described by Russ *et al.*[6] The specific activity of the preparation was 5μ Ci/μg. The binding was monitored with a Tesla-NZQ714T Gamma-counter.

Cytotoxicity of Macrophages

The sensitivity of cells to the cytotoxic activity of macrophages was tested by a slightly modified version of the method of Schultz and Chirigos.[7]

Chromosome Analysis

Chromosomes of cultured cells were analyzed by the method of Rothfels and Siminovitch.[8]

Expression of H-2 Specificities

The absorbing capacity of cells for H-2.23 and H-2.32 specificities was essayed in the microdroplet cytotoxicity test according to Wigzell[9] and in the ^{51}Cr-labeled target cell cytotoxicity test according to Micková and Ivanyi.[10] C3H target cells and monospecific antisera against H-2.23 and H-2.32 antigens were employed.

Interferon

Mouse interferon was induced in LG-cells with NDV and was partially purified by Zn-acetate precipitation and column chromatography on SP-Sephadex C-25, as described previously.[11] Interferon used for comparative analysis of various fractions represented a preparation further purified by polyacrylamide gel electrophoresis (PAGE) according to Stanček and Paucker[12] and Kawade.[13] The human interferon employed in these studies was of the leukocyte type.[14] For AV assay of IF, the cytopathic effect inhibition method was used.[15] EMC and vesicular stomatitis virus VSV were used for challenge of rodent and human cells, respectively. The CGIE of IF in cells was estimated by comparing the cell number in IF-treated and control (untreated) cell cultures 4–5 days after seeding 10^5 cells per ml in at least three parallel tubes.[11]

Immunoelectrophoresis of Interferon Preparations

The method introduced by Laurell[16] and applied to interferon assay by Fuchsberger and Borecký[17] was used with a modification. This consisted in using two layers of agarose (one containing IF fractions, the other containing anti-IF globulin). The agarose plates were brought in contact immediately before electrophoresis.

Chemicals

Cyclic 3′5′ adenosine-monophosphate (c-AMP) was a product of Fluka (Switzerland). Prostaglandin E2 (PGE2), a product of Chinoin (Hungary), was stored at −70° C as a stock solution containing 0.33 mg of the substance per ml of ethanol.

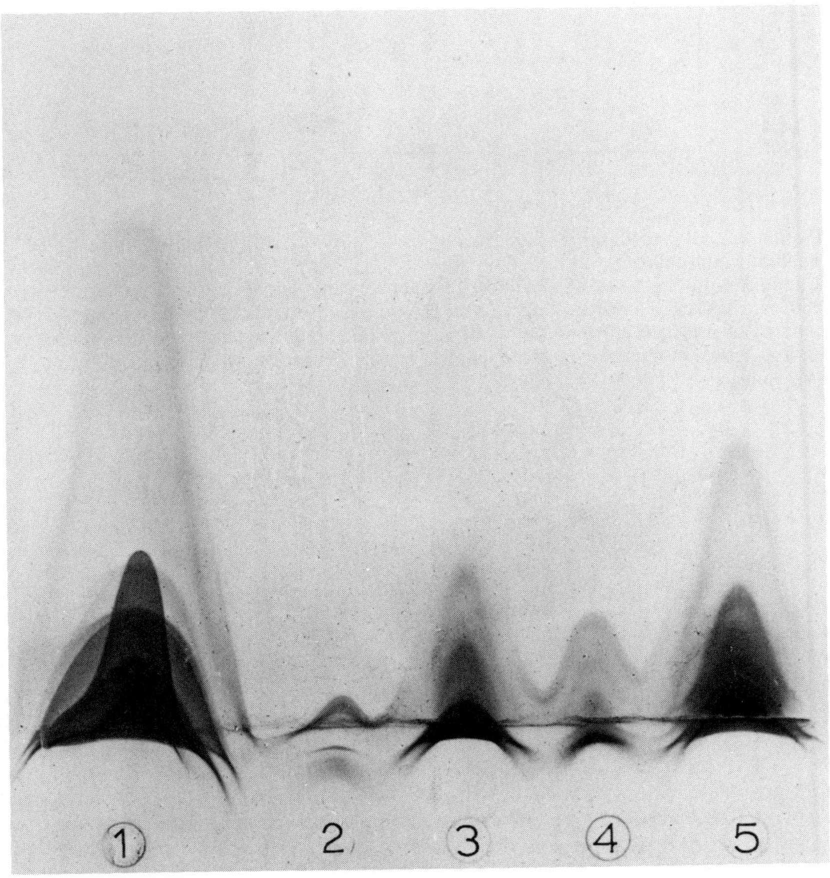

FIGURE 1. Immunoelectrophoretic profiles of mouse interferon during purification. 1: Cultivation medium (2180 μg protein per ml). 2: IF-crude preparation (IF-titer 5.1 × 10^3, protein 790 μg per ml, specific activity 6.5 × 10^3). 3: IF-Zn-acetate-precipitated preparation (IF titer 8.2 × 10^4, protein 705 μg per ml, specific activity 1.2 × 10^5) 4: Nonadsorbed fraction from SP-Sephadex (IF titer 3.2 × 10^2, protein 420 μg per ml, specific activity 7.8 × 10^5) 5: IF-fractions eluted from SP-Sephadex (IF titer 1.3 × 10^6, protein 820 μg per ml, specific activity 1.6 × 10^6).

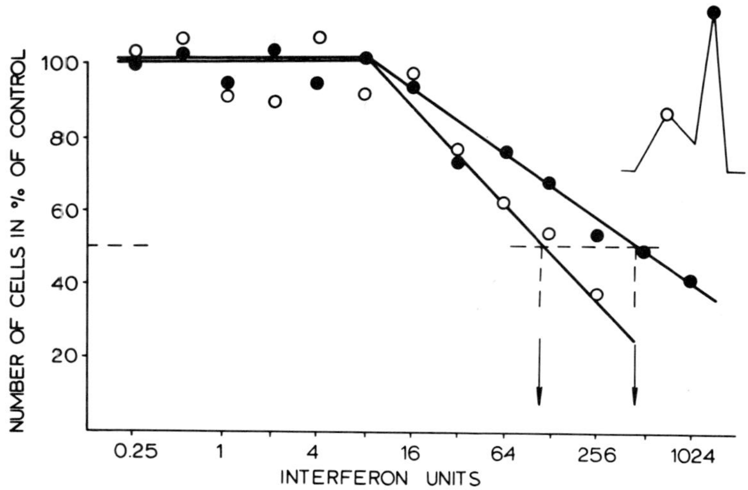

FIGURE 2. Cell-growth inhibitory effect of graded amounts of the "slow" (○) and "fast" (●) molecular species of purified L-cell interferon.

Abscissa: Antiviral units of interferon. *Ordinate:* Number of cells in percent of control. Arrows indicate the relative amounts of PAGE fractions that were necessary for 50% inhibition of multiplication of L-cells. *Insert in the upper right corner:* PAGE fractions used for examination. (From Fuchsberger *et al.*[11] Reproduced from *Acta Virol.* with permission.)

Theophylline ethylenediamine (Aminophyllin) was purchased from Sigma (USA). cAMP and theophylline were kept at 4° C until used.

RESULTS

Studies in L-929 Mouse Fibroblasts and Other Rodent Cells

The Problem of Homogeneity of Interferon Preparation

The mouse IF preparation obtained by induction of LG cells (a substrain of L-929) in a serum-free medium with NDV was purified by a combined proce-

TABLE 1

ANTIVIRAL ACTIVITY OF TWO ELECTROPHORETIC FRACTIONS OF MOUSE INTERFERON IN "FRESHLY" EXPLANTED (A) AND "AGED" (B) L-929 CELLS*

Experiment No.	Titers in L cells per ml			
	"Slow" Fraction		"Fast" Fraction	
	A	B	A	B
I.	5,120	6,400	20,000	1,310,720
II.	1,280	1,280	5,120	40,000
III.	1,280±	2,560	1,280	20,000

*From Fuchsberger *et al.*[11] Used with permission of the Editor of *Acta Virol.*

dure.[11] Such a preparation was used for examination of the CGIE and AV activities of the "fast" and "slow" molecular species of IF obtained in PAGE. In most of subsequent studies, however, partially purified preparations not subjected to electrophoretic separation were used. Although the specific activity of such preparations was relatively high, i.e. 1.6×10^6 units per mg protein, in a modified immunoelectrophoretic assay using a potent sheep anti-IF serum, heavy contamination with non-IF constituents could be visualized (FIGURE 1). Examination of IF fractions separated by PAGE revealed a quantitative discrepancy between the CGI and AV activities in the molecular species constituting the "fast" peak (specific activity 2.62×10^6 units per mg protein). Thus, when compared with the CGI activity of the "slow" peak of IF, a further "intraspecies" molecular heterogeneity could be registered.[11] This discrepancy (FIGURE 2) could be partially explained by the different binding avidities of the "fast" molecular

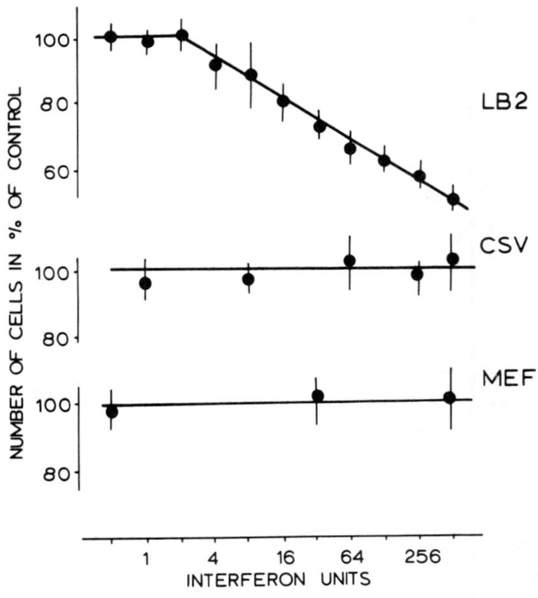

FIGURE 3. Quantitative relations between the antiviral and cell-growth inhibitory activities of interferon in LB2, CSV-21 and mouse embryonic fibroblast cells (MEF).

Ordinate: Number of cells in percent of control. *Abscissa:* Antiviral units of interferon.

(From Borecký *et al.*[4] Reproduced from *Neoplasma* with permission.)

species of IF for the "young," i.e. freshly explanted LB2-cells (as used in the CGI test), and "aged" cells, i.e. treated with IF after achieving confluency on glass and used in AV-tests (TABLE 1).

Independent Modulation of Cell-sensitivity to Various Interferon Activities

A clear dichotomy between two IF activities (i.e. CGI and AV) was achieved by long-term cultivation of LB2 cells in the presence of homologous IF.[3] The resulting cell line (CSV-21) retained its sensitivity toward the AV effect of IF but proved to be completely resistant to its CGIE (FIGURE 3). Although by electronmicroscopic examination the CSV-21 cells showed cytological alterations, the modified cells did not differ from the parent strain in gross morphology (FIGURE

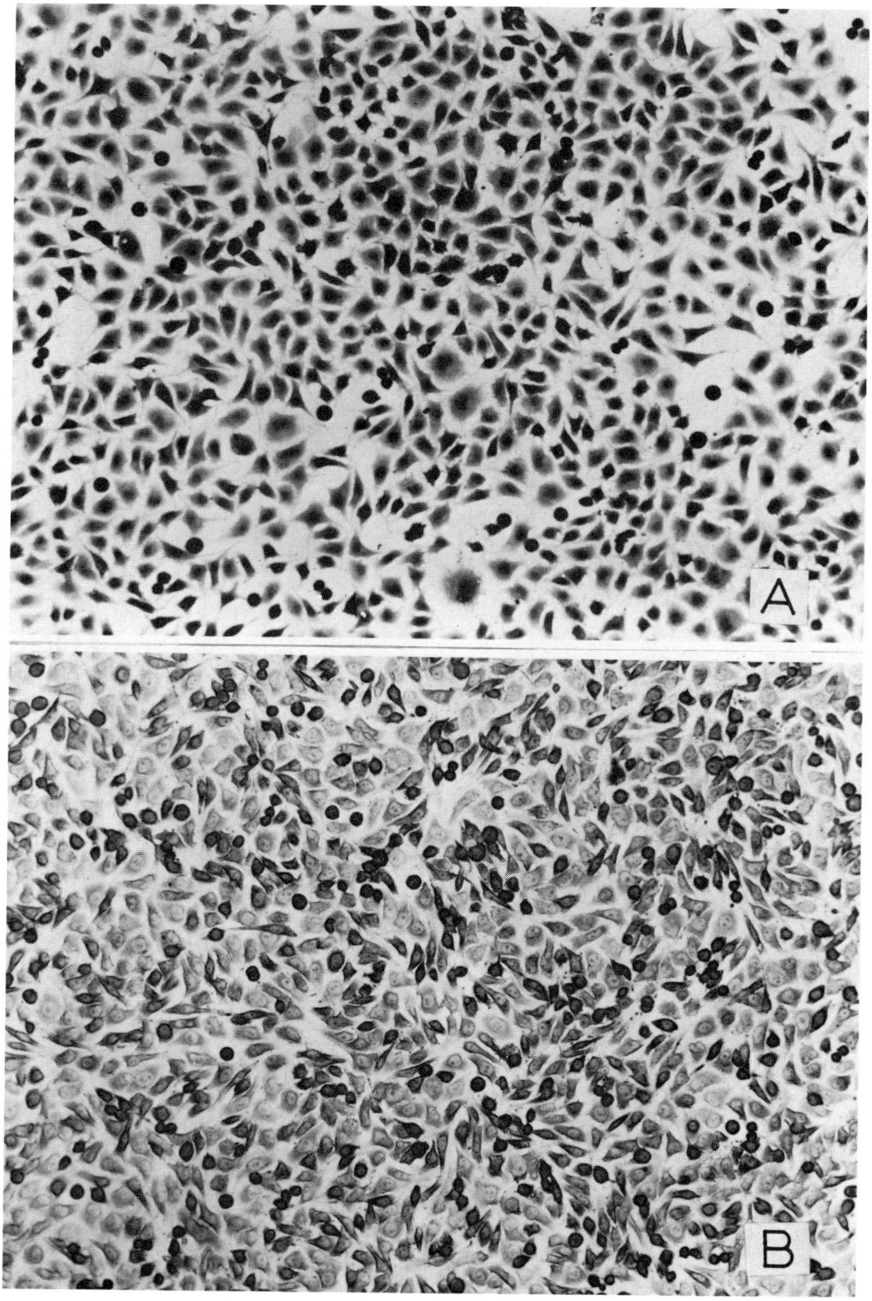

FIGURE 4. Interferon resistant CSV-21 cells (B) derived from LB2 cells (A) by continuous cultivation in the presence of homologous interferon. Giemsa-stain, enlargement 120×.

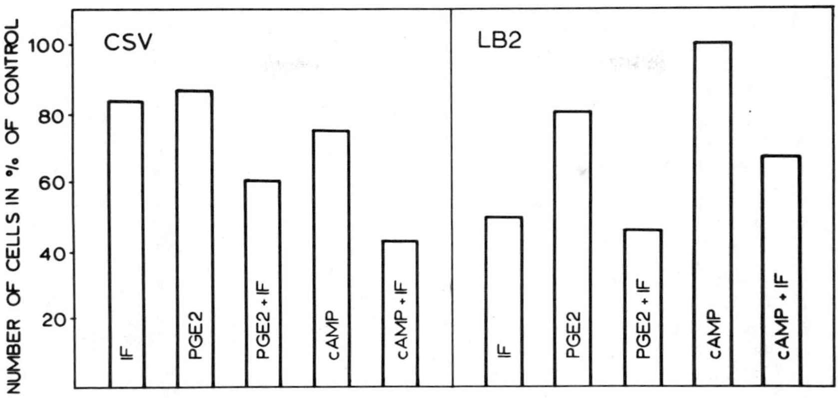

FIGURE 5. Effect of cyclic AMP, prostaglandin E2, and, theophylline on the sensitivity of CSV-21 and LB2 cells to the cell-growth inhibitory effect of interferon.

Ordinate: Number of cells in percent of control. *Abscissa:* Substances tested in cell-growth inhibitory test. Average from two experiments. After 16 hr of incubation the cells (10^5 per ml) were treated with 256 units of interferon per ml and either 30–50 μg of cAMP, or, 0.75–1 μg of PGE2 (with 20.5 μg of theophylline). The number of cells was estimated after 3–4 days when the control cells achieved confluency. (From Borecký *et al.*[4] Reproduced from *Neoplasma* with permission.)

4). Recently, it has been found that the CSV-21 cells also show an increased resistance to the toxic effect of dsRNA.[18] This IF-resistant subline resembles the human IF-resistant subline obtained by Kuwata *et al.*[19] and differs from the IF-resistant L-1210 subline described by Gresser *et al.*[20] Attempts to enhance the sensitivity of the CSV-21 subline to the CGIE of IF by PGE2 (plus theophylline) or cAMP were partially successful although ineffective in the parent LB2 strain (FIGURE 5).

Species Differences in Sensitivity of Cells to Various Activities of Interferon

Several years ago we reported that human IF effectively inhibited the multiplication of mouse L-cells, whereas it was inactive in this respect in BHK-21

TABLE 2

CELL-GROWTH INHIBITORY ACTIVITY OF HUMAN INTERFERON IN CELLS FROM THREE SPECIES*

Cells	Species	Antiviral Units† of Interferon (cell line/ challenge virus)	No. of Cells in % of Control
U	Human	1,280 (U/VSV)‡	27
LB2	Mouse	1,280 (LB2/EMC)	60
BHK-21	Hamster	1,280 (BHK-21/EMC)	100

*From Borecký *et al.*[21] Reproduced with permission of the Editor of *Intervirology*.
†Calculated from titration in homologous cells, as indicated in parentheses.
‡Indicates the system used for calculation of "antiviral" units.

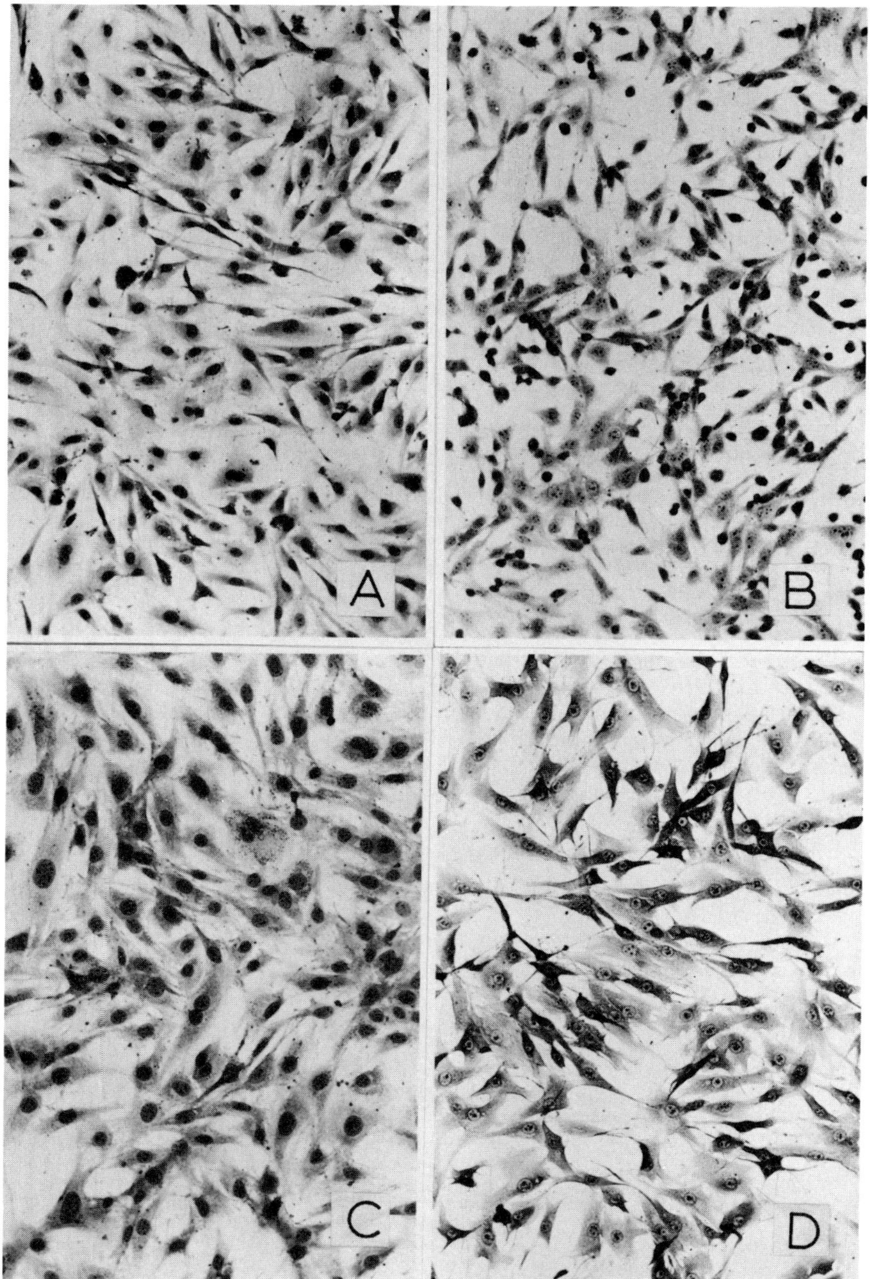

FIGURE 6. Morphological appearance of (A) mouse embryonic cells (2nd passage) after treatment with (B) SV40 (13th passage), (C) MSV (6th passage), and (D) 20-methylcholanthrene (8th passage). Giemsa-stain, enlargement 90×.

cells.[21] Since the actual number of IF units applied to human, mouse, or hamster cells was carefully calculated from the results of titration of the AV activity of human IF preparation in each of these cells separately, the results of CGI tests in heterologous rodent cells can be taken as evidence that species differences determine the CGI response of cells to a greater deal than in the case of AV activity (TABLE 2).

Studies in Cells Transformed by Carcinogenic Viruses or 20-Methylcholanthrene

Establishment of Transformed Cell Lines

Treatment of cultures of C3H mouse embryonic fibroblasts with two different viruses (SV40 or MSV), or 20-methylcholanthrene resulted in the appearance of

TABLE 3

GROWTH CHARACTERISTICS OF MOUSE EMBRYONIC FIBROBLASTS TREATED WITH SV40, MSV (HARVEY), AND 20-METHYLCHOLANTHRENE, RESPECTIVELY

Cells	Passage	Agglutination with Concanavalin A 500	100 μg per ml	50	Growth in Semisolid Agar	Population Density per $cm^2 \times 10^3$ After 72 Hours	Tumorigenicity for C3H Mice[2]
MEF (Parent)	2	+	−	−	−	49	0/3
MEF-SV40	8	++++	++	+	+	200	0/3 (18)‡
MEF-SV40	21	ND	ND	ND	+	560	ND
MEF-MSV*	15	++++	+++	++	−	150	3/3 (17)
MEF-MSV*	26	ND	ND	ND	−	510	6/6 (35)
MEF-MCH*	9	++++	++	+	−	100	0/3
MEF-MCH*	32	ND	ND	ND	+	410	ND

*Cell-lines obtained after treatment of the parent embryonic cell population with SV40 (MEF-SV40), or mouse sarcoma virus (MEF-MSV), or 20-methylcholanthrene (MEF-MCH).

†Mice with tumors: mice inoculated.

‡The passage in which oncogenicity was tested is shown in parentheses.

ND: Not done.

foci of multilayered cells 3 to 6 weeks later (FIGURE 6). In contradistinction to untreated primary C3H fibroblasts, the cultures with foci of transformed cells were capable of *in vitro* passages. This made it possible to study three different cell lines derived from a common parent population. After establishment of "morphological" transformation, the cells were examined in successive passages for agglutinability with Concanavalin A, ability to grow in soft agar, and tumorigenicity in newborn C3H mice. In addition, the population density after 72 hours of growth and, occasionally, the chromosome number were examined (TABLE 3, FIGURE 7). Only the MSV-transformed cells proved to be oncogenic for newborn C3H mice when assayed in the 8th and 35th passage before cloning. However, the MSV cells did not grow in semisolid agar. The chromosome number of MSV cells was 63 ± 3.3, while control MEF cells contained 38 ± 0.51 chromosomes. On the other hand, the SV40 cells grew relatively well in

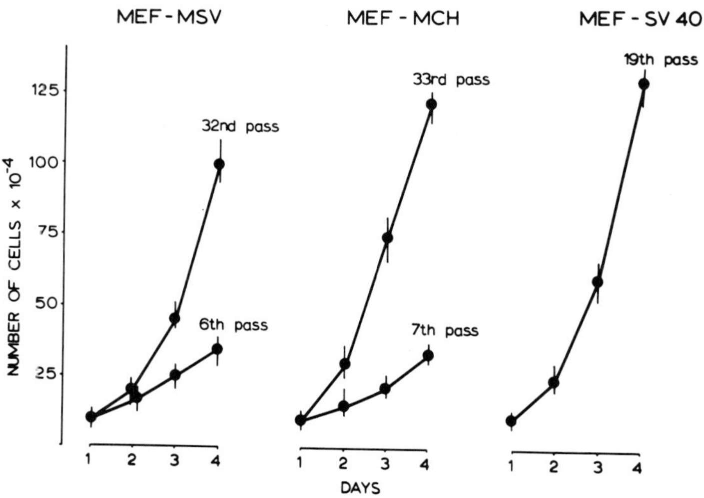

FIGURE 7. Growth curves of MSV-, SV40- and MCH-transformed cell-lines *in vitro*. *Ordinate:* Days of cultivation *Abscissa:* Number of cells × 10^{-4}.

semisolid agar but did not induce tumors in mice. These cells were T-antigen positive by the immunofluorescence technique. Their chromosome number was 46 ± 3.1. In MCH-transformed cells, the ability to grow in semisolid agar was detected in the 32nd passage. All morphologically transformed cell lines were agglutinated by 100 μg per ml of Concanavalin A, which did not agglutinate parent cells. The population density of subculturable cells after 3 days of cultivation was 2 to 10 times higher than in parent cells.

The Antiviral and the Cell-growth Inhibitory Effects of Interferon in Transformed Lines

When compared with the parental non-transformed cells, in the MSV line mouse interferon exerted a decreased antiviral activitity against EMC virus

TABLE 4

SENSITIVITY OF TRANSFORMED FIBROBLAST LINES TO THE ANTIVIRAL EFFECT OF MOUSE INTERFERON

Cells	Passage	$TCID_{50}$ of EMC Virus Used in Test	Interferon Titer per ml
MEF (Parent)	2	100	20,000
MEF-MSV	20	100	2,560
MEF-MCH	22	100	40,000 ±
MEF-SV40	25	≃I*	160,000 ±

*The actual $TCID_{50}$ of EMC virus used in test. The MEF-SV40 line was resistant to EMC virus.

while the estimation of AV activity of IF in SV40 cells often was unreliable since the SV40-line showed an increased resistance against the cytopathic effect of EMC virus (TABLE 4).

Also, the SV40 cells differed from MSV cells in being completely unable to produce IF when stimulated with NDV. In contradistinction, the MCH-transformed cells after 35 passages *in vitro* regained the ability to produce IF, which was undetectable in the first passages after transformation. (Compare passages 9 and 35 in TABLE 5).

Assay of the CGI activity of mouse IF in the transformed lines showed that the SV40 cells in the 7th passage were resistant to more than 3000 units of IF while both the MCH-line (22nd passage) and the MSV-line (22nd passage) proved to be more sensitive (FIGURE 8).

TABLE 5

INTERFERON PRODUCTION* IN CELL LINES TRANSFORMED WITH SV40, MSV (HARVEY), AND 20-METHYLCHOLANTHRENE, RESPECTIVELY

Cells	Passage	Interferon Titer per ml
MEF (Parent)	2	320
MEF-SV40	14	<10
MEF-SV40	37	<10
MEF-MCH	9	<10
MEF-MCH	35	80
MEF-MSV	8	320
MEF-MSV	12	320±
MEF-MSV	28	640

*Newcastle disease virus was used for IF induction.

The Antiviral and the Cell-growth Inhibitory Effects of Interferon in Cloned Transformed Cells

Altogether, 8 clones and 2 subclones of SV40-transformed cells and 7 clones and one subclone of MCH-treated cells were analyzed for sensitivity to the CGI and AV effects of IF. The cloning of SV40 line was started in the 8th passage after transformation.

As shown in TABLE 6, when tested in the 18th passage, the SV40 clones can be divided into three groups according to their sensitivity to the CGI effect of IF. While some of the clones were inhibited by as little as 24 to 110 units of IF (clones No. 5, 27, 35), others required more than 3000 units for the same effect (clones No. 31 and 53). Since the clones from the SV40-treated cells retained their relative resistance against EMC virus, the actual amount of EMC virus used in the AV test was in the majority of cases below 100 $TCID_{50}$. This led to an enhanced sensitivity of IF titration but, in general, the differences among clones do not seem significant. The SV40 clones, like the SV40-line, did not produce detectable levels of IF when stimulated with NDV.

The MCH clones were started after 30 passages of the MCH line *in vitro* since the cells underwent a growth crisis before a stabilized MCH line appeared. The clones showed a relatively uniform IF-producing capacity (TABLE 7) and did not differ significantly in sensitivity to the AV activity of IF. Their sensitivity to

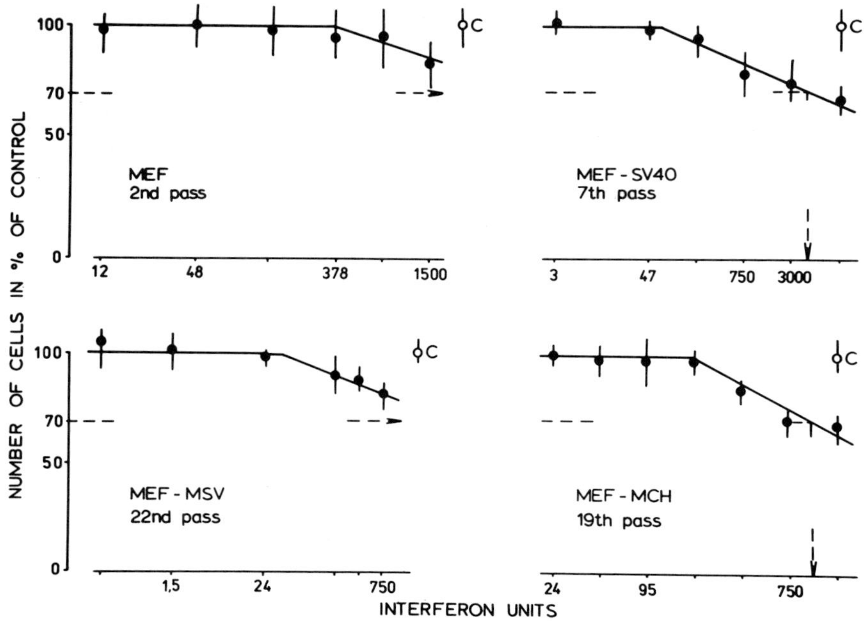

FIGURE 8. The cell-growth inhibitory effect of mouse interferon in embryonic cells (MEF) and cell-lines transformed by SV40, MSV, and MCH, respectively.

Ordinate: Number of cells in percent of control. *Abscissa:* Antiviral units of interferon applied to cells C: Number of cells in control nontreated culture. Average from 3 parallel tubes.

TABLE 6

SENSITIVITY OF THE MEF-SV40 CLONES TO THE CELL-GROWTH INHIBITORY AND ANTIVIRAL EFFECT OF INTERFERON AND THE INTERFERON-PRODUCING CAPACITY OF CLONES

Group	Clone No.	Passage	CGI Titer*	AV Titer† × 10^3	IF Production‡
I	5	18	24	160	<10
	27	18	110	160	<10
	35	18	50	40	<10
	35-4§	39 (+3)	50	80	ND
	35-8§	39 (+3)	50	80	ND
II	3	39	2,200	640	<10
	30	39	1,540	20	<10
	44	39	1,400	320	<10
III	31	39	3,000	320	<10
	63	39	3,000	320 ±	<10

*Interferon units required for a 30% inhibition of growth.

†Highest dilution of IF that inhibits the cytopathic effect of 10 $TCID_{50}$ EMC virus in the clones. (In tests with clones 35 and/or 30 the actual number of $TCID_{50}$ was ≃ 100.)

‡AV-titer detected in the medium after stimulation of the clone with NDV.

§Subclone. The number of passages of the subclone *in vitro* is given in parentheses.

TABLE 7

SENSITIVITY OF THE MEF-MCH CLONES TO THE CELL-GROWTH INHIBITORY AND ANTIVIRAL EFFECT OF INTERFERON AND THE INTERFERON-PRODUCING CAPACITY OF CLONES

Group	Clone No.	Passage	CGI Titer*	AV Titer† $\times 10^3$	IF Production‡
I	36	20	640	64	80±
	43	11	400	128±	80
	49	16	700	128	80±
	52	17	580	64	160
II	41	11	1,300	64	ND
	57	22	2,500	64	80
	57-5§	32(+2)	2,500	80	ND
	73	12	2,500	128	160±

*Interferon units required for a 30 per cent growth inhibition.

†Highest dilution of IF that inhibits the cytopathic effect of 100 $TCID_{50}$ of EMC virus in the clone.

‡AV-titer detected in the medium after stimulation of the clone with NDV.

§Subclone. The number of *in vitro* passages of the subclone is given in parentheses.

ND: Not done.

the CGI of IF seems to be, in general, lower than of SV40 clones and they can be divided into two groups in this respect. Three of four tested MCH clones (No. 36, 49 and 57) in the 15th to 20th passage produced tumors in C3H mice. During two additional passages *in vitro*, the tumor cells retained the sensitivity of the parent clones to the AV effect of IF. The MCH clones and subclones seem to have a stabilized average number of chromosomes (85 to 95) (TABLE 8).

TABLE 8

INTERFERON SENSITIVITY, TUMORIGENICITY, AND CHROMOSOME NUMBER OF MEF-MCH CLONES IN VARIOUS PASSAGES

Clone No.	Passage	AV Titer§ $\times 10^3$	CGI Titer§	Tumorigenicity in C3H Mice¶	Chromosome Number (Mean)
36	15–20	64	640	3/5	87 ± 4.6
36/1	25 (+1)‡	64	640	3/3	85 ± 4.8
36/2	25 (+2)	64	640	ND	86 ± 4.5
49	16–18	128±	700	1/3	93 ± 6.7
49/1*	21 (+1)	128	700	ND	94 ± 6.1
52	17	64	580	0/5	87 ± 4.9
57	20–29	64	2,500	3/6	85 ± 4.2
57-5†	32 (+2)	128	2,500	ND	85 ± 4.2

*Cells from tumors induced in mice by the clone 36 or 49.

†Subclone.

‡The number of passages of the subclone *in vitro* is shown in parentheses.

§See TABLES 6 and 7.

¶Mice with tumors: mice inoculated.

ND: Not done.

Examination of Surface Differences Between Clones

Three types of tests were used. Two selected MCH clones (No. 57 and 36) differing in sensitivity to the CGIE of IF were, tested for their ability to (1) bind soybean lectin, (2) absorb monospecific anti-H-2 sera directed against the anti-H-2.32 and/or anti-H-2.23 specificities present on parent C3H cells, and (3) to react with syngeneic (C3H) or heterogeneic (Swiss) macrophages.

It can be seen in FIGURE 9, that the IF-resistant (No. 57) and IF-sensitive (No. 36) clones differ in their avidity for binding soybean lectin but this avidity does not parallel the IF sensitivity of clones. On the contrary, the clone No. 57 with lower sensitivity toward IF binds significantly more of this lectin reacting with *N*-acetyl-galactosamine residue than the IF-sensitive clone No. 36. IF treatment did not enhance the lectin-binding capacity of treated clones.

The enhancing effect of IF on expressivity of two selected H-2 specificities (H-2.23 and H-2.32) in these clones seemed comparable suggesting that, in this effect, IF does not clearly discriminate between CGIE-sensitive and nonsensitive cells. FIGURE 10 shows the results of cytotoxicity tests with ^{51}Cr-labeled C3H target cells. Similar results were obtained in the microdroplet cytotoxicity test (not shown). However, these tests also indicate that transformation alone can lead to an enhanced expression of some of H-2 specificities.

On the other hand, both the syngeneic and heterogeneic macrophages proved to be capable of distinguishing the IF-sensitive and resistant MCH clones. IF treatment enhanced the cytotoxicity of macrophages for the IF-sensitive clone as well as for the "sensitive" L-cells, while the number of "resistant" cells surviving the cocultivation with macrophages remained significantly higher (FIGURE 11). This suggests that the IF- and the macrophage-sensitivity of a cell might be codetermined by the same marker.

DISCUSSION

In these studies, established mouse cell lines (L-929) and their sublines (LB2, LG, CSV-21), primary or secondary Swiss mouse embryonic cells, as well as secondary C3H embryonic cells transformed by an RNA virus (MSV), a DNA

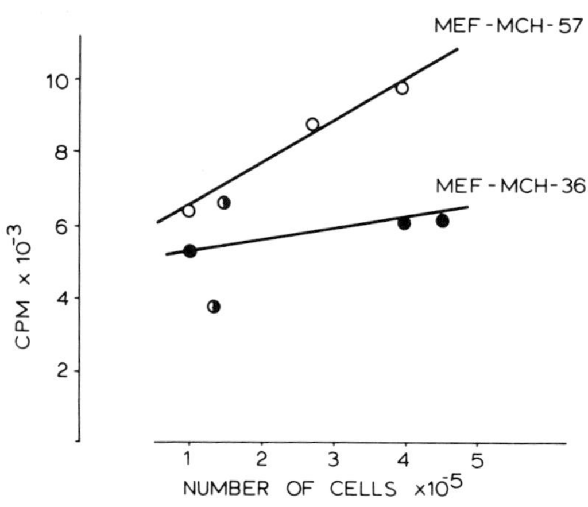

FIGURE 9. Binding of ^{125}I-labeled soybean lectin to interferon-sensitive (No. 36) and resistant (No. 57) MCH cells. *Ordinate:* cpm × 10^{-3} *Abscissa:* Number of cells treated × 10^{-5} ○——○: Clone No. 57, ●——●: Clone No. 36. ◑: Binding of lectin after treatment of cells with interferon.

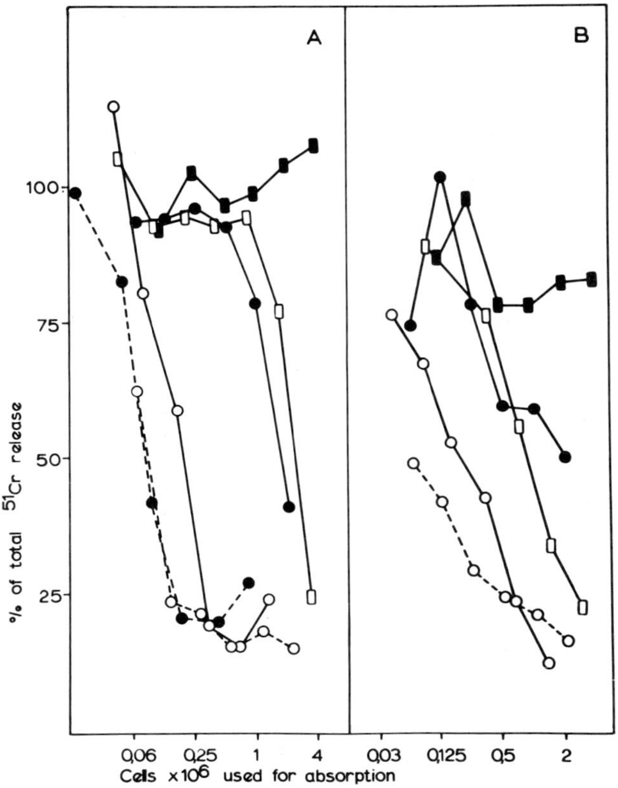

FIGURE 10. Residual cytotoxic activities of anti-H-2.23 (anti-K) and anti-H-2.32 (anti-D) sera for ^{51}Cr-labeled C3H fibroblasts after absorption with MCH-36 or MCH-57 cells.

Panel A: Anti-H-2.23 serum. *Panel B:* Anti-H-2.32 serum. *Ordinate:* Percent of total ^{51}Cr release *Abscissa:* Number of cells × 10^6 used for absorption. ○——○: MCH-36 cells; ○---○: MCH-36 cells treated with interferon; ●——●: MCH-57 cells; ●---●: MCH-57 cells treated with interferon; □——□: C3H cells (control): ■——■: control for unabsorbed serum. 12 × 10^3 units of interferon were used for treatment of 10^6 cells.

virus (SV40), or 20-methylcholanthrene were used. Transformed C3H cells were employed for two reasons. First, to show whether the transforming agent exerts a specific influence on the behavior of cells toward IF and, second, because transformed cells made possible the isolation of subculturable clones and registration of the effect of prolonged subcultivation on the response of cells to IF. The cells originating from a common C3H parent culture were considered "transformed" by either agent on the grounds of such criteria as focus formation in tissue culture, growth in semisolid agar and agglutinability by Concanavalin A. As auxiliary criteria, tumor production in newborn C3H mice and changes in chromosome number were examined. Since MSV-transformed cells, even after 26 passages *in vitro* did not grow in semisolid agar, as yet, no clones were obtained from this cell line. In contradistinction, clones were easily obtained from SV40-transformed cells, but they remained during at least 21 passages

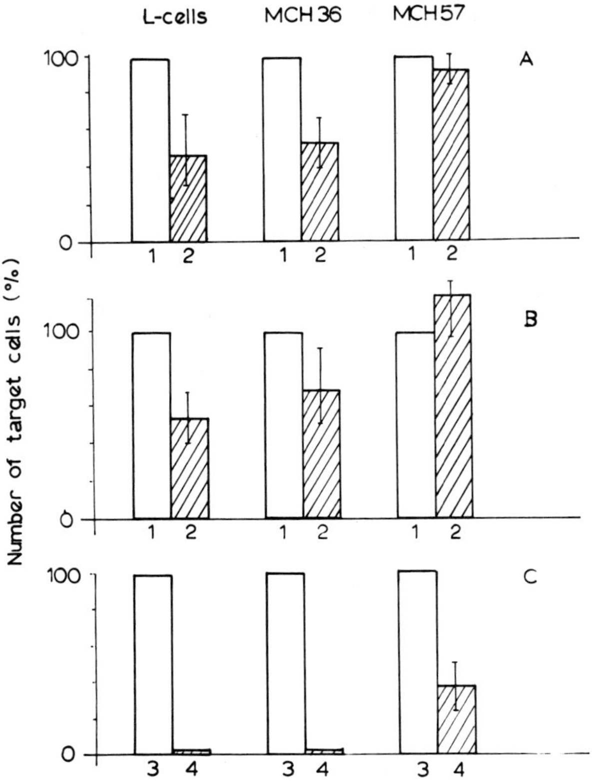

FIGURE 11. Growth inhibition of L-cells and 2 methylcholanthrene-transformed clones (No. 57 and 36) by activated peritoneal macrophages. A. Allogeneic (Swiss) macrophages 1: Target cells alone 2: Target cells with macrophages. B. Syngeneic (C3H) macrophages 1,2: As in A. C. Allogeneic (Swiss) macrophages 3: Target cells in the presence of macrophages 4: Interferon-treated target cells in the presence of macrophages.

Macrophages were activated with phage f2 ds-RNA (10 μg per 2×10^6 cells for 2 hr at 37° C). The target cells were preincubated with 100 units per ml of interferon (2 hr at 37° C). The number of surviving target cells was estimated in 3 parallels after 72 hr of contact with macrophages.

nontumorigenic for C3H mice. In this respect, the MCH-transformed cells occupy an intermediate position since they acquired both the ability to grow in semisolid agar and tumorigenicity after prolonged (32) passages *in vitro*. Concurrently, the MCH cells regained the IF-producing capacity, which was transiently lost after MCH-treatment of parent cells. Our experience with the MCH-transformed cells supports the view of Heidelberger,[22] O'Neill,[23] and others that expression of tumorigenicity in transformed cells requires prolonged passages *in vitro*, but is at variance with Barretts and Tso's[24] view that growth in soft agar correlates with tumorigenicity.

Eight clones and two subclones of SV40-transformed cells and seven clones and one subclone of MCH-transformed cells were obtained and used in comparative tests. While the sensitivity of clones to the AV activity of IF seems to be similar to that found in the parent lines, and their IF-producing capacity after stimulation with NDV was also comparable to the parent lines, i.e. it was either undetectable (SV40 clones) or retained (MCH clones), the sensitivity to the CGIE of IF in SV40 clones showed a more than 100-fold variation. The MCH clones on the basis of their sensitivity to the CGIE of IF can be divided into two groups. The variations in CGI sensitivity show no correlation with other parameters tested in this study. As follows from examination of a few subclones, the tested properties seem to be stable characteristics of the clone.

In order to gain some insight in the surface differences between clones, selected MCH clones were examined for their binding capacity of lectins, expression of H-2 specificities present on the surface of parent C3H cells, and destruction by macrophages. It has been found that the binding avidity for soybean lectin of the untreated "less" sensitive clone was significantly higher than that of the CGIE-sensitive clone. These results indicate differences in the concentration of *N*-acetyl-galactosamine on the surface of the clones examined and suggest that this sugar might hinder the CGIE of IF.[25]

The two MCH clones (No. 36 and 57) were tested by two methods also for expression of two H-2 specificities (H-2.32 and H-2.23) by their ability to absorb monospecific antisera after IF treatment. The results indicate that IF enhances the expression of both specificities on both cell-types in partial agreement with the report of Vignaux and Gresser.[26] The differences could be caused by the fact that the tested H-2 specificities were on transformed cells used in our study enhanced already before IF-treatment.

Finally, the cells of the IF-sensitive and the relatively insensitive MCH clones No. 36 and 57, respectively, were exposed to phagocytosis by allogeneic and/or syngeneic mouse peritoneal macrophages.

In this test, the sensitivity of the clone to the cytotoxic effect of macrophages was found to parallel its sensitivity to the CGIE of IF. This finding suggests that, at least in MCH-transformed cells, resistance to CGIE of IF and to cytotoxic effect of macrophages might be codetermined by the same surface component (*N*-acetyl-galactosamine).

Friedman and Pastan[27] reported that the AV activity of IF can be enhanced by pretreatment of chicken cells with cyclic nucleotides. Accordingly, the CGI resistance of the IF-resistant CSV-21 subline of LB2 cells was lowered by pretreatment of cells with PGE2 plus theophylline and/or cAMP.[4] However, no enhancement of CGIE was achieved by this treatment of the IF-sensitive parent LB2 line and the effect of PGE2 or cAMP in the CSV-21 cells in the absence of IF was marginal. This finding does not exclude the possibility that the expression of CGIE of IF in the cell might be determined by the level of the "second messenger," but the mechanism of this regulation remains unclear. First, in addition to cAMP and PGE2, other substances with cell-growth inhibitory activity, such as chalones, α-globulins etc., were found recently.[28] But as yet these inhibitors were not shown to exert a virus-suppressive effect.[29] Second, if we consider IF a hormone[30] requiring a second messenger of cAMP–cGMP type, then these substances after addition to the cells should mimic the CGIE of IF themselves.[31] Such an effect of cAMP was, however, not observed in cells used in our experiments and the cAMP sensitivity of cells did not parallel their IF sensitivity. Alternatively, the CGIE might be mediated by a special type of the second messenger. Interestingly, as yet, no report appeared on a transfer of CGIE from IF-treated to nontreated cells and there is no indication for participation of the presumed antiviral protein in CGIE.[10]

Taken together, these results suggest that the CGIE of IF might be mediated through receptors which differ from those mediating the AV effect.[32] Independent variation of CGIE in the clones and the relative uniformity of AV effect in these cells lend support to this hypothesis. Probably, a cooperation of receptors is required for a demonstrable CGIE since, in contradistinction to the AV effect, greater amounts of IF, longer contact and exponentially growing cells are long known prerequisites for its demonstration.[33] The suggested role of the *N*-acetyl-galactosamine residues in the functioning of these receptors remains to be confirmed by further studies.

These studies demonstrated also a functional "intraspecies" heterogeneity of the purified mouse IF that—with the results of clonal analysis of transformed cell—makes the attempts to unify the concept of IF presently premature. However, it seems safe to say today that should the CGIE activity of IF be effectively exploited in cancer therapy, a pretherapeutic *in vitro* testing of target cells is inevitable.

Summary

Eight clones and two subclones of SV40- and seven clones and one subclone of 20-methylcholanthrene-transformed C3H mouse embryonic fibroblasts were compared in tests for sensitivity to the antiviral and cell-growth inhibitory activities of a partially purified mouse L-cell interferon. While the sensitivity of clones and subclones to the antiviral activity of interferon was comparable to that of parent lines, the cell-growth inhibitory activity of interferon in the SV40 clones showed a more than 100-fold variation and the methylcholanthrene-transformed cells could be divided into two groups in this respect. No correlation of sensitivity to the cell-growth inhibitory effect of interferon with the chromosome number, interferon-producing capacity or tumorigenicity of clones could be detected. However, the cells of the interferon-sensitive clones No. 36 of the methylcholanthrene-transformed line were destroyed by macrophages at higher percentage than the cells of the resistant clone, and the resistant cells showed an increase binding of ^{125}I-labeled soybean lectin. These results suggest that (1) the cell-growth inhibitory effect of interferon might be mediated by a specific type of receptors, and (2) *N*-acetyl-galactosamine present on the surface of interferon-resistant cells in a higher concentration than on interferon-sensitive cells hinders the recognition of cells both by macrophages and by interferon.

References

1. Gresser, I. 1977. Cell. Immunol. **34:** 406–415.
2. Finter, N. B., Ed. 1973. Interferons and Interferon Inducers. 2nd edit. North-Holland, Publishing Co. Amsterdam and London.
3. Fuchsberger, N., L. Borecký, & V. Hajnická. 1974. Acta Virol. **18:** 85–87.
4. Borecký, L., N. Fuchsberger, V. Hajnická-Gondová, F. Čiampor & Č. Altaner. 1977. Neoplasma **24:** 125–137.
5. Macpherson, I. & L. Montagnier. 1964. Virology **23:** 291–294.
6. Russ, G., B. Styk & K. Poláková. 1978. Acta Virol. **22:** 1–10.
7. Schultz, R. M. & M. A. Chirigos. 1978. Cancer Res. **38:** 1003–1007.
8. Rothfels, K. H. & L. Siminovitsch. 1958. Stain. Technology **33:** 73–77.
9. Wigzell, H. 1965. Transplantation **3:** 423–431.
10. Mičková, M. & P. Ivanyi. 1973. Transplant. Proc. **5:** 1423–1425.

11. FUCHSBERGER, N., V. HAJNICKÁ & L. BORECKÝ. 1975. Acta Virol. **19:** 59–66.
12. STANČEK, D. & K. PAUCKER. 1970. Acta Virol. **14:** 125–132.
13. KAWADE, Y. 1973. Jap. J. Microbiol. **17:** 129–131.
14. CANTELL, K. 1970. Preparation of human leukocyte interferon. *In* International Symp. on Interferon and Interferon Inducers. Symp. Ser. Immunobiol Standards. **14:** 6–8. Karger, Basel, Switzerland.
15. LACKOVIČ, V. & L. BORECKÝ. 1965. Arch. Ges. Virusforsch. **17:** 619–624.
16. LAURELL, C. B. 1966. Analyt. Biochem. **15:** 45–51.
17. FUCHSBERGER, N. & L. BORECKÝ. 1978. Acta Virol. **22:** 238–240.
18. LACKOVIČ, V. & L. BORECKÝ. 1976. Acta Virol. **20:** 347–348.
19. KUWATA, T., A. FUSE & N. MORINAGA. 1976. J. Gen. Virol. **33:** 7–15.
20. GRESSER, I., M. T. BANDU & D. BRUOTY-BOYÉ. 1974. Jour. Nat. Cancer Inst. **52:** 553–559.
21. BORECKÝ, L., N. FUCHSBERGER & V. HAJNICKÁ. 1974. Intervirology **3:** 369–377.
22. HEIDELBERGER, C. H. 1977. Cancer **40:** 430–433.
23. O'NEILL, F. J. 1978. Exp. Cell. Res. **117:** 393–401.
24. BARRETT, J. C. & P. O. P. TS'O. 1978. Proc. Nat. Acad. Sci. USA **75:** 3297–3301.
25. JANKOWSKI, W. J., M. W. DAVEY, J. A. O'MALLEY, E. SULKOWSKI & W. A. CARTER. 1975. J. Virol. **16:** 1124–1130.
26. VIGNAUX, F. & I. GRESSER. 1978. Proc. Soc. Exp. Biol. Med. **157:** 456–460.
27. FRIEDMAN, R. M. & I. PASTAN. 1969. Biochem. Biophys. Res. Commun. **36:** 735.
28. LIPKIN, G., M. ROSENBERG & M. E. KNECHT. 1976. Biochem. Pharmacol. **25:** 1333–1337.
29. KARINIEMI, A. L. 1977. Acta Derm. Venereol. (Stockholm) **57**(Suppl.): 1–26.
30. HUANG, K. 1977. Texas Res. Biol. Med. **35:** 350–356.
31. MALKINSON, A. M. 1975. Hormone Action. Outline in Studies in Biology. :10–37. Chapman and Hall. London.
32. CHANY, C. 1976. Biomedicine **25:** 148–157.
33. RILEY, F. L. & H. B. LEVY. 1977. Effect of interferon on cellular RNA synthesis and structure. *In* the Interferon System. A Current Review to 1978. S. Baron & F. Dianzani. Eds. Texas Rep. Biol. Med. **35:** 239–246.

DOES HUMAN LEUKOCYTE INTERFERON INFLUENCE THE RESTRICTION POINT CONTROL IN CULTURED CELLS?

Abla A. Creasey,* James C. Bartholomew,†
and Thomas C. Merigan*

**Division of Infectious Diseases*
Department of Medicine
Stanford University School of Medicine
Stanford, California 94305

†Laboratory of Chemical Biodynamics
Lawrence Berkeley Laboratory
University of California
Berkeley, California 94720

Inteferons display a tumor-reducing effect in a number of human tumors *in vivo*.[1-3] In cell culture, interferons inhibit the proliferation of both normal and malignant cells.[4-7] The mechanism of this inhibition of growth is unclear. Normal cells in culture can be shifted between proliferation and quiescence, depending of the accomplishment of a specific event in G_1 called restriction point.[8,9] One of many possibilities as to the mechanism of the antiproliferative action of interferon is that interferons may influence that event in a manner which limits cell cycling. We therefore used two indirect approaches to test this hypothesis:

1. We studied the effect of interferon on the growth of a number of human melanoma cell lines. Some of these lines have maintained the restriction point control and others seem to have altered regulation of that control mechanism.
2. We studied the kinetics of transition of cells out of the quiescent state into the proliferative phase in the presence of interferon.

Effect of Interferon on the Growth of the Melanoma Cells

Human leukocyte interferon preparations (specific activity of 10^6 reference units per milliliter) in concentrations of 25 to 10^3 U/ml were used to determine the growth inhibitory dose for each of the melanoma cell lines. Using viable cell counts, lines with growth reduction of 40% or less with 10^3 U/ml of interferon were considered interferon resistant. The inhibition of growth was not associated with a direct toxic effect as determined both by 0.1% trypan blue exclusion and plating cells previously exposed to interferon for colony counts. Melanoma cell lines with restriction point control (i.e., those which reside in G_0-G_1 at saturation density) are more susceptible to growth inhibition by interferon than those which seem to have altered regulation of that transition (Table 1). The distribution in the cell cycle was determined by flow cytometry and autoradiography;[10,11] when greater than 90% of the cells had G_1 DNA content at saturation density the cultures were considered blocked in G_0-G_1.

It was interesting to find out that the observed correlation between behavior at saturation density and interferon sensitivity holds true for cell lines other than melanoma (Table 1).

TABLE 1

RELATIONSHIP OF CELL CYCLE BEHAVIOR TO INTERFERON SENSITIVITY

Human Cell Lines	Growth Inhibition by Interferon (U/ml) 25	250	1000	Antiviral Activity of Interferon (250 U/ml)	Restriction Point Control*
Hs294T	+†	+	+	+‡	+
Hs852T	−§	+	+	+	+
Hs939T	−	+	+	+	+
M3	−	+	+	+	+
SH4	−	−	+	+	+
Hs294T-Clone 6 revertant	−	+	+	+	+
GM37	−	−	+	+	+
Hs294T-Clone 6	−	−	−	−¶	−
GM637-SV40 transformed	−	−	−	−	−
Hs695T	−	−	−	+	−
HeLa	−	−	−	+	−

*Only cell lines that block in G_0–G_1 at saturation density were considered to have the restriction point control. Populations with greater than 90% G_1 cells were considered blocked in G_0–G_1.

†+ means greater than 40% reduction in cell number as compared to control.

‡+ means virus titer was reduced by interferon treatment of the cells.

§− means less than 40% reduction in cell number as compared to control.

¶− means virus titer was *not* reduced by interferon treatment of the cells.

EFFECTS OF INTERFERON ON THE CELL CYCLE

Interferon treatment (250 U/ml) of actively growing melanoma cells (Hs294T) impeded their progression from one phase of the cell cycle to another. Indeed, the fraction of the population in each of the phases of the cell cycle essentially remained constant over the 4-day period. Control cells, however, progressed towards residence in G_1, which is consistent with their behavior at saturation density.

Constant cell cycle distribution as a function of time could have meant that interferon had no effect on the cell cycle or that it slowed the cells in all phases of the cell cycle. The first alternative, however, is not consistent with the growth response of these cells (TABLE 1) to interferon. It is then more likely that interferon blocks movement through all phases of the cell cycle. We therefore tested the latter possibility by using colcemid (0.2 μg/ml for 16 hours) to impose a specific block in mitosis to see if interferon-treated cells would accumulate behind the block. Control cells were trapped behind the block, while almost none of the interferon-treated cells accumulated in mitosis. We concluded that in growing populations interferon hindered the progress of cells through all phases of the cell cycle.

The effect of interferon (250 U/ml) on the progress of quiescent, serum-stimulated (G_0-G_1) cells into S was studied kinetically. Under these conditions, we found that interferon does not block the serum stimulation of the cells; however, it did decrease the transition rate of the cells out of G_0-G_1, and increased the dispersion in the transit time from the beginning of serum stimulation to the entrance of cells into S. Furthermore, movement through S was extended by several hours. In those experiments where the progress of interferon-treated cells through the cell cycle was followed for 2 to 3 days, there was little evidence of a start of a new movement into S in the presence of interferon.[12]

Time of interferon treatment of cells seems to be a critical factor in the expression of many of the cell cycle perturbations caused by interferon. We have found that interferon treatment of cells 4 to 6 hours before commencement of DNA synthesis perturbs cycling through S for those cells already committed to make DNA before interferon was added. However, treatment of cells in early G_1 seems to influence the commitment step itself, because the transition probability of the cells out of G_0-G_1 into S is greatly decreased. Treatment of cells in S has minimal inhibitory effects on DNA synthesis during that division cycle.

Relationship of Antiviral and Anticellular Effects of Interferon

The association of the antiviral and antiproliferative activities of interferon in the same molecule has been a subject of controversy in the literature. The availability of a number of cell lines with various growth responses to interferon allowed us to investigate this issue. A summary of the ability of interferon to inhibit VSV replication in cells used in this study is shown in Table 1. Most cell lines, except two (Hs294T-clone 6 and GM637), were sensitive to the antiviral action of interferon. Of interest is the association of the two activities of interferon in all but two of the cell lines (Table 1).

References

1. Strander, J. K., K. Cantell & C. Carstrom. 1973. J. Nat. Cancer Inst. **51:** 733–742.
2. Merigan T. C., K. Sikora, J. Breeden, R. Levy & S. Rosenberg. 1978. New Engl. J. Med. **299:** 1449–1453.
3. Merigan, T. C. 1979. New Engl. J. Med. **300:** 42–43.
4. Paucker, K., K. Cantell & W. Henle. 1962. Virology **7:** 324–334.
5. Balkwill, F. R. & R. T. D. Oliver. 1977. Int. J. Cancer **20:** 500–505.
6. Strander, H. & S. Einhorn. 1977. Int. J. Cancer **14:** 468–473.
7. Lundgren, E., I. Larsson, H. Miorner, & O. Strannegard. 1979. J. Gen. Virol. **42:** 589–595.
8. Temin, H. 1971. J. Cell. Physiol. **78:** 161–170.
9. Pardee, A. B. 1974. Proc. Natl. Acad. Sci. USA **71:** 1286–1290.
10. Bartholomew, J. C., H. Yokota & P. Ross. 1967. J. Cell Physiol. **88:** 277–286.
11. Bartholomew, J. C., A. L. Pearlman, J. R. Landolph & K. Straub. 1979. Cancer Res. **39:** 2538–2543.
12. Creasey, A. A., J. Bartholomew & T. C. Merigan. 1980. Proc. Natl. Acad. Sci. USA **77:** 1471–1475.
13. Dahl, H. & M. Degre. 1975. Nature **257:** 799–801.
14. Knight, E., Jr., 1976. Nature **262:** 302–303.

EFFECTS OF CONCANAVALIN A ON THE ANTIVIRAL AND CELL GROWTH INHIBITORY ACTION OF HUMAN INTERFERONS

T. Kuwata,* A. Fuse,* N. Takayama,† and N. Morinaga*

**Department of Microbiology*
School of Medicine, Chiba University
Chiba 280, Japan
†Tokyo Metropolitan Komagome Hospital
Tokyo 113, Japan

In addition to its antiviral activity, pleiotypic actions of interferon have been reported in recent years.[1-3] However, it is not yet clear whether such actions are based on the common mechanism or not. We examined the effect of cycloheximide and puromycin on the antiviral and cell growth-inhibitory action of human and mouse interferon.[4] These protein inhibitors partly inhibited the antiviral action of human leukocyte interferon (Le-IF) in our RSa and RSb cell lines, as already reported in other cells.[3] However, when these agents were applied to cells together with Le-IF, they suppressed the multiplication of cells to a remarkably greater degree than when applied singly. Such results may suggest that protein synthesis is required for the expression of the antiviral action of interferon but, for the suppression of cell growth, protein synthesis might not be needed. A discrepancy between the effects on antiviral and cell growth-inhibitory actions was also demonstrated by using ouabain[5] and cholera toxin.[6]

On the other hand, Besançon and Ankel[7] reported that when Sepharose-bound mouse interferon was pretreated with concanavalin-A (Con A), its antiviral action was abolished. In addition, when mouse L cells were pretreated with phytohemagglutinin (PHA) or Con A, then antiviral action of interferon was also partially suppressed. Thus, Con A seemed to be bound to the mouse interferon molecule or to the interferon receptor on the cell surface. Therefore, we studied the effect of lectins on the antiviral and anticellular action of human interferons. In this report, we describe the effect of Con A on the antiviral and cell-growth-inhibitory action of human interferons by using human transformed cell line, RSa, and its variant cell lines.

Materials and Methods

Cells

Human transformed cell line RSa and its interferon-resistant variant IF^r were used as before.[4,5,8] Con A-resistant cell lines, Con A^r-1 and Con A^r-3, were isolated by treating RSa cells with 100 μg/ml of ethylmethane sulfonate for 24 hours and selected with 20 μg/ml of Con A. Details of biological characteristics of these cell lines will be reported separately. Human uterine adenocarcinoma cell line HEC-1B was supplied by Dr. S. Sekiya of the Department of Gynecology and Obstetrics of our Medical School. Human cell line VA-13, which was transformed by simian virus 40, was obtained, through Dr. T. Oda, Cancer Institute, Okayama University. All these cell lines were maintained by using Eagle's

0077-8923/80/0350-0211 $01.75/0 © 1980, NYAS

minimal essential medium (MEM) supplemented with 10% calf serum at 37°C in 5% CO_2 in air. For the experiments using Con A, serum concentration was reduced to 5% in the culture medium.

Estimation of Cell Multiplication

About 2×10^5 cells were seeded into 60 mm plastic dishes in 5 ml of culture medium. After 24 hours, the culture medium was changed for that with or without Con-A and then the culture medium was changed every other day. On the sixth day, Con A-treated cells were at first treated with 10 mM α-methyl-D-mannoside at 37°C and then detached from dishes with 2 mM EDTA. Control cells were detached with the mixture of EDTA-trypsin solution. Viable cells were determined by dye exclusion test with 0.4% trypan blue solution.

Measurement of DNA and Protein Synthesis

DNA and protein synthesis were measured as described before.[6,9] Cells in Linbro multi-well plate (No. 76-033-05) were refed with MEM containing various concentrations of Con A. Monolayers were rinsed twice with MEM after 24 hours incubation and incubated in 0.2 ml of MEM (minus amino acids) containing 0.1 μCi of ^{3}H-thymidine (20 Ci/mmol) and 0.05 μCi of ^{14}C-amino acid mixture (50 mCi/milliatom carbon). After one hour of incubation cells were washed three times with cold calcium- and magnesium-free phosphate buffered saline (PBS) and lysed by adding 0.5 ml of 0.5% sodium dodecyl sulfate (SDS) solutions. Then, 0.5 ml of 20% trichloroacetic acid solutions were added and the radioactivity of acid-precipitable materials was measured in a Beckman LS-235 liquid scintillation counter.

Virus

Vesicular stomatitis virus (VSV), Indiana strain, was used for the assay of interferon and measurement of antiviral state in the cells. Virus titers were estimated by using RSa cells cultured in Linbro multi-well plate (No. 76-003-05) and 50% tissue culture infectious dose ($TCID_{50}$) was calculated.

Interferons

Human leukocyte interferon (Le-IF) was kindly provided by Dr. K. Cantell, Central Public Health Laboratory, Helsinki. Its specific activity was 4×10^6 U/mg protein. Human fibroblast interferon (F-IF) was the gift of Dr. A. Billiau, Rega Institute, Leuven, Belgium. Its specific activity was 6.5×10^5 U/mg protein. Interferons were assayed by estimating 50% inhibition of cytopathic changes in RSa cells caused by about 80 $TCID_{50}$ of VSV, and expressed as reference units/ml.

Lectin

Con A was purchased from Pharmacia Fine Chemicals AB, Uppsala, Sweden. Con A was dissolved in PBS at the concentration of 1 mg/ml and aliquots were stored at −20°C.

Cell Agglutination Assay

The cells were washed three times with PBS and then harvested with 2 mM EDTA. After the cells were washed once with PBS, cell suspensions were prepared with PBS at the concentration of 10^6 cells/ml. Equal volumes of cell suspension and Con A solution were put into wells of Linbro multi-well plate (No. 76-033-05) and gently shaken for 30 minutes at room temperature. Cell agglutination was examined by an inverted microscope and scored from 0 to ++++.

Con A-binding Assay

^{125}I-labeled Con A (specific activity, 4.2×10^4 cpm/μg) was prepared by using chloramine T as described by Hunter,[10] and unbound iodine was removed by chromatography on a column of Biogel-P60. More than 95% of labeled Con A was bound to chick erythrocytes.

The cells were cultured in the wells of Linbro multi-well plate (No. 76-033-05). After being washed twice with PBS, ^{125}I-Con A was added to a total volume of 0.2 ml of PBS containing 0.25% bovine serum albumin. After 30 min of incubation at room temperature, the cell monolayers were washed three times with PBS (0.25% BSA) and removed from the wells with 0.5% SDS solution. Radioactivity bound to the cells was determined directly by a gamma-counter. Nonspecific binding of ^{125}I-labeled Con A was less than 10% of the total radioactivity bound in the absence of α-methyl-D-mannoside.

Electron Microscopy

After incubation with Le-IF (100 U/ml) or mock-IF for 20 hours, the cells were fixed with 2.5% glutaraldehyde in PBS at 4°C overnight. After being washed with 0.2 M cacodylate buffer (pH 7.6), the monolayers were incubated with cacodylate buffer (pH 7.6) containing 100 μg/ml of Con A for 30 min at room temperature. The dishes were washed three times with 0.2 M cacodylate buffer (pH 7.2) and then incubated with peroxidase in 0.2 M cacodylate buffer (pH 7.2) at the concentration of 1 mg/ml for 40 min.[11] The diaminobenzidine (DBA) reaction was performed by incubation of the cells with 3,3′-diaminobenzidine (1 mg/ml) in 0.05 M Tris buffer (pH 7.6) containing 0.01% H_2O_2 for 15 min at room temperature, and then cell layers were postfixed with 1% OsO_4 in PBS for 60 min. Thin sections were stained with lead citrate for 2 min, and examined with a Hitachi H300 electron microscope.

RESULTS

Cytotoxicity of Con A to RSa and Its Variant Cell Lines

In order to examine correlation between sensitivity of cells to interferon and to cytotoxicity of Con A, RSa and its variant cell lines, IF^r and Con A^r-3, were compared for their sensitivity to Con A. As shown in FIGURE 1, RSa cells were sensitive to Con-A cytotoxicity and the Con A concentration that suppressed the cell number to 10% of control was about 25 μg/ml. In contrast, Con A^r-3 cells were fairly resistant to 80 μg/ml of Con A. Unexpectedly, interferon-resistant IF^r cells were partially resistant to Con A and the dose necessary to suppress to 10% of control was about 35 μg/ml. These results were confirmed by the inhibition of DNA and protein synthesis by Con A in these three cell lines (FIGURE 2). Relative

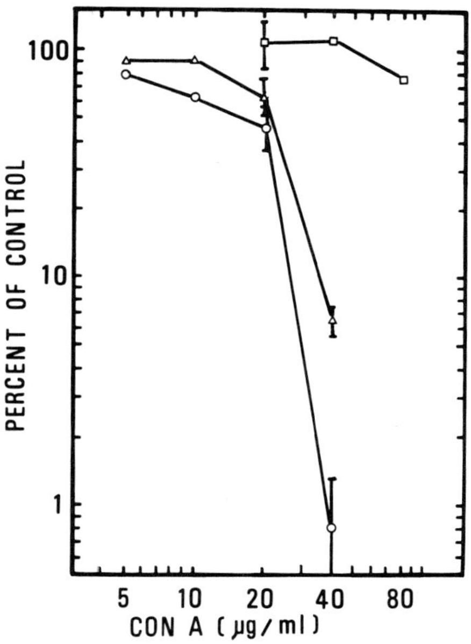

FIGURE 1. Cytotoxicity of Con A for RSa (○——○), IF^r (△——△), and Con A^r -3 (□——□) cells. After treatment with Con A for 6 days, viable cells were counted and the ratio of numbers of Con A-treated and not treated cells were calculated. Con A was diluted with MEM with 5% calf serum.

resistance of IF^r cells suggests that variation from interferon sensitivity to resistance elicited some changes in plasma membrane of IF^r cells.

Agglutination of Cells by Con A

It has been well established that Con A agglutinates transformed cells preferentially.[12] Therefore, Con A agglutinabilities of RSa, IF^r, and Con A-resistant cells were compared (TABLE 1). In this test, almost no difference was detected in the agglutinability between RSa and IF^r cells. In disagreement with the results already reported by others,[13,14] Con A^r-1 and Con A^r-3 were also sensitive to Con A agglutination. RSa cells treated with 100 U/ml of Le-IF were agglutinated by Con A as nontreated cells.

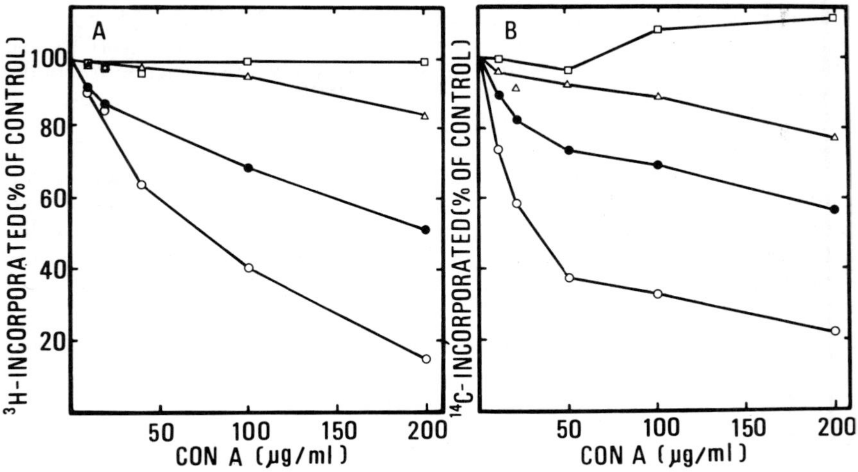

FIGURE 2. Effect of Con A on DNA and protein synthesis of cells. Procedures of measurement of DNA and protein synthesis were described in MATERIALS AND METHODS. ○——○, RSa; ●——●, IF^r; △——△, Con A^r −3; □——□, Con A^r−1.

Combined Effect of Con A and Interferon on Multiplication and Viability of RSa and IF^r Cells

RSa cells are quite sensitive to the cell growth-inhibitory action of Le-IF and F-IF. Therefore, RSa cells were treated with Con A and Le-IF, and their effect on the growth of cells was examined (FIGURE 3A). The number of viable cells 6 days after Con A or Le-IF treatment was 45% and 29% of control, respectively, but in the case of combined treatment, surviving cells were about 2.0% of control. The same kind of experiment using Con A and F-IF (FIGURE 3B) showed that combined treatment also markedly inhibited cell multiplication, and Con A and interferon seemed to act on cells synergistically.

In the next experiment, Con A concentration was maintained at 20 μg/ml and

TABLE 1
AGGLUTINATION OF CELLS BY CON A

	Con A Concentration (μg/ml)									
Cells	320	160	80	40	20	10	5	2.5	1.25	0
RSa	++++	++++	++++	+++	+++	+++	++	+	−	−
RSa*	++++	++++	++++	+++	++	++	+	±	−	−
IF^r	++++	++++	++++	+++	+++	+++	++	+	−	−
Con A^r − 3	++++	++++	++++	+++	+++	+++	++	+	−	−
Con A^r − 1	NT	+++	+++	++	++	+	+	−	−	−
Con A^r − 1†	NT	+	−	−	−	−	−	−	−	−

*Treated with 1000 U/ml of Le-IF for 24 hours.
†In the presence of 10 mM α-methyl-D-mannoside.
NT: not tested.

units of interferon applied were changed from 10 to 200 U/ml, and combined effect of Con A and Le-IF was examined (FIGURE 4). When the cells were treated with 20 μg/ml Con A for 6 days, survival of viable cells was 61% of control. In the case of combined treatment, however, a marked decrease in viable cells was evident with increasing units of Le-IF.

To determine whether these results were due chiefly to the effect of interferon or Con A, IF^r cells were used and the combined effect of Con A and interferon was examined (FIGURE 5A). In this case, 400 U/ml of Le-IF was applied, and the effect of combined treatment was slightly lower than was the case with RSa cells (FIGURE 3A) but, such an effect was apparent. IF^r cells were partially resistant to F-IF,[15] and combined treatment of cells with F-IF and Con A

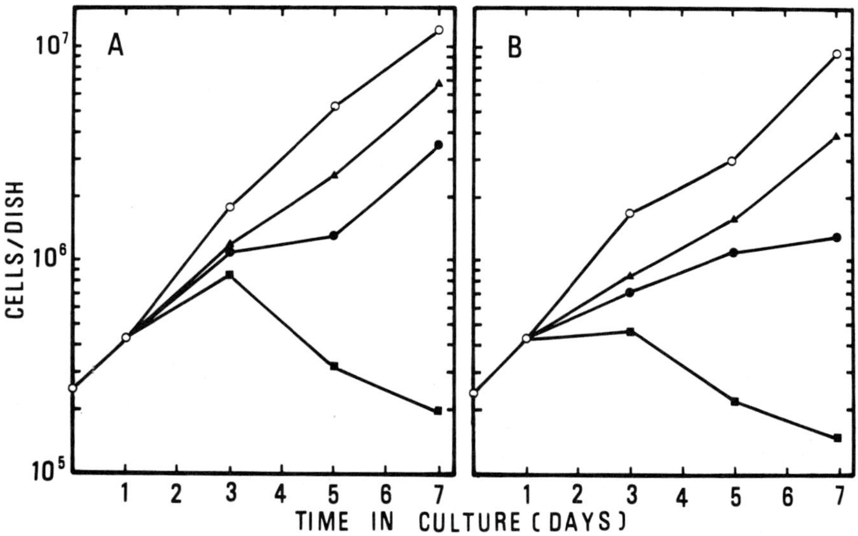

FIGURE 3. Combined treatment of RSa cells with Con A and Le-IF (A) or F-IF(B). ○——○, control cells; ●——●, treated with 200 U/ml of Le-IF(A) or 20 U/ml of F-IF(B); ▲——▲, treated with 20 μg/ml of Con A; ■——■, treated with 200 U/ml of Le-IF(A) or 20 U/ml of F-IF(B) and 20 μg/ml of Con A. In the case of combined treatment, interferon and Con A were mixed and preincubated in a water bath at 37°C for 1 hr and the cells were then treated with such mixtures.

also showed a synergistic effect (FIGURE 5B). As shown in the later experiments, only slight, if any, enhancement of Con A binding by interferon was observed in IF^r cells. Therefore, the enhanced effect of cell growth inhibition by combined treatment might not be considered to be due to enhanced Con A binding by interferon.

Effect of Con A and Interferon on Con A^r Cells

The effect of combined treatment with Con A and interferon was also examined by using Con A-resistant Con A^r cells. We found the sensitivity of this cell line to the anticellular action of interferon to be slightly greater than that of

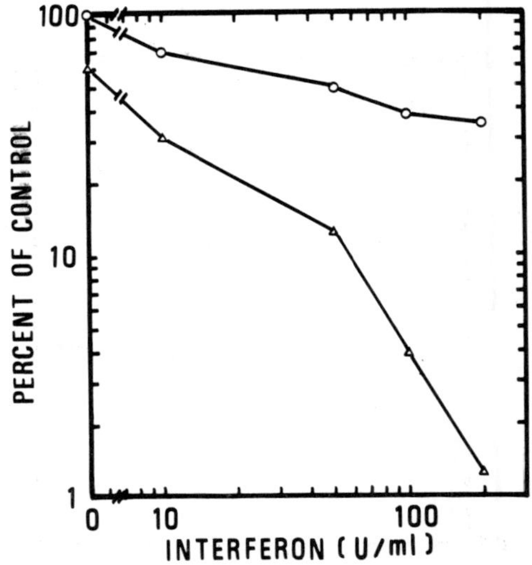

FIGURE 4. Comparison of viable cells after combined treatment with 20 μg/ml of Con A and varying doses of Le-IF. ○——○, treated with Le-IF alone; △——△, treated with 20 μg/ml of Con A and Le-IF.

RSa (FIGURES 3A and 6A). When 200 U/ml of Le-IF and 20 μg/ml of Con A were combined, their effect was almost equal to the results obtained after treatment with Le-IF alone (FIGURE 6A), probably because the dose of Con A was too low. A similar result was also obtained with F-IF and Con-A (FIGURE 6B). When combined treatment with 200 U/ml of Le-IF and 100 μg/ml of Con A was performed in these cells, a synergistic effect was also observed (FIGURE 6C).

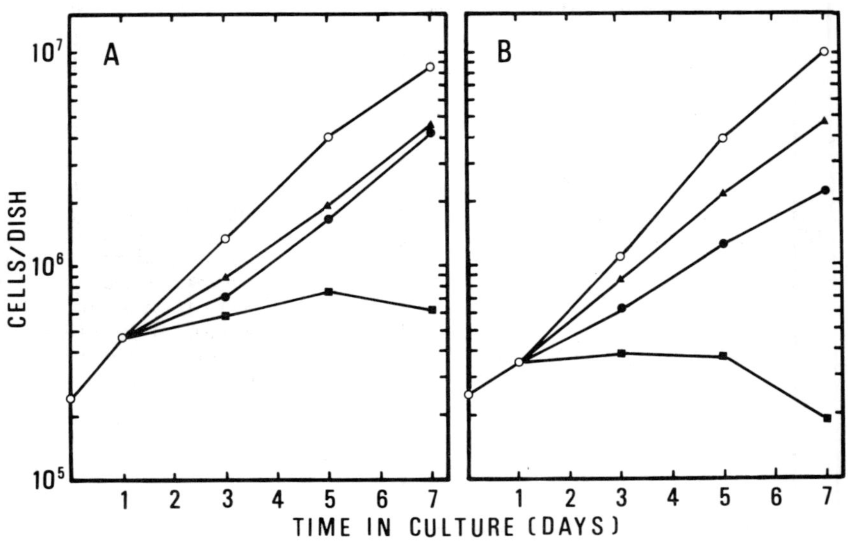

FIGURE 5. Combined treatment of IF^r cells with Con A and Le-IF(A) or F-IF(B). ○——○, control cells; ●——●, treated with 400 U/ml of Le-IF(A) or 100 U/ml of F-IF(B); ▲——▲, treated with 20 μg/ml of Con A; ■——■, treated with 400 U/ml of Le-IF(A) or 100 U/ml of F-IF(B) and 20 μg/ml of Con A.

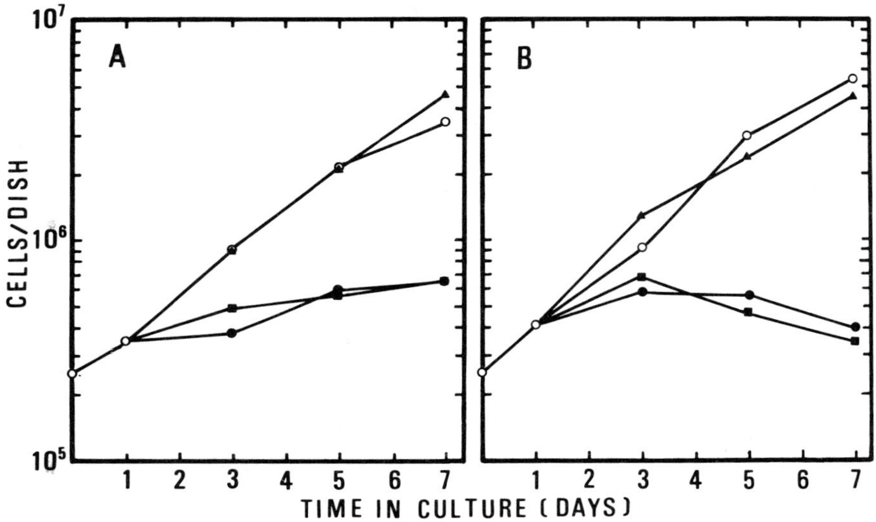

FIGURE 6A & B. Combined treatment of Con A^r-3 cells with Le-IF (A) or F-IF (B) and Con A. ○——○, control cells; ●——●, treated with 200 U/ml of Le-IF (A) or 20 U/ml of F-IF (B); ▲——▲, treated with 20 μg/ml of Con A; ■——■, treated with 200 U/ml of Le-IF (A) or 20 U/ml of F-IF (B) and 20 μg/ml of Con A.

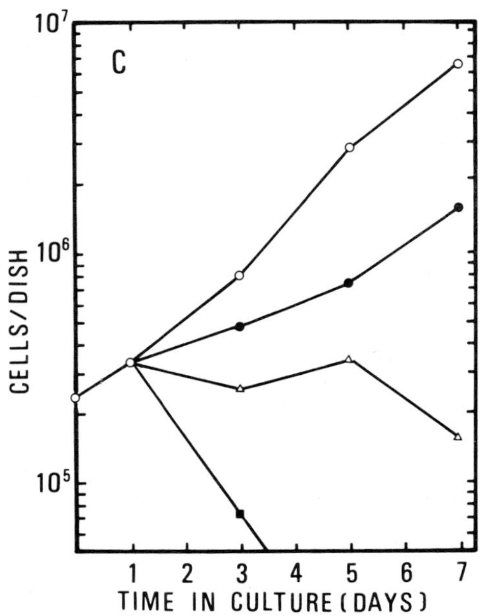

FIGURE 6C. Combined treatment of Con A^r-3 cells with Le-IF and Con A. ○——○, control cells; ●——●, treated with 200 U/ml of Le-IF; △——△, treated with 100 μg/ml of Con A; ■——■, treated with 200 U/ml of Le-IF and 100 μg/ml of Con A.

TABLE 2
EFFECT OF INTERFERON AND CON A ON DNA SYNTHESIS IN RSa AND CON A^r CELLS

Cells	Treatment* Interferon (U/ml)	Con A (μg/ml)	^{3}H-Thymidine Incorporated	% Of Control
RSa	0	0	21800 19323	100
	0	20	11039 12308	58
	Le-IF 200	0	5972 4224	25
	F-IF 20	0	8934 8488	43
	Le-IF 200	20	4163 3274	18
	F-IF 20	20	7283 6526	34
Con A^r−3	0	0	21975 19852	100
	0	20	21245 21996	102
	Le-IF 200	0	7927 6113	33
	F-IF 20	0	13109 11993	60
	Le-IF 200	20	6031 5542	29
	F-IF 20	20	11637 11195	55

*Cells were treated with interferon or Con A or with both for 26 hours.

Since the cells were treated with Con A and interferon continuously for 6 days in the above experiments, the effect of these agents on the cells was estimated in a shorter period by measuring the rate of incorporation of ^{3}H-thymidine (TABLE 2). These results show that treatment with Con A and interferon suppressed thymidine incorporation more than that with Con A or interferon

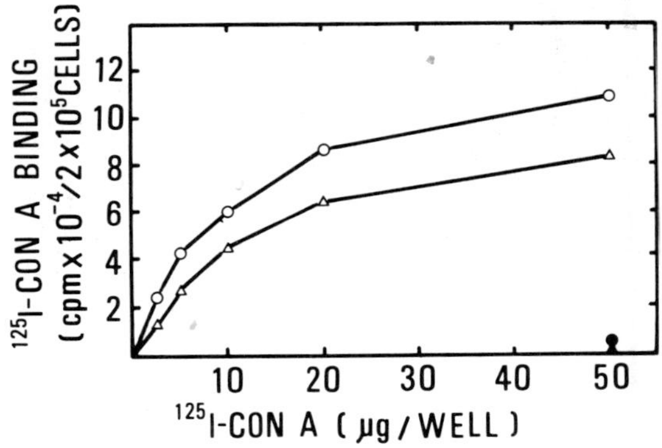

FIGURE 7. Binding of Con A to RSa (O——O) and Con A^r−3 cells (Δ——Δ). Experimental procedure was described in MATERIALS AND METHODS. At the same time RSa cells (●) and Con A^r−3 cells (▲) were also treated with ^{125}I-labeled Con A in the presence of 0.1 M α-methyl-D-mannoside.

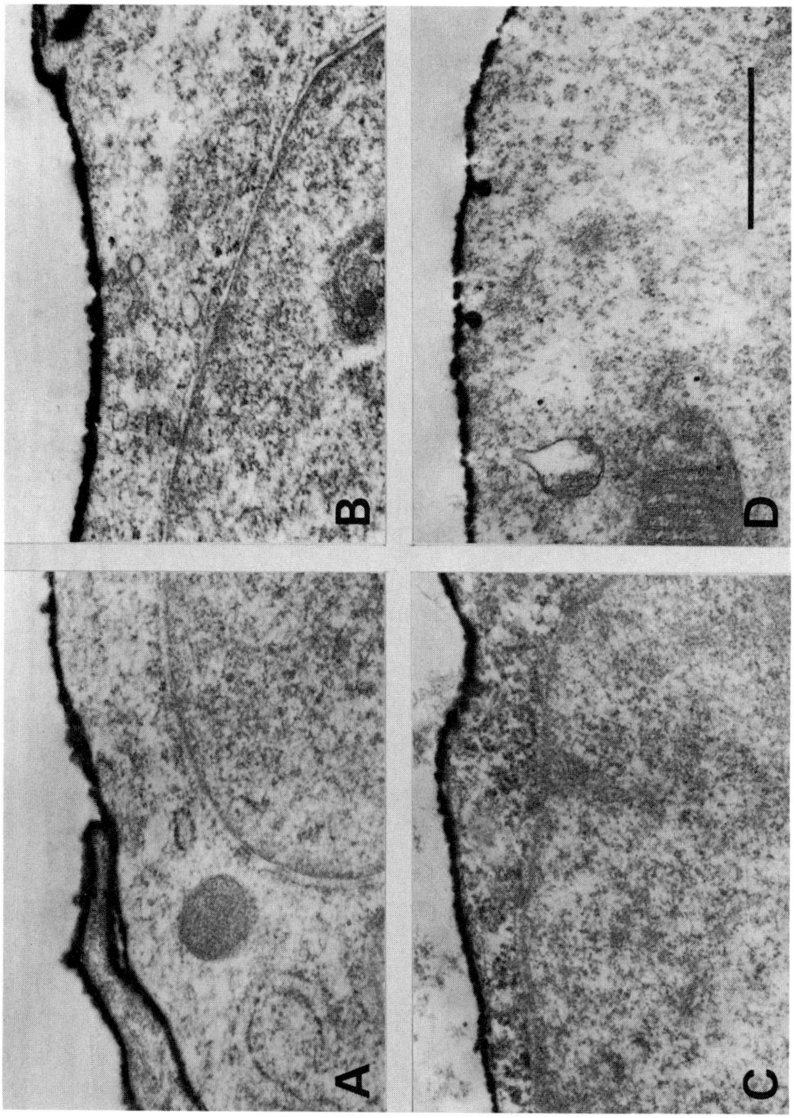

FIGURE 8. Binding of Con A to the surface of RSa and Con A^r-3 cells. The bar indicates 1 μm. A: Con A^r-3 cell treated with 100 U/ml of Le-IF; B: RSa cell treated with 100 U/ml of Le-IF; C: Con A^r-3 cell treated with mock Le-IF; D: RSa cell treated with mock Le-IF.

alone in RSa and to a lesser degree in Con A^r−3 cells. These results are different from the effect of Con A on the antiviral action of interferon, as will be shown in the later experiments described in this paper.

Con A Binding to RSa and Con A^r Cells

To analyze the effect of Con A on the growth of cells, binding of Con A to the cell was measured by using ^{125}I-labeled Con A (FIGURE 7). Con A^r−3 cells were resistant to the cytotoxicity of Con A (FIGURE 1), but they also adsorbed Con A in about 73% of RSa (FIGURE 7). These results suggest that there is no direct correlation between the grade of binding and sensitivity of cells to cytotoxicity of Con A. Localization of Con A adsorbed to the cells was demonstrated in electron micrographs (FIGURE 8). These pictures also indicate that Con A was adsorbed to the cell surface of Con A^r cells as in the case of RSa cells. In control cells, which

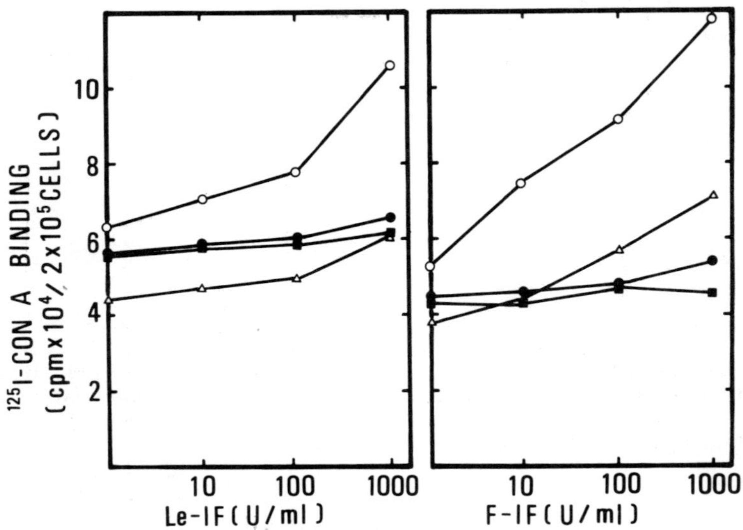

FIGURE 9. Effect of Le-IF(A) and F-IF(B) on the Con A binding to cells. O——O, Rsa; ●——●, IF^r; Δ——Δ, Con A^r−3; □——□, HEC. Cells were treated with either Le-IF or F-IF for 40 hr. After the cells had been washed twice with PBS, 50 μg of ^{125}I-Con A were added to each well. Con A binding was measured as in FIGURE 7.

were treated with Le-IF but not treated with Con A, there were no such deposits on the cell surface.

Enhancement of Con A Binding by Interferon

It has been reported that mouse interferon increased the binding of Con A to mouse leukemic cells L 1210.[16] Therefore, attempts were made to examine whether human Le-IF or F-IF could enhance Con A binding in our cell system. As shown in FIGURE 9A, treatment with 1000 U/ml of Le-IF enhanced Con A binding to RSa by 65% and also to Con A^r-3 cells by about 35%. This enhancement depended on the dose of interferon applied. However, in IF^r cells, enhancement was about 10% and in HEC cells, which are quite resistant to the cell growth-inhibitory action of interferon (unpublished data), little, if any, enhancement of Con A binding was detected. Same kind of experiments were performed by using F-IF (FIGURE 9B). In this case F-IF enhanced more markedly than in the case of Le-IF and 1000 U/ml of F-IF enhanced Con A binding by 120% in RSa and in Con A^r-3 cells enhancement by over 80% was detected. However, IF^r cells were rather resistant to enhancement of Con A binding by F-IF as in the case of Le-IF.

TABLE 3

EFFECT OF SUCCESSIVE TREATMENT OF RSa CELLS WITH INTERFERON AND CON A ON THE ANTIVIRAL ACTION OF INTERFERON

Treatment*			
Le-IF (U/ml)	Con A (μg/ml)	VSV Titer (log $TCID_{50}$/0.2 ml)	Inhibition
0	0	7.5	
200	0	3.2	4.3
0	500	6.2	
200	500	2.0	4.2
0	250	6.5	
200	250	2.2	4.3
0	100	6.7	
200	100	2.2	4.5
0	50	7.0	
200	50	3.0	4.0

*RSa cells were treated with 200 U/ml of Le-IF for 22 hours, once washed with MEM, and then treated with Con A for 1 hour. After having been washed once with MEM, cells were infected with VSV at approximately 1 $TCID_{50}$/cell. Medium samples were taken 16 hours after infection and assayed for infectious VSV. In this and the following experiments, Con A was diluted with PBS and interferon with MEM.

Effect of Con A on the Antiviral Action

RSa cells were pretreated with 200 U/ml of Le-IF, then treated with various concentrations of Con A for 1 hour and then challenged with VSV (TABLE 3). It was verified above that interferon treatment enhances Con A binding to the cell surface, but there was almost no effect of Con A on the antiviral state of the cells induced by Le-IF. When the cells were treated first with Con A and then with interferon, the effect of Con A was slightly suppressive in RSa cells, but not so in Con A^r-3 (TABLE 4). This TABLE also indicates that RSa and Con A^r-3 cells had almost the same sensitivity to the antiviral action of Le-IF or F-IF.

On the other hand, when Con A and interferon were preincubated at 37°C for 1 hour and then added to the cell cultures and kept for 22 hours, the antiviral action of interferon was reduced, depending on the concentration of Con A (TABLE 5). In other experiments, Con A and interferon were mixed and added to the cell sheets without preincubation. In these cases, inhibition of interferon action was also observed (data not shown).

TABLE 4

EFFECT OF PRETREATMENT OF CELLS WITH CON A ON THE ANTIVIRAL ACTION OF INTERFERON

Cells	Treatment* Con A (μg/ml)	Le-IF (U/ml)	VSV Titer (log $TCID_{50}$/ml)	Inhibition
RSa	0	0	6.7	
	0	200	3.0	3.7
	500	0	4.7	
	500	200	1.5	3.2
	250	0	4.7	
	250	200	1.7	3.0
	100	0	5.7	
	100	200	2.5	3.2
	50	0	6.0	
	50	200	2.0	4.0
Con A^r−3	0	0	6.5	
	0	200	2.5	4.0
	500	0	5.5	
	500	200	2.2	3.3
	250	0	5.7	
	250	200	1.7	4.0
	100	0	6.5	
	100	200	2.5	4.0
	50	0	6.0	
	50	200	≦2.0	4.0≦

*RSa and Con A^r−3 cells were pretreated with Con A for 8 hours, washed once with MEM, and then treated with Le-IF for 22 hours.

TABLE 5

EFFECT OF COMBINED TREATMENT WITH CON A AND INTERFERON ON THE ANTIVIRAL ACTION OF INTERFERON IN RSa CELLS

Treatment* Con A (μg/ml)	Le-IF (U/ml)	VSV Titer (log $TCID_{50}$/0.2 ml)	Inhibition
0	0	7.5	
0	200	3.7	3.8
500	0	3.7	
500	200	2.0	1.7
250	0	4.0	
250	200	2.0	2.0
100	0	4.0	
100	200	2.0	2.0
50	0	6.0	
50	200	2.2	3.8

*Equal volumes of interferon and Con A solution were mixed and incubated in a 37°C water bath for 1 hour and then RSa cells were treated with such mixtures for 22 hours.

Discussion

Lectins have been used as probes to analyze the surface structures of cell membranes.[12,17] We found the IF^r cell line, which is resistant to human interferons, to be somewhat more resistant to Con A than its parental RSa cell line. Such a result may suggest some common membrane receptors between human interferons and Con A. It was reported recently that L-1210R cells resistant to mouse interferon are partially resistant to the toxic effect of ricin and abrin.[18] Previously, we compared the ganglioside composition of RSa and IF^r cells, and found no detectable difference in them.[19] Gangliosides have been considered to be a part of the interferon receptor,[19–21] but there still remains a possibility that a specific glycoprotein may compose a part of receptors for both human interferons.[22]

Human interferon and Con A have the capacity to suppress the growth of RSa cells. When these cells were treated with interferon and Con A simultaneously, multiplication of the cells was suppressed more markedly than treatment with either of them alone. Such results were confirmed by using another cell line, VA-13 cells, (data not shown) and also in short-term experiments by measuring DNA synthesis in RSa after combined treatment (TABLE 2). In connection with these results, it should be noted that, when mouse spleen cells were first primed with small dose of homologous interferon, the amount of interferon required to cause inhibition of Con A-induced blastogenesis was considerably reduced.[23]

On the other hand, it was reported that treatment of leukemia L-1210 cells with mouse interferon increased the binding of Con A to the cell membrane.[16] In human lymphocytes, the binding of Con A as well as PHA was also significantly enhanced by human Le-IF.[24] We also observed the same phenomenon by using human transformed cell line RSa with Le-IF or F-IF. RSa cells are characterized by their sensitivity to antiviral and especially to anticellular action of interferon.[8,25] Now they have been found to be sensitive to the enhancing effect of interferon on Con A binding. On the other hand, IF^r and HEC cells were not sensitive to such action of interferon. HEC cells are resistant to both the antiviral and anticellular action of interferon (unpublished data), whereas IF^r cells are resistant to the anticellular action, but only slightly resistant to the antiviral action of interferon. Considering these facts, the combined effect of Con A and interferon on RSa and IF^r cells may not be due to the mere enhancement of Con A binding by interferon treatment. As a plausible explanation, interferon *per se* might have acted on the cells and suppressed the cell growth synergistically with Con A. We have already reported that human interferon given at late G_1 phase inhibits DNA synthesis in synchronized RSa cells.[9,26] Moreover, it has been amply verified that interferon suppresses DNA synthesis elicited by mitogenic actions of Con A and PHA in mouse spleen cells and human lymphocytes.[27–31] On the other hand, molecular mechanisms underlying cytotoxicity of Con A have been not yet clarified.[32] A recent report suggests that activity of DNA polymerase is inhibited in human neuroblastoma cells.[33] It may be necessary to confirm this action in other systems.

Concerning Con A resistance of cells, two types have been reported.[13,34–37] One of them bound Con A to almost the same degree as did Con A-sensitive parental cells.[13,24] Therefore, mere enhancement of Con A binding to cell membrane by interferon treatment does not always indicate increase of Con A cytotoxicity.

As discussed above, Con A and interferon suppressed the growth of RSa and IF^r cells synergistically. Such results were also confirmed in short-term experiments by measuring DNA synthesis after combined treatment (TABLE 2). On the contrary, when Con A and interferon were mixed at 37°C and then applied to the cells, the antiviral action of interferon was not enhanced but suppressed. When the cells were treated with Con A before or after interferon, slight, if any, effect on interferon action was detected (TABLES 3 and 4). The latter procedure was expected to enhance Con A binding to the cell membrane and subsequently modify cellular response to interferon and viral infection. Overall results suggest that mechanisms underlying the anticellular and antiviral actions of interferons may not be the same.

Recently antiviral actions of interferon were attributed to the enhancement of 2′−5′A-dependent endonuclease and protein kinase and subsequent inhibition of protein synthesis in the interferon-treated cells.[38] Whether these enzymes also play a key role in the anticellular action of interferon is a important problem and awaits further investigation. It is at present unclear what effects Con A might give on such enzyme actions.

SUMMARY

Sensitivities of human transformed cell line RSa and its variant cell line IF^r to the cytotoxicity of Con A were compared. IF^r cells were more resistant than RSa to Con A. Con A-resistant cell lines, Con A^r-1 and Con A^r-3, were isolated from RSa, and they were slightly more sensitive than RSa cells to the cell growth-inhibitory actions of interferons. Agglutinability of RSa, IF^r, and Con A^r cells by Con A was compared and found to be almost equal.

The combined effects of Con A and interferon upon growth and viability of these cell lines were tested. When RSa and IF^r cells were treated simultaneously with Con A and Le-IF, growth of the cells was suppressed more markedly than when treatment was with Con A or Le-IF alone. To clarify the mechanism of this phenomenon, binding of ^{125}I-labeled Con A was examined. Though there were some differences, both leukocyte and fibroblast interferon enhanced the binding of Con A to RSa cells and also to Con A^r cells but, in interferon-resistant IF^r and HEC cells, enhancement of Con A binding was low or not observed. Therefore, the combined effect of Con A and interferon on the inhibition of cell growth is not considered to be merely due to the enhanced binding of Con A by interferon action.

Successive treatment of RSa or Con A^r cells with Con A and interferon did not enhance the antiviral action of interferon at all. On the contrary, simultaneous treatment with Con A and interferon suppressed the antiviral action of interferon, depending on the concentration of Con A used. Thus, the effect of Con A on the antiviral and cell growth-inhibitory action of interferon seems rather different.

ACKNOWLEDGMENTS

The authors are grateful to Dr. N. Suzuki for his stimulating discussion, and Mr. S. Fukuda and Mr. T. Suzuki, Central Laboratory for Electron Microscopy, University of Tokyo Hospital, for their help in performing electron microscopy. This work was supported by a Grant from the Ministry of Education, Science and Culture, Japan.

REFERENCES

1. DE CLERCQ, E. & W. E. STEWART II. 1973. The breadth of interferon action. *In* Selective Inhibitors of Viral Functions. W. A. Carter, Ed.: 81–106. CRC Press. Cleveland.
2. GRESSER, I. 1977. On the varied biologic effect of interferon. Cellular Immunol. **34:** 406–415.
3. STEWART, W. E., II. 1979. The Interferon System.: 1–421. Springer-Verlag. Vienna & New York.
4. KUWATA, T., A. FUSE & N. MORINAGA. 1977. Effects of cycloheximide and puromycin on the antiviral and anticellular activities of human interferon. J. Gen Virol. **37:** 195–198.
5. KUWATA, T., A. FUSE & N. MORINAGA. 1977. Effects of ouabain on the anticellular and antiviral activities of human and mouse interferon. J. Gen. Virol. **34:** 537–540.
6. FUSE, A. & T. KUWATA. 1979. Effect of cholera toxin on the antiviral and anticellular activities of human leukocyte interferon. Infect. Immun. In Press.
7. BESANÇON, F. & H. ANKEL. 1974. Inhibition of interferon action by plant lectins. Nature **250:** 784–786.
8. KUWATA, T., A. FUSE & N. MORINAGA. 1976. Effects of interferon on cell and virus growth in transformed human cell lines. J. Gen. Virol. **33:** 7–15.
9. FUSE, A. & T. KUWATA. 1978. Inhibition of DNA synthesis and alteration of cyclic AMP level in RSa cells by human leukocyte interferon. J. Nat Cancer Inst. **60:** 1227–1232.
10. HUNTER, W. M. 1978. Radioimmunoassay. *In* Handbook of Experimental Immunology. D. M. Weier, Ed.: 14. 1–40. Blackwell Scientific Publications. Oxford.
11. BERNHARD, W. & S. AVRAMEAS. 1971. Ultrastructural visualization of cellular carbohydrate components by means of concanavalin A. Exp. Cell Res. **64:** 232–236.
12. NICOLSON, G. L. 1974. The interactions of lectins with animal cell surfaces. Int. Rev. Cytol **39:** 90–190.
13. OZANNE, B. & M. LURYE. 1974. Isolation and characterization of two classes of Con A resistant SV3T3 cells. *In* Control of Proliferation in Animal Cells. B. Clarkson & R. Baserga, Eds.: 177–190. Cold Spring Harbor Laboratory.
14. GUERIN, C., A. ZACHOWSKI, B. PRIGENT, A. PAPAF, I. DYNIA, M.-A. DIAWARA & E. L. BENEDETH. 1974. Correlation between the mobility of inner plasma membrane structure and agglutination by concanavalin A in two cell lines of MOPC 173 plasmocytoma cells. Proc. Nat. Acad. Sci. USA **71:** 114–117.
15. KUWATA, T., A. FUSE, N. SUZUKI & N. MORINAGA. 1979. Comparison of the suppression of cell and virus growth in transformed human cells by leukocyte and fibroblast interferon. J. Gen. Virol. **43:** 435–439.
16. HUET, C. I. GRESSER. M.-T. BANDU & P. LINDAHL. 1974. Increased binding of concanavalin A to interferon-treated murine leukemia L 1210. Proc. Soc. Exp. Biol. Med. **147:** 52–57.
17. NOONAN, K. D. 1978. Lectins as probes of the transformed cell surface. *In* Virus-Transformed Cell Membranes. C. Nicolau, Ed.: 281–371. Academic Press. London, New York & San Francisco.
18. BESANÇON, F. & H. ANKEL. 1979. Decreased sensitivity of an interferon-resistant subline of murine leukemia L-1210 cells to toxic effects of ricin and abrin. Biochem. Biophys. Res. Commun. **88:** 818–825.
19. KUWATA, T., S. HANDA, A. FUSE & N. MORINAGA. 1978. Effect of glycolipids detectable in transformed human cells on interferon activities. Biochem. Biophy. Res. Commun. **85:** 77–84.
20. BESANÇON, F. & H. ANKEL. 1977. Membrane receptors for interferon. Texas Rep. Biol. Med. **35:** 282–292.
21. VENGRIS, V. E., F. H. REYNOLDS, JR., M. D. HOLLENBERG & P. M. PITHA. 1976. Interferon action: Role of membrane gangliosides. Virology **72:** 486–493.
22. FRIEDMAN, R. M. 1978. The mechanism of action of interferon: Possible primary effects on membranes. Horizons Biochem. Biophys. **5:** 281–313.
23. ROZEE. K. R., S. H. S. LEE & J. NGAN. 1973. Effect of priming on interferon inhibition of Con A induced spleen cell blastogenesis. Nature New Biol. **245:** 16–18.

24. MIORNER, H., L. E. LANDSTROM. E. LARNER, I. LARSSON, E. LUNDGREN & O. STRANNEGARD. 1978. Regulation of mitogen-induced lymphocyte DNA synthesis by human interferon of different origins. Cell. Immunol. **35:** 15–24.
25. KUWATA, T., T. ODA, S. SEKIYA & N. MORINAGA. 1976. Characteristics of a human cell line successively transformed by Rous sarcoma virus and simian virus 40. J. Nat. Cancer Inst. **56:** 919–926.
26. FUSE, A. & T. KUWATA. 1977. Inhibition of DNA synthesis of synchronized RSa cells by human leukocyte interferon. J. Nat. Cancer Inst. **58:** 891–897.
27. LINDAHL-MAGNUSON, P., LEARY & I. GRESSER. 1972. Interferon inhibits DNA synthesis induced in mouse lymphocyte suspension by phytohemagglutinin or by allogenic cells. Nature New Biology **237:** 120–121.
28. BLOMGREN, H., H. STRANDER & K. CANTELL. 1974. Effect of human leukocyte interferon on the response of lymphocytes to mitogenic stimuli in vitro. Scand. J. Immunol. **3:** 697–705.
29. WEINSTEIN, Y., B. R. BRODEUR, K. L. MELMON & T. C. MERIGAN. 1977. Interferon inhibition of lymphocyte mitogenesis. Immunology **33:** 313–319.
30. PACHECO, D., R. FALCOFF, L. CATINOT, F. FLOCH, G. H. WERNER & E. FALCOFF. 1976. Inhibitory effect of interferon on DNA and RNA synthesis in murine spleen cells stimulated by lectins. Ann. Immunol. **127C:** 163–171.
31. GURARI-ROTMAN, D., M. REVEL, B. TARTAKOVSKY, S. SEGAL, T. HAHN, Z. HANDZEL & S. LEVIN. 1978. Lymphoblastogenisis in Down's syndrome and its inhibition by human interferon. FEBS Lett. **94:** 187–190.
32. BRILES, E. B. & S. KORNFELD. 1978. Lectin-resistant cell surface variants of eukaryotic cells. Trends Biochem. Sci. **3:** 223–227.
33. BHATTACHARYA, P., I. SIMET & S. BASU. 1979. Inhibition of human neuroblastoma DNA polymerase activities by plant lectins and toxins. Proc. Nat. Acad. Sci. USA **76:** 2218–2221.
34. WRIGHT, J. A. 1973. Evidence for pleiotropic changes in lines of Chinese hamster ovary cells resistant to concanavalin A and phytohemagglutin-P. J. Cell Biol. **56:** 666–675.
35. WRIGHT, J. A. & H. CERI. 1977. The concanavalin A binding properties of concanavalin A-resistant and sensitive hamster cell lines. Biochim. Biophys. Acta **469:** 123–136.
36. GOTTLIEB, C., A. M. SKINNER & S. KORNFELD. 1974. Isolation of a clone of Chinese hamster ovary cells deficient in plant lectin-binding sites. Proc. Nat. Acad. Sci. USA **71:** 1078–1082.
36. STANLEY, P. & J. P. CARVER. 1977. Lectin receptors and lectin resistance. Adv. Exp. Med. Biol. **84:** 265–282.
37. BAGLIONI, C. 1979. Interferon-induced enzymatic activities and their role in the antiviral state. Cell **17:** 255–264.

SENSITIVITY OF HUMAN OVARIAN CARCINOMA CELLS TO INTERFERON AND OTHER ANTITUMOR AGENTS AS ASSESSED BY AN *IN VITRO* SEMI-SOLID AGAR TECHNIQUE*

Lois B. Epstein, Jen-Ta Shen, John S. Abele, and Constance C. Reese

Cancer Research Institute and Departments of Pediatrics, Obstetrics and Gynecology, and Pathology University of California, San Francisco San Francisco, California, 94143

Introduction

There has been considerable recent interest in the antiproliferative and antitumor effects of interferon on the part of both basic scientists and clinicians. Based on the results of *in vitro*, and *in vivo* experiments in animals,[1] *in vitro* experiments with human cells or cell lines,[2-4] and early results of therapeutic trials in malignancy in man,[5,6] interferon (IF) appears to hold promise as a therapeutic agent for the treatment of malignancy.

After cancer of the breast, colon, and lung, carcinoma of the ovary follows as the fourth leading cause of cancer deaths among American women, and is the leading cause of death from gynecological neoplasia.[7,8] A new technique for the culture of human tumor stem cells in semi-solid agar has recently been described,[9] and the most extensive progress has been made with tumor cells from patients with carcinoma of the ovary,[10] multiple myeloma,[11,12] and lymphoma.[13] The test system is such that it permits the use of freshly explanted tumor cells from individual patients obviating the need for deriving long-term lines, an often frustrating and unsuccessful task. Also, the test system permits the evaluation of the sensitivity of individual patient's tumors to the antiproliferative effects of numerous chemotherapeutic agents.[14] The assay used for various types of tumors has been shown to be predictive of drug resistance *in vivo* with 97% accuracy and predictive of drug sensitivity *in vivo* (in heavily pretreated patients) with 64% accuracy.[15]

Since this technique was employed so successfully with human ovarian carcinoma and conventional antitumor agents we were prompted to do similar studies to evaluate the effects of IF in this system. Specifically we desired to determine whether human ovarian carcinoma cells were sensitive to the antiproliferative effects of IF and whether such sensitivity could be related to the histology or grade of the tumor or to the stage of the patient's disease. In addition we hoped also to obtain information that would pertain to the relative potencies of IF and the more conventional antitumor agents for ovarian carcinoma cells.

Methods

Ascitic fluid samples were obtained in heparinized vacuum bottles from 15 patients with ovarian carcinoma, 3 of whom were studied on two separate

*This work was supported by a grant from the Cancer Research Coordinating Committee of the University of California and by National Institutes of Health Grant AI-12481.

0077-8923/80/0350-0228 $01.75/0 © 1980, NYAS

occasions. The semi-solid agar culture technique of Hamburger and Salmon was employed.[9] The samples were usually processed within several hours after receipt and always within 24 hours. As depicted in FIGURE 1, the cells were washed, triturated, counted, and aliquots were prepared for determination of viability by trypan blue dye exclusion and for Pap smears as an independent analysis for the proportion of tumor cells. The washed cells were then incorporated into 0.3% agar with CMRL 1066 medium enriched with 15% horse serum to yield a final concentration of cells of 2×10^5/ml. One ml aliquots of the agar-cell mixture were then pipetted into 35 mm plastic petri dishes previously prepared with an underlayer that contained 0.5% agar enriched with conditioned medium.

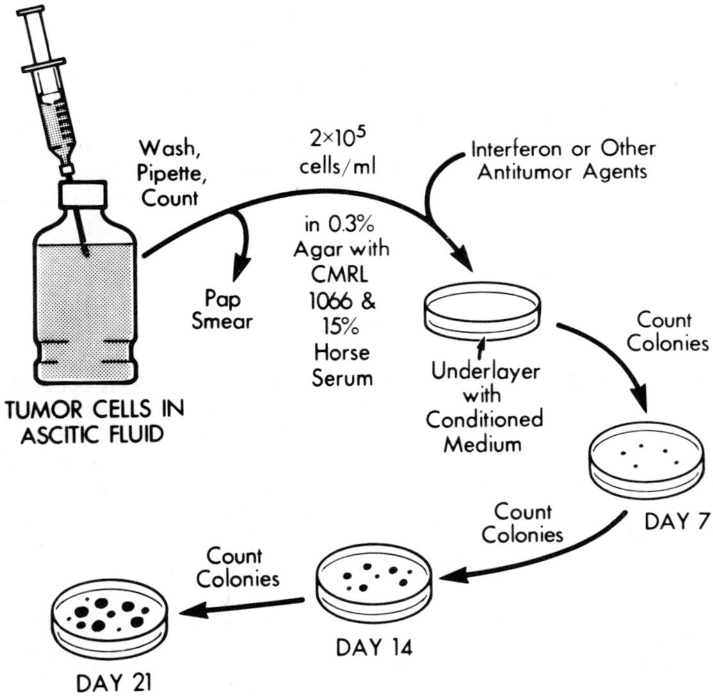

FIGURE 1. Method for growing human tumor cells in semi-solid agar.

The latter was obtained from the supernatant culture fluids of adherent murine spleen cells previously primed by the intraperitoneal injection of mineral oil.

Agents to be evaluated for their antiproliferative capacity were either incorporated into the upper layer of the culture system for the duration of culture or preincubated with the cells in Hanks balanced salt solution for one hour at 37°C. For the latter type of experiments, the cells were washed twice after the preincubation and then incorporated into the upper layer of the culture system.

Human leukocyte interferon (specific activity 2.3×10^5 units/mg protein) and antiserum to human leukocyte interferon were obtained through the courtesy of the Viral Resources Branch, NIAID, NIH, Bethesda, MD. All other antitumor agents were obtained in pure form through the courtesy of the Drug Synthesis and Chemistry Branch and the Natural Products Branch of the Division of Cancer Treatment of NCI, NIH, Bethesda, MD. The drugs were dissolved in either sterile buffered saline or water and stored at $-70°C$ in small aliquots. The final concentrations of each agent employed were: Interferon, 30, 100, and 300 units/ml; Adriamycin, .05, 0.1, and 0.5 μg/ml; Cis Platinum, .01, 0.1, and 1.0 μg/ml; Hexamethylmelamine, 0.1, 0.5, 1.0, and 5.0 μg/ml; Melphalan .04, 0.1, 0.2, and 0.4 μg/ml; and Velban .05, 0.1, and 0.2 μg/ml. Three culture dishes were prepared for each concentration of agent employed, and six were prepared as controls, with no antitumor agent added. In some experiments, IF was combined with antiserum to IF for one hour at room temperature prior to inclusion in the upper layer.

The cultures were maintained at 37°C in a humidified CO_2 incubator and the plates examined with a Tiyoda inverted microscope at weekly intervals (usually at 7, 14, and 21 days) after initiation of the cultures. Tumor cell colonies were scored in three categories: (1) those containing 10–30 cells; (2) those containing >30 cells; and (3) those containing 10 or more cells of which more than half showed evidence of degeneration by virtue of their darkened appearance. In addition, serial photomicrographs of representative fields from several experiments were made with the camera attachment on a Zeiss inverted microcsope.

RESULTS

Patient and Culture Characteristics

A summary of the important clinical and histological data concerning the patients employed in this study is given in TABLE 1. Patients ranged in age from 29–76 years, and all presented initially in either Stage III or IV of the disease. Most of the patients were evaluated in our culture system many months after the resection of their primary tumor, but information concerning the histology and degree of cellular differentiation was available from the referring physicians. Two of the primary tumors were undifferentiated, three were classified as mucinous, and ten were classified as serous with either good, moderate, or poor degree of differentiation.

Our study was conducted over a 2-year period, and during that time ascitic fluid samples were obtained from the fifteen patients, twice in three instances. Viability of the ascitic fluid cells ranged from 86 to 97%, with the exception of one sample which had a viability of 23% (KL-1). The proportion of tumor cells as assessed by Pap smear ranged from 0 to 84%, with 4 of the 15 patients having 1% or less tumor cells.

Growth in culture, as defined by an increase in total cell colony number and/or increase in colonies with >30 cells/colony with increasing duration of culture occurred in eight samples, giving a success rate of 53% when calculated from the number of patients, 45% when calculated from the number of samples studied, or 67% when calculated from the number of samples known to contain tumor cells. All of the samples that grew were shown to contain tumor cells when Pap smears were performed. Six of the eight patients had had no chemotherapy prior to the paracentesis. Two of the eight had chemotherapy previously but not within one month of the tap. The mean age of the patients whose tumor cells grew successfully in culture was 52.

By contrast, the mean age of the patients whose tumor cells did not grow in

TABLE 1

SOURCES OF ASCITIC FLUID SAMPLES USED FOR OVARIAN CARCINOMA CULTURES

Patient	Age	Stage of Disease*	Histology	Primary Tumor: Degree of Cellular Differentiation	Primary Tumor: Therapy Prior to Tap†	Ascitic Fluid Per cent Tumor Cells‡ (%)
Samples that grew in culture§						
JE	32	III	Serous	Good	None	N.D.
PU	29	III	Serous	Poor	None	4
HO	66	III	Serous	Poor	None	N.D.
BE	46	IV	Mucinous	Moderate	CP, HMM > 1 mo; A, C, M, > 6 mo	20
KU	46	III	Serous	Moderate	C, A, V > 1 mo	15
CA	72	IV	Mucinous	Moderate	None	84
VA	65	IV	Serous	Moderate	None	38
BK	58	IV	—	Undifferentiated	None	27
Samples that did not grow in culture						
BR¶	70	III	—	Undifferentiated	C, HMM, < 2 wk	79, 50
DO	62	III	Serous	Poor	M < 1 wk.	39
SL¶	70	III	Serous	Poor	Mi, FU, Rad > 1 mo	1
KL¶	60	III	Serous	Moderate	None	0, 0
DL	57	III	Serous	Moderate	FU, C, < 1 mo	65
RI	76	III	Mucinous	Poor	M < 2 wk	0, 0
UI	66	IV	Serous	Moderate	CP < 3 wk	1

*Stage III, Growth involving one or both ovaries with widespread intraperitoneal metastasis to the abdomen. Stage IV, Growth involving one or both ovaries with distant metastases outside the peritoneal cavity.

†A, Adriamycin; CP, Cis Platinum; C, Cytoxan; FU, 5-Fluourouracil; HMM, Hexamethylmelamine; M, Melphalan; Mi, Mitomycin; V, Vincristine.

‡Percent tumor cells as determined by Pap smears.

§Growth is defined as increase in total cell colony number and/or increase in colonies with >30 cells per colony with increasing duration of culture.

¶Donors studied on two occasions, each time resulting in no growth.

this culture system was 66. Lack of ability to grow in culture was confirmed for three patients on whom repeat attempt at culture also failed. In each instance in which growth did not occur in these seven patients, either ≤1% tumor cells were found on Pap smear of the ascitic fluid cells, or the patients had a history of previous chemotherapy up to 1–2 weeks prior to the paracentesis. Thus successful growth of ovarian carcinoma in this culture system is more likely to occur when one employs ascitic fluid of younger patients who have had no previous chemotherapy and have demonstrated Pap-smear-positive tumor cells in their ascitic fluid.

The patterns of growth of the tumors from individual donors are depicted in FIGURE 2. Growth was reflected by an increase in total colony number with time and/or by an increase in the number of colonies that contained >30 cells. In several instances the number of colonies with 10–30 cells also increases with time, but this was not a constant phenomenon. Obviously the increase in size of a colony is a reflection of a balance between proliferation and eventual death of the cells, and after 4–5 weeks, most of the colonies had perished.

Serial photomicrographs depicting the actual growth of a colony of ovarian carcinoma cells with time are shown in FIGURE 3. Increase in the size and volume of the colony was observed with time. Also we frequently observed the formation of cystic-like structures within the colonies with degeneration of the central cells and overgrowth of the outermost layers. Scattered throughout the agar were small cells which under the inverted microscope appeared to be lymphocytes and macrophages. Collections of these same cells were also often seen at the outer margins of the tumor colonies.

The patterns observed in cultures in which no growth occurred are depicted in FIGURE 4. Although tumor cells were present in the initial inoculum of BR, DO, and DL, by 21 days only sparse evidence of viable tumor cells was noted.

Effect of Interferon

Of the eight patients whose tumor cells grew, the cultures of seven were studied in the presence of various concentrations of IF incorporated into the upper layer of the semi-solid agar culture system (TABLE 2). Response to interferon was defined as a ≥50% reduction in total tumor colony number that persisted for the duration of culture, with concentrations of interferon of ≤300 units/ml. Response to IF was observed in cultures of four of the seven patients studied, and a partial response, defined as reduction in total colony number by greater or equal to 25%, was observed for one other donor, giving an overall response rate of 71%. The sensitivity to the antiproliferative effects of IF did not appear to be related to the histology or grade of the tumor or to the stage of the disease.

FIGURE 5 is illustrative of a patient whose tumor cells responded well to the antiproliferative effects of interferon. Only 30 units/ml was effective in reducing tumor colony number by ≥50%. With increasing concentrations of IF, increasing amounts of degeneration were observed. Reduction was observed not only in the total colony number, but also in the number of colonies which contained 10–30 cells and >30 cells.

In samples from three patients in whom a response to IF was observed, parallel cultures were prepared in which 100 units/ml of IF and sufficient antiserum to neutralize that amount of IF were incorporated into the upper layer of agar in the culture system. The antiserum neutralized the antiproliferative

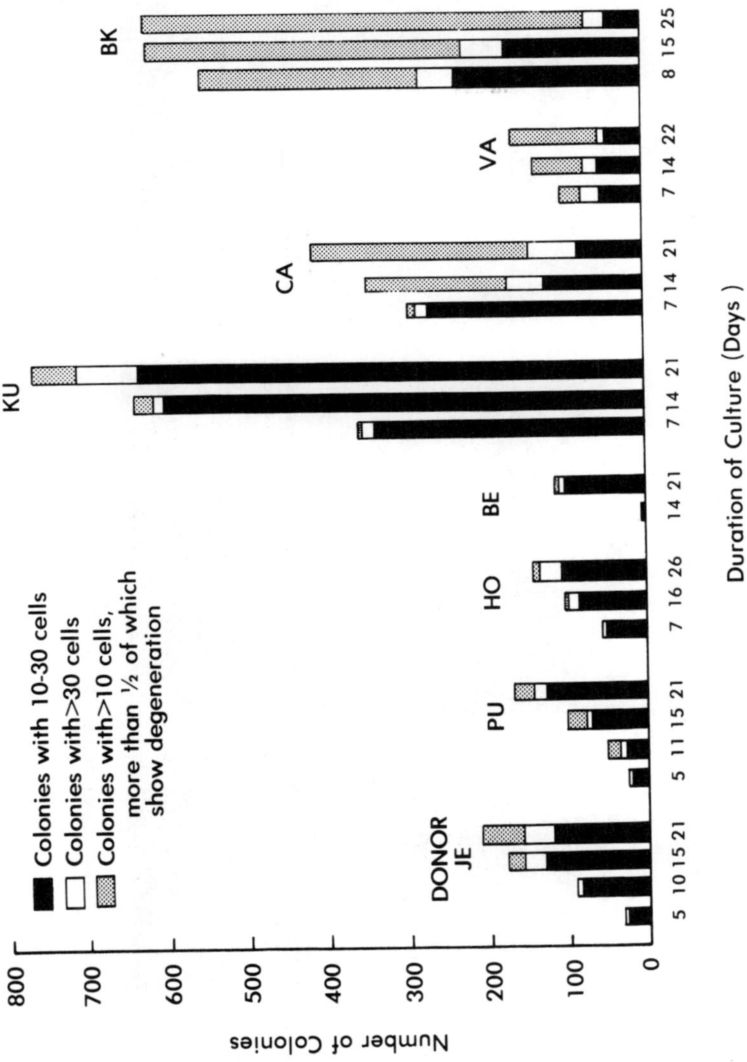

FIGURE 2. Human ovarian carcinoma cells: patterns of growth *in vitro* in semi-solid agar.

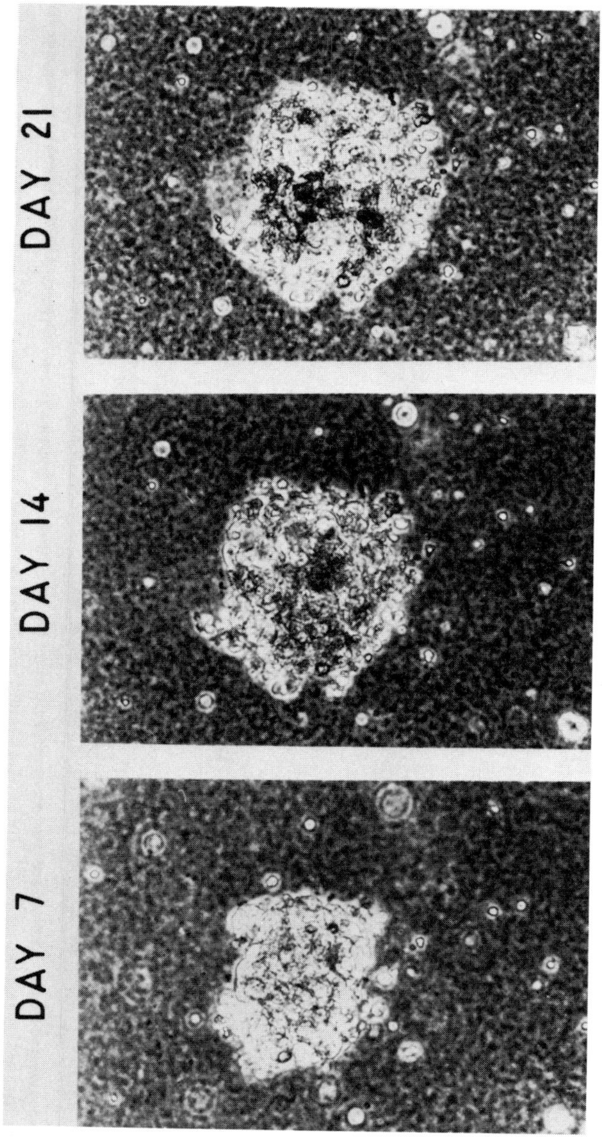

FIGURE 3. Growth of ovarian carcinoma cells *in vitro*. Serial photomicrographs of a single colony. Magnification 400×.

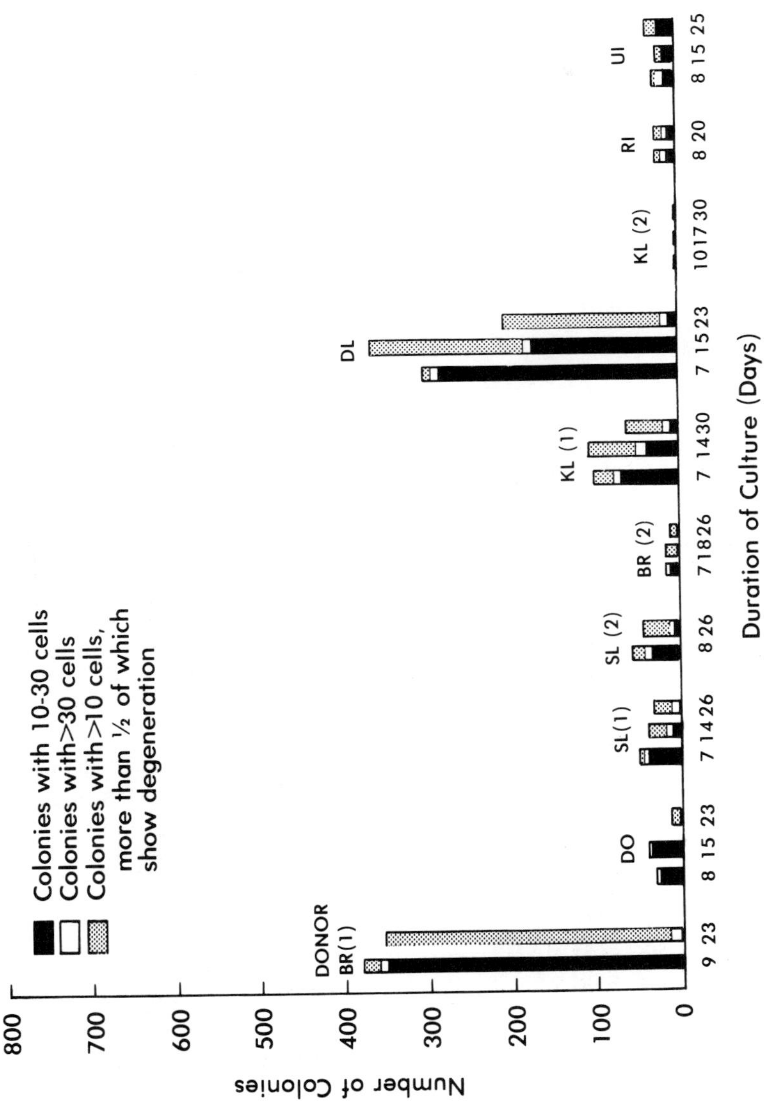

FIGURE 4. Human ovarian carcinoma cells: patterns of nongrowth *in vitro* in semi-solid agar.

TABLE 2
RESPONSE OF OVARIAN CARCINOMA TUMOR COLONIES TO INTERFERON INCORPORATED INTO AGAR CULTURES

Sample	Response to Interferon*	Response Rate
Samples that grew in culture		
PU	−	
HO	++	
BE	++	
KU	++	*71%*
CA	+	
VA	−	
BK	++	
Samples that did not grow in culture but were known to contain > 1% tumor cells		
BR-1	++	
DO	++	75%
BR-2	−	
DL	+	

*−, No response to interferon; +, ≥25% reduction in total tumor colony number; ++, ≥50% reduction in total tumor cell colony number.

effects of the interferon, and in each instance the total number of colonies and the number of colonies with >30 cells were restored to the level of the non-IF-treated control cultures. This is supportive evidence that the antiproliferative effects of the IF are due to the IF itself, and not to some contaminant of the IF preparation. FIGURE 6 is illustrative of one of the two patients whose tumor cells did not respond to interferon, despite growth of the tumor cells in culture.

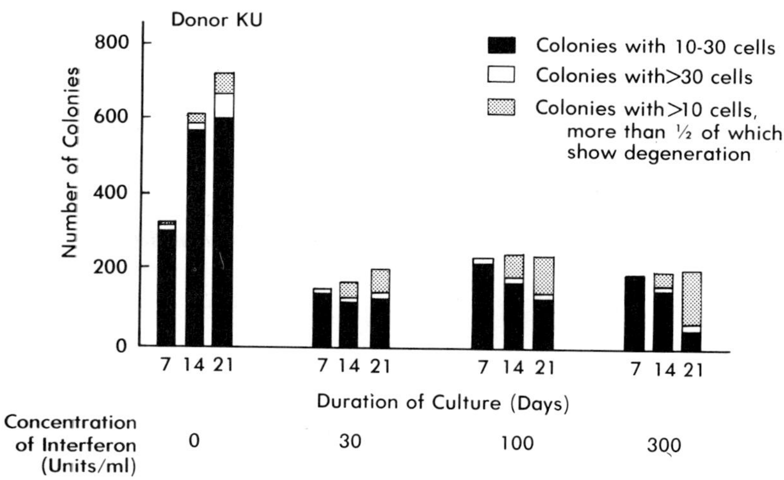

FIGURE 5. Sensitivity of ovarian carcinoma cells to interferon *in vitro*.

An interesting phenomenon with regard to assessment of the antitumor effects of IF was observed when we summarized the colony count data from the cultures that did not meet our criteria for growth (TABLE 2). We found that, despite lack of objective evidence of tumor cell colony growth, of four samples from three patients known to contain >1% tumor cells, IF treatment of the tumor cells resulted in ≥50% reduction of tumor colony number in two samples, and ≥25% reduction in another. Thus a 75% response rate to IF was observed in tumor cell containing samples which did not grow in culture. Judging from the history of these three patients, all of whom had received chemotherapy up to 1–2 weeks prior to paracentesis, recent therapy appears to inhibit growth of tumor cells in culture, but in 75% of cases does not impede the expression of the antiproliferative effects of interferon.

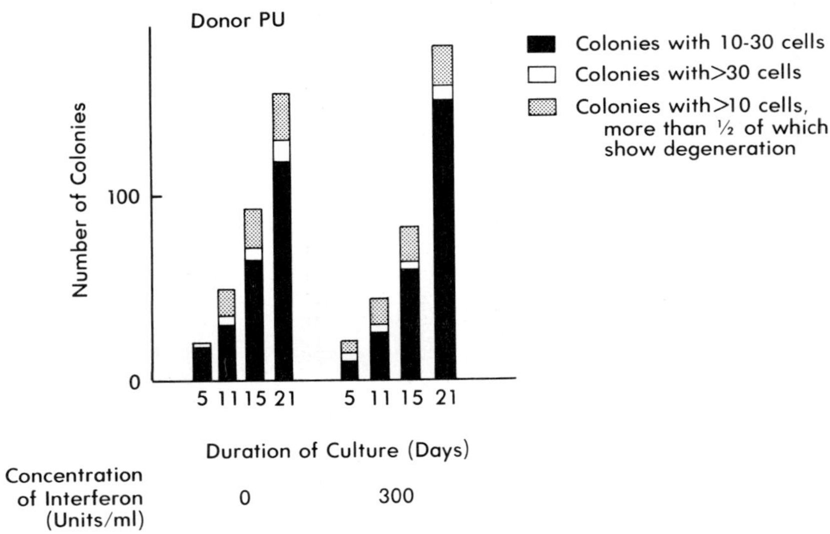

FIGURE 6. Lack of sensitivity of ovarian carcinoma cells to interferon *in vitro*.

Comparison of Effects of Interferon with Effects of Other Antitumor Agents

The data summarized in TABLE 3 and TABLE 4 illustrate the results obtained from experiments in which we studied the comparative efficacy of interferon and other antitumor agents either incorporated into the agar of the culture system or preincubated with the cells prior to their incorporation into agar. Examination of the data from both tables in which interferon and the antitumor agents were run in parallel for a given donor indicates that IF and the other drugs appear to have the same degree of effectiveness. In the four experiments in which the cells were preincubated with the antitumor agents excellent responses were noted with interferon, Cis Platinum, Melphalan, and Velban (TABLE 4). In the five experiments in which the antitumor agents were incorporated into the agar, a unique profile was observed for each tumor. In general, tumors that were sensitive to interferon were also sensitive to at least one other agent.

TABLE 3

COMPARISON OF RESPONSE OF OVARIAN CARCINOMA TUMOR COLONIES TO INTERFERON AND OTHER ANTITUMOR AGENTS INCORPORATED INTO AGAR CULTURES

		Dose, Extent, and Time of Response to																	
		Interferon (units/ml)			Adria* (μg/ml)			Cis Pt (μg/ml)			HMM (μg/ml)			Melph (μg/ml)			Velban (μg/ml)		
Sample	Day	300	100	30	0.5	0.1	0.005	1.0	0.1	0.01	5.0	1.0	0.5	0.4	0.2	0.04	0.2	0.1	0.05
PU†	5	–																	
	11	–																	
	15	–																	
	21	–																	
HO†	7	+¶																	
	16	++																	
	26	++																	
BE†	14	++	++	++															
	21	++	++	++															
KU†	7	+	+	++															
	14	++	++	++															
	21	++	++	++															

CA†	7	+	−	−	−	−		−	−	−				−	−	−			
	14	+	−	−	+	+		−	−	−				−	−	−			
	21	−	−	−	+	+		+	−	−				−	−	−			
VA†	7	−	−	−	+		+	−	−	−	−		−	+	−				
	14	−	−	−	+		+	−	−	−	−		−	+	−				
	22	−	−	−	++		++	+	−	−	−		−	+	−				
BK†	8	+		+	−	+		−	++		−				−				
	15	++	+	−	+	−		+	++		−				−				
	25	++	+	−	+	−		+	++		−				−				
BR-1§	9	++	++	++															
	23	++	++	++															
DO§	8	++	−	−															
	15	++	+	+															
BR-2§	7	−	−	−				−	−	−	−	−	−				−	−	−
	18	−	−	−				−	−	−	−	−	−				−	−	−
	26	−	−	−				−	−	−	−	−	−				−	−	−
DL§	7	+	−	+				−	−		−	−	−				−	−	−
	15	+	−	++				+	−		−	−	−				−	−	−
	23	++	+	++															

*Abbreviations for antitumor agents: Adria, Adriamycin; Cis Pt, Cis Platinum; HMM, Hexamethyl melamine; Melph, Melphalan.
†Samples in which the control, nontreated grew in culture.
¶+, > 25% reduction in total tumor colony number; ++, ≥50% reduction in total tumor colony number; −, no response to agent.
§Samples in which the control, nontreated did not grow in culture but which were known to contain >1% tumor cells.

TABLE 4
COMPARISON OF RESPONSE OF OVARIAN CARCINOMA TUMOR COLONIES TO PREINCUBATION OF CELLS FOR ONE HOUR WITH INTERFERON AND OTHER ANTITUMOR AGENTS

		Dose, Extent, and Time of Response to																				
		Interferon (units/ml)			Adria* (μg/ml)			Cis Pt (μg/ml)			HMM (μg/ml)			Melph (μg/ml)			Velban (μg/ml)		
Sample	Day	300	100	30	0.5	0.1	0.05	1.0	0.1	0.01	5.0	1.0	0.5	0.4	0.2	0.04	0.2	0.1	0.05
BE†	14	++	++	++	−	−	−	−	−	−	−	−	−	−	−	−	−	−	−
	21	++	++	++	++	++	++	++	++	++	++	++	++	++	++	++	++	++	++
KU†	7	−	−	+				+	−	+	−	−	−	−	−		−	+	
	14	+	−	+				++	+	+	−	+	+	+	+	+	++	++	+
	21	++	++	++				++	++	++	++	++	++	++	++	++	++	++	++
BR-1§	9	+		−	+	−			++	++	+	+	+	++	++	++	++	++	++
	23	++		−						+				+		+	++	+	
DO§	8	++		−	−	−	−	+	+	+				++	++	++	++	++	−
	15	++		−	−	−	−	++	++	++				++	++	++	++	++	+
	23	++		−	−	−								++	++	++	++	++	

*Abbreviations for antitumor agents: Adria, Adriamycin; Cis Pt, Cis Platinum; HMM, Hexamethyl melamine; Melph, Melphalan.
†Samples in which the control, nontreated grew in culture.
‡+, ≥25% reduction in total tumor colony number; ++, ≥50% reduction in total tumor colony number; −, no response to agent.
§Samples in which the control, nontreated did not grow in culture but which were known to contain >1% tumor cells.

It is important to note, however, that in no instance, did IF or the other antitumor agents completely destroy all of the tumor colonies for any of the patients.

Discussion

We have confirmed the efficacy of the semi-solid agar culture technique for the *in vitro* growth of human ovarian carcinoma cells from ascitic fluid samples. Using this culture technique, we have demonstrated for the first time that human ovarian carcinoma cells are sensitive to the antiproliferative effects of human leukocyte interferon *in vitro*.

There is no doubt that this culture technique originally described by Hamburger and Salmon,[9,10] is time consuming, tedious, and demanding. It would greatly benefit by the application of modern electronic counting devices for scoring the number and size of each individual colony. Nevertheless the technique has been successful in our hands, and could in the future have numerous other applications for the study of various aspects of the biology, biochemistry, and growth potential of individual human tumors.

In terms of growth and proliferation of the tumor cells in culture, we achieved our best results when the ascitic fluid samples were obtained from women with a mean age of 52, who had received no chemotherapy within the past month prior to the paracentesis, and whose ascitic fluid samples had >1% tumor cells demonstrable by Pap smear. It was clear that those ascitic fluid samples which did not show evidence of growth and proliferation were from patients who had received chemotherapy within 1–2 weeks of the paracentesis or had no demonstrable tumor cells in their ascitic fluid, the latter representing 4 of 15 patients that we studied.

In previous studies using this system for ovarian carcinoma cells Hamburger and Salmon *et al.*[9,10] have shown that the tumor cell colonies consisted of cells with the same characteristics of the original tumor, as demonstrated by morphological, histochemical and cytogenetic techniques. These authors stress that this culture system is a primary bioassay for tumor stem cells, and that each tumor colony represents the progeny of a single tumor stem cell.

In our minds, however, there still is a question as to whether single cell preparations can be obtained uniformly at the initiation of the culture system. Although some tumor cells do exist in ascitic fluid as individual cells, more often they occur in clumps, often associated with the other cells found in ascitic fluid such as lymphocytes, polymorphs, macrophages, and mesothelial cells. Despite earnest efforts to dissociate such clumps into single cells prior to initiation of the cultures it was not always possible to do so, and we frequently observed what appeared to be lymphocytes and macrophages at the periphery of good-sized viable tumor colonies. The question arose as to whether such cells were in intimate association with nondissociated tumor cell clumps at the time of initiation of culture or whether they migrated through the agar secondary to some chemotactic factor elaborated by the tumor cell colonies. Depletion of the macrophage population (by phagocytosis of carbonyl iron) from the ascitic fluid of patients with ovarian carcinoma has been shown to greatly reduce the growth of the tumor colonies,[10] and suggests that such macrophages might play an important role in affecting tumor growth.[16]

Another puzzling aspect of this system is that given equivalent viability of various ascitic fluid cell preparations, the number of colonies observed did not always correlate with the proportion of tumor cells as determined by Pap smear analysis. This perhaps was a reflection of the unique clonigenic potential of individual tumors, and we recognize that colony number and size reflect the interplay of intrinsic cloning efficiency, growth rate, and effects of prior therapy on viability during the duration of culture.

The response of the human ovarian cells to the antiproliferative effects of interferon was quite marked, with a response rate of 71% in samples in which the control, nontreated cultures showed evidence of growth with time, and 75% in samples in which tumor cells were observed, but no overall growth occurred. The responses occurred in the range of final concentrations of IF of 30–300 units/ml, levels well within the range observed in the serum of patients on clinical trials with interferon.[17] Sensitivity to interferon did not appear to be related to the histology or grade of the tumor or to the stage of the disease. Furthermore recent therapy may have acted to inhibit growth of the tumor cells in culture, but it did not appear to interfere with the expression of the antitumor effects of the interferon. This observation could have profound implications for clinicians involved with therapeutic trials of interferon.

We recognize that the response was not an all or none phenomenon, as our endpoint was $\geq 50\%$ reduction in overall tumor colony number. In each case in which sensitivity to IF was demonstrated, residual tumor colonies were still present, presumably resistant to the antiproliferative effects of the interferon. Neutralization of these antiproliferative effects of IF with antiserum directed against human leukocyte IF suggested strongly that the antiproliferative effects are due to IF itself, and not a contaminant of the interferon preparation.

The mechanism underlying the antiproliferative effect of IF in this system is not known. It is not possible at this time to ascertain whether the IF had a direct effect on the tumor cells or whether its antiproliferative effect was mediated via an effect on the lymphocytes and macrophages that were intimately associated with many of the tumor colonies. There are numerous precedents in the literature demonstrating the multifaceted effects of IF on various aspects of the immune response and its cellular components, the lymphocyte and the macrophage,[18–20] and several other reports in this volume are pertinent to this aspect of interferon action.

We are aware that the *in vitro* conditions of culture employed in our study do not duplicate the complexity of the *in vivo* situation, but we feel that our study indicates for the first time that human ovarian carcinoma cells are sensitive to the antiproliferative effects of interferon. In general, the responsiveness of the tumor cells to IF ran parallel to the overall response to a variety of other chemotherapeutic agents. However, it is of interest that in subsequent studies we have shown that ascitic fluid-derived colonies are more sensitive to the antiproliferative effects of IF than are colonies derives from solid tumors.[21]

Whether the *in vitro* culture system we have employed will prove to be predictive of *in vivo* response to IF, just as it has been demonstrated to be for other antitumor agents,[15] remains to be seen. Such information could be obtained by the simultaneous performance of combined clinical and culture studies. With antitumor agents and ovarian carcinoma Salmon *et al.*[15] have found this *in vitro* culture system to predict drug resistance with 99% accuracy and drug sensitivity with 64% accuracy. In view of the acute shortages of human leukocyte interferon the importance of developing a predictive assay for resistance or response to interferon for individual tumors is obvious.

SUMMARY

To determine the sensitivity *in vitro* of human ovarian carcinoma cells to the antiproliferative effects of human leukocyte interferon, 18 samples of ascitic fluid from 15 affected patients were cultured in semi-solid agar by the technique of Hamburger and Salmon. Cultures were examined at weekly intervals after initiation and the number and size of each tumor colony recorded. Growth as defined by increase in total tumor colony number with time was obtained in 45% of the samples, or 53% of the patients, or 67% of the ascitic fluid samples with tumor cells demonstrated by Pap smear. No growth occurred in samples from recently treated patients or in samples devoid of tumor cells as assessed by Pap smear.

Response to interferon directly incorporated into the agar culture system or preincubated with cells prior to their inclusion in culture was defined as reduction in total tumor colony number by ≥50% and partial response by ≥25% reduction. The response rate for samples, the nontreated controls of which showed evidence of growth, was 71%, and that of samples that contained tumor colonies with no increase in growth during the culture period was 75%. Sensitivity to interferon was not related to the histology or grade of the tumor or to the stage of the disease. In general the responsiveness of the tumor cells to interferon ran parallel to the overall responsiveness to a variety of other chemotherapeutic agents.

As this culture system has been proven by other investigators[15] to be predictive of *in vivo* resistance to antitumor drugs with considerable accuracy and also to be predictive of *in vivo* response to a lesser degree, it will be important to determine whether similar relationships between *in vitro* and *in vivo* sensitivity obtain for interferon.

ACKNOWLEDGMENTS

We thank Drs. Howard Jones, Michael Friedman, Ernest Rosenbaum, Richard Cohen, Samuel Spivak, George Hulme, Myron Turbow, and Paul Fraser for helping us to obtain ascitic fluid samples.

We thank Dr. Charles Epstein for thoughtful discussions, Bruce Travis for preparing the photomicrographs, Nancy H. McManus for editorial assistance, and Diana Zawacki and Mary Joan E. Fredette for typing the manuscript.

REFERENCES

1. Gresser, I. 1977. *In* Cancer—A Comprehensive Treatise. F. Becker, Ed.: 521–571. Plenum. New York.
2. Balkwill, F. R. & R. T. D. Oliver. 1977. Int. J. Cancer. **20:** 500–505.
3. Hilfenhaus, J., H. Damin & R. Johannsen. 1977. Arch. Virol. **54:** 271–277.
4. Einhorn, S. & H. Strander. 1978. Adv. Exp. Med. Biol. **110:** 159–174.
5. Strander, H., K. Cantell, S. Ingimarsson, P. A. Jakobsson, U. Nilsonne & G. Soderberg. 1977. Fogerty Intern. Center Proc. **28:** 377–381.
6. Merigan, T. C., K. Sikora, J. H. Breeden, R. Levy & S. A. Rosenberg. 1978. New Engl. J. Med. **299:** 1449–1453.
7. Griffiths, C. T. 1974. *In* Cancer Medicine. J. F. Holland & E. Frei III, Eds.: 1710–1720. Lea and Febiger. Philadelphia.

8. IOACHIM, H. L., B. H. DORSETT, M. SABBATH, B. ANDERSSON & H. R. K. BARBER. 1973. Gyn. Oncology. **1:** 130–142.
9. HAMBURGER, A. W. & S. E. SALMON 1977. Science **197:** 461–463.
10. HAMBURGER, A. W., S. E. SALMON, M. B. KIM, J. M. TRENT, B. J. SOEHNLEN, D. S. ALBERTS & H. J. SCHMIDT. 1978. Cancer Res. **38:** 3438–3444.
11. HAMBURGER, A. W. & S. E. SALMON. 1977. J. Clin. Invest. **60:** 846–854.
12. HAMBURGER, A. W., M. B. KIM & S. E. SALMON. 1979. J. Cell Physiol. **98:** 371–376.
13. JONES, S. E., A. W. HAMBURGER, M. B. KIM & S. E. SALMON. 1979. Blood **53:** 294–303.
14. SALMON, S. E., A. W. HAMBURGER, B. SOEHNLEN, B. G. M. DURIE, D. S. ALBERTS & T. E. MOON. 1978. New Engl. J. Med. **298:** 1321–1327.
15. SALMON, S. E., D. S. ALBERTS, F. L. MEYSKENS, B. G. M. DURIE, S. E. JONES, B. J. SOEHNLEN, L. YOUNG, H.-S. G. & T. E. MOON. 1980. *In* Cloning of Human Tumor Stem Cells. S. E. Salmon, Ed. Chapter 18. Alan R. Liss, Inc. New York.
16. SALMON, S. E. & A. W. HAMBURGER. 1978. Lancet **1:** 1289–1290.
17. JORDON, G. W., R. P. FRIED & T. C. MERIGAN. 1974. J. Infect. Dis. **130:** 56–62.
18. EPSTEIN, L. B. 1977. *In* Interferons and Their Actions. W. E. Stewart II, Ed.: 91–132. CRC Press. Cleveland.
19. HERBERMAN, R. B., J. Y. DJEU, J. R. ORTALDO, H. T. HOLDEN, W. H. WEST & G. D. BONNARD. 1978. Cancer Treatment Rep. **62:** 1893–1896.
20. HERBERMAN, R. B., J. R. ORTALDO & G. D. BONNARD. 1979. Nature **277:** 221–223.
21. EPSTEIN, L. B., J. T. SHEN, J. S. AGELE & C. C. REESE. 1980. *In* Cloning of Human Tumor Stem Cells. S. E. Salmon, Ed. Chapter 21. Alan R. Liss, Inc. New York.

DIFFERENTIAL EFFECT OF HUMAN INTERFERON ON NORMAL AND NEOPLASTIC T- AND B-CELL LYMPHOCYTES

A. M. Attallah,* T. Fleischer,† J. R. Neefe,‡ A. Kazakis,*
and T. J. Yeatman*

**Division of Pathology*
Bureau of Biologics
Bethesda, Maryland 20205

†Metabolism Branch, National Cancer Institute
National Institutes of Health
Bethesda, Maryland 20205

‡Division of Immunologic Oncology
Lombardi Cancer Center
Georgetown University School of Medicine
Washington, D.C. 20007

INTRODUCTION

Interferons are a unique set of proteins that possess potent antiviral, antiproliferative, and immunoregulatory activities. The encouraging trials of interferon (IF) in osteosarcoma and non-Hodgkin's lymphoma have led to widespread interest by clinical oncologists in the potential antitumor effect of human interferon.[1,2]

We have examined the effect of IF in an *in vitro* system using proliferating normal and neoplastic T and B cells. Pertubations in the cell cycle by IF were measured by flow cytometry and effects on antibody production were measured by plaque-forming cell analysis and IgM biosynthesis.

MATERIALS AND METHODS

Proliferating Normal T and B Cells

Continuous T-cell cultures were prepared as previously described. Briefly, heparinized whole blood was obtained from normal donors and mononuclear cell suspensions were isolated by the Ficoll-Hypaque method. The cells were washed twice and resuspended in RPMI 1640 media (GIBCO, Grand Island, NY) containing 20% heat-inactivated fetal bovine serum (FBS) (Reheis Chemical Co., Phoenix, AZ), glutamine, penicillin, and streptomycin. The cultures (5×10^6 cells/ml) were then incubated at 37°C in a 5% CO_2 humidified atmosphere. The cultures were supplemented with 20% concentrated conditioned media (CM) to induce continuous growth. The conditioned media was prepared from normal human lymphocytes from a single donor by incubating the cultures for 24–72 hr at 37°C in 5% CO_2 humidified atmosphere. CM were concentrated by dialysis against polyethylene-glycol powder to ¼ of the original volume and dialysis against PBS overnight at 4°C, then filter-sterilized and frozen at −70°C until use.[3,4] For assessment of B-cell proliferation, mononuclear cells were separated

0077-8923/80/0350-0245 $01.75/0 © 1980, NYAS

from heparinized venous blood obtained from normal adult donors by Ficoll-Hypaque density-centrifugation. Cells from the interface were collected and after two washings were resuspended in RPMI 1640 medium. (Grand Island Biological Co., Grand Island, NY) and 10% human AB serum. Cultures were stimulated with polyclonal activator PWM (GIBCO) in a concentration range from 1/50 to 1/1000 final dilution.

Proliferating Neoplastic T and B Cells

MOLT 4 is an established cell line with T-cell characteristics derived from the peripheral blood of a patient during a relapse of acute lymphoblastic leukemia (ALL). Daudi is an established cell line with B-cell characteristics derived from a patient with Burkitt's lymphoma. Both neoplastic cell lines were cultured in RPMI 1640 medium containing 20% heat-inactivated FBS, 200 mM glutamine and 100 units/ml each of penicillin and streptomycin.

Immunoglobulin Biosynthesis in Vitro

Lymphocytes (2×10^6) from normal volunteers were cultured in the presence of pokeweed mitogen for 12 days. This lectin is known to induce polyclonal immunoglobulin production *in vitro*. The techniques used for immunoglobulin measurement have been described in detail elsewhere.[5] The cumulative secretion of IgM, IgG, and IgA was determined by double-antibody radioimmunoassays essentially as previously described for IgE.[6]

Assay for PFC

Culture conditions for the generation of anti-sheep red blood cell (SRBC) PFC after polyclonal stimuation of human peripheral blood lymphocytes have been described.[7] At termination of culture (6 days), cell suspensions were assayed for direct PFC against SRBC as previously described.[8]

Flow Cytometry (FCM)

Two $\times 10^5$ cells in 0.2 ml RPMI 1640 media were added to 1 ml of staining solution consisting of 0.1% sodium citrate, 50 μg/ml propidium iodide, 10 mM NaCl, and 0.1% Nonidet P40. After allowing the stained cells to equilibrate for 10 min at 0°C, they were analyzed for cellular fluorescence on a Cytofluorograph Model FC-200 (Ortho Instruments, Westwood, MA). In this instrument, individual cells are illuminated by a 50 mW argon laser (488 nm); the fluorescence signal of each cell is amplified and fed into a pulse height analyzer (Ortho Instruments Model 2102) to generate a DNA histogram. Each histogram was analyzed for the percentage of cells in $S+G_2+M$ phase as previously described. Briefly, the number of cells that were visually judged to lie outside the G_1 peak were divided by the total number of cells in the histogram. For consistency, the same channel numbers of the cells outside the G_1 peak in experimental cultures. All results are expressed as the mean of duplicate cultures.

Human Interferon (HIF)

Namalva cells suspended in RPMI 1640 with 2% heat-inactivated fetal bovine serum were treated with Sendai virus. The induced IF was separated from the cells and partially purified and concentrated by treatment with 2–5% trichloroacetic acid (TCA) and ethanol (essentially as described by Cantell *et al.*,[9] but using TCA instead of 0.5M KScN). This partially purified human lymphoblastoid IF induced in Namalva cells[10] with specific activity, 1.25×10^5 reference units/mg protein, was a gift from Wellcome Research Laboratories, England. Residual Sendai virus was not detected in the preparation.

RESULTS

Effect of Human Interferon on the Cell Cycle of Proliferating T Cells

Cellular DNA analysis by flow cytometry has proven to be an extremely reliable and reproducible technique for analyzing cell cycle progression. In FIGURE 1 the histogram on the left side of each graph represents the DNA histogram of proliferating normal T cells and the right side represents the same T

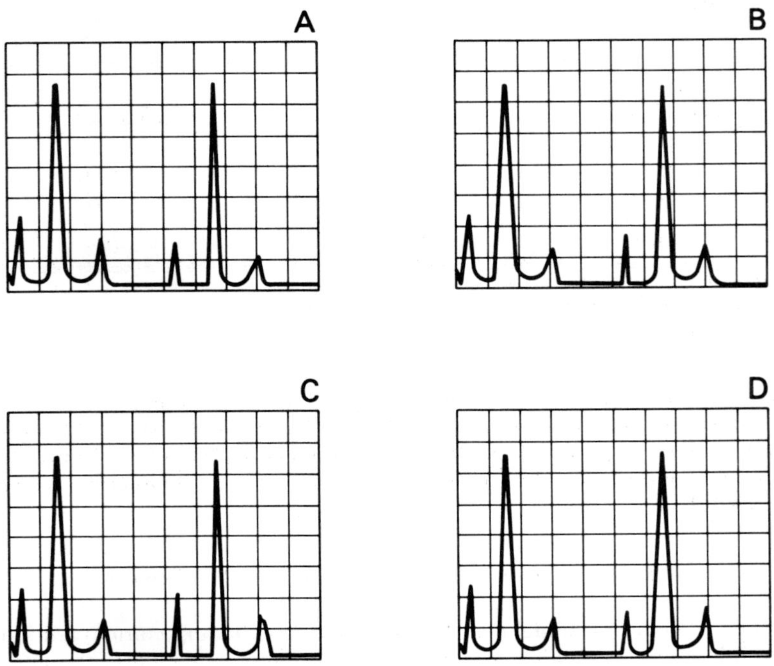

FIGURE 1. Effect of HIF on FCM patterns of a continuous T-cell culture. Each graph represents two histograms; the small peak to the left of each histogram represents cellular debris. The large peak represents cells in G_1, while the smaller peak to the right represents cells in G_2; cells in S phase lie between the two peaks.

cells with IF added to the culture medium. The large peak to the left in each histogram represents cells in G_1 while the smaller peak to the right represents cells in G_2; cells in S phase fall between the two peaks. The histograms are essentially identical suggesting that HIF had little effect on cell cycle progression. At 2000 units/culture (1A) there is some suppression of cells in $S+G_2+M$. TABLE 1 summarizes the data derived from the histograms. HIF up to 2000 units/culture caused only a modest decrease in the % $S+G_2+M$. In contrast, FIGURE 2 shows the effect of 500 units of HIF on the neoplastic T-cell line, while on the left side (control), 60.9% of the cells are in the $S+G_2+M$ phase, while on the right side (culture with 500 units HIF for 48 hr) only 38.8% of the cells are in $S+G_2+M$, a reduction of 36.3%. Fifty units of HIF reduced the $S+G_2+M$ of MOLT by 23.0% (data not shown).

Effect of Human Interferon on the Cell Cycle of Proliferating B Cells

The effect of HIF on B cells was more striking. Histograms of PWM-stimulated lymphocytes treated with HIF showed modest increases in percent $S+G_2+M$ (figure not shown); in marked contrast, only 1 unit HIF caused a

TABLE 1

EFFECT OF HUMAN INTERFERON (HIF) ON CELL CYCLE PROGRESSION OF A CONTINUOUS T-CELL LINE (CTCL)

HIF* (units/culture)	CTCL	
	% $S+G_2+M$	% Δ from control†
50	11.0‡	—
100	9.7	−11.8
500	10.5	−4.5
1000	8.9	−19.1
2000	9.0	−18.2

*HIF added for 48 hr of culture.
†% Δ from control = percentage change from control.
‡Mean of duplicate cultures.

marked change in the DNA histogram of Daudi cells (figure not shown). TABLE 2 shows the quantitative FCM results. Whereas 125 units of HIF on up caused a modest increase in proliferation of PWM-stimulated lymphocytes, 1 unit caused nearly 40% suppression in Daudi cells, which was not increased by higher amounts of HIF.

Effect of Human Interferon on Antibody Production

Pokeweed mitogen stimulated B cells in culture to undergo terminal differentiation into immunoglobulin-producing plasma cells. Evaluation of the effect of HIF on PWM-induced SRBC antibody production is shown in TABLE 3. HIF tends to modestly increase the number of PFC at lower doses (100–250), while at higher doses there are only minimal changes from the control. In addition, PWM-induced polyclonal IgM production by normal lymphocytes was only minimally changed by HIF at concentrations up to 500 units (TABLE 4).

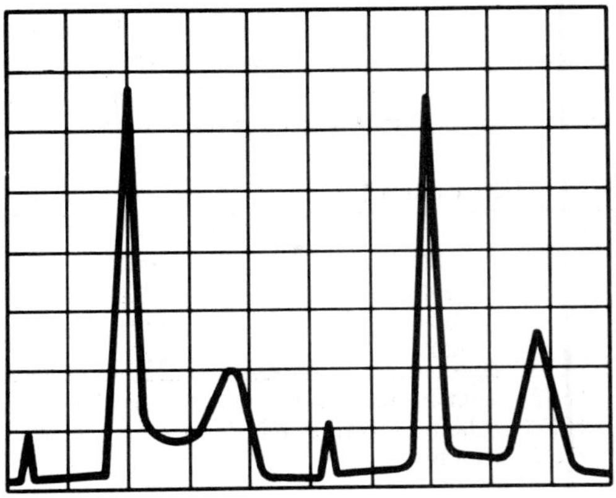

FIGURE 2. Effect of HIF on MOLT cells. The histogram on the right are MOLT cells treated with 500 units HIF for 48 hours; there is a marked reduction in the S-phase fraction.

DISCUSSION

The exact mechanism(s) by which IF exerts its *in vivo* antitumor effect is, at present, unknown; it is certain to be complex because of the broad spectrum of effects mediated by IF. In this study we chose to examine lymphoid cells *in vitro* in order to examine separately the effects of IF on cell cycle progression and antibody biosynthesis. In other studies, we[11] and others[12] have found that FCM analysis of proliferating cells shows very good correlation with tritiated thymidine uptake measurements of DNA synthesis. The recent demonstration that normal T cells can be maintained in continuous culture for more than 1 year[4] enabled us to directly compare the effects of HIF on normal and neoplastic T cells. When we used FCM to examine these proliferating T cells, we found that both a normal and a neoplastic cell line were inhibited to some degree by HIF; the neoplastic T-cell line was somewhat more sensitive in that only 50 units caused 23% inhibition while 1000 units of HIF were needed to suppress the CTCL by 19%. One possible reason that HIF had little effect on the normal cells is that the percentage of proliferating cells is rather low (11%). In previous studies

TABLE 2

EFFECT OF HUMAN INTERFERON (HIF) ON CELL CYCLE PROGRESSION OF PROLIFERATING NORMAL AND NEOPLASTIC B CELLS

HIF* (units/culture)	PWM		Daudi	
	% S+G$_2$+M	% Δ from control	% S+G$_2$+M	% Δ from control
C$_0$	21.0	—	35.4	—
1			21.8	−38.4
10			18.3	−48.3
100			21.3	−39.8
125	27.4	+30.4		
250	29.2	+39.0		
500	29.1	+38.6	20.9	−40.1
1000	29.8	+41.9	20.1	−43.2

*HIF added at the same time of PWM stimulation, or for 48 hours for Daudi cells.
†% Δ from control = percentage change from control S+G+M value.

TABLE 3

EFFECT OF HUMAN INTERFERON (HIF) ON THE NUMBER OF PLAQUE-FORMING CELLS (PFC) OF PWM-STIMULATED HUMAN LYMPHOCYTES

HIF/Culture*	PFC/Culture†		
	Exp 1	Exp 2	Exp 3
0	260	32	54
100	366	46	155
250	N.T.‡	N.T.	178
500	189	31	171
1000	195	29	118

*HIF = human interferon in international units.
†PFC = plaque-forming cells determined as previously described.[7]
‡N.T. = not tested.

using CTCL with a proliferating fraction of 30%, however, 2000 units of HIF caused only 9% inhibition.[13] FCM analysis of proliferating B cells showed a different picture. All doses of HIF from 125 to 2000 units caused a modest increase in proliferation of PWM-stimulated lymphocytes; as little as 1 unit HIF caused 40% inhibition of the neoplastic B-cell line Daudi. The inhibition seen was not dose-dependent in that up to 1000 units HIF did not cause any substantial increase in inhibition. Thus, a subpopulation of Daudi cells may be resistant to the antiproliferative effect of IF, a result similar to that found previously[14] with L1210 mouse cells. It should be stressed that these results are for only one cell line and should not be taken as representing the response of all neoplastic B-cell lines to HIF; other studies have shown that lymphoblastoid B-cell lines are extremely heterogeneous in their response to HIF.[15]

In addition to the FCM analysis on proliferation, we performed studies on cell function of plasma cells generated by pokeweed mitogen stimulation of human peripheral blood lymphocytes. Immunoglobulin production by PWM-stimulated lymphocytes was not significantly suppressed using relatively high concentrations of HIF, nor was the number of plaque-forming cells induced by PWM markedly affected by HIF. These results contrast with previous studies in which PFC response to sheep red blood cells (SRBC) by mouse spleen cells was reduced by mouse IF.[16,17] PWM is a polyclonal stimulator whereas SRBC is a T-dependent antigen; our lack of inhibition may reflect a difference in polyclonal induction of antibody production compared to antigen specific induction. In addition, the IF preparation used in these studies is relatively free of non-IF protein and it is possible that an unidentified product such as lymphocyte

TABLE 4

THE EFFECT OF HUMAN INTERFERON (HIF) ON THE BIOSYNTHESIS OF IGM OF POKEWEED MITOGEN-STIMULATED PERIPHERAL HUMAN LYMPHOCYTES

HIF/Culture	IgM/Culture (ng/ml)
C_0	1446
5	1391
50	1186
500	1610

chalone[18] was present in the previous studies. Finally, our results may simply reflect a species difference in response to IF. In other studies, in which a patient with Hodgkin's disease was treated with HIF, serum IgG, IgA and IgM were not decreased by HIF therapy;[19] additionally, response to PWM and other mitogens was moderately increased.

This study shows that at least one Burkitt's lymphoma cell line is exquisitely sensitive to the anitproliferative effects of HIF. Whether this sensitivity is also reflected *in vivo* remains to be seen, but the demonstration that FCM analysis can be used for assessing the effects of HIF suggests that patients' hematopoetic diseases could be easily evaluated for response to IF on a serial basis.

In addition to antiproliferative effects seen here, HIF shows many other effects that make it attractive as a potential antineoplastic agent. The known antiviral activity of HIF *in vitro* and *in vivo* might be useful to prevent opportunistic viral diseases such as *Herpes zoster* that often accompany malignancy. The lack of inhibition of immunoglobulin biosynthesis of PFC-formation of normal cells shown in this study also suggests that resistance to bacterial infections would not be compromised by HIF therapy. Finally, HIF has been reported to exert other effects[20,21] besides cell-growth inhibition which might further augment the clinical usefulness of HIF. We [22] and others[23,24] have recently shown that antibody-dependent cell-mediated cytotoxicity and natural killer cytotoxicity are markedly augmented by HIF. These cell-mediated immune responses are thought to play some role in tumor rejection; this HIF might not only slow down neoplastic growth but might also activate and enhance immune rejection mechanisms in the host.

Summary

The effect of human interferon (HIF) on the growth and function of normal and neoplastic proliferating human T and B cells was studied. Cell cycle analysis by flow-cytometry showed that up to 2000 units of HIF had little effect on the proliferating fraction (that is, the percent $S+G_2+M$ phases of the cell cycle) of normal T cells grown continuously with growth-promoting factor from PHA-stimulated lymphocytes, while 500 units of HIF suppressed the percent $S+G_2+M$ of the acute lymphocytic leukemia (ALL) T-cell line, MOLT, by 36%. Up to 2000 units of HIF had a moderate enhancing effect on the percent $S+G_2+M$ of PWM-stimulated lymphocytes. In striking contrast, a single unit of HIF caused nearly 40% suppression of the percent $S+G_2+M$ of Daudi, a Burkitt's lymphoma cell. One-thousand units of HIF did not decrease the number of antibody-forming normal cells, and up to 500 units of HIF did not inhibit the total Ig secreted by these cells. These results suggest that amounts of HIF affecting the proliferation of some neoplastic lymphoid cells has little effect on the proliferation of normal T and B cells. In addition, HIF does not appear to affect polyclonal induction of B-cell differentiation.

Acknowledgments

We thank J. E. Sullivan for technical assistance, Dr. S. P. D. Noguchi and J. C. Petricciani for assistance, and E. Kirshbaum for typing this manuscript.

REFERENCES

1. STRANDER, H. 1977. Interferons: Anti-neoplastic drugs? Blut **35:** 277–288.
2. MERIGAN, T. C., K. SIKORA, J. H. BREEDEN, R. LEVY & S. A. ROSENBERG. 1978. Preliminary observations on the effect of human leukocyte interferon in non-Hodgkin's lymphoma. New Engl. J. Med. **299**(No. 26): 1449–1453.
3. BONNARD, G. D., D. J. SCHENDEL, W. H. WEST, J. M. ALVAREZ, R. D. MACA, K. YASAKA, R. L. FINE, R. B. HERBERMAN, M. O. DELANDAZ URI, & D. A. MORGAN. 1978. Continued growth of normal human T lymphocytes in culture with retention of important function. *In* Human Lymphocyte Differentiation: It's Application to Cancer. B. Serrou & C. Rosenfeld, Eds.:319–326. Elsevier North-Holland Biochemical Press, USA.
4. RUSCETI, F. W., D. A. MORGAN & R. C. GALLO. 1977. Functional and morphologic characterization of human T cells continuously grown *in vitro*. J. Immunol. **119:** 131–138.
5. WALDMANN, T. A., M. DURN, S. BRODER, M. BLACKMAN, R. M. BLAESE & W. STROBER. 1974. Role of suppressor T cells in pathogenesis of common variable hypogammaglobulinemia. Lancet **2:** 609–613.
6. WALDMANN, T. A., S. H. POLMAR, S. T. BALESTRA, M. C. JOST, R. M. BRUCE & W. D. TERRY. 1972. Immunoglobulin E in immunologic deficiency diseases. II. Serum IgE concentration of patients with acquired hypogammaglobulinemia, thymoma, and hypogammaglobulinemia, myotonic dystrophy, intestinal lymphangiectasis and Wiskott-Aldrich syndrome. J. Immunol. **109:** 304–310.
7. FAUCI. A. S. & K. R. PRATT. 1976. Polyclonal activation of bone marrow derived lymphocytes from human peripheral blood measured by a direct plaque-forming cell assay. Proc. Nat. Acad. Sci. USA **73:** 3676.
8. FAUCI, A. S., K. R. PRATT & G. WHALEN. 1976. Activation of human B lymphocytes. II. Cellular interactions in the PFC response of human tonsillar and peripheral blood B lymphocytes to polyclonal activation by pokeweed mitogen. J. Immunol. **117:** 2100.
9. CANTELL, K., S. HIRVONEN, K. E. MOGENSEN & L. PYHALA. 1973. Human leukocyte interferon: Production, purification, stability and animal experiments. In Vitro Monogr. **3:** 35–38.
10. JOHNSTON, M. D., K. H. FANTES, N. B. FINTER & B. CHIR. 1978. Factors influencing production of interferon by human lymphoblastoid cells. *In* Human Interferon, Production and Clinical use. W. R. Stinebring & P. J. Chapple, Eds. Advan. Exp. Med. Biol. **110:** 61–75. Plenum Press. New York and London.
11. ATTALLAH, A. M., T. J. YEATMAN, P. D. NOGUCHI & J. C. PETRICCIANI. 1979. Is DNA synthesis a requisite for the differentiation of B lymphocytes into immunoglobulin-secreting plasma cells? Int. Arch. Allergy. Appl. Immunol. **60:** 132–139.
12. RUCKDESCHEL, J. C., J. G. DOUKAS, N. P. DRAKE & M. R. MARDINEY, JR. 1977. Application of laser cytometry to the analysis of immunologically induced *in vitro* lymphocyte responsiveness. Transplantation **23:** 396–403.
13. ATTALLAH, A. M., T. FLEISHER, R. KHALIL, P. D. NOGUCHI & A. URRITIA-SHAW. 1980. Proliferative and functional aspects of interferon-treated human normal and neoplastic T and B cells. Br. J. Cancer. In press.
14. GRESSER, I., M. T. BANDU & D. BROUTY-BOYE. 1974. Interferon and cell division. IX. Interferon-resistant L1210 cells: Characteristics and origin. J. Nat. Cancer Inst. **52:** 553–559.
15. EINHORN, S. & H. STRANDER. 1978. Interferon therapy for neoplastic diseases in man *in vitro* and *in vivo* studies. *In* Human Interferon, Production and Clinical Use. W. R. Stinebring & P. J. Chapple, Eds. Advan. Exp. Med. Biol. **110:** 159–171. Plenum Press. New York and London.
16. BRODEUR, B. R. & T. C. MERIGAN. 1974. Suppressive effect of interferon on the humoral response to sheep red blood cells in mice. J. Immunol. **113:** 1319.
17. JOHNSON, H. M., B. G. SMITH & S. BARON. 1975. Inhibition of the primary *in vitro* antibody response by interferon preparations. J. Immunol. **114:** 403–409.
18. ATTALLAH, A. M. 1979. Lymphocyte chalone and lymphoid disease. *In* Naturally

Occurring Biological Immunosuppressive Factors and Their Relationship to Disease. R. H. Neubauer, Ed.:175–187. CRC Press, Inc. Boca Raton, Florida.
19. BLOMGREN, H., K. CANTELL, B. JOHANSSON, C. LAGERGREN, U. RINGBORG & H. STRANDER. 1976. Interferon therapy in Hodgkin's disease. Acta Med. Scand. **119:** 527–532.
20. ATTALLAH, A. M. & D. M. STRONG. 1979. Differential effects of interferon on the MHC expression of human lymphocytes: Enhanced expression of HLA without effect on Ia. Int. Arch. Allergy Appl. Immunol. **60:** 101–105.
21. STEWART II, W. E. 1979. The Interferon System. Springer-Verlag. Vienna-New York.
22. ATTALLAH. A. M. & T. FOLKS. 1979. Interferon-enhanced human natural killer and antibody-dependent cell-mediated cytotoxic activity. Int. Arch. Allergy Appl. Immunol. **60:** 377–382.
23. TRINCHIERI, G., D. SANTOLI & J. KOPROWSKI. 1978. Spontaneous cell-mediated cytotoxicity in humans: Role of interferon and immunoglobulin. J. Immunol. **121:** 1849–1855.
24. HERBERMAN, R., R. J. ORTALDO & G. D. BONNARD. 1979. Augmentation by interferon of human natural killer and antibody-dependent cell-mediated cytotoxicity. Nature (London) **277:** 221–223.

ROLE OF RECEPTORS AND THE CYTOSKELETON IN REVERSE TRANSFORMATION AND STEROIDOGENESIS INDUCED BY INTERFERON

C. Chany, S. Rousset, M. F. Bourgeade, D. Mathieu, and A. Grégoire

Institut National de la Santé et de la Recherche Médicale, U.43
Hôpital St. Vincent de Paul
Paris, France

Institut de Recherches Scientifiques sur le Cancer
Villejuif, France

INTRODUCTION

Interferon, originally described as an antiviral substance, is more and more considered to be a messenger molecule having a much broader but as yet incompletely defined significance. In this presentation we explore the different biological effects of interferon (IF) in transformed cells, either those that are undifferentiated or that have, on the contrary, conserved functional markers of the original tissue (the capacity to produce steroids).

The common link between these different IF effects is the modulation of the cell membrane components which appears shortly after treatment.[1,2] We have postulated that this modification is due to cooperative interactions between a nonspecific binding site made up of gangliosides,[3] and an IF species-specific activator site consisting of glycoproteins and interferon itself.[1,2] Available data indicate that the IF-governed modulating state has to be preserved for the maintenance of the antiviral state and perhaps for other metabolic effects of this substance.[4]

MATERIALS AND METHODS

Cells

Two cell model systems are studied: (1) BALB/c mouse cells transformed by the Moloney strain of Sarcoma virus (MSV). In parallel, cells carried for more than 200 passages in the presence of 56 units of mouse IF are studied.[5] As reported in 1968, these cells underwent reverse transformation and in spite of the presence of the transforming virus, they recovered many of the phenotypic expressions usually attributed to normal cells. The cells are resistant to the antiviral effect of exogenous IF and are not refractory to repeated inductions of this substance by viruses. (2) The Y1 mouse adrenal tumor cell line established by Buonassisi *et al.*[6] was obtained from the American Type Culture Association (Bethesda, MD).

0077-8923/80/0350-0254 $01.75/0 © 1980, NYAS

Medium

Mouse MSV and MSV-IF+ cells are carried in Eagle's minimum essential medium (MEM) plus 10% newborn calf serum. Mouse Y1 cells are grown in Ham's medium (F10) containing 12.5% horse serum and 2.5% calf serum.

Interferon Preparations

Interferon, induced in mouse L, MSV-IF+, or Ehrlich ascites cells, is obtained using standard procedures. Purification was performed according to procedures of De Maeyer-Guignard *et al.*[7] and Chelbi-Alix and Thang.[8] Specific activity of purified preparation is 5×10^8 reference units/mg of protein.

Human leukocyte interferon (Hu Le IF) is prepared according to the method of Falcoff *et al.*[9] and, as modified by Cantell *et al.*[10] The purification procedure is that of Cantell *et al.*[10] The specific activity of the preparation is 10^7 units/mg of protein. The antiviral effect of the IF is estimated either by the 50% inhibition of CPE or the 90% inhibition of vesicular stomatitis virus (VSV) in appropriate cell systems.

Steroid Secretion of Y1 Cells

Steroid secretion into culture medium is measured by a fluorometric method described by Braunsberg and James.[11] The results are expressed for 10^6 cells suspended in 2 ml of tissue culture medium.

Estimation of cAMP Content

Suspensions containing 10^6 cells from different preparations are sonicated for 6 sec at 0°C. Thereafter the cells are extracted by ethyl alcohol and evaporated to dryness at 4°C. The extract is resuspended in an acetate buffer 0.05 M pH 6.2. The amount of cAMP is measured by radioimmunoassay described by Steiner *et al.*[12] and purchased from the Pasteur Institute (Paris, France).

Chemicals

Cytochalasin B, colchicine, vinblastine, and actinomycin D were purchased from Sigma (St. Louis, MO) and used at a 5 μg concentration. Sodium butyrate was obtained from E. Merck (Darmstadt, West Germany) and used as indicated.

Preparation for Electron Microscope Studies

MSV mouse BALB/c and MSV-IF+ cells, grown in 60 ml plastic flasks, are treated or not with interferon and/or sodium butyrate. They are then detached mechanically, centrifuged, and fixed with glutaraldehyde 2.5% in Sörensen

TABLE 1

EFFECT OF CYTOCHALASIN B (CB), VINBLASTINE (VB) AND ACTINOMYCIN D (ACT D) ON THE DECAY OF ANTIVIRAL PROTECTION INDUCED BY INTERFERON (IF)

Hours of Treatment			
5 hr 30	1 hr	18 hr	EMC Yield*
IF	MEM	MEM	1.90
IF	Act D†	MEM	2.68
IF	MEM	CB + Vb	0.47
IF	Act D	CB + Vb	2.70

*The results are expressed as the log EMC yield in control/treated cells after 18 hr at 37°C.

†Actinomycin D at the concentration employed inhibits 93% of transcription.

As shown by adequate controls, none of these drugs affect significantly virus replication.

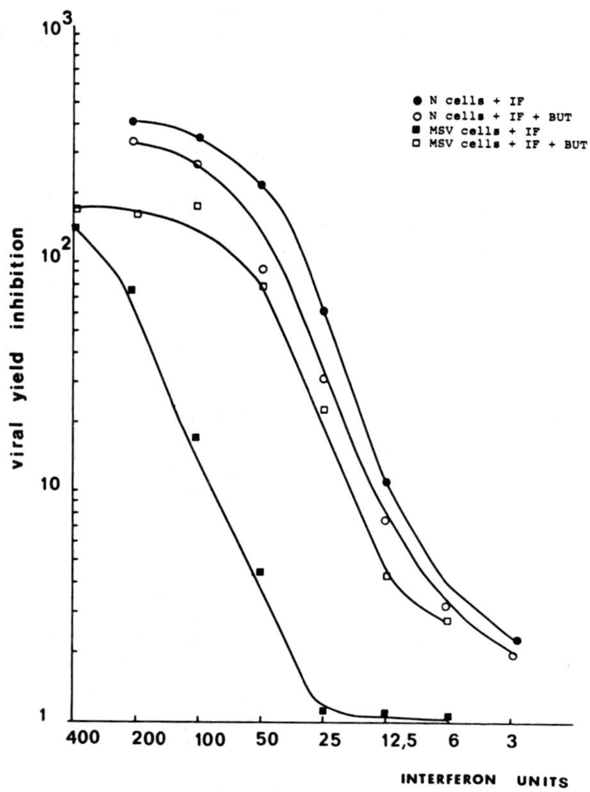

FIGURE 1. Effect of butyrate (BUT) and interferon (IF) antiviral action in normal (N) and MSV-transformed murine cells. This illustration is reproduced from Bourgeade & Chany[18] by permission of the *Int. J. Cancer*.

phosphate buffer 0.1 M pH 7.5. They are subsequently postfixed by osmium tetraoxide (1%), dehydrated and embedded in epon. Ultrathin sections are contrasted with uranylacetate and lead citrate. They are viewed in a Siemens Elmiskop 101 at an accelerating voltage of 80 kV.

RESULTS

Transformed Cells That Do Not Express Any Differentiated Cell Function

Previous studies have shown that in different cells the integrity of the cytoskeletal system is prerequisite for the expression of the antiviral effect of interferon. This is true for both type I and type II interferons.[13,14] As here shown, cytoskeleton disrupting drugs (cytochalasin B and vinblastine) not only prevent the establishment of antiviral protection in the cell, but also induce its rapid decay when added after a 5 hr 30 min IF treatment and maintained for a further 18 hr at 37°C. It is of interest that actinomycin D added at the same time as cytochalasin B will prevent this decay, thus showing the necessity of intact transcription for the effect of this drug (TABLE 1).

It is known that BALB/c mouse cells transformed by MSV are less sensitive to IF than normal cells. It has been shown that in Rous Sarcoma-transformed cells, the expression of the Sarc gene induces a disappearance of filamentous structures in the cell.[15] On the other hand, sodium butyrate, which can restore at least in part the synthesis of microfilaments, induces reverse transformation[16,17] and increases in parallel IF sensitivity.[18] Sodium butyrate, however, is only effective when the cells are pretreated for at least 16 hr prior to the addition of IF, thus indicating that an incubation period is necessary for restoration of cell processes. No change in IF sensitivity is observed in normal cells (FIGURE 1).

Effect of Interferon on the Cytoskeleton in MSV-transformed Cells

MSV-transformed cells are kept in the presence of sodium butyrate (2 mM) for 48 hr, and IF (500 units) is then added for 24 hr. In parallel control preparations, sodium butyrate, interferon, or both, are replaced by MEM. The ultrastructural aspect of these control cells is shown in FIGURE 2. Treatment of the cells either with butyrate (FIGURE 3) or IF (FIGURE 4) increases the amount of filamentous structures and the number of desmosomes or hemidesmosomes. Combination of the treatments increases additively the two effects (FIGURE 5). The semiquantitative analysis of these results is presented in Table 2. The chemical nature of these filamentous structures, considered as part of the cytoskeleton, is under investigation.

MSV-IF$^+$ cells carried for long periods in the presence of interferon have been shown to express properties of normal cells in spite of the continued presence of the transforming virus. When studied in ultrathin sections, an impressive extension of the microfilamentous network located under the cytoplasmic membrane is observed (FIGURE 6). The fibronexus is clearly detectable, thus indicating that these cells probably produce fibronectin.

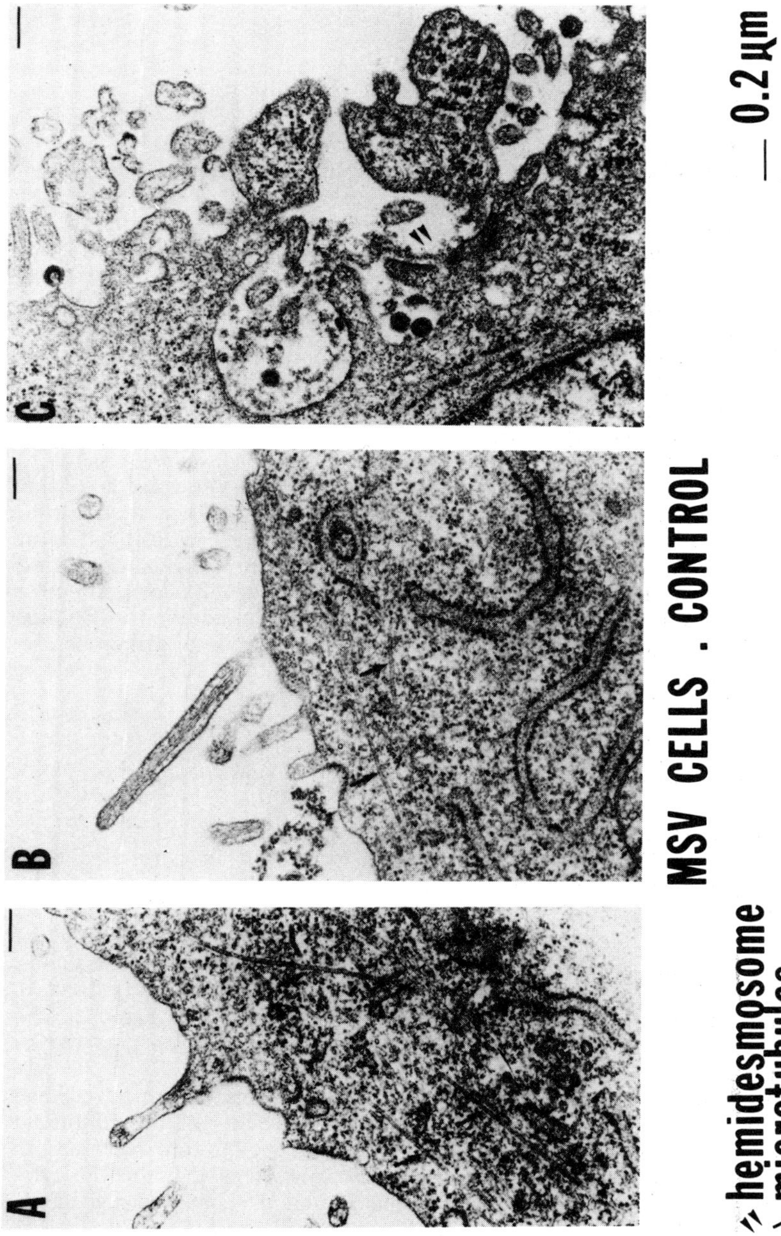

FIGURE 2. A, B: Microtubules and intracytoplasmic filaments; C: Hemidesmosomes and C-type particles.

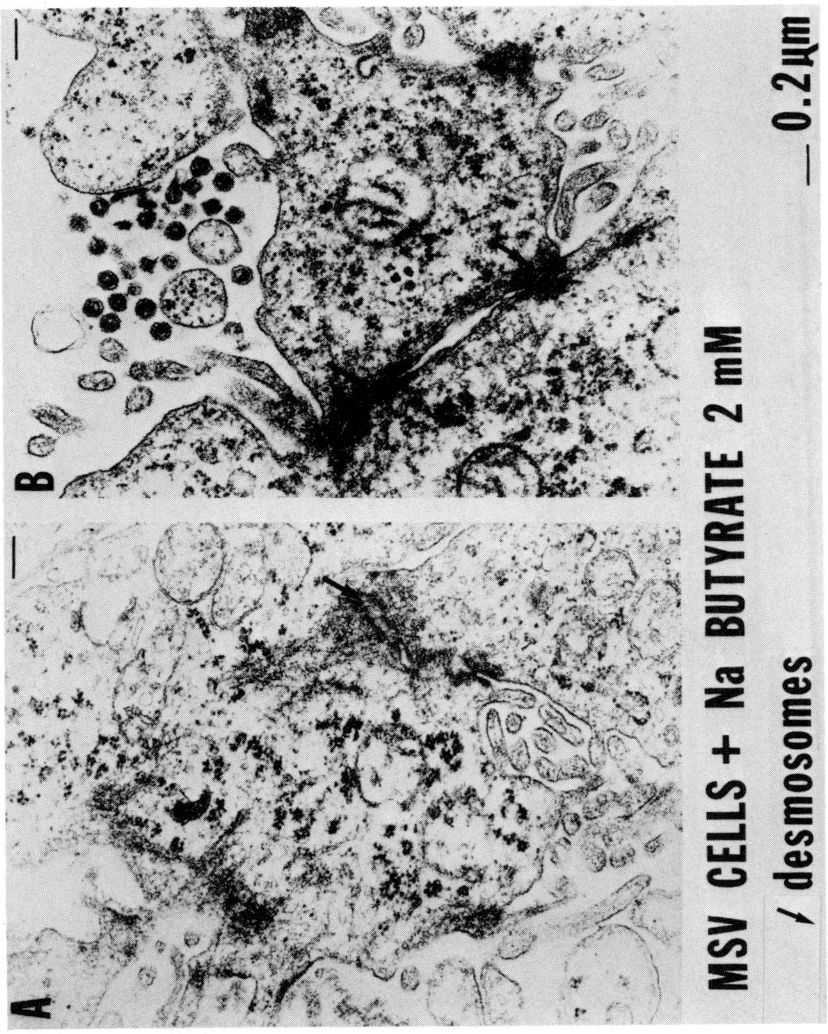

FIGURE 3. A: Desmosomes and related filaments; B: Increased number of desmosomes and C-type particles.

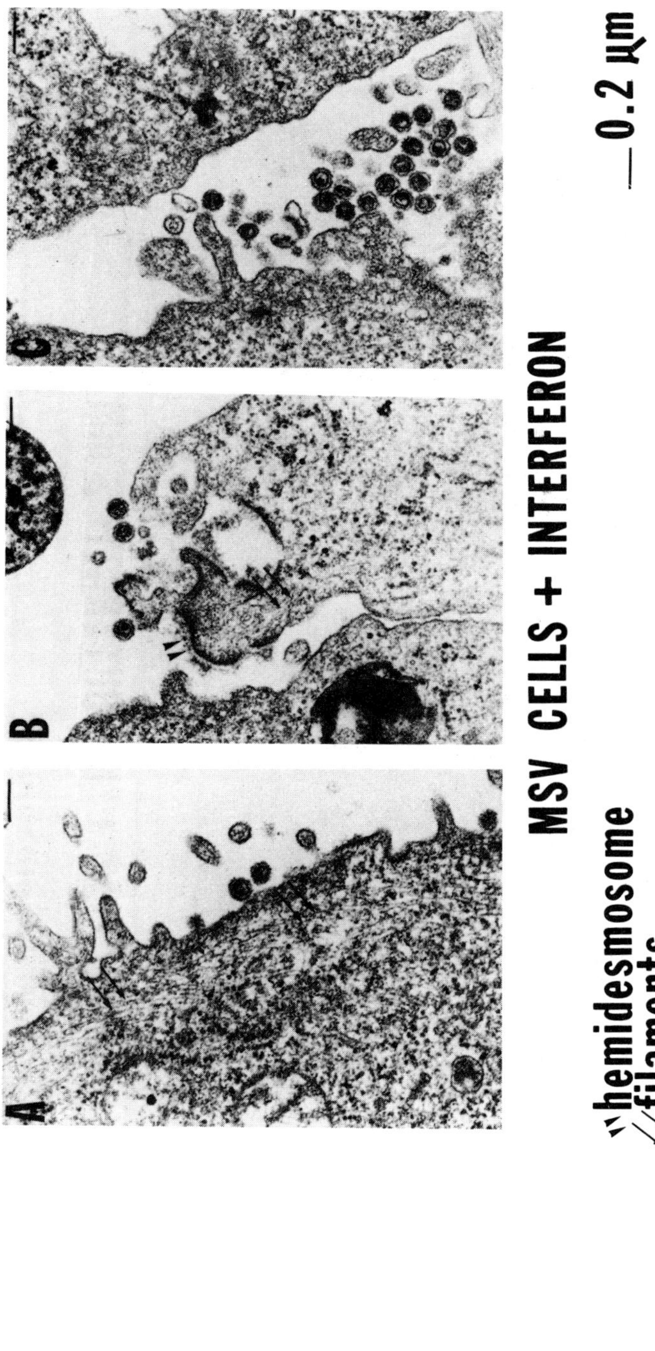

FIGURE 4. A: Increased number of intracytoplasmic filaments; B: Hemidesmosomes and related filaments; C: C-type particles.

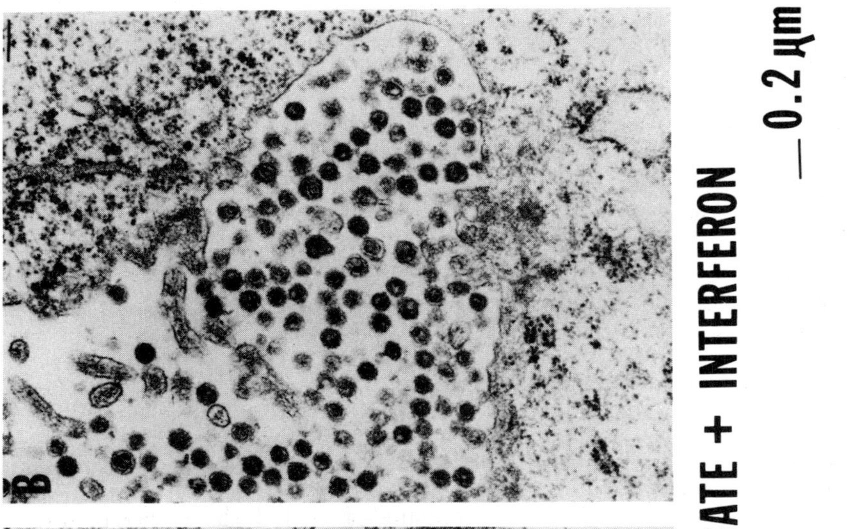

FIGURE 5. A: Extension of a hemidesmosome and related filaments; B: C-type particles.

TABLE 2

EFFECT OF INTERFERON AND/OR SODIUM BUTYRATE (SEMIQUANTITATIVE ULTRASTRUCTURAL STUDY) COUNT/100 CELLS

Cells	Experiment 1*		Experiment 2†		Experiment 3†	
	Desmosomes	Hemidesmosomes	Desmosomes	Hemidesmosomes	Desmosomes	Hemidesmosomes
MSV control	9	45	11	57	29	61
MSV + BUT (2 mM)	78	60	79	42	ND	ND
MSV + IF	85	85	24	82	52	102
MSV + IF – BUT (2 mM)	132	156	64	107	ND	ND

*Murine IF (500 units/ml).
†Purified murine IF (1000 units/ml).

Effect of Interferon in Transformed Cells Expressing Differentiated Cell Functions: The Synthesis of $\Delta^4$3 Ketocorticosteroids

Adrenal Y1 cells are treated by increasing concentrations of highly purified mouse interferon. As shown in FIGURE 7, 18-hr treatment of the cells results in ketosteroid production comparable to the one obtained with cholera toxin. The comparison of the dose-response curves shows a complete dissociation between the antiviral effect and steroidogenesis induced by interferon. Human IF at concentrations 100 times higher does not produce similar effects. Steroid production is preceded by a rapid increase of cAMP yield, which in 1 hr rises from 55 picomols to 205 picomols and decreases thereafter.

The synthesis of steroids is associated to a cell rounding effect comparable to the one observed after cholera toxin treatment (data to be published elsewhere).

It is of interest that in preliminary studies with the electron microscope, no detectable modification of the microfilamentous structure is observed. In contrast, microtubules seen in control cells are no longer present after interferon treatment. Further investigations will confirm or not this first impression.

DISCUSSION

The data here presented show that the IF response can differ according to the capacity (or lack of capacity) of the transformed cell to express differentiated cell functions.

As shown earlier in normal or transformed cells, cytoskeleton-disrupting drugs block the development of the antiviral mechanism in the cell. Here we show that in addition they might accelerate the decay of the same mechanism when added 5 hr 30 min after interferon. Since actinomycin D blocks this decay, restores and even increases the IF-induced antiviral state, it is likely that this decay involves cell transcription[19,20] and does not result because of drug toxicity. In MSV-transformed cells in which the cytoskeleton is altered, sodium butyrate partly restores it and raises the number of desmosomes and hemidesmosomes. These cells become more sensitive to interferon. In the same cells, IF also induces a restoration of the cytoskeleton, and the combined action of the two is

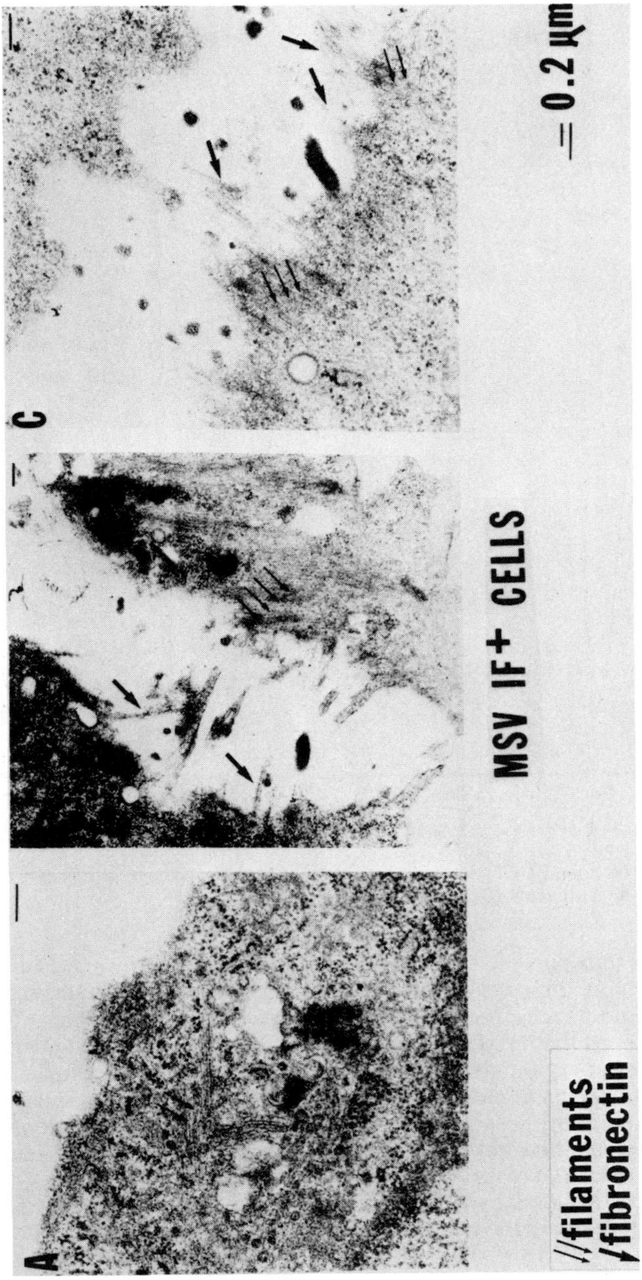

FIGURE 6. A: Numerous intracytoplasmic filaments; B, C: Intracytoplasmic filaments and fibronectin.

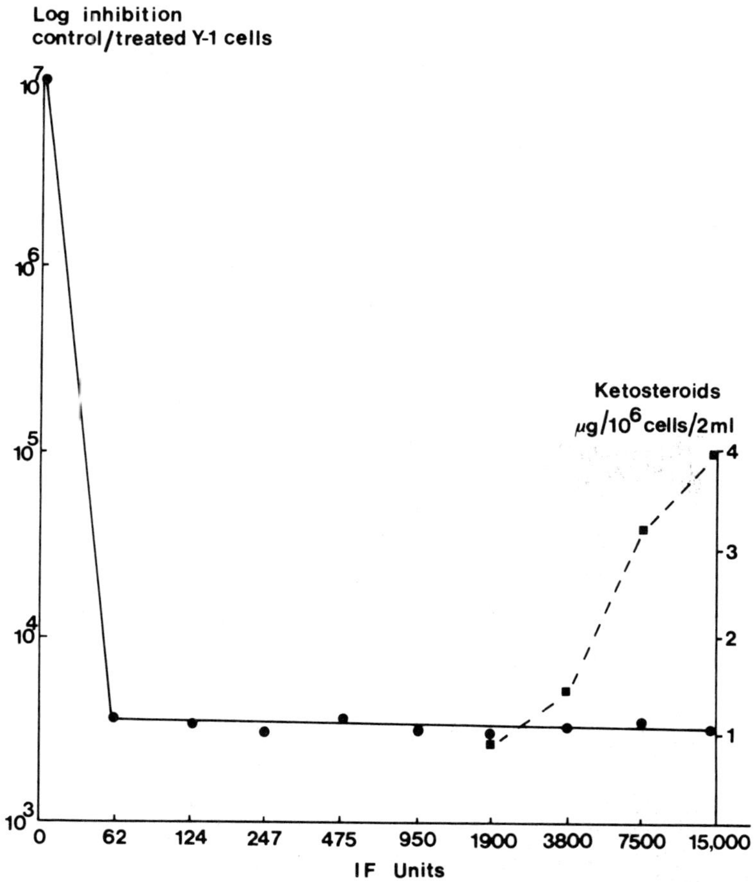

FIGURE 7. Treatment of Y1 cells with increasing concentrations of highly purified mouse interferon. ●, Antiviral effect; ■, Ketosteroids.

additive. It is thus possible that sodium butyrate improves receptor functions by the restoration of the cytoskeleton, by the increase of ganglioside synthesis as shown for cholera toxin,[21] or by other not yet detected mechanisms.

It is of interest that in MSV-transformed cells carried for a long period in the presence of IF, an intensive increase of the microfilamentous network is observed. The chemical nature of these structures is presently under investigation. It is likely that there is a relationship between this observation and the reverse transformation reported already in 1968. Thus, this change in the phenotypic expression of the cell (which recovers characteristics of a normal cell) could contribute to explain the antitumor effect of this substance. The presence of clearly detectable fibronexus suggests that these cells could also elaborate fibronectin.

In contrast, IF affects differently differentiated adrenal cells. In this system, interferon triggers ketosteroid synthesis in a manner comparable to cholera toxin, with a significant increase of cAMP. The cell rounding effect of both IF and cholera toxin suggests that no important proliferative effect on the intracytoplasmic filamentous structures is induced. The effects of IF and cholera toxin on the cytoskeleton of these cells will be analyzed elsewhere. Preliminary observations show, however, that after interferon treatment microtubules are no longer seen in the cells. This observation is in line with a report by Temple and Wolff[22] showing that antimicrotubular agents also induce steroidogenesis in these cells, however, in the absence of adenylate cyclase activation.

Finally, the question arises as to what extent these unusual IF-induced cell modifications are related to the molecule itself. This is obviously difficult to estimate for older experiments mentioned in this article. The recent experiments are performed however with highly purified mouse IF (specific activity between 10^8 and 5×10^8 units/mg of protein) which diminishes the chances of impurities being involved. Nevertheless, in spite of these arguments, the role of impurities in some of the here reported metabolic changes cannot be completely excluded.

References

1. Chany, C., A. Gregoire, M. Vignal, J. Lemaitre-Moncuit, P. Brown, F. Besançon, H. Suarez & R. Cassingena. 1973. Proc. Nat. Acad. Sci. USA **70:** 557–561.
2. Chany, C. 1976. Biomedicine **24:** 148–157.
3. Besançon, F. & H. Ankel. 1974. Nature **252:** 478–480.
4. Pauloin, A., F. Chany-Fournier, L. Epstein & C. Chany. 1977. C. R. Acad. Sci. Paris **284:** 1119–1122.
5. Chany C. & M. Vignal. 1968. C. R. Acad. Sci. Paris **267:** 1798–1800.
6. Buonassisi, V., G. Sato & A. Cohen. 1962. Proc. Nat. Acad. Sci. USA **48:** 1184–1190.
7. De Maeyer-Guignard, J., Minh Nguy Thang & E. De Maeyer. 1977. Proc. Nat. Acad. Sci. USA **74:** 3787–3790.
8. Chelbi-Alix, M. D. & Minh Nguy Thang. 1980. *In* Methods in Enzymology. S. Tetska, Ed. In press.
9. Falcoff, E., R. Falcoff, F. Fournier & C. Chany. 1966. Ann. Inst. Pasteur **111:** 562–584.
10. Cantell, K., S. Hirvonen, K. E. Mogensen, L. Pyhala. 1974. *In* The Production and Use of Interferon for the Treatment and Prevention of Human Virus Infections. In Vitro Monograph. C. Waymouth, Ed. Vol. **3:** 35–38. Tissue Culture Association, Rockville, Maryland.
11. Braunsberg, H. & V. H. T. James. 1960. Anal. Biochem. **1:** 452–468.
12. Steiner, A. L., D. M. Kipnis, R. Utiger & C. Parker. 1969. Proc. Nat. Acad. Sci. USA **64:** 367–373.
13. Bourgeade, M. F. & C. Chany. 1976. Proc. Soc. Exp. Biol. Med. **153:** 501–504.
14. Bourgeade, M. F., C. Chany & T. Merigan. 1980. J. Gen. Virol. **46:** 449–454.
15. McClain, D. A., P. F. Maness & G. M. Edelman, 1978. Proc. Nat. Acad. Sci. USA **75:** 2750–2754.
16. Altenburg, B. C., D. P. Via & S. H. Steiner. 1976. Exp. Cell Res. **102:** 223–231.
17. Storrie, B., T. T. Puck & L. Wenger. 1978. J. Cell. Physiol. **94:** 69–76.
18. Bourgeade, M. F. & C. Chany. 1979. Int. J. Cancer **24:** 314–318.
19. Chany, C., F. Fournier & S. Rousset. 1971. Nature New Biol. **230:** 113–114.
20. Lab, M. & F. Koehren. 1972. Ann. Inst. Pasteur **122:** 567–573.
21. Fishmann, P. H. & E. Atikkane. 1979. J. Biol. Chem. **254:** 4342–4344.
22. Temple, R. & J. Wolff. 1973. J. Biol. Chem. **248:** 2691–2698.

THE EFFECT OF INTERFERON ON CYCLIC NUCLEOTIDES*

Michael G. Tovey

Institut de Recherches Scientifiques sur le Cancer
94800 Villejuif, France

Cécile Rochette-Egly

Unité 61
Institut National de la Santé et de la Recherche Médicale
67200 Strasbourg, France

The effect of interferon on cells can become manifest in a variety of ways including: a reduction in the rate of cell multiplication,[1-3] resistance to virus replication,[4] specific enhancement or inhibition of specialized cellular functions,[3,5-10] and modifications of the cell surface.[3,11-14] Interferon also exhibits a marked antitumor action,[3] and can influence the immune system.[3,15] By analogy with the established mode of action of certain polypeptide hormones,[16] it is possible that cyclic nucleotides may play a role in the development of some of the diverse effects of interferon on cells. Thus, treatment of cells with various derivatives of adenosine 3',5' cyclic monophosphate (cAMP),[17-19] or compounds that increase the intracellular levels of cAMP,[20] has been shown to potentiate the antiviral action of interferon. Similarly, it has been reported that increased levels of cAMP precede the establishment of the antiviral state,[20,21] or occur concomitantly with the inhibition of cell multiplication[22] in interferon-treated cells. However, these studies were undertaken in conventional batch culture in which the environment is continuously changing, rendering the interpretation of changes in intracellular cAMP concentration difficult. These difficulties can be overcome by the use of chemostat culture, in which cell multiplication occurs at a constant rate and in a constant environment. We have recently described the establishment of steady-state cultures of animal cells in the chemostat and the application of this technique to the investigation of the effect of interferon on tumor cell multiplication.[23]

The use of this sensitive and controlled system has enabled us to show that treatment of steady-state chemostat cultures of mouse leukemia L1210 cells with interferon results in a rapid increase in the intracellular concentration of guanosine 3',5' cyclic-monophosphate (cGMP), which precedes by several hours an increase in the concentration of cAMP and an inhibition of cell multiplication.[26] We show herein that a rapid increase in the intracellular concentration of cGMP also occurs in conventional batch cultures of L1210 cells treated with interferon, and that this effect is also obtained with electrophoretically pure interferon. We also show that differences are observed in the response of cAMP in batch and chemostat cultures of L1210 cells treated with interferon.

*This work was aided in part by grants from the Direction des Etudes Recherches et Techniques (78-34-210), the Centre National de la Recherche Scientifique (ATP 3231) and the Institut National de la Santé et de la Recherche Médicale (ATP 76-72).

0077-8923/80/0350-0266 $01.75/0 © 1980, NYAS

MATERIALS AND METHODS

Chemostat Cultures

Mouse leukemia L1210 cells were cultivated under glucose limitation in a chemostat (300 ml working volume) in Eagle's minimal essential medium supplemented with 10% heat-inactivated horse serum as previously described.[23]

The dilution rate (D) is defined as the quotient:

medium flow rate (ml/day)/culture volume (ml).

In the steady-state

$$\mu = \frac{\ln 2}{\text{Td}} = \text{D (day}^{-1}\text{)}$$

where μ = specific growth rate and Td = doubling time of cells. Samples (< 1% of culture volume) were removed directly from the culture vessel via a sampling port.

Batch Cultures

Mouse L1210 cells were cultivated in stirred suspension culture in the same medium used for chemostat culture but with a non-growth-limiting glucose concentration of 2 mg/ml.

Cyclic Nucleotide Determinations

One milliliter of cell suspension was extracted with 1 ml of 12% trichloroacetic acid for 15 min at 0°C. The suspension was then centrifuged (2,000 × g, 10 min) and the supernatant was extracted twice with 10 volumes of water-saturated ether, purified on a column of Dowex AG1 × 8[27] and assayed for cAMP content as previously described,[28] and for cGMP content with Boehringer test kits (Mannheim, Germany). Results were calculated from the mean of four replicates in pmoles per 10^6 cells. Alternatively, the intracellular concentrations of the cyclic nucleotides were determined on 1.0 ml of cell suspension after centrifugation (800 × g, 5 min) and extraction with 2 ml of 6% trichloroacetic acid at 0°C. The suspension was then centrifuged (2,000 × g, 10 min) and the supernatant was extracted with ether and assayed for cAMP and cGMP content as described above. Recovery (70–80%) was monitored with 1 m μCi of [^{3}H]cAMP or [^{3}H]cGMP. The acid-precipitable material was dissolved in 1.0 ml of 0.6 N. NaOH and assayed for protein content by the method of Lowry *et al.*[29] Results are expressed as the mean of four replicates in pmoles per mg of protein. In the majority of experiments the concentration of cyclic nucleotides was determined without prior separation of cAMP and cGMP since this procedure was found to give the most consistant results. The recovery of cAMP and cGMP after separation on AG 1 × 8 has been shown to depend upon the molar quantities of the cyclic nucleotides applied.[30]

[^{3}H]Thymidine Incorporation

Samples were removed directly from the chemostat and pulse-labeled with 5 μCi [^{3}H]TdR (25 Ci/mmol, CEA France) for 30 min at 37°C. Incorporation of [^{3}H]thymidine into cellular material was determined by measuring the radioactivity in the trichloroacetic acid insoluble material retained on a Millipore filter, as previously described.[24]

Interferon Preparations

Interferon was prepared from suspension cultures of mouse sarcoma C243-3 cells inoculated with Newcastle disease virus. The methods of production, partial purification, and assay of the interferon have previously been described.[31] Mock interferon was prepared and purified in a manner identical to interferon,[31] with the exception that the virus inducer was added just prior to harvesting the culture supernatant. Two types of interferon preparations were used in this study. Partially purified interferon of specific activity 2×10^7 reference units/mg protein and interferon which had been further purified by sequential affinity[32,33] and ion exchange[34] chromatography to a specific activity of 7.5×10^8 reference units/mg protein. The highly purified interferon was prepared by Dr. Michel Aguet in our laboratory. When the purified interferon with an activity of 7.5×10^8 reference units/ml was subjected to electrophoresis in polyacrylamide gels containing SDS, only three bands corresponding to apparent molecular weights of 35,000, 28,000 and 22,000 were observed after staining with Coomassie Blue. Biological activity of interferon was found only in elutes of gel slices corresponding to these bands.

Experimental Procedure

Interferon was introduced into the chemostat by injection into the culture vessel and by simultaneous addition to the inflowing medium to maintain a constant concentration for the duration of each experiment (2 to 4 days). A single interferon concentration of 6400 units/ml, corresponding to between 1 and 2 units of interferon per 10^3 cells in the chemostat, was used throughout this study.

RESULTS

Establishment of Steady-State Concentrations of Cyclic Nucleotides

Constant intracellular concentrations of cAMP and cGMP were obtained after a period of adjustment ranging from approximately 200 to 500 hours of continuous operation of the chemostat. Once a steady-state became established, the intracellular concentration of both cAMP and cGMP remained constant during the steady-state, so that the standard deviation of the mean concentrations of cAMP and cGMP was the same as the standard deviation of replicates of individual points (FIGURE 1).

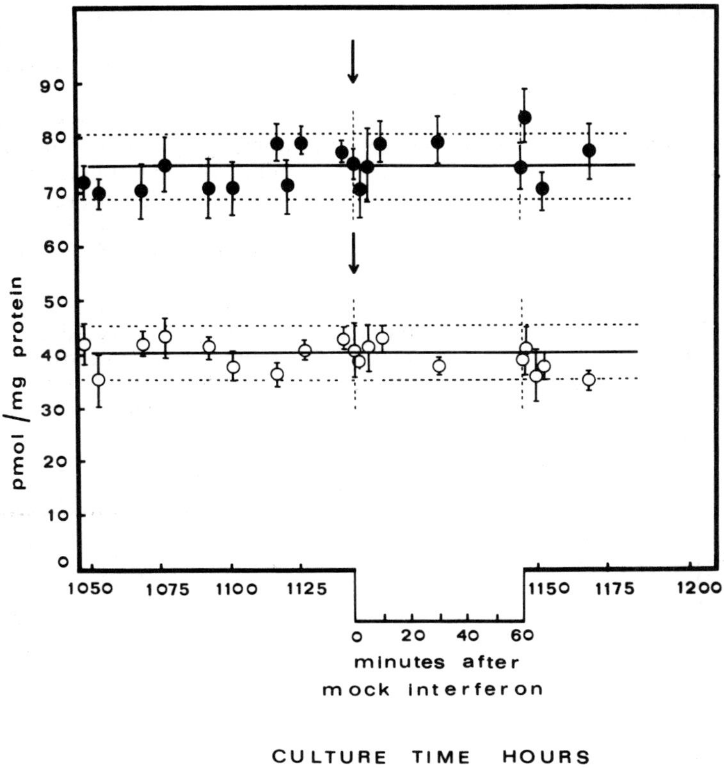

FIGURE 1. A chemostat culture of L1210 cells under steady-state conditions at a growth rate of 1.5 day^{-1} (Td 11.1 hours). ●, Intracellular concentration of cAMP (steady-state mean value: 74.7 ± 6.0 pmol/mg protein); ○, Intracellular concentration of cGMP (steady-state mean value: 40.5 ± 3.46 pmol/mg protein).

The horizontal solid lines with broken lines above and below represent the steady-state mean value with standard deviation. The error bars represent the standard deviation of the replicates for a particular point.

↓ Time of addition of mock interferon.

Effect of Interferon on the Intracellular Concentrations of cGMP

A rapid increase in the intracellular concentration of cyclic GMP was observed 1 to 5 minutes after the addition of interferon to steady-state chemostat cultures of mouse L1210 cells (FIGURE 2). The increase in the intracellular concentration of cGMP was maximal between 1 and 10 minutes after the addition of interferon and then returned to its previous steady-state value between 10 and 300 minutes later (FIGURES 2 and 3). The increase in cGMP in response to interferon treatment appeared to be more rapid when L1210 cells were cultivated at a fast growth rate than at a slow growth rate in the chemostat. Thus at a growth rate of 1.5 day^{-1} (Td 11.1 hours) a maximal increase in the concentration of cGMP occurred 1 minute after the addition of interferon and then returned to its previous steady-state level by 10 minutes, whereas at a growth rate of 0.5 day^{-1} (Td 33.2 hours) the maximum increase in cGMP did not occur until 5 to 10 minutes and then did not return to the previous steady-state level until 60 (FIGURE 3) to 300 minutes (FIGURE 2) later.

The increase in the concentration of cGMP in the chemostat after addition of interferon was followed 2 hours later by an inhibition of [^{3}H]thymidine incorporation (30–50%), that is, 22 hours prior to an inhibition of cell multiplication.[24] We have previously shown that the inhibition of thymidine incorporation in the chemostat results from an inhibition of thymidine transport rather than from an inhibition of DNA synthesis,[35] and it may reflect an effect of interferon on the cell surface.

A rapid increase in the intracellular concentration of cGMP was also observed when L1210 cells cultivated in batch culture were treated with interferon. Thus a threefold increase in the intracellular concentration of cGMP occurred 1 to 5 minutes after the addition of interferon (FIGURE 4). The concentration of cGMP remained elevated for 20 min and then declined rapidly between

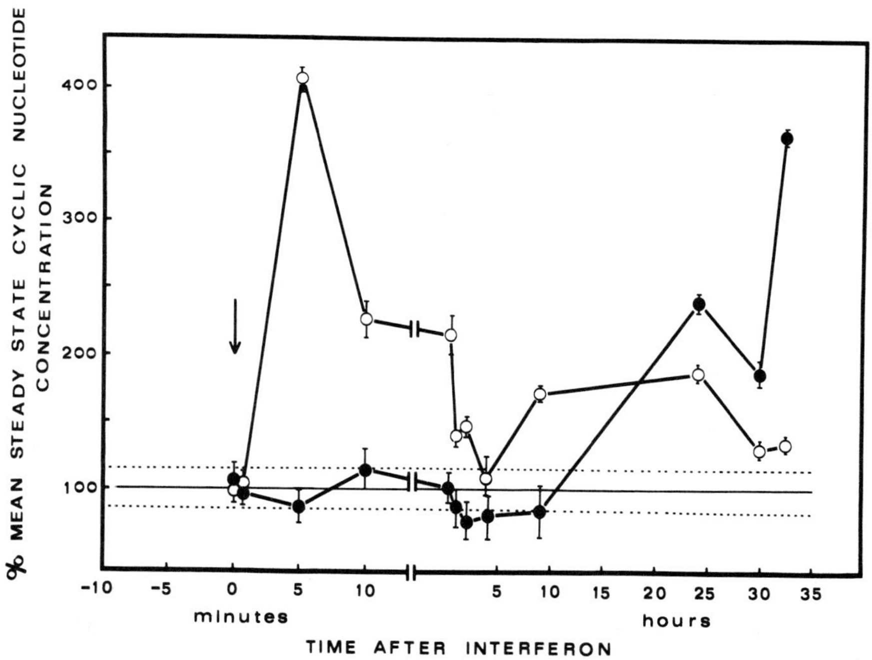

FIGURE 2. The effect of interferon on the steady-state intracellular concentrations of cAMP and cGMP in a chemostat culture of mouse L1210 cells Growth rate 0.5 day^{-1} (Td 33.2 hours). ●, Intracellular concentration of cAMP; ○, Intracellular concentration of cGMP.

The horizontal solid lines with broken lines above and below represent the steady-state mean value with standard deviation. The error bars represent the standard deviation of the replicates for a particular point.

↓ Time of addition of interferon.

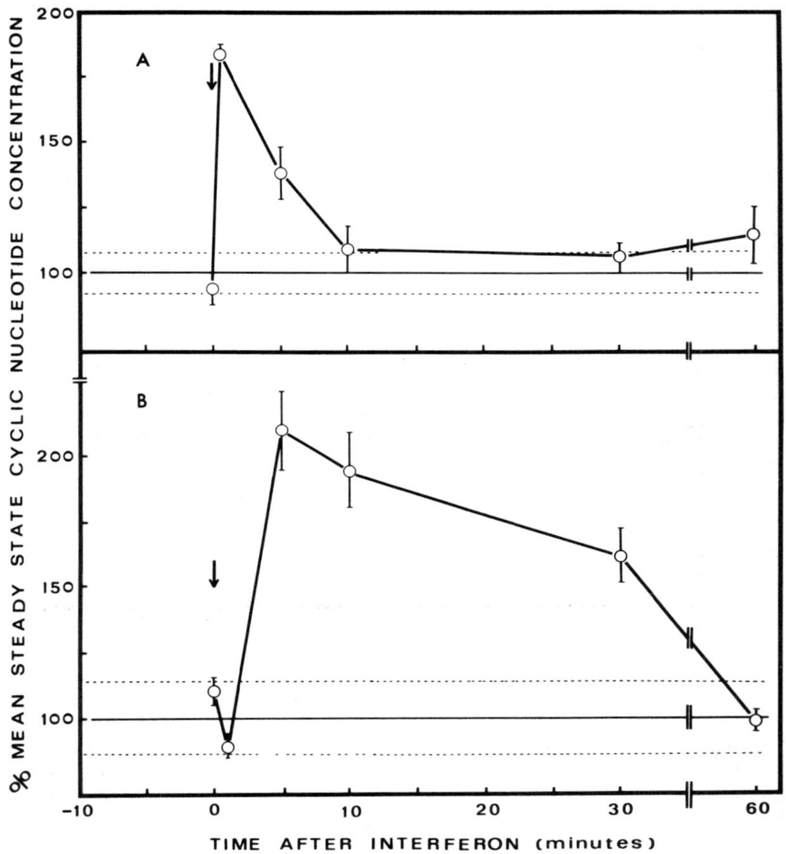

FIGURE 3. The effect of interferon on the steady-state intracellular concentration of cGMP in chemostat cultures of mouse L1210 cells. (*A*) = Growth rate 1.5 day^{-1} (Td 11.1 hours); (*B*) = Growth rate 0.5 day^{-1} (Td 33.2 hours).

The horizontal solid lines with broken lines above and below represent the steady-state mean value with standard deviation. The error bars represent the standard deviation of the replicates for a particular point.

↓ Time of addition of interferon.

20 and 25 min returning to approximately the same level as that prior to the addition of interferon (FIGURE 4).

Effect of Interferon on the Intracellular Concentration of cAMP

No increase in the intracellular concentration of cAMP was observed during the first 5 hours after the addition of interferon to steady-state chemostat cultures of mouse L1210 cells (FIGURE 2). A slight increase (35–64 %) in the concentration of cAMP was observed at 6 and 9 hours in one experiment, and at 9 hours only in

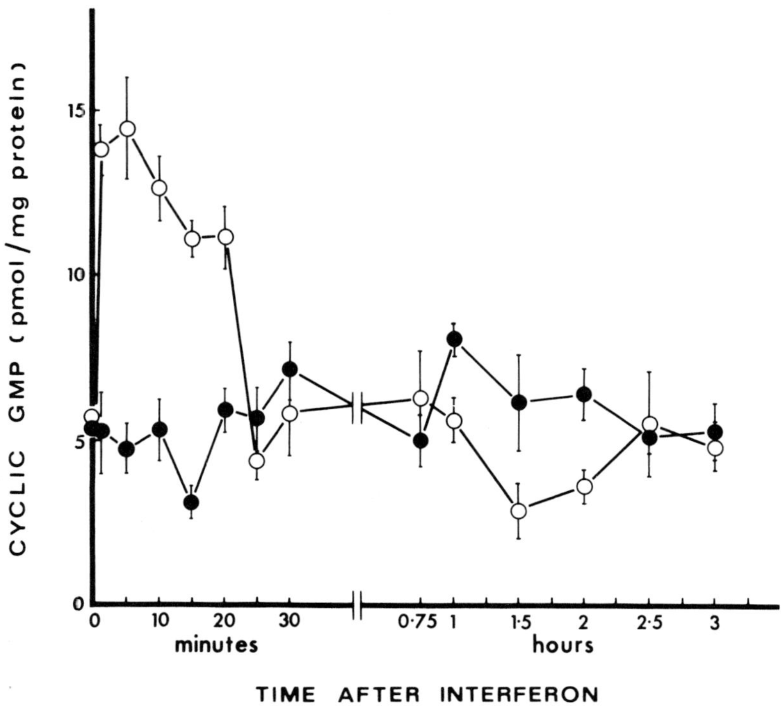

FIGURE 4. The effect of interferon on the intracellular concentration of cGMP in a batch culture of mouse L1210 cells. ○, Treated with 6400 u/ml of electrophoretically pure interferon (specific activity 7.5 × 10^8 units/ml) in phosphate buffered saline (PBS); ●, Treated with an equal volume of PBS.

a second experiment, whereas in a third experiment no increase in the concentration of cAMP occurred until 24 hours after interferon. In all three chemostat experiments the first pronounced increase (2 to 3.8 fold) in the concentration of AMP occurred 24 hours after the addition of interferon (FIGURE 2) concomitantly with the first significant inhibition of cell multiplication. Contrastingly, however, in batch culture a progressive increase in the intracellular concentration of cAMP was observed between 2 and 3 hours after the addition of interferon (FIGURE 5).

Effect of Prostaglandin E_1 on Steady-State Intracellular Concentrations of cAMP and cGMP

In order to determine the sensitivity of chemostat cultures of L1210 cells to substances known to enhance cAMP levels, the effect of prostaglandin E_1 (PGE_1) on the steady-state concentration of cAMP was compared to that of interferon. Treatment of chemostat cultures of L1210 cells with PGE_1, in agreement with its previously reported action,[36] caused a marked and rapid (5 to 10 min) increase in the steady-state concentration of cAMP without exerting a pronounced effect on the intracellular concentration of cGMP (FIGURE 6). A marked inhibition (45 to

60%) of [^{3}H]thymidine incorporation was observed two hours after the addition of PGE_1 to chemostat cultures of L1210 cells followed by an inhibition of cell multiplication at 24 hours (data not shown).

Effect of Interferon on the Ratio of cAMP to cGMP

Treatment of steady-state chemostat cultures of mouse L1210 cells with interferon resulted in a rapid decrease in the ratio of cAMP to cGMP at 1 to 30 minutes followed by a recovery and an increase in the ratio from 5 to 24 hours later (FIGURE 7). In contrast, treatment of steady-state cultures of L1210 cells with PGE_1 caused a rapid increase in the ratio of cAMP to cGMP at 5 to 10 minutes. The ratio then decreased progressively to reach the previous steady-state value at 5 hours followed by a further decrease at 26 and 31 hours (FIGURE 7).

Evidence That Interferon Is the Factor Responsible for the Effects Observed.

Treatment of L1210 cells with the same number of units of either partially purified (specific activity 2×10^7 units/mg protein) or electrophoretically pure

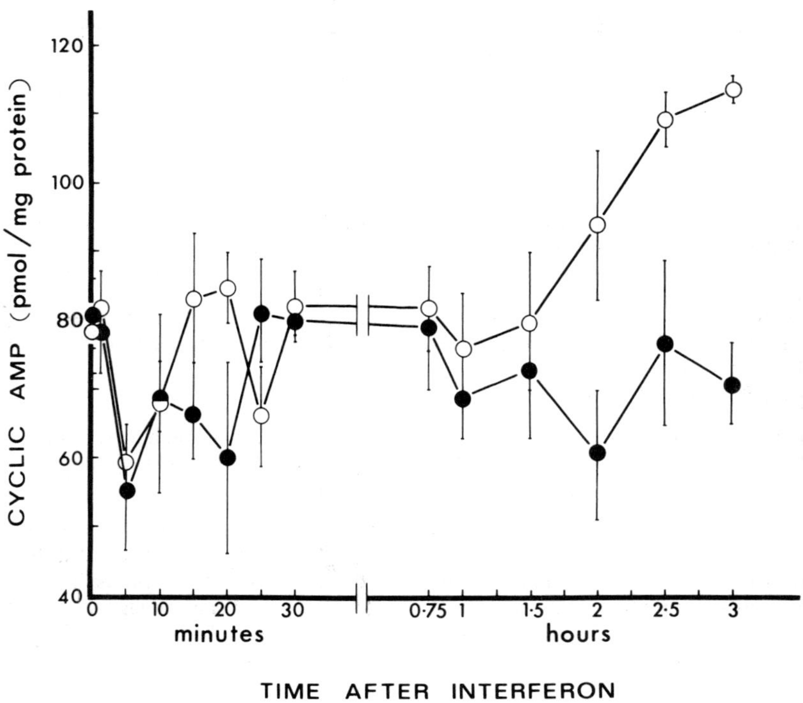

FIGURE 5. The effect of interferon on the intracellular concentration of cAMP in a batch culture of mouse L1210 cells. ○, Treated with 6400 units/ml of electrophoretically pure interferon (specific activity 7.5×10^8 units/ml) in PBS; ●, Treated with an equal volume of PBS.

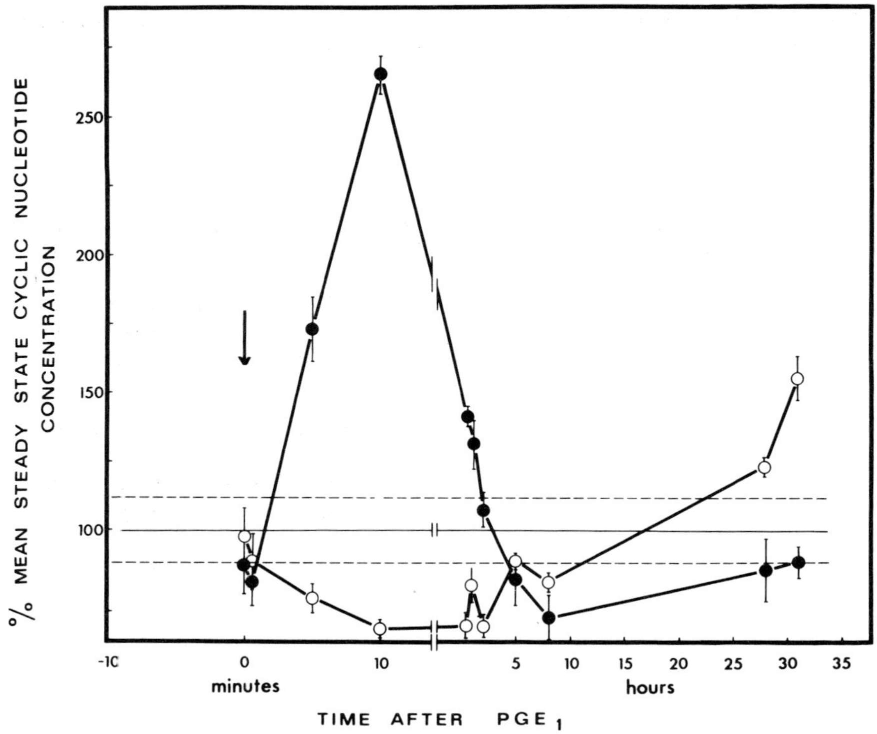

FIGURE 6. The effect of prostaglandin E_1 on the steady-state intracellular concentrations of cAMP and cGMP in a chemostat culture of mouse L1210 cells. Growth rate 1.0 day^{-1} (Td 16.6 hours). ●, Intracellular concentration of cAMP; ○, Intracellular concentration of cGMP.

The horizontal solid lines with broken lines above and below represent the steady-state mean value with standard deviation. The error bars represent the standard deviation of the replicates for a particular point.

↓ Time of addition of PGE_1.

PGE_1 (Sigma, USA) was introduced directly into the culture vessel and added continuously to maintain a final concentration of 10^{-5} molar for the duration of the experiment.

(specific activity 7.5×10^8 units/mg protein) interferon both gave a similar increase in the intracellular concentration of cGMP, strongly suggesting that the effects observed were indeed due to interferon. Furthermore, mock interferon, prepared and purified in the same manner as interferon, had no significant effect on the steady-state intracellular concentration of either cAMP or cGMP (FIGURE 1).

DISCUSSION

The intracellular concentrations of cAMP and cGMP have been found to change as cells in multiply in culture, and both cell density and cell growth rate

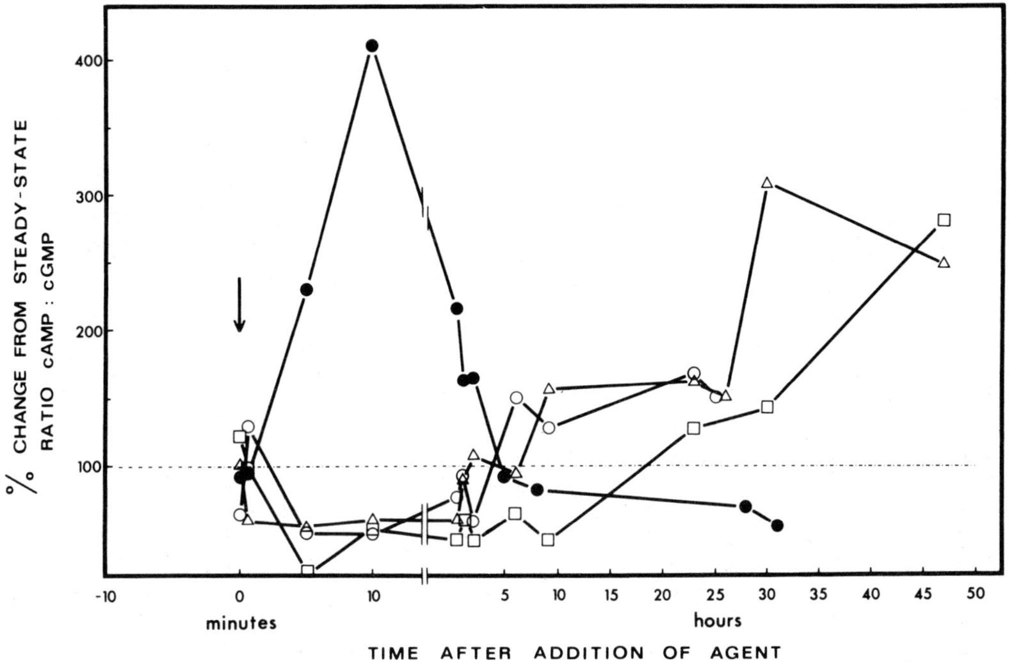

FIGURE 7. The effect of interferon and prostaglandin E_1 on the steady-state ratio of cAMP: cGMP in chemostat cultures of L1210 cells. ●, PGE_1 (10^{-5} molar). Growth rate 1.0 day^{-1} (Td 16.6 hours); ○, Interferon (6400 units/ml). Growth rate 0.5 day^{-1} (Td 33.2 hours); □, Interferon (6400 units/ml). Growth rate 0.5 day^{-1} (Td 33.2 hours); **Δ**, Interferon (6400 units/ml). Growth rate 1.5 day^{-1} (Td 11.1 hours).

The horizontal broken line represents the steady-state mean value.

are thought to influence and in turn be influenced by the intracellular levels of the two cyclic nucleotides.[37,38] We have shown however that when mouse leukemia L1210 cells are cultivated under steady-state conditions in the chemostat the intracellular concentrations of both cAMP and cGMP remain constant.[26] Under such conditions it is very much easier to determine the effect of interferon on cyclic nucleotides than in the continuously changing environment of batch culture. The use of the chemostat has enabled us to detect a rapid increase in the intracellular concentration of cGMP as soon as 1 minute after the addition of interferon. However, the effect of interferon on cGMP is not confined to the particular conditions pertaining in the chemostat since this effect is also observed in batch cultures of L1210 cells treated with interferon. Furthermore, our results strongly suggest that this effect is indeed due to interferon since the same number of units of either partially purified (specific activity 2×10^7 units/mg protein) or electrophoretically pure (specific activity 7.5×10^8 units/mg protein) interferon both gave a similar increase in the intracellular concentration of cGMP.

The effect of interferon on the intracellular concentration of cGMP occurring at 1 to 5 minutes is the earliest effect of interferon on cells described to date and suggests a very rapid interaction of interferon with the cell surface.

A number of the effects of interferon on cells that occur within a few hours suggest an action of interferon on the cell surface,[3,15] and indeed interferon has been reported to induce alterations in the plasma membrane[40] and to affect certain membrane-dependent processes.[35,41] The transitory elevation of cGMP in interferon-treated cells may also reflect an interaction of interferon with the cell surface and may play a role in the development of some of the effects of interferon on cells. Thus, interferon has been reported to stimulate a number of processes that are also influenced by agents that increase cGMP levels, such effects include enhancement of lysosomal enzyme release,[41,43] cytotoxicity of sensitized T lymphocytes,[44,45] benz(a)anthracene-induced synthesis of aryl hydrocarbon hydroxylase,[6,45] interferon production,[8,47] histamine release,[7,48] and the excitability of neurons.[38,49]

Interferon is not unique in affecting the concentration of cGMP. Similar rapid yet transitory effects on the intracellular concentration of cGMP have been observed in cells treated with mitogens,[38,50] transfer factor,[51] cholinergic agents,[37] and imidazole[38]; these effects are thought to reflect a "membrane to nuclear signal."[50] Although the increase in the concentration of cGMP is associated with a stimulation of cell division in lymphocytes treated with mitogens,[38] some substances such as carbamoylcholine and imidazole increase the concentration of cGMP without stimulating cell division.[38]

Cyclic AMP has been shown to enhance the antiviral action of interferon,[17] although cAMP alone does not exhibit antiviral activity.[17] Increased levels of cAMP have also been shown to precede the development of the antiviral state in interferon-treated cells,[20,21] although increased adenylate cyclase activity was not observed.[21]

In agreement with previous reports, we have shown that a significant increase in the intracellular concentration of cAMP occurs 2 to 3 hours after the treatment of batch cultures of mouse L1210 cells with interferon. We have shown that electrophoretically pure interferon enhances cAMP levels, strongly suggesting that the observed effect is indeed due to interferon rather than to a contaminant of the interferon preparation. However, when mouse L1210 cells were treated with interferon under controlled steady-state conditions in the chemostat, the first pronounced effect on the intracellular concentration of cAMP occurred concomitantly with the first detectable inhibition of cell multiplication 24 hours after the addition of interferon. This is in contrast to the action of PGE_1, a known inducer of cAMP, which caused a rapid (5 to 10 minutes) and pronounced increase in the intracellular concentration of cyclic AMP in chemostat cultures of L1210 cells (FIGURE 6).

The opposing influences of cAMP and cGMP are thought to play an important role in the regulation of cell proliferation.[52] Thus it has been shown that when the intracellular concentrations of the cyclic nucleotides are expressed as the ratio of cAMP to cGMP a close correlation exists between changes in this ratio and the progression of cells through the various stages of the cell cycle.[53] Our results show that interferon treatment causes an initial rapid decrease in the ratio of cAMP to cGMP followed by an increase in this ratio which parallels the inhibition of cell multiplication in the chemostat (FIGURE 7). In contrast, treatment of L1210 cells with PGE_1 causes a rapid and marked increase in the ratio of cAMP to cGMP (FIGURE 7). The temporal association between elevated levels of cyclic AMP and an inhibition of cell multiplication in interferon-treated chemostat cultures of L1210 cells suggests that the effect of interferon on cyclic AMP may at least in part, be secondary to an inhibition of cell multiplication.

ACKNOWLEDGMENTS

We thank Dr. Ion Gresser for his advice and encouragement and Miss J. Begon-Lours for her skilled technical assistance.

REFERENCES

1. GRESSER, I., D. BROUTY-BOYE, M-T. THOMAS & A. MACIEIRA-COELHO. 1970. Proc. Nat. Acad. Sci. USA **66:** 1052–1058.
2. KNIGHT, E., Jr. 1976. Nature (London) **262:** 302–303.
3. GRESSER, I. & M. G. TOVEY. 1978. Biochim. Biophys. Acta **516:** 231–247.
4. ISAACS, A. & J. LINDENMANN. 1957. Proc. Royal Soc. B **147:** 258–267.
5. LIEBERMAN, D., Z. VOLOCH, H. AVIV, U. NUDEL & M. REVEL. 1974. Mol. Biol. Rep. **1:** 447–451.
6. NEBERT, D. W. & R. M. FRIEDMAN. 1973 J. Virol. **11:** 193–197.
7. IDA, S., J. J. HOOKS, R. P. SIRAGANIAN & A. I. NOTKINS. 1977. J. Exp. Med. **145:** 892–906.
8. STEWART, W. E., II, I. B. GOSSER & R. Z., LOCKHART, Jr. 1971. J. Virol. **7:** 792–801.
9. YARON, M., I. YARON, D. GURARI-ROTMAN, M. REVEL, H. R. LINDNER & U. ZOR. 1977. Nature (London) **267:** 457–459.
10. ROZEE, K. R., L. J. KATZ & E. S. MCFARLANE. 1969. Can. J. Microbiol. **15:** 969–971.
11. LINDAHL, P., P. LEARY & I. GRESSER. 1973. Proc. Nat. Acad. Sci. USA **70:** 2185–2188.
12. HUET, C., I. GRESSER, M-T. BANDU & P. LINDAHL. 1974. Proc. Soc. Exp. Biol. Med. **147:** 52–57.
13. KNIGHT, E., Jr. & B. C. KORANT. 1977. Biochem. Biophys. Res. Commun. **74:** 707–713.
14. CHANG, E. H., F. T. JAY & R. M. FRIEDMAN. 1978. Proc. Nat. Acad. Sci. USA **75:** 1859–1863.
15. GRESSER, I. 1977. Cell Immunol. **34:** 406–415.
16. ROBINSON, G. A., R. W. BUCHTER & E. W. SUTHERLAND. 1971. Cyclic AMP. Academic Press. New York.
17. FRIEDMAN, R. M. & I. PASTAN. 1969. Biochem. Biophys. Res. Commun. **36:** 735–740.
18. ALLEN, L. B., N. C. EAGLE, J. H. HUFFMAN, D. A. SHUMAN, R. B. MEYER & R. W. SIDWELL. 1974. Proc. Soc. Exp. Biol. Med. **146:** 580–584.

19. MECS, I., M. KASLER, A. LOZA & G. KOVACS. 1974. Acta Microbiol. Acad. Sci. Hung. **21:** 265–268.
20. WEBER, J. M. & R. B. STEWART. 1975. J. Gen. Virol. **28:** 363–372.
21. MELDOLESI, M. T., R. M. FRIEDMAN & L. D. KOHN. 1977. Biochem. Biophys. Res. Commun. **79:** 239–246.
22. FUSE, A. & T. KUWATA. 1978. J. Nat. Cancer Inst. **60:** 1227–1232.
23. TOVEY, M. G. & D. BROUTY-BOYE. 1976. Exp. Cell Res. **101:** 346–354.
24. TOVEY, M. G., D. BROUTY-BOYE & I. GRESSER. 1975. Proc. Nat. Acad. Sci. USA **72:** 2265–2269.
25. TOVEY, M. G. & D. BOUTY-BOYE. 1979. Exp. Cell Res. **118:** 383–388.
26. TOVEY, M. G., C. ROCHETTE-EGLY & M. CASTAGNA. 1979. Proc. Nat. Acad. Sci. USA **76:** 3890–2893.
27. MURAD, F., V. MANGANIELLO & M. VAUGHAN. 1971. Proc. Nat. Acad. Sci. USA **68:** 736–739.
28. ROCHETTE, C. & M. CASTAGNA. 1977. Biochem. Biophys. Res. Commun. **74:** 1287–1296.
29. LOWRY, O. H., N. J. ROSEBROUGH, A. L. FARR & R. J. RANDALL. 1951. J. Biol. Chem. **193:** 265–275.
30. DE HAEN, C., T. L. EGGERMAN, M. OSE & R. H. WILLIAMS. 1978. *In* Advances in Cyclic Nucleotide Research. Vol. **9:** 767. Raven Press. New York.
31. TOVEY, M. G., J. BEGON-LOURS & I. GRESSER. 1974. Proc. Soc. Exp. Biol. Med. **146:** 809–815.
32. SIPE, J. D., J. DE MAEYER-GUIGNARD, B. FAUCONNIER & E. DE MAEYER. 1973. Proc. Nat. Acad. Sci. USA **70:** 1037–1040.
33. DE MAEYER-GUIGNARD, J. M. G. TOVEY, I. GRESSER & E. DE MAEYER. 1978. Nature **271:** 622–625.
34. IWAKURA, Y., S. YONEHARA & Y. KAWADE. 1978. J. Biol. Chem. **253:** 5074–5079.
35. BROUTY-BOYE, D. & M. G. TOVEY. 1977. Intervirology **9:** 243–252.
36. MAKMAN, M. H., B. DVORKIN & E. KEEHN. 1974. *In* Control of Proliferation In Animal Cells. B. Clarkson & R. Baserga, Eds.: 649–663. Cold Spring Harbor Laboratory. Cold Spring Harbor, N.Y.
37. CHLAPOWSKI, F. J., L. A. KELLY & R. W. BUTCHER. 1975. *In* Advances in Cyclic Nucleotide Research. P. Greengard & G. A. Robinson, Eds. Vol. **6:** 245–338. Raven Press. New York.
38. GOLDBERG, N. D. & M. K. HADDOX. 1977. Ann. Rev. Biochem. **46:** 823–896.
39. AHN, H. S., S. G. HOROWITZ, H. EAGLE & M. H. MAKMAN. 1978. Exp. Cell Res. **114:** 101–110.
40. CHANG, E. H., F. T. JAY & R. M. FRIEDMAN. 1978. Proc. Nat. Acad. Sci. USA **75:** 1859–1863.
41. GROLLMAN, E. F., G. LEE, S. RAMOS, P. S. LAZO, R. KABACK & R. M. FRIEDMAN. 1978. Cancer Res. **38:** 4172–4185.
42. HALBACH, M., K. KOSCHEL & C. JUNGWIRTH. 1978. J. Gen. Virol. **39:** 387–390.
43. IGNARRO, L. J., N. KRASSIKOFF & J. SLYWKA. 1973. J. Pharmacol. Exp. Ther. **186:** 86–89.
44. LINDAHL, P., P. LEARY & I. GRESSER. 1972. Proc. Nat. Acad. Sci. USA **69:** 721–725.
45. GAROVOY, M. R., R. B. STROM, M. KALINER & C. B. CARPENTER. 1975. Cell. Immunol. **20:** 197–204.
46. RUDDON, R. W., D. E. LUNDEEN & L. E. RIKANS. 1973. Mol. Pharmacol. **9:** 686–691.
47. YOSHIDA, I., M. AZUMA, T. SUENAGA & F. MIZUNO. 1978. J. Gen. Virol. **39:** 303–310.
48. KALINER, M., R. P. ORANGE & K. F. AUSTEN. 1972. J. Exp. Med. **136:** 556–567.
49. CALVET, M-C & I. GRESSER. 1979. Nature(London) **278:** 558–560.
50. HADDEN, J. W., E. M. HADDEN, M. K. HADDOX & N. D. GOLDBERG. 1972. Proc. Nat. Acad. Sci. USA **69:** 3024–3027.
51. KIRKPATRICK, C. H. & T. K. SMITH. 1976. *In* Transfer Factor: Basic Properties and Clinical Applications. M. S. Ascher, A.A. Gottlieb & C. H. Kirkpatrick, Eds.: 161–172. Academic Press, New York.
52. GOLDBERG, N. D., M. K. HADDOX, E. DUNHAM, C. LOPEZ & J. W. HADDEN. 1975. *In* Control of Proliferation in Animal Cells. B. Clarkson & R. Baserga, Eds.: 609. Cold Spring Harbor Laboratory. Cold Spring Harbor, N.Y.
53. ZEILIG, C. E. & N. D. GOLDBERG. 1977. Proc. Nat. Acad. Sci. USA **74:** 1052–1056.

INTERACTIONS OF INTERFERON WITH *IN VITRO* MODEL SYSTEMS INVOLVED IN HEMATOPOIETIC CELL DIFFERENTIATION*

Giovanni B. Rossi,† Antonina Dolei,‡ Maria R. Capobianchi,‡
Cesare Peschle,§ and Elisabetta Affabris†

†Laboratorio di Malattie Batteriche e Virali
Istituto Superiore di Sanità
Rome, Italy

†Cattedra di Microbiologia
University of Rome
Rome, Italy

‡Istituto di Virologia
University of Rome
Rome, Italy

§Istituto di Patologia Medica and ICHO
University of Naples
Naples, Italy

INTRODUCTION

The Systems

Erythropoiesis has been a suitable tool for defining several aspects of the regulation of eukaryotic cell differentiation. The control of red blood cell formation involves a number of critical steps, which include proliferation of pluripotent hemopoietic stem cells, their commitment to erythropoiesis, the proliferation of committed precursor cells, and, finally, the expression of several biosynthetic and morphogenetic activities characteristic of terminally differentiated erythroid cells.[1,2]

The *in vitro* development of clonal short-term cell cultures in semi-solid medium permitted identification of the precursors at different stages of the erythroid pathway. The most immature, pluripotent hemopoietic stem cell is the so-called CFU-S (spleen colony-forming unit),[3] which is capable of both self-renewal and differentiation to various precursors of the erythroid myelomonocytic, megakaryocytic and lymphoid lineages.[4-7] Two erythroid progenitors have been identified in mammals, the erythroid burst- (BFU-E) and colony- (CFU-E) forming-unit; the former represents an early progenitor, which differentiates into the late one, i.e. CFU-E.[8]

This schematic classification includes precursors at several stages of differentiation, which sequentially evolve one into the other, in a process regulated *via* both long- and short-range mediators.[9,10] These include hormones such as erythropoietin and microenvironmental influences, respectively.

*This work was supported in part by Grants from Consiglio Nazionale delle Ricerche (Progetti Finalizzati Virus, NN. 79.00420.84, 79.00424.84 and Controllo della Crescita Neoplastica N. 78.02858.96) and from N.A.T.O. (N. 1152).

0077-8923/80/0350-0279 $01.75/0 © 1980, NYAS

Studies with normal erythropoietic cells have been limited by several factors, including inability to establish normal erythroid precursor cells in long-term cultures, limited availability of genetic variants of significance to differentiation, and difficulties in obtaining differentiating populations synchronized with respect to events critical for the differentiation process. For these reasons, a useful model for studying the control mechanisms involved in the regulation of the expression of erythroid cell differentiation, is represented by the murine erythroleukemia cell system (Friend Leukemia Cells, FLC). These cells have been isolated by C. Friend (reviewed in ref. 11) from mice inoculated with the Friend virus (FLV) complex.

This complex is a Friend virus strain capable of inducing an erythroleukemia accompanied by polycythemia and is now designated FLV-P, whereas another strain, the original isolate of C. Friend, induces the same type of erythroleukemia but accompanied by anemia, and is thus, designated FLV-A. Until 1977, most studies on Friend virus were carried out on the FLV-P strain that was taken to represent the whole system. FLV-P consists of a defective spleen focus-forming virus (SFFV)[11,12] and a replication-competent leukemogenic agent (LLV). The FLV-A appears to lack the SFFV component as judged by the *in vivo* assay, but recent molecular studies have revealed that also FLV-A contains a highly defective component. The two defective virus genomes appear to be related, although not identical to one another.[13]

FLC are established cell lines growing in suspension, with a doubling time of about 12 hr during the logarithmic phase of growth. They are chronically infected by FLV, which is continuously shed from the cells, with a maximum of virus production in the log growth phase. Different FLC sublines vary with respect to the relative proportions of the FLV component produced.

FLC are erythroid precursors blocked in their differentiation pathway at the stage of proerythroblast (late CFU-E). The majority of the clones available show a low (0.5-2%) but definite level of spontaneous differentiation. The addition of dimethyl sulfoxide (DMSO) to FLC cultures causes, in a stochastic way,[14] a massive shift towards more differentiated stages of erythropoiesis.[11] The precise mechanism of this phenomenon is still unknown. Yet the availability of a cell population whereby 70–90% of the cells may be induced at will to a quasi-terminal erythroid differentiation, immediately prompted an avalanche of studies dealing with several aspects of erythropoiesis.[1] This included synthesis of heme, hemoglobin (Hb), globin mRNA, changes of chromatin and of erythrocyte-specific membrane parameters (reviewed in ref. 11). DMSO is no longer the only agent known to promote such changes as an endless list of unrelated compounds has been uncovered. In most cases treatment with the inducer results also in enhancement of virus production, as well as in a modification of the ratio between the components of the FLC complex.[15] It must be pointed out that the relationship between the stimulation of the differentiation and that of the virus production is not univocal, as some compounds can stimulate only one of the two phenomena. A large number of FLC variants have been developed so far, that may differ with respect to (1) inducibility versus resistance to a given inducer; (2) the range of differentiated function(s) expressed upon induction by a given inducer; (3) constitutive production of a differentiation parameter; and (4) the amount of virus components produced as well as the ratios thereof, (i.e. *high* versus *low* virus producers; SFFV-negative clones). (See ref. 16 for review.) Taken together, these features are indicative of a system that can be largely modulated at will.

The above-mentioned characteristics are self-explanatory with respect to the rationale of studying interferon (IF) effects on these systems. For instance FLC provide an additional opportunity for studying IF effects on the expression of integrated retrovirus genomes (reviewed in ref. 17) that can in turn be modulated by treatment with the various inducers. At the same time, it is possible to assess IF actions on cellular parameters and to determine possible relationships between the differential expression of virus genomes and that of erythroid markers.

The great bulk of evidence accumulated recently on the pleiotypic nature of IF actions makes it tempting to suggest its possible role as a physiologically ubiquitous mediator of cell interactions. To test this hypothesis, systems such as FLC, whereby well-defined functions are being expressed at a level modifiable at will, represent an ideal experimental tool.

We shall discuss here the results of our work on the multifaceted relationships between IF and FLC,[18-25] and present some additional data pertaining to both FLC and normal hemopoietic cells.

Materials and Methods

Cells

Friend leukemia cells, clone 745A, obtained from Dr. C. Friend (New York, NY), were grown in Eagle's Minimum Essential Medium (Flow, Irvine, Scotland) supplemented with 10% fetal calf serum (Flow). The cells were routinely seeded at 10^5/ml in 250 ml flasks or in 60 mm Petri dishes from Falcon Plastic and kept at 37°C in a humidified 5% CO_2 atmosphere with or without DMSO added at the indicated concentrations. The various doses of IF were added either at the time of cell seeding or as noted in the text. Cells were counted daily with a hemocytometer; their viability, assessed by the trypan blue exclusion, was never below 90%. Percentages of Hb-producing cells were determined by the wet benzidine staining method according to the procedure described in ref. 26.

Interferon

Mouse IF was prepared by infecting aged mouse L_{929} or C_{243} (a Moloney Sarcoma virus-transformed cell line) fibroblasts with 1–10 HAU/10^6 cells of Newcastle disease virus. The virus was removed after 1 hour of adsorption, monolayers washed with PBS and incubated with medium containing 3% fetal calf serum for 18 hr. Clarified supernates were brought to pH 2.0 with 6N HCl, kept at 4°C for 5 days, neutralized to pH 7.0 and stored at −80°C. Partial purification by ammonium sulfate precipitation and/or chromatography on Poly (U)- Sepharose (Farmacia, Uppsala, Sweden) was carried out according to the method given in ref. 27. The specific activities of IF preparations ranged from 4×10^4 to 4×10^7 units/mg protein. Amounts of IF are given throughout this paper in mouse units, i.e. the amount of IF reducing by 50% plaque production by vesicular stomatitis virus (VSV). This unit equals 4 research reference units of the National Institute of Health Search Standard Preparation, code G-002-904-511.

RNA Extraction from Nuclear and Cytoplasmic Fractions

Pellets of 5 to 10 × 10^7 cells were used. Nuclear and cytoplasmic fractions were obtained by subcellular fractionation according to the procedure described in ref. 28; nuclei were found to be free of cytoplasmic residues by phase contrast microscope examination. After digestion with proteinase K[29], the RNAs were extracted using the phenol/chloroform/isoamyl alcohol technique.

Globin ^{3}H-cDNA-RNA Hybridization

Full length ^{3}H-labeled DNA complementary (^{3}H-cDNA) to globin RNA (specific activity 10^7 cpm/μg) was prepared as described.[19] All hybridizations were performed in 0.2 M sodium phosphate buffer (pH 6.8) and 0.5% sodium dodecyl sulfate, containing 1000 cpm cDNA and different amounts of RNAs in a final volume of 22 μl. Reaction mixtures were sealed in capillary tubes, heated at 100°C for 10 min, and incubated for 43 hr at 68°C. The amount of ^{3}H-cDNA hybridized was determined by S_1 nuclease (Miles Laboratories) digestion, with each sample diluted into 3 ml 0.1 M sodium acetate, pH 4.5, 1 mM $ZnSO_4$, and 10 μg/ml calf thymus DNA (heat denatured, Sigma). Digestion was carried out for 40 min at 45°C, and then the trichloroacetic acid-precipitable radioactivity of samples was determined. Background radioactivity (always less than 3%) was determined by S_1 nuclease digestion of an RNA-free hybridization mixture. Glassware was treated with a silane and heated at 180°C for 3 hr.

Results and Discussion

Interferon Ability to "Induce" Globin mRNA and Hemoglobin Synthesis in Untreated FLC

Untreated 745A cells differentiate very poorly along the erythroid pathway, as only 0.5–2% of the cells will become benzidine-positive (B+) over a 4-day culture period. This low percentage may vary with the different clones of cells tested in various laboratories. There has been a report of a spontaneously differentiating clone endowed with the ability of producing 70% or more B+ cells without any treatment.[30]

We have tested the effects of low doses (5-250 U/ml) of IF on the erythroid differentiation of FLC. These doses fully induce an antiviral state with respect to both exogenous infection with VSV and endogenous production of reverse transcriptase-containing particles in the supernates. As shown in FIGURE 1 (*left panel*), there is a good correlation between IF doses and percent B+ determined on day 3 of culture in the presence of IF. Determination of percent B+ values is not a very sensitive assay, as it will score as positive only a cell that has already accumulated 20% of its maximal Hb content. The magnitude of the effect is not striking, but reproducible. Its dose-response relationship holds true also when globin mRNA amounts have been measured in the cytoplasms of the same FLC preparations (FIGURE 1, *right panel*).

The kinetics of the IF effects is shown in TABLE 1. Percent B+ values reach a plateau at 72 hr after cell seeding, whereas globin mRNA amounts peak at 48 hr and decline thereafter. The plateau phase reached by the B+ values is not in

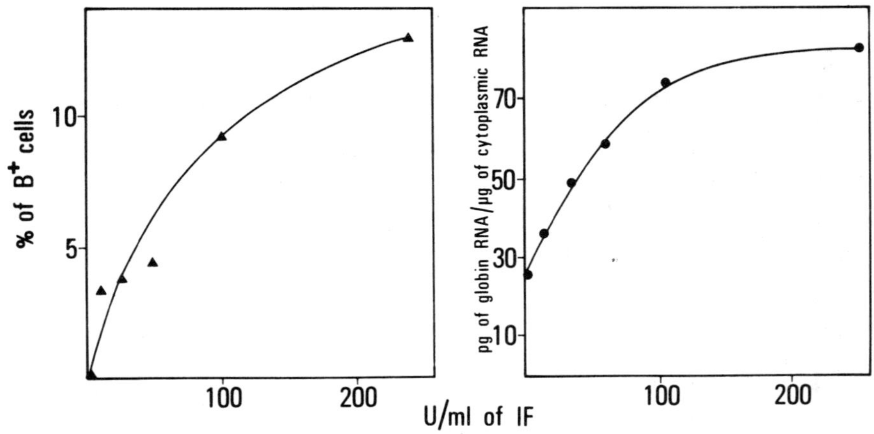

FIGURE 1. Dose-dependence of erythroid differentiation in unstimulated FLC given IF. Cells were harvested on day 3. *Left panel:* percent B+ cells; *right panel:* picograms of globin mRNA/microgram cytoplasmic RNA, measured by molecular hybridization as in MATERIALS AND METHODS.

contrast with the globin mRNA decline at the same time intervals, since it is conceivable that a B+ cell may remain so even if globin mRNA production is not going on any more. Hemoglobin is, in fact, a very stable protein. The reasons for the globin mRNA decline in IF-treated FLC remain to be determined. One obvious possibility is that IF is degraded or inactivated and therefore unable to further induce growing cells; under these conditions, therefore, globin mRNA molecules would be diluted out or degraded (globin mRNA half-life = 17.5 hr[31]). In this regard we emphasize that we have observed a slight "comeback" of reverse transcriptase activity in the fluids at 72 and 96 hr after treatment with IF doses lower than 100 U/ml. If IF is added again at 48 hr after cell seeding, the values of reverse transcriptase in the fluids do not increase at all but remain at the levels typical for IF-treated FLC, i.e. almost zero.

TABLE 1

TIME-COURSE OF THE STIMULATION OF FLC DIFFERENTIATION BY LOW DOSES OF INTERFERON*

Time (hours)	%B+		Globin mRNA (pg/μg)	
	Untreated	IF-treated	Untreated	IF-treated
12	ND	ND	49	57
24	ND	ND	57	68
48	1.4	5.9	66	148
72	3.6	15.2	34	127
96	2.5	15.9	17	39

*Cells were seeded in the presence of 50 U/ml of IF. At the indicated time intervals replicate cultures were harvested to assess cell counts, viability, percentage of B+ cells, and globin mRNA content. Cytoplasmic RNAs were extracted as in MATERIALS AND METHODS, and hybridized to globin cDNA. Results are expressed as picograms/microgram of cytoplasmic RNA.

Effects of Low Doses on FLC Erythroid Differentiation Stimulated by DMSO

As already described elsewhere,[22-24] low doses of IF are able to "enhance" the expression of the globin gene "induced" by DMSO, as measured by the B+ assay. The data from a dose-response experiment are shown in TABLE 2. The effect is best visualized on day 3 as opposed to day 4 of culture and, most importantly, under nonsaturating DMSO conditions, i.e. 0.8–1.2% versus 1.5%, which is the routine DMSO concentration (v/v) used for optimal induction in our hands. Experiments are in progress to determine whether or not the "enhanced" effect is additive or synergistic. Data available to date suggest that IF addition apparently results in a more efficient FLC induction by DMSO. Accordingly, on day 3 of culture, 0.8% and 1.2% DMSO will induce 50 and 64% B+ respectively; replicate cultures seeded in the presence of 30 U/ml of IF will show 60 and 72% B+, respectively. On day 4, the differential between DMSO+IF-treated and DMSO-treated FLC is appreciable only at the 0.8% DMSO concentration (82% versus 73% B+), whereas data obtained with higher DMSO concentrations are superimposable (ca. 87% B+) regardless of IF treatment. In other words, when the DMSO-treated cultures express their maximal potential for differentiation under given experimental conditions (roughly 90%, in our hands), the addition of IF does not further increase that potential.

Influence of Cholera Toxin on Interferon Effects on FLC

Pre- or cotreatment with $10^{-7} - 10^{-9}$ M cholera toxin (CT) effectively reduces the magnitude of the antiviral state established by IF treatment of animal cells.[32] VSV yields after cotreatment of cells with IF + CT were at least 1-log higher than those found after treatment with IF alone.[32]

FLV chronic infection of FLC results in abundant production of reverse transcriptase-containing particles into the supernates. Although IF effects on retroviruses life cycle are multifaceted (reviewed in ref. 17), the production of infectious virus in the supernates of the various retrovirus-infected and IF-treated cell systems studied is consistently suppressed. This is also the case for the FLV system,[21,24] where we observed a block of both infectious virus release and reverse transcriptase-containing particles in the supernate.

Pretreatment, as well as cotreatment, of FLC with the above doses of CT

TABLE 2

ENHANCING EFFECT OF LOW DOSES OF PURE INTERFERON ON GLOBIN GENE EXPRESSION OF FLC STIMULATED WITH DMSO

Treatment*	Day 3		Day 4	
(IF U/ml)	% B+	% Increase†	% B+	% Increase†
0	20	0	38	0
6	19	0	39.2	3
12	26	27	39.2	3
24	36	76	47	24

*All FLC cultures were seeded in the presence of 105% DMSO. IF, at the indicated doses, was added 8 hr later, and cells were scored on days 3 and 4. Values reported are the mean of duplicate cultures.

†Percent increase of B+ cells with respect to DMSO controls, taken as 100.

significantly reduces the IF inhibitory effect on both chronic production of FLV and VSV yields.[33] This phenomenon is not apparently mediated by adenylate cyclase activation by CT. In fact, pretreatment of FLC with the purified B subunit of CT (which is unable to activate this enzymatic system, yet binds to plasma-membrane receptors for CT just as well) also reduces IF effects on virus production.

Similar studies have also been performed with respect to the "enhancement" of DMSO-induced erythroid differentiation caused by low doses of IF. Preliminary data suggest that pretreatment with 10^{-9} M CT of FLC cultures, subsequently seeded in the presence of DMSO + IF, results in fully effacing the "enhancement" of erythroid differentiation. The percent B+ values in CT + DMSO + IF-treated FLC were superimposable to those detected in FLC treated with DMSO alone.[33]

These data are not taken to imply that IF and CT share the same receptors on the plasma membrane. As a matter of fact, an IF receptor has not as yet been conclusively identified. The data merely indicate that binding of CT (or, in some instances, of its B subunit) to the plasma membrane deranges the subsequent establishment of IF-mediated antiviral state and/or its effect on cell functions.

Studies with Pure Interferon Preparations: Low Doses

Murine IF has been purified to homogeneity by at least two independent groups.[27,34] Both reported a final specific activity of 1–2 × 10^9 international reference units/mg protein. One of these preparations has been tested in several systems to find out whether cell-related effects observed with crude or less purified IF preparations were also induced by such pure IF.[35] This was, indeed, the case.

We have been able to do the same in our systems through the generosity of both Dr. P. Lengyel (Yale Univ., New Haven, CT) and I. Gresser (Institut des Recherches sur le Cancer, Villejuif, France) who have provided us with samples of their pure IF preparations.

In TABLE 2 are shown the data obtained with low IF doses on FLC differentiation induced by 1.05% DMSO. Both on day 3 and 4 after seeding, IF treatment results in increased B+ values when compared with DMSO-treated controls. As already mentioned, the effects are more readily observed on day 3 than on day 4. These findings show conclusively that the effects observed upon treatment of DMSO-induced FLC with low doses of IF are indeed due to IF itself.

Inhibition of FLC Erythroid Differentiation in DMSO-treated Cells Given High Interferon Doses

In previous studies[18–20,22] we reported the inhibition of both cell growth and erythroid differentiation in untreated and, respectively, DMSO-induced FLC given high doses of IF either at time zero or at sequential time intervals after cell seeding (up to 48 hr later). The marked inhibition of cell growth curves is characterized by a significant prolongation of G_1 and G_2 phases of the cell cycle.[20] Cell growth is also reduced in DMSO-treated FLC, but not to such an extent that DMSO induction is prevented. In other words, DMSO + IF-treated FLC still go through at least 3 cell doublings thus fulfilling the cell cycle requirements for

DMSO imprinting (see review in ref. 36). In recent studies we have noticed that the IF dose-response curve with respect to the inhibitory effect on FLC differentiation has shifted to the right, i.e. larger IF doses than those previously mentioned are now needed to obtain the same effects. This is probably due to a number of concomitant changes that have occurred in the FLC system in our hands. Namely, the adoption of serum batches selected on the basis of prolonged (5-week) pretesting for both FLC growth and differentiation in the presence of DMSO resulted in substantially modified culture conditions. Cells attain saturation density levels much sooner (day 3 versus day 5) and much higher (3.5–4 versus 1.5–2 $\times$ 10^6/ml) than before. Under these conditions also the induction of erythroid differentiation by DMSO has been accelerated and quantitatively improved. A representative dose-response in such conditions is shown in the lower portion of TABLE 3 and may be compared with that obtained with a pure IF preparation (TABLE 3, upper portion). It is apparent that a semipurified IF preparation (sp. act. 10^5 mouse U/mg protein) must be given at doses as high as 25,000–50,000 U/ml to achieve a substantial reduction of percent B+ values. Conversely, 1-log lower doses of pure IF preparations are sufficient to cause the same effect. It may be concluded (1) that the IF-mediated inhibition of FLC erythroid differentiation is due to IF itself, and (2) that, if anything, less purified IF preparations seem to contain factors antagonistic to IF rather than contaminant proteins possibly responsible for the observed effects. It must also be emphasized that such high doses of IF are not necessarily "toxic" nor unphysiological. On one hand, they do not affect overall protein synthesis.[18,22] On the other hand, Dianzani and Baron[37] reported that pericellular concentrations of IF may be even higher than the dose levels used in our experiments. They also pointed out that pericellular concentrations may be more meaningful in physiological

TABLE 3

COMPARISON OF THE INHIBITORY EFFECTS OF PURE AND PARTIALLY PURIFIED INTERFERON PREPARATIONS ON GLOBIN GENE EXPRESSION OF FLC TREATED WITH DMSO

Treatment* (IF U/ml)	Day 3		Day 4	
	% B+	% Inhibition†	% B+	% Inhibition†
Pure IF‡				
0	38	0	58	0
1000	20.8	45	37	36
2000	21	45	30	48
2500	14	63	27	53
Partially Purified IF§				
0	71.3	0	83.7	0
4500	ND	ND	67.7	19
9000	ND	ND	58.0	31
25000	23.2	67	52.5	37
50000	7.5	89	36.0	57
90000	1.5	97	8.2	90

*All FLC cultures were seeded in the presence of 1.5% DMSO. IF, at the indicated doses, was added 8 hr later and cells were scored on days 3 and 4. Values reported are the mean of duplicate cultures.

†Percent decrease of B+ cells with respect to DMSO control, taken as 100.

‡Specific activity: 2 $\times$ 10^9 international reference units/mg protein.[27]

§Specific activity: 10^5 international reference units/mg protein.

terms than IF levels in the sera, which may only reflect an equilibrium rate between production and clearance.

Block of FLC Differentiation is Reversible upon Removal of Interferon

An additional argument against the supposed toxicity by which IF effects could be mediated, is provided by reversibility experiments. One set of such experiments were carried out in cells pretreated for 3 days with DMSO or DMSO + IF (50,000 U/ml). Cells were counted, % B+ was determined, then both compounds were washed out, and cultures reseeded at a cell density of 5×10^5/ml either in the presence or in the absence of DMSO. The reseeding time was designated time *zero* and all cell samples were diluted 1:2 daily thereafter. As shown in FIGURE 2, cells previously treated with DMSO, washed and reseeded once again in 1.5% DMSO showed a further increase of B+ values. In replicate cultures reseeded in the absence of DMSO, B+ cells decreased as they were progressively diluted by the expanding population of uninduced FLC. It is noteworthy, though, that in the first 24 hr after washing out DMSO, there was an increase of B+ cells also in the DMSO-free sample. This increase is probably due to residual translation of globin mRNA molecules that accumulated prior to the removal of DMSO.

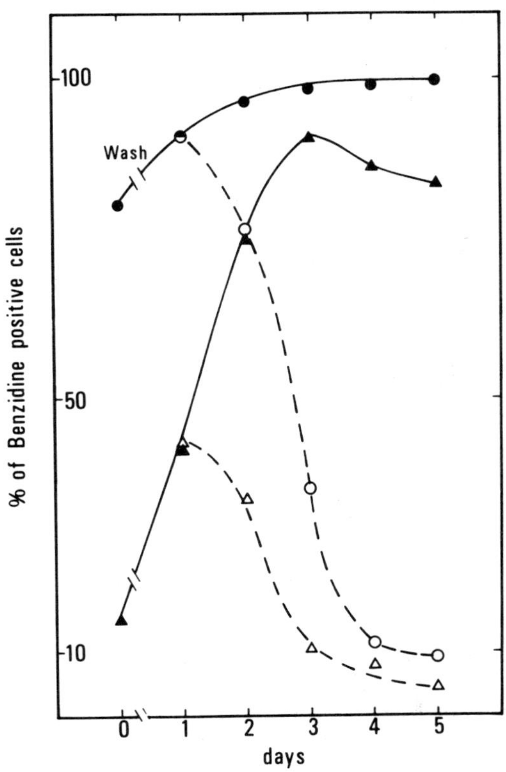

FIGURE 2. Reversibility of the IF-mediated block of erythroid differentiation. FLC were pretreated for 3 days with 1.5% DMSO alone (*circles*) or DMSO+IF, 50,000 U/ml (*triangles*). Cells were then washed and reseeded in fresh medium either in the presence (*filled symbols*) or in the absence (*open symbols*) of DMSO. Cultures were diluted 1:2 every day and sampled for cell counts and percent B+ determinations.

Cultures pretreated with DMSO+IF showed a pronounced reduction of B+ cell (12% versus 75% in DMSO-treated controls). When DMSO and IF were washed out, and cells were reseeded in the presence of DMSO, percent B+ cells increased sharply as to reach plateau values similar to those shown by cells not previously exposed to IF. On the other hand, replicate DMSO + IF-treated FLC, washed and reseeded in the absence of both compounds, showed in the first 24 hr an increase of B+ cells and then a progressive decline thereof. The quasi-optimal inducibility by DMSO of FLC previously exposed to DMSO + IF and blocked in the expression of differentiation, is taken to mean that IF treatment of FLC had not selected a DMSO-resistant subpopulation thus unable to differentiate. The sharp rise of B+ cells during the first 24 hr following removal of DMSO + IF and reseeding with/without DMSO deserves some further comments. In the former case, it is unlikely that this early rise of B+ cells is due to induction events occurring after IF removal and cell reseeding, as it is known that B+ cells begin to appear only 48 hr after DMSO addition. In the latter instance, moreover, cells were no longer exposed to DMSO and thus no further induction could take place. These data suggest, instead, that the early hemoglobinization of poorly differentiated FLC could be accounted for by translation of previously accumulated globin mRNA molecules, which were unable to promote globin synthesis in the presence of IF.

To further prove this point, experiments were carried out in the presence of 8 μg/ml of α-amanitin. This drug specifically inhibits cell RNA Polymerase II, and, given at this dosage, completely prevents in our hands any *de novo* synthesis of globin mRNA.[22] Cells were given DMSO or DMSO + IF (50,000 U/ml) in a standard type of experiment. Percent B+ cells were determined on day 3 and 4, showing once more a pronounced inhibition of differentiation in the DMSO + IF-treated FLC. Replicate cultures were harvested on day 3, washed free of DMSO and/or IF, and reseeded at 10^6/ml in fresh medium to which was added 8 μg/ml of α-amanitin. Data not shown indicate that B+ values observed at 20 hr after removal of DMSO and IF and addition of α-amanitin were slightly incresed in the DMSO-treated sample (from 66 to 78%) and more substantially so in the DMSO + IF-treated cells (from 7 to 25%).

These experiments appear to have multifaceted implications:

(1) The IF-mediated inhibition of DMSO-induced differentiation occurs at a step subsequent of DMSO imprinting;

(2) This block is fully reversible;

(3) There is no need for *de novo* globin mRNA synthesis to express the differentiated phenotype upon IF removal; and

(4) The pattern of FLC inducibility by DMSO is not altered by IF treatment.

Inhibition of Globin Gene Expression in FLC Treated with DMSO and High Doses of Interferon: Molecular Aspects

As mentioned before, treatment of DMSO-stimulated FLC with high doses of IF results in a pronounced decrease of erythroid differentiation, as measured by B+ values. This effect could have been due to a number of intracellular events taking place at any step of the metabolic pathway leading to Hb synthesis. The rate of heme synthesis is only marginally affected by IF,[19] therefore it does not appear to be the limiting factor. Thus we focused our attention on the pathway of globin gene expression as the likeliest site of IF action(s). We first analyzed the globin chains synthesized in FLC treated with DMSO + IF. Chromatography analysis in carboxymethylcellulose (CM-52) columns under denaturing conditions (8 M urea) revealed that these cells do not synthesize appreciable amounts of DBA/2 mouse adult β- and α-chains, whereas control DMSO-induced FLC have considerable amounts of radiolabeled material that cochromatographs with carrier adult mouse globin chains.[19] It was also shown that DMSO + IF-treated FLC synthesize protein component(s) which are eluted from CM-52 columns with lower ionic strength than β chains; this material is also present in DMSO-treated cells, but to a lesser extent. Similar proteins have been observed by others in extracts from mouse normal reticulocytes[38] and in erythroleukemic cells,[39] and they were thought to be related to Hb. In fact, these proteins from DMSO + IF-treated FLC are immunoprecipitated by a rabbit serum against DBA/2 mouse globin, and will be subjected to thorough investigations. Their presence could be due to an altered assembly of α-chains (as in human β-thalassemia), or, alternatively, they could reflect the "switched-on" synthesis of globin chains other than β and α, which would also occur during DMSO induction and could be amplified by IF action.

Next, we investigated whether and how globin mRNA synthesis and accumulation was affected. As already observed,[19] DMSO + IF-treated FLC do contain smaller amounts of globin mRNA than DMSO-treated controls. There is no evidence of nuclear storage of globin transcripts in DMSO + IF-treated FLC, as the majority of globin sequences are found into the cytoplasms in both experimental conditions. Moreover globin mRNA molecules made in DMSO + IF-treated FLC do not differ from those in DMSO-induced FLC with respect to other parameters. The mRNA populations from the two experimental conditions are indistinguishable from each other by base sequence: the melting curves of the hybrids of labeled cDNA with RNAs extracted from the two cell cultures are identical. T_m is about 75.5°C in both, so that major alterations of base sequence can be excluded. The possibility of increased degradation of globin mRNA molecules in DMSO + IF treated cells was ruled out in an indirect way by molecular hybridization of RNAs fractionated by PAGE under denaturing conditions (99.9% formamide); both preparations peak at the same fraction. On the other hand, the peak profile of mRNAs from DMSO + IF-treated cells is steeper than that from DMSO-treated cells. This indicates that the former mRNAs are, if any, less degraded than the latter ones. Moreover, the reversibility of the effect in the absence and in the presence of α-amanitin also seems to argue against major globin mRNA degradation.

mRNAs from both experimental conditions were also tested for their translatability in cell-free protein synthesizing systems. In the heterologous wheat germ cell-free system, no detectable differences were observed, as judged by the electrophoretic mobility of the product. When S_{30} lysates of the DMSO- and DMSO + IF-treated FLC were tested for the endogenous capacity to synthesize globin-sized proteins, essentially the same picture was obtained, i.e. comparable ability for protein synthesis of normalized amounts of globin mRNA. Addition of tRNA did not result in an increased efficiency of the system. The overall picture of transcription in DMSO + IF-treated FLC can, thus, be summarized as follows:

(1) There is a reduction in the accumulation of globin mRNA molecules;

(2) These appear to be very similar to the corresponding ones in DMSO-treated cells with respect to size, base sequence, ability to act as template in cell-free protein-synthesizing systems;

(3) There is no evidence for preferential globin mRNA degradation in DMSO + IF-treated cells when compared with DMSO-induced cells; and

(4) Under conditions where even reduced globin mRNA amounts should lead to sizable synthesis and accumulation of globin, neither one takes place. (Heme is not the limiting factor as its synthesis is only reduced twofold). In contrast there appear to be increased amounts of a more cationic protein material immunologically related to globin, the nature of which remains to be determined.

We have carried out some preliminary experiments aimed at elucidating further the molecular levels at which IF action is being implemented. Cytoplasmic RNAs have been fractionated into "membrane" (the material sedimented after centrifugation at 10,000 g of nuclei-free cell lysates), cytosol and polysome preparations. Globin mRNA amounts were then measured in each of these fractions. The data (to be published elsewhere) suggest that the relative ratios of globin mRNA found in the cytosol versus polysomes are inverted in DMSO- versus DMSO + IF-treated FLC. In the former cell population, 90% was found on the polysomes and the remaining 10% in the cytosol, the amount found in the "membrane" fraction being negligible. In DMSO + IF-treated FLC only 30% globin mRNA was found on the polysomes as opposed to almost 70% detected in the cytosol. Replicate cultures were treated exactly as described above for the reversibility experiment in the presence of α-amanitin (*vide supra*), and globin mRNA amounts were measured in the same fractions obtained from the cytoplasmic RNAs. The ratio of globin mRNA between the polysome and the cytosol fractions of DMSO-induced FLC (9:1 before washing out DMSO) decreased (5.8 versus 4.2, 20 hr after DMSO removal). In contrast, the ratio between the corresponding fractions from DMSO + IF-treated FLC (3:7 before washing out DMSO + IF) reverted to almost the opposite figures (6.5 versus 3.5) 20 hr after removing both compounds. Much more work needs to be done to fully substantiate these findings, that appear to suggest, for the time being, a much lower "binding" of globin mRNA molecules to polysomes in the presence of IF.

This could of course be due to altered poly(A) stretches or to modifications of the "cap" structure at the 5′ end of the molecule. Work is in progress to answer these questions.

Effects of Interferon on the Levels of Ornythine-Decarboxylase in Untreated as well as in DMSO-induced FLC

Gazitt and Friend[40] presented evidence with regard to the induction of the enzyme L-ornythine-decarboxylase (ODC) soon after DMSO administration to FLC.

This enzyme is crucial in the pathway leading to polyamines, which may play a role in the mechanism of induction of erythroid differentiation in FLC.[40] Gazitt and Friend have shown that DMSO administration "enhances" significantly ODC activity in FLC with a peak 3 hr after induction. The activity goes back to control values at 9 hr. From their studies, which were extended to all known inducers, it appears that this assay may divide all FLC inducers into two groups, i.e. those which do increase ODC activity, and those which do not. In collaboration with these investigators, we have carried out preliminary studies on ODC activity in FLC treated with DMSO and low or high doses of IF. The data are apparently well in line with those described above with respect to IF effects on FLC differentiation, i.e. low IF doses (36, 60 and 500 U/ml) stimulate ODC activity levels in both untreated and DMSO-induced FLC. Conversely, high IF doses (50,000 U/ml) have an inhibitory effect since they reduce by almost 50% ODC activity levels detected between 2.5 and 6 hr after DMSO induction of FLC. From the interesting parallelism between IF effects on ODC levels and those on eyrthroid differentiation in the FLC system one could infer that the action(s) of IF on the FLC differentiation could be mediated via the stimulation or the inhibition of ODC activity. Some observations, on the other hand, are in contrast to this:

(1) IF acts on ODC quite early (2–3 hr after seeding in the presence of IF), which is slightly surprising if compared to the longer time interval (at least 8 hr) generally required for the establishment of the "classical antiviral state." On the other hand, it has been shown that IF can affect retrovirus replication with a kinetics different from that of the conventional "antiviral state." In fact, as soon as 30 min after treatment with IF, cell cultures exogenously infected with murine leukemia virus, in the presence of cycloeximide, show a delay in virus uncoating,[41] which appears to result from an interaction of IF with the cell membrane, independent from any *de novo* protein synthesis.

It would appear, then, that the modulation of ODC activity by IF is not necessarily mediated by the same cascade of molecular events that takes place with respect to the "classical antiviral" activity.

(2) In untreated as well as in DMSO and/or IF-treated cultures ODC activity peaks 3 hr after cell seeding,[40] whereas the action of IF on FLC differentiation can be observed also when IF is given to the cells 8–24 hr after cell seeding in the presence of DMSO, i.e. when ODC activity is already back at base levels.

Preliminary Data on Interferon Effects in Vitro *on Normal Hemopoietic Precursors*

We have carried out preliminary experiments to assess the effects of partially purified as well as pure IF preparations on the clonogenic capacity *in vitro* of monomyelocytic (CFU-C), early (BFU-E) and late (CFU-E) erythroid precursors in mouse bone marrow cells. These experiments have been carried out in C. Peschle's laboratory in Naples according to methods described elsewhere.[42,43] Ortega *et al.*[44] reported inhibition of murine CFU-E and human BFU-E upon treatment *in vitro* of marrow cells with crude preparations of homologous IFs. Smith *et al.*[45] also observed inhibition by IF of the proliferative-differentiating response evoked by erythropoietin on normal erythroid precursors.

The data, shown in TABLE 4, are suggestive of generalized effects of IF on murine hemopoietic precursors. BFU-E appear to be the most sensitive to IF addition, since 10 U/ml already induce 50% reduction of BFU-E number. It is also noteworthy that this inhibition is exerted by both semipurified and pure IF preparations. CFU-C show an intermediate degree of sensitivity as 50% reduction of their number is achieved only with 60–100 U/ml. It is also interesting to point out that CFU-E, i.e. the most advanced erythroid precursor, is the least sensitive to IF as 12% and 7%, respectively, of control CFU-E colonies are still observed in plates given 1,000 and 10,000 U/plate of IF. At these dosages no BFU-E or CFU-C were detected.

Even though the experiments done with pure versus semi-purified IF preparations did not quite overlap in terms of dose range, they are still comparable. In fact, one could draw a single dose-response curve by employing the data from the two independent experiments. These data, therefore, represent a novelty with respect to IF effects on murine BFU-E and CFU-C. Finally, they provide a

TABLE 4

EFFECTS OF SEMIPURIFIED AND PURE INTERFERON PREPARATIONS ON THE CLONOGENIC CAPACITY OF MURINE BONE MARROW CELLS*

	CFU-E/ 2 × 10^5 Cells		BFU-E/ 2 × 10^5 Cells		CFU-C/ 1 × 10^5 Cells	
Treatment	A†	B‡	A†	B‡	A†	B‡
none	1,300	978	46	48	185	142
10	1,140	876	21	24	183	135
20	1,210	ND	16	ND	137	ND
40	1,190	ND	10	ND	131	ND
60	1,120	ND	9	ND	77	ND
100	ND	558	ND	8	ND	72
1,000	ND	120	ND	1	ND	ND
10,000	ND	66	ND	ND	ND	ND

*A single experiment per given IF preparation is presented; two plates/point.
†Experiment carried out with pure IF.[27]
‡Experiment carried out with semipurified IF (see TABLE 3).

preliminary confirmation that these effects are once again attributable to IF itself, as also shown for other nonantiviral effects (see review in ref. 46).

ACKNOWLEDGMENTS

We acknowledge the generosity of Drs. P. Lengyel (Yale Univ., New Haven, CT) and I. Gresser (Institut des Recherches sur le Cancer, Villejuif, France) who made available to us fully purified mouse interferon preparations.

REFERENCES

1. PESCHLE, C. 1980. Ann. Rev. Med. **31:** 303–314.
2. CLINE, M. J. & D. W. GOLDE. 1979. Nature **277:** 177–181.
3. TILL, J. E. & E. A. MCCULLOCH. 1961. Rad. Res. **14:** 213–222.
4. METCALF, D. 1977. Hemopoietic colonies. In vitro cloning of normal and leukemic cells. *In* Recent Results in Cancer Research. Springer-Verlag. Berlin.
5. MURPHY, M. J., C. Peschle, A. S. GORDON & E. A. MIRAND, Eds. 1978. In Vitro Aspects of Erythropoiesis. Springer-Verlag. New York.
6. GOLDE, D. W., J. M. CLINE, D. METCALF, C. F. FOX, Eds. 1978. Hemopoietic Cell Differentiation. Academic Press. New York.
7. STAMATOYANNOPOULOS, G., A. W. NIENHUIS, Eds. 1979. Cellular and Molecular Regulation of Hemoglobin Switching. Grune and Stratton. New York.
8. AXELRAD, A. A., D. L. MCLEOD, M. M. SHREEVE & D. S. HEATH. 1974. *In* Hemopoiesis in Culture. W. A. Robinson, Ed.: 226–234. U.S. Government Printing Office. Washington.
9. FILMANOWICZ, E. & C. W. GURNEY. 1961. J. Lab. Clin. Med. **57:** 65–72.
10. KURLAND, J. J., I. A. BROXMEYER, L. M. Pelus, R. S. BOCKMAN & M. A. MOORE. 1978. Blood **52:** 388–407.
11. FRIEND, C. 1978. Harvey Lectures, Series **72:** 253–281.
12. FRIEND, C., W. SCHER, D. TSUEI, J. HADDAD, J. C. HOLLAND, N. SZRAJER & H. HAUBENSTOCK. 1979. *In* Oncogenic Viruses and Host Genes. Y. Ikawa, Ed.:279–301. Academic Press. New York.

13. DUESBERG, P., L. EVANS, M. NUNN, D. LINEMEYER, D. TROXLER & E. SCOLNICK. 1980. *In* In vitro and in vivo erythropoiesis. The Friend System. G. B. Rossi, Ed.:353–371. Elsevier. Amsterdam.
14. GUSELLA, J., R. GELLER, B. CLARKE, V. WEEKS & D. HOUSMAN. 1976. Cell **9:** 221–230.
15. OSTERTAG, W. & I. B. PRAGNELL. 1978. Proc Nat. Acad. Sci. USA **75:** 3278–3282.
16. HARRISON, P. R. 1977. *In* Biochemistry of cell differentiation MPT International Review of Science, Ser. II. J. Paul, Ed. University Park Press. London.
17. FRIEDMAN, R. M. 1977. Bacteriological Review **41:** 543–567.
18. ROSSI, G. B., G. P. MATARESE, C. GRAPPELLI, A. BENEDETTO & F. BELARDELLI. 1977. Nature **270:** 50–52.
19. ROSSI, G. B., A. DOLEI, L. CIOÈ, A. BENEDETTO, G. P. MATARESE & F. BELARDELLI. 1977. Proc. Nat. Acad. Sci. USA **74:** 2036–2040.
20. MATARESE, G. P. & G. B. ROSSI. 1978. J. Cell. Biol. **75:** 344–355.
21. RAMONI, C., G. B. ROSSI, G. P. MATARESE & A. DOLEI. 1977. J. Gen. Virol. **37:** 285–296.
22. CIOÈ, L., A. DOLEI, G. B. ROSSI, F. BELARDELLI, E. AFFABRIS, R. GAMBARI & A. FANTONI. 1978. *In* In vitro Aspects of Erythropoiesis. M. J. Murphy, Ed.:159–171. Springer-Verlag. New York.
23. DOLEI, A., M. R. CAPOBIANCHI, L. CIOÈ, G. COLLETTA, G. VECCHIO, G. B. ROSSI, E. AFFABRIS & F. BELARDELLI. 1978. *In* Antiviral Mechanisms in the Control of Neoplasia. P. Chandra, Ed.: 729–739. Plenum Press. New York.
24. DOLEI, A., G. COLLETTA, M. R. CAPOBIANCHI, G. B. ROSSI & G. VECCHIO. 1980. J. Gen. Virol. **46:** 227–236.
25. DOLEI, A., M. R. CAPOBIANCHI, G. B. ROSSI, F. TITTI & E. AFFABRIS. 1980. In vitro and in vivo erythropoiesis. The Friend System. G. B. Rossi, Ed.: 563–575. Elsevier. Amsterdam.
26. ORKIN, S. H., F. I. HAROSI & P. LEDER. 1975. Proc. Nat. Acad. Sci. USA **72:** 98–102.
27. DE MAEYER-GUIGNARD, J., M. G. TOVEY & I. GRESSER. 1978. Nature **271:** 622–625.
28. PENMAN, S. 1969. Fundamental Techniques in Virology. K. Habel & N.P. Salzman, Eds. Academic Press. New York.
29. COLLETTA, G., F. FRAGOMELE, M. L. SANDOMENICO & G. VECCHIO. 1979. Exp. Cell. Res. **119:** 253–264.
30. ROVERA, G. & S. SURREY. 1977. Cancer Res. **37:** 4211–4219.
31. BASTOS, R. N., Z. VOLLOCH & H. AVIV. 1977. J. Mol. Biol. **110:** 191–203.
32. FRIEDMAN, R. M. & L. D. KOHN. 1976. Biochem. Biophys. Res. Commun. **70:** 1078–1081.
33. BELARDELLI, F., C. AUSIELLO, M. TOMASI & G. B. ROSSI. 1980. Virology. In press.
34. KAWAKITA, M., B. CABRER, H. TAIRA, M. REBELLO, E. SLAPTERY, H. WEIDELI & P. LENGYEL. 1978. J. Biol. Chem. **253:** 598–602.
35. GRESSER, I., J. DE MAEYER-GUIGNARD, M. G. TOVEY & E. DE MAEYER. 1979. Proc. Nat. Acad. Sci. USA **76:** 5308–5312.
36. MARKS, P. A. & R. A. RIFKIND. 1978. Ann. Rev. Biochem. **47:** 419:448.
37. DIANZANI, F. & S. BARON. 1975. Nature **257:** 682–683.
38. BOYER, S. H., K. D. WUN, A. N. NOYES, R. YOUNG, W. SCHER, C. FRIEND, H. D. PREISLER & A. BANKS. 1972. Blood **40:** 823–835.
39. OSTERTAG, W., T. CROZIER, N. KLUGE, H. MELDERES & S. DUBE. 1973. Nature New Biol. **243:** 203–205.
40. GAZITT, J. & C. FRIEND. 1980. In vitro and in vivo erythropoiesis. The Friend System. G. B. Rossi, Ed.:209–218. Elsevier. Amsterdam.
41. ABOUD, M., R. SHOOR, D. MOLDOVAN & S. SALZBERG. 1979. 12th Meeting of the European Tumor Virus Group. Spa. Belgium. Abstr.
42. PESCHLE, C., G. MIGLIACCIO, F. LETTIERI, A. R. MIGLIACCIO, R. CECCARELLI, P. BARBA, F. TITTI & G. B. ROSSI. 1980. Proc. Nat. Acad. Sci. USA **77:** 2054–2058.
43. ROSSI, G. B. & C. Peschle. 1980. *In* Experimental Hematology Today. S. J. Baum & G. D. Ledney, Eds. Springer-Verlag. New York.
44. ORTEGA, J. A., M. A. ANDREW, N. A. SCHORR, P. P. DUKES & T. C. MERIGAN. 1979. Exp. Hematol. **7:** 145–150.
45. SMITH, K. A., T. N. FREDRICKSON, L. E. MOBRAATEN & E. DE MAEYER. 1976. Exp. Hematol. **14:** 164–168.
46. STEWART, W. E. II. 1979. The Interferon System. Springer-Verlag. New York.

THE EFFECTS OF INTERFERON ON 3T3-L1 CELL DIFFERENTIATION*

Sidney E. Grossberg and Susan Keay†

Department of Microbiology
The Medical College of Wisconsin
Milwaukee, Wisconsin 53226

INTRODUCTION

The biological role(s) of interferon (IF), in eukaryotic cell physiology remains uncertain. The varied cellular effects of interferons that have been described include stimulatory as well as inhibitory actions on animal cells.[1,2] Interferons have recently also been reported to modify cell surfaces[3] and inhibit the developmental process in Friend virus-transformed cells[4] as well as influence the expression of developmentally regulated[5] or serum-stimulated[6] cell enzyme activity.

Our studies have been directed toward understanding the possible role of IF in regulating the process of eukaryotic cell differentiation. Mouse 3T3-L1 fibroblasts that differentiate into adipose cells were chosen as the model system. The parent 3T3 cell line was derived from tissues of late fetuses by Todaro and Green.[7] A clone, designated 3T3-L1, subsequently obtained by Green and Kehinde[8] undergoes the conversion process over a period of about three weeks, changing from flattened cells with extended processes to large, rounded cells containing great amounts of refractile material. The conversion begins when cultures become confluent and growth is reduced. The merits of this system include the fact that during differentiation the cells undergo a very distinctive morphological alteration, synthesize new enzymes, increase the number of cell membrane insulin receptors, and show altered cellular metabolism. An additional virtue is that the system is uncomplicated by viral infection. Further, the cells undergo differentiation in culture without added chemical stimuli, although serum factors, insulin, or caffeine analogs added to the culture medium will hasten the process.[9,10]

MATERIALS AND METHODS

Cell Cultures

3T3-L1 cells were kindly provided by Dr. Howard Green (Massachusetts Institute of Technology, Cambridge) and propogated in plastic culture flasks with Dulbecco's modified Eagle's medium containing 10% calf serum, 100 units/ml penicillin and 100 μg/ml streptomycin. Differentiation experiments were carried out with cells first grown to confluence in propagation medium in 25 cm² plastic flasks or 24-well plastic culture plates. Cells were stimulated to differentiate by

*These studies were supported in part by National Institutes of Health Grant R01-AI 13818.

†Scholar of the Insurance Medical Scientist Scholarship Fund (North American Reassurance Company).

0077-8923/80/0350-0294 $01.75/0 © 1980, NYAS

increasing the concentration of calf serum to 20% or 30% and/or by adding crystalline bovine insulin (provided by Eli Lilly Company, Indianapolis). Mouse L_{929} cells were grown in Eagle's minimal essential medium (MEM) in Hanks' balanced salt solution containing 10% fetal bovine serum, penicillin and streptomycin, as above, in glass culture bottles of approximately one-liter capacity.

Interferons

Mouse fibroblast interferon was induced with Newcastle disease virus in L_{929} cells maintained in MEM containing 2% serum. The IF in the 24-hour-cell-culture supernatant was precipitated by trichloracetic acid, resuspended in 0.1 M KCl-HCl, pH2, and chromatographed on Sephadex G-100 equilibrated with the same buffer. The pooled fractions from a single peak of antiviral activity underwent a final TCA precipitation and the resuspended interferon had a specific activity of about 10^5 units/mg protein.

Interferon Assay

The antiviral activity of mouse IF was measured in L_{929} cells and 3T3-L1 cells by the hemagglutinin yield-reduction method employing either GDVII[11] or encephalomyocarditis[12] virus. The former assay measures the same unitage assigned to the NIH standard, G002-904-511, and the latter assay about one-third as much.

Lipid Extraction and Assay

Cell lipids were extracted by the method of Folch using chloroform/methanol 2:1 v/v.[13] Major lipid classes were separated by silica-gel thin-layer chromatography and the amounts measured by rhodamine dye fluorometry against appropriate standards simultaneously chromatographed.[14] Standards for triglycerides, cholesterol, cholesterol esters, and free fatty acids were more than 99% pure. Lipid biosynthesis was measured after a 6-hour pulse by following the incorporation of [1-^{14}C]acetate (New England Nuclear) (specific activity 50 μCi/μM) into Folch-extractable lipids.

Protein Assay

Protein concentrations of the sonicates of cultured cells were measured by the perchloric acid Coomassie blue G250 method,[15] using bovine serum albumin as the standard.

RESULTS

To determine the possible effect mouse interferon might have on the differentiation of 3T3-L1 fibroblasts into adipose cells, the fibroblasts were given 20% calf serum medium containing 1,000 units/ml of partially purified interferon plus

100 μg/ml of insulin. Control cells were given the same medium containing the same concentration of insulin or calf serum alone and no other additives. The medium in each set of cultures was replenished three times a week, and by day 14 insulin-stimulated cultures contained many cells undergoing the conversion to adipose cells. These cells progressively withdrew their processes, became nearly spherical, and underwent adipose cluster formation (FIGURE 1). Control cultures, however, maintained their endothelioid or fibroblastic flattened appearance with greatly extended cellular processes. The cultures stimulated to differentiate by insulin but treated simultaneously with IF more closely resembled the control fibroblastic cultures, although some differentiating cells could be identified in the IF-treated cultures. Such cells were far fewer in number and contained fewer lipid granules than those in the insulin-stimulated controls. At no time was there any morphological evidence of cell killing.

Biochemical changes in the presence of insulin or insulin plus IF were also monitored during the period of differentiation. Cultures grown in 25 cm^2 flasks were given medium (20% calf serum) containing insulin, or insulin plus IF, as above. On day 14, cells were rinsed with Hanks' balanced salt solution, scraped into 2 ml of the solution, and the lipids extracted into chloroform/methanol. The analysis of cellular lipid content following separation of the major lipid classes by thin-layer chromatography is summarized in TABLE 1. Insulin-stimulated cultures showed a general increase in cellular lipids, particularly triglycerides, cholesterol, and cholesterol esters. In cultures stimulated to differentiate but exposed to interferon, triglyceride levels were similar to the unstimulated control cultures given serum alone; cholesterol content, instead of increasing 6-fold following insulin stimulation, only increased about 2-fold, and the amount of cholesterol esters similarly increased only 2.5-fold. Thus, IF greatly inhibited the accumulation of intracellular lipids.

The above experiment was repeated with cultures labeled with 2.5 μCi of [1-^{14}C]acetate for 6 hours prior to harvest to determine the relative levels of lipid biosynthetic activity in cultures treated with interferon. The results are shown in TABLE 2. It is clear that IF, even at doses less than one antiviral unit/ml, inhibits the insulin-stimulated increase in [1-^{14}C]acetate incorporation into cellular lipids.

Treatment of 3T3-L1 cells with mouse IF at doses clearly inhibitory to [1-^{14}C]acetate incorporation into lipids did not inhibit the incorporation of radiolabeled leucine into trichloracetic acid-precipitable protein. Also, total DNA content of these cells did not differ from controls (data not shown).

A number of experiments were done to determine whether the agent in IF preparations responsible for the inhibition of adipose cell formation was indeed IF. Mock IF had no inhibitory effect as determined by observation of morphological changes or by following the incorporation of radio-labeled acetate into Folch-extractable lipids. Partially purified mouse fibroblast interferon, which was treated with trypsin to destroy all of its antiviral activity, failed to inhibit the differentiation stimulated by insulin. Antibody to mouse fibroblast IF (obtained from Dr. Dunnick at the National Institutes of Health) completely abolished the interferon inhibitory effect on this differentiation. Heterologous species' interferons that failed to show antiviral activity in 3T3-L1 cells also failed to exhibit antidifferentiation activity; these included partially purified human leukocyte, human fibroblast, and chicken IF. Two highly purified mouse IF, (the first with a specific activity of 1.2×10^9 units/mg protein and the second 5×10^7 units/mg protein) obtained from Dr. Edward DeMaeyer (Orsay, France) and Dr. Robert

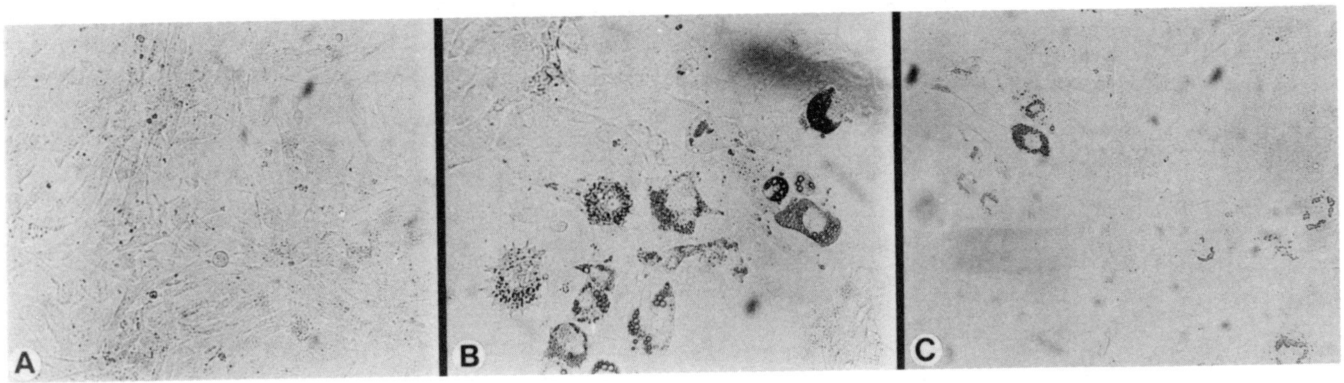

FIGURE 1. Photomicrographs (120 x) of 3T3-L1 cell cultures were taken 14 days after monolayers grown to confluence had been fed with medium containing 20% calf serum as the control (A), plus insulin 100 μg/ml (B), or plus insulin 100 μg/ml and L-cell interferon (specific activity = 2.4×10^4 units/mg) 1,000 units/ml (C). Note the relatively undifferentiated appearance of the culture in panel A, compared with the enlarged, rounded, differentiating cells with cytoplasmic lipid inclusions in panel B. Cells stimulated to differentiate but inhibited by interferon show only an occasional differentiating cell with fewer lipid inclusions, as shown in panel C.

TABLE 1
CHEMICAL EVIDENCE OF THE INHIBITION BY INTERFERON OF THE DIFFERENTIATION OF 3T3-L1 FIBROBLASTS INTO ADIPOSE CELLS

Cell Treatment	Lipid Content (μg) 14 Days After Treatment		
	Triglycerides	Cholesterol	Cholesterol Esters
Unstimulated control*	525.0	14.2	199.5
Insulin†-stimulated control	989.6	85.5	930.8
Insulin† + interferon‡	524.6	34.4	526.8

*20% calf serum.
†100 μg/ml.
‡1000 units/ml L-cell interferon (specific activity = 2.4×10^4 units/mg).

Friedman (Bethesda, MD), respectively, also showed antidifferentiation effects in stimulated cells. Finally, antidifferentiation activity was demonstrable in the same fraction having the peak of antiviral activity following isoelectric focusing (data not shown).

DISCUSSION

The evidence presented clearly indicates that interferon can inhibit the conversion of one cell type into another. The different parameters of the differentiation of 3T3-L1 fibroblasts into adipose cells, namely, altered microscopic morphology, lipid accumulation, and increased *de novo* lipid biosynthesis were all inhibited by interferon. Inhibition is not a result of nonspecific toxicity since total DNA content and protein synthesis of cells were not altered by IF treatment. The properties of the factor responsible for the antidifferentiation effects correspond to those attributed to IF, namely, sensitivity to trypsin, neutralization by antibody to L-cell IF, and no activity by either mock IF preparations or by heterologous species' IF derived from human fibroblast, human leukocyte, or chicken cells. Moreover, antiviral and antidifferentiation

TABLE 2
ENZYMIC EVIDENCE FOR THE INHIBITION OF DIFFERENTIATION BY INTERFERON OF 3T3-L1 FIBROBLASTS INTO ADIPOSE CELLS

Treatment*	Interferon† Unitage in		[^{14}C]Acetate Incorporation into Cellular Lipids DPM/μg Protein (range)
	L Cells	3T3-L1	
Insulin-stimulated control	0	0	152.3 (132.8–159.8)
Interferon	0.15	0.03	73.6 (64.8–82.5)
Interferon	4.0	0.8	58.8 (52.1–60.4)
Interferon	100.0	20.0	53.4 (44.3–70.1)

*All cultures were fed with medium containing 20% dialyzed calf serum and 10 μg/ml insulin. On day 11 monolayers were scraped off, sonicated, and extracted into chloroform/methanol 2:1. The lipid extracts were then counted by scintillation spectrometry.
†L-cell interferon (specific activity = 5×10^5 units/mg).

activities could be found at the same isoelectric point following isoelectric focusing of L-cell interferon.

The 3T3-L1 model of conversion of fibroblast to adipose cells appears to have important *in vivo* physiological correlates. Adipose tissue is composed of adipocytes, capillaries, endothelial cells, and pre-adipose fibroblasts. This tissue acts as a hormonally controlled energy storage bank for the organism. It develops late in embryonic life and mostly in early post-natal stages; pre-adipose cells persist and convert to adipocytes later (Green, 1978). Besides the fundamental roles that IF may play during embryonic differentiation and organogenesis, it is tempting to speculate that the conversion of fibroblasts into adipose cells or the accumulation of intracellular lipids manifest in aging or obesity might be affected by IF.

The mechanism by which IF achieves its antidifferentiation effects may be through actions on cell membranes. Loss of integrity of microfilament structure underlying cell membranes appears to be a feature of the 3T3-L1 differentiation process, and interferon treatment stimulates an increase in these elements of the cytoskeleton (Keay, Kushnaryov, and Grossberg, manuscript in preparation). Interferon action in 3T3-L1 cells does not appear to depend upon the competition for free receptor sites on the cell surface for hormone (insulin) binding. If 3T3-L1 cells are stimulated first by insulin and then treated hours or even days afterward with IF, differentiation is arrested just as when insulin and IF are simultaneously applied.[16] Moreover, we have recently shown that IF will inhibit the differentiation of 3T3-L1 cells treated with a xanthine analog in the absence of serum, a circumstance which will make possible further refined analysis of the effect of interferon on the cellular differentiation process.

Summary

Mouse 3T3-L1 fibroblasts, after attaining confluence, slowly differentiate functionally and morphologically into adipose cells. This conversion, characterized by a great accumulation of lipids, mostly triglycerides, is hastened by added insulin. The cells are relatively sensitive to the antiviral action of mouse fibroblast interferon (IF). Most cells treated with insulin in the presence of partially or highly purified interferon fail to differentiate. IF-treated cell cultures have far fewer adipose cells and much less lipid than replicate control cultures likewise stimulated to differentiate. The greatest differences are noted in the intracellular levels of triglycerides, cholesterol, and cholesterol esters, as well as in the incorporation of [^{14}C]acetate into Folch-extractable lipids. Variously inactivated or mock IF preparations as well as several heterologous species interferons fail to inhibit 3T3-L1 differentiation. Thus, interferon appears to alter the program of events involved in the conversion of 3T3-L1 fibroblasts into adipose cells.

Acknowledgments

We gratefully acknowledge the gifts of 3T3-L1 cells from Dr. Howard Green (Massachusetts Institute of Technology, Cambridge), of highly purified mouse interferons from Dr. Edward DeMaeyer (University of Paris, Orsay) and Dr. Robert Friedman (National Institutes of Health, Bethesda, MD), and of purified human leukocyte interferon from Dr. Kari Cantell (State Serum Institute, Helsinki, Finland).

References

1. Baron, S., P. A. Brunell & S. E. Grossberg. 1979. Mechanisms of action and pharmacology—Immune and interferon systems. *In* Antiviral Agents and Viral Diseases of Man. G. Galasso, T. C. Merigan & R. Buchanan, Eds.: 151. Raven Press. New York.
2. Gresser, I. 1978. Antitumor effects of interferon. *In* Cancer. A Comprehensive Treatise. F. F. Becker, Ed.: 521. Plenum Press. New York.
3. Grossman, E. F., G. Lee, S. Ramos, P. S. Lazo, H. R. Kaback, R. M. Friedman & L. D. Kohn. 1978. Relationships of the structure and function of the interferon receptor to hormone receptors and establishment of the antiviral state. Cancer Res. **38:** 4172.
4. Rossi, G. B., G. P. Matarese, C. Grapelli & F. Bellardelli. 1977. Interferon inhibits dimethylsulphoxide-induced erythroid differentiation of Friend leukemia cells. Nature **267:** 50.
5. Matsuno, T., N. Shirasawa & S. Kohno. 1976. Interferon suppresses glutamine synthetase induction in chick embryonic neural retina. Biochem. Biophys. Res. Commun. **70:** 310.
6. Sreevalsan, T., J. Taylor-Papadimitriou & E. Rozengurt. 1979. Selective inhibition by interferon of serum stimulated biochemical events in 3T3 cells. Biochem. Biophys. Res. Commun. **87:** 679.
7. Todaro, G. & H. Green. 1963. Quantitative studies of the growth of mouse embryo cells in culture and their development into established lines. J. Cell Biol. **17:** 299.
8. Green, H. & O. Kehinde. 1974. Sublines of mouse 3T3 cells that accumulate lipid. Cell **1:** 113.
9. Green, H. 1978. The adipose conversion of 3T3 cells. *In* Differentiation and Development. Miami Winter Symposia. Vol. **15.** F. Ahmad, T. R. Russell, J. Schultz & R. Werner, Eds.: 13. Academic Press. New York.
10. Russell, T. R. 1978. Regulation of the conversion of 3T3-fibroblasts into adipose cells. *In* Differentiation and Development. Miami Winter Symposia. Vol. **15.**F. Ahmad, T. R. Russell, J. Schultz & R. Werner, Eds.: 37. Academic Press. New York.
11. Oie, H. K., C. E. Buckler, C. P. Uhlendorf, D. A. Hill & S. Baron. 1972. Improved assays for a variety of interferons. Proc. Soc. Exp. Biol. Med. **140:** 1178.
12. Jameson, P., M. A. Dixon & S. E. Grossberg. 1977. A sensitive interferon assay for many species of cells: Encephalomyocarditis virus hemagglutinin yield reduction. Proc. Soc. Exp. Biol. Med. **155:** 173.
13. Folch, J., M. Lees & G. H. Stanley. 1957. A simple method for the isolation and purification of total lipides from animal tissues. J. Biol. Chem. **226:** 497.
14. Roch, L. A. & S. E. Grossberg. 1971. Rapid fluorometric micromethod for *in situ* quantitation of lipids on thin-layer chromatograms. Anal. Biochem. **41:** 105.
15. Sedmak, J. J. & S. E. Grossberg. 1977. A rapid, sensitive, and versatile assay for protein using Coomassie brilliant blue G250. Anal. Biochem. **79:** 544.
16. Keay, S. & S. E. Grossberg. 1980. Interferon inhibits the conversion of 3T3-L1 mouse fibroblasts into adipocytes. Proc. Nat. Acad. Sci. USA In press.

THE EFFECTS OF INTERFERON IN MOUSE CELLS INFECTED WITH MuLV*

Paula M. Pitha

Oncology Center
The Johns Hopkins University School of Medicine
Baltimore, Maryland 21205

The mechanism of the antiviral effect of interferon has not been clarified as yet; however, with most viruses studied (exceptions seem to be oncornaviruses), interferon seems to inhibit selectively the translation of viral mRNA, while the translation of cellular mRNA is not affected. The mechanism by which interferon inhibits replication of oncornaviruses seems to be very unusual. In this viral system, the interferon effect is not an early event, but the block occurs after the synthesis of viral proteins at the level of virus assembly and maturation.[1-15] It seems that the inhibition of the oncornavirus maturation and assembly in interferon-treated cells may be a manifestation of interferon-induced changes in plasma membrane physiology. These changes, however, are probably very subtle and difficult to monitor and therefore are detectable only with systems involving amplification of this effect—such as in a membrane-associated process of virus assembly and budding.

Recent evidence from many different laboratories indicates that apart from its antiviral effect interferon has a definite anticellular effect.[16-20] This effect has been demonstrated with purified interferon (both human and mouse) and appears to be a property of the interferon molecule and not to be caused by impurities in interferon preparations. There is no experimental evidence to indicate that the cellular effect of interferon is based, as the antiviral effect, on the inhibition of protein synthesis. It is rather believed to be a manifestation of the pleiotropic action of interferon such as an action of interferon on the physiology of cellular membranes.[20,21]

The present paper summarizes our knowledge of the interferon effect on different types and parameters of MuLV infection and describes our recent study in which we examined the effect of interferon on the total cellular protein synthesis and the distribution of the cellular and viral proteins in the plasma membrane.

Effect of Interferon on MuLV Replication

Our results indicated[10,22] that AKR-leukemia virus (AKR-L1 virus), exogenous, IdUrd-induced endogenous, and chronic MuLV infection were all comparably sensitive to interferon. Interferon, however, did not block viral protein synthesis or prevent the establishment of infection by exogenous MuLV genome. With all three types of infection the amount of infectious virus in culture fluids was markedly reduced by interferon, and in all three cases the effect was temporary.

*This work was supported by Grant CA-19061 from the National Cancer Institute. P.M.P. is a scholar of the Leukemia Society of America.

0077-8923/80/0350-0301 $01.75/0 © 1980, NYAS

In general there was no difference in the effect of interferon on the acute, exogenous, and endogenous infection; there was a proportional reduction in virus infectivity and reverse transcriptase activity in the culture fluids, and reduction in the number of cell-producing virus. In chronically infected cells, however, there was a disproportionate decrease in infectivity as compared to reverse transcriptase activity in the culture fluids, suggesting the formation of defective particles. These results were somewhat at variance with the studies of Friedman and Ramseur[3] and Billiau *et al.*,[6] who did not find any disproportion between infectivity and reverse transcriptase activity in their experiments with chronically infected cells, but were recently confirmed by both these groups.

We next studied the effect of interferon on exogenous MuLV infection by examining additional parameters of virus replication.[11] We chose to study the acute MuLV infection since we believed that the localization of the interferon block can be determined more precisely in this system than in chronic infection. We found, as measured by hybridization with AKR-L1 ^{3}H-DNA probe, that the whole AKR virus genome was transcribed in interferon-treated cells and the amount of virus-specific RNA was reduced only by twofold. The synthesis of gp71 glycoprotein as determined by radioimmunoprecipitation and radioimmunoassay with anti-AKR-gp71 serum was inhibited 2–5 fold and both cellular and soluble gp71 were affected comparably. The synthesis of viral protein (or glycoprotein) required for virus-induced XC cell fusion was not critically affected by interferon treatment, while under these conditions interferon reduced the amount of cell associated virus by more than 100-fold. Thus, neither the reduction in synthesis of viral RNA, nor gp71 glycoprotein or p30 core protein was sufficient to explain the magnitude of inhibition in the particle production. These results suggested, however, that the interferon-induced inhibition of MuLV replication occurs in two steps (FIGURE 1). The first block, which is relatively inefficient, affects an early step in the virus replication, while the major interferon effect is on late events in the virus development. Recently, the effect of interferon on the synthesis of viral RNA in exogenous MuLV infection was studied by the Salzberg group,[23] who confirmed our data, while the majority of studies by other groups were focused on chronic infection in which the early block of MuLV replication would not be observed.

It has been suggested by other groups that the interferon block is due to the inhibition of release or "trapping" of the virus from the cell membranes of the infected cells. Our results, however, pointed more to a defect in virus maturation and assembly. Since in our system (SC-1 cells infected with AKR-L1 virus) interferon treatment led to the formation of defective particles, we compared the virions produced in the presence and absence of interferon for infectivity, content of viral RNA, and morphology.[12] The amount of virions produced in the presence and absence of interferon was compared both in the cellular and extracellular components. It was found that the amount of cell-associated infectious virus was not greatly affected in interferon-treated cells; under the same conditions, the number of cell associated virions quantitated by electron microscopy was twofold higher in interferon treated cells than in the controls. In culture medium, however, the majority of particles released were noninfectious. The particles produced in the presence and absence of interferon were morphologically indistinguishable.

The infectious virus assembled on the cell membranes of interferon-treated cells had lower stability at 37°C than the cell-associated virus grown in the absence of interferon. The release of infectious virus from interferon-treated cells was not inhibited by actinomycin D and cycloheximide, while both these

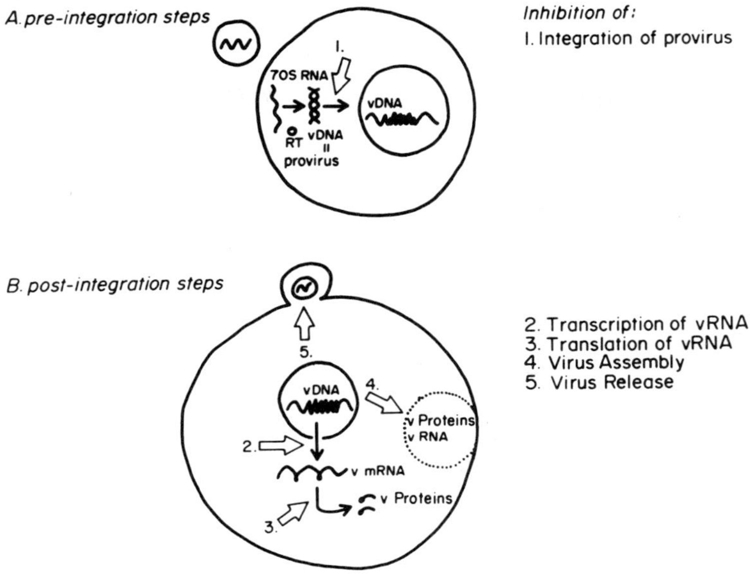

FIGURE 1. MuLV (MSV) replication—possible location of interferon block.

drugs significantly inhibited virus production in the controls. The virus produced both in the presence and absence of interferon contain the same amount of virion 70S RNA. The results show that the interferon inhibition of MuLV replication is due to a deficiency in virion assembly, which leads both to the formation of noninfectious particles and to reduced virions production.

The biochemical basis for the loss of virus infectivity in the presence of interferon was studied both with AKR-L1 virus and Rauscher murine leukemia virus (RLV) (in JLSV-6 cells).[14,15] Interferon treatment of JLSV-6 cells chronically infected with RLV leads to the formation of noninfectious particles containing in addition to the structural proteins of env and gag genome additional polypeptides (90k, 65k, 55k, 40k) which are precipitable with anti-RLV serum (FIGURE 2). The 90k dalton [^{3}H]glucosamine-containing fucose-deficient glycoprotein is antigenically different from gp71, but precipitable and anti-MuLV serum. The presence of 90k glycoprotein in the virions seems to be related to the loss of virus infectivity; virus production in NIH 3T3 cells chronically infected with RLV was found to be rather insensitive to interferon treatment, and the particles produced in the presence of interferon did not contain 90k glycoprotein.

To examine how the presence of 90k glycoprotein in the interferon virions affects their membrane topology, surface proteins of purified virions produced in the presence and absence of interferon were analyzed (FIGURE 3). Surface iodination[24] of the control virions revealed the presence of one major surface protein with the mobility of gp71. To confirm its relationship to gp71, immunoprecipitation was done with the anti gp71 serum. When the precipitate was analyzed under reducing conditions, gp71 was detected as a major labeled band; under nonreducing conditions part of the gp71 is associated with p15E and the gp90 complex is detected.[25]

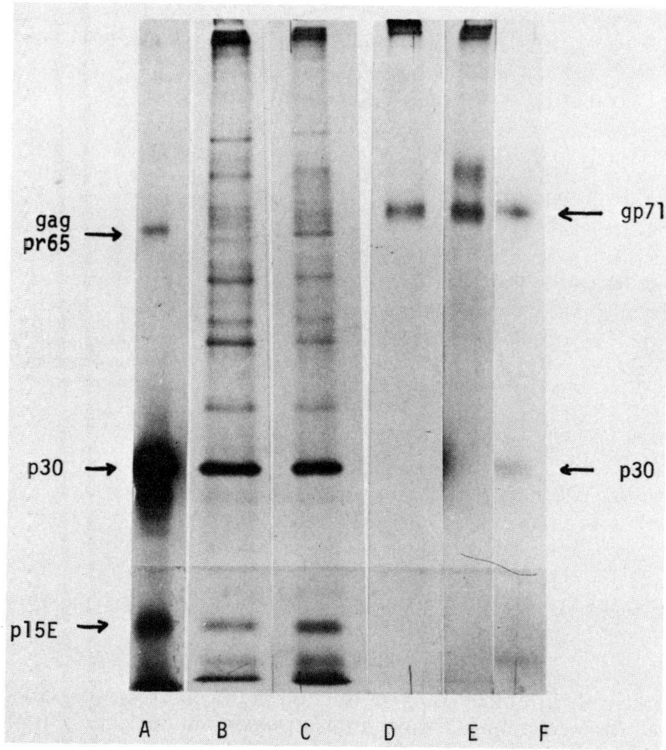

FIGURE 2. Polypeptide pattern of MuLV synthesized in the presence and absence of interferon. ^{125}I-labeled gag pr65, p30, and p15 (A); ^{3}H-amino acid-labeled proteins of control virions (B); virions produced in the presence of interferon (C); [^{3}H]glucosamine-labeled glycoproteins of control virions (D); virions produced in the presence of interferon (E); and ^{125}I-labeled gp71 and p30 (F).

Surface iodination of the intact interferon virions revealed patterns different from those of the control virions and both gp71 and 90k glycoprotiens are detected. Analysis of the iodinated proteins after precipitation with gp71 antiserum under both nonreducing and reducing conditions revealed only the presence of a gp71, indicating that in these virions gp71 does not form a complex with p15E. These data provide evidence that the mature MuLV produced in the presence and absence of interferon differ in their surface morphology, which could explain the observed difference in infectivity between these two types of virions. Whether the 90k glycoprotein is a viral or cellular protein remains to be established.

EFFECT OF INTERFERON ON MSF-INDUCED TRANSFORMATION

It has been suggested by others[26] and by us[22] that the observed late block of the MuLV replicative cycle may reflect changes in the cells surface caused by interferon. Transformation by sarcoma viruses causes significant changes[27] in the cell surface, which are probably expressed in the changes in the cell morphology accompanying transformation. It was therefore of interest to examine whether the presence of interferon would affect the morphology of previously transformed cells. The effect of interferon on viral transformation has been examined in a system where helper leukemia virus is not required for focus formation.[13] No alteration in the morphology of foci was observed. A small reduction in the number of foci was observed with concentrations of interferon that did not affect cell growth. This reduction was observed only when interferon was present early in the infection. The failure of interferon to affect the transformed phenotype suggests that the membrane effect of interferon has little consequence for the membrane changes involved in focus formation, despite their postulated effect on MuLV replication.

Effect of Interferon on the Rate of Synthesis of Viral Proteins

We have shown previously that the synthesis of p30 and gp71 was not inhibited by the interferon treatment in AKR-2B cells chronically infected with MuLV.[10,11] These experiments, however, did not eliminate the possibility of an

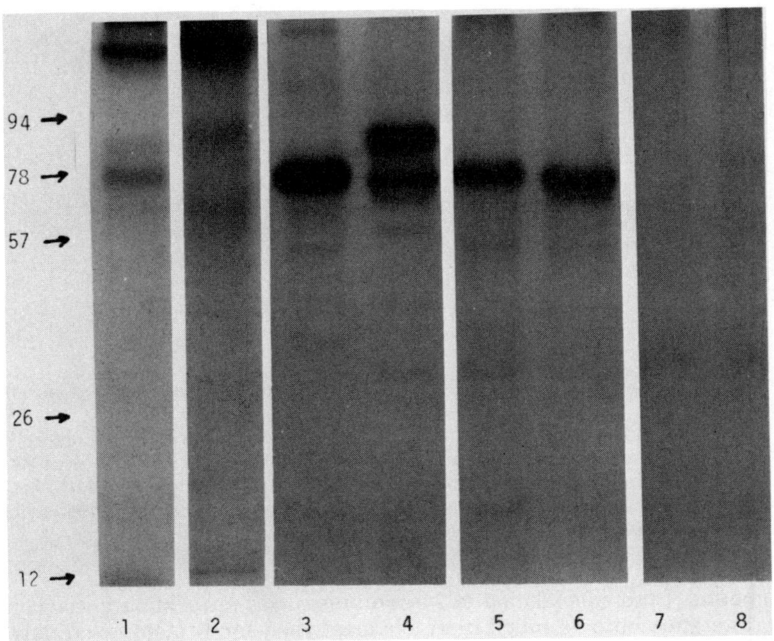

FIGURE 3. Accessibility of viral glycoproteins on the surface of virions produced in the presence and absence of interferon. Unprecipitated samples (0.1 μg of protein) control virions (1), interferon virions (2), immunoprecipitation (2 × 10[6] cpm) anti-gp71 serum controls (3,4), interferon (5,6), reducing conditions (3,5), nonreducing conditions (4,6), anti-p30 serum controls (7), and interferon (8).

alteration or a defect in the viral protein synthesis. To determine whether the observed lack of fidelity in the virus assembly could be explained by the slow-down in the rate of viral protein synthesis or its processing, the interferon-treated cells were pulsed for short periods of time with ^{3}H-labeled amino acids and then the radioactivity was chased for 3 and 6 hr in the presence of interferon. The ^{3}H-labeled proteins were analyzed on SDS page before and after immunoprecipitation with anti MuLV, gp71, and p30 serum. The analysis of the labeled proteins (FIGURE 4) on acrylamide gels indicated that in interferon-treated cells

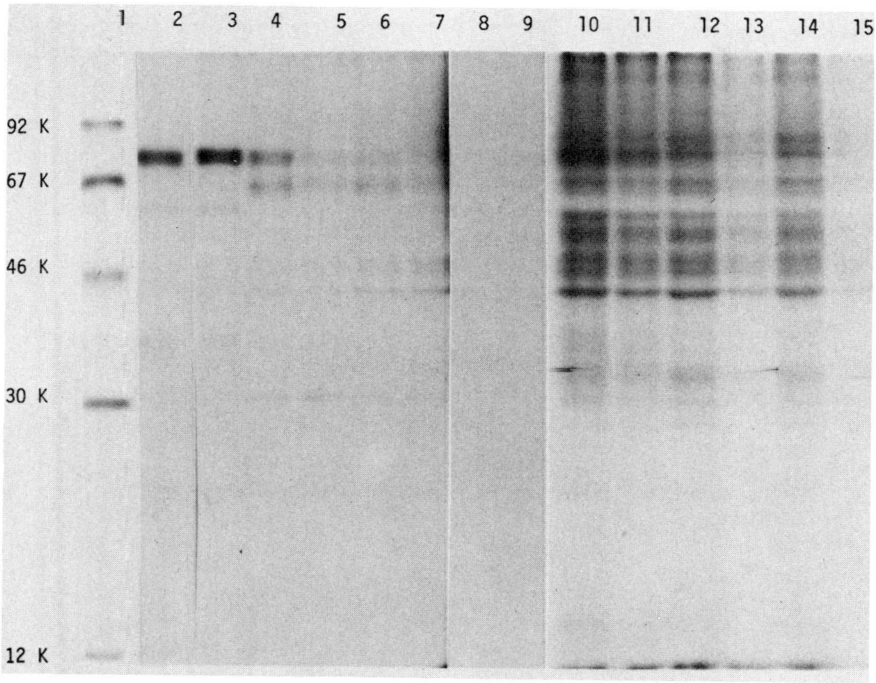

FIGURE 4. Synthesis of viral proteins in the cells in the presence and absence of interferon.

The ^{3}H-labeled proteins of JLSV-6 cells infected with RLV were analyzed before (10–15) and after (2–7) immunoprecipitation with the anti-RLV serum. Controls: 20-min pulse (2,10), 3-hr chase (4,12), and 6-hr chase (6,14). Interferon-treated cells: pulse (3,11), 3-hr chase (5,13) and 6-hr chase (7,15). Nonimmunized serum controls (8), interferon (9), radioactive molecular weight markers (1).

the amount of proteins labeled in 20-min pulses was lower than in the controls. This difference became much more obvious when the proteins were analyzed after a 3 and 6 hour chase, indicating faster turn over of labeled proteins in MuLV-infected interferon-treated cells. No qualitative difference in the pattern of labeled proteins was however observed (FIGURE 4). In the cells labeled for a short period of time with ^{3}H-amino acid in the presence and absence of interferon, the anti-MuLV serum precipitated env pr85 and gag pr65, and these were further processed into gp71 and p30 respectively, in comparable rates, both in the interferon-treated cells and controls. We have shown that the virions from interferon-treated cells contain 90k glycoprotein, which is antigenically unrelated to gp71 but is recognized by the anti-MuLV serum. The env pr85 synthesized in the interferon-treated cells is identical to that synthesized in the controls and thus probably unrelated to 90k glycoprotein detected in the virions.

These results indicate that the rate of synthesis and processing of viral proteins in interferon-treated cells is comparable to that in the control cells.[15]

Effect of Interferon on the Cell Protein Synthesis

Although we did not observe any difference in the rate of synthesis of viral proteins or their processing when analyzed after immunoprecipitation, the possibility that interferon treatment alters the synthesis of either nonconstitutive viral protein(s) or cellular protein(s) required for virus assembly has not been eliminated. To examine this possibility the interferon-treated and untreated (SC-1) cells infected with AKR virus were pulse labeled with radioactivity for a short period of time, the radioactivity was chased off in the presence and absence of interferon, and the labeled proteins were analyzed on two-dimensional gel electrophoresis (FIGURE 5). It can be seen that using this method, which offers a much higher degree of resolution than the one-dimensional gel electrophoresis, we were able to identify proteins in the range of 15,000–85,000 daltons synthesized in the control cells but not present in the cells treated with interferon.

These results indicate in cells chronically infected with MuLV, interferon treatment may lead to a selective inhibition of synthesis or faster turn over of proteins. Further studies have to establish whether these proteins are of cellular or viral origin and what are their function(s) (if any) in virus assembly.

In interferon-treated cells, on the other hand, we detected synthesis of 90k and 30k dalton proteins that were not labeled under identical conditions in the untreated controls. It has been reported recently by Farrell *et al.*[28] that interferon treatment of mouse ascite cells leads to a synthesis of a 14,000 dalton protein. Failure to detect this protein in our system may be due to a pulse-chase condition compared to a long time labeling period in ascite cells.

The Effect of Interferon on the Distribution of Cellular and Viral Proteins in Plasma Membranes

Although there are many indications that the interferon treatment induces changes in plasma membranes, the biochemical bases of this effect are not known. We attempted to compare the distribution of the cellular and viral protein in plasma membranes of cells treated with interferon and compared them to the untreated controls. Mouse lymphocyte cell lines chronically infected with AKR-L1 virus were used for these studies. These cells, when infected with AKR-L1 virus express viral antigen but produce relatively low amounts of viral particles (10^3–10^4 Pfu/ml). Treatment with interferon produced reduction in infectious virus comparable to that observed with mouse fibroblast (150 units/ml – 100-fold decrease). This system is very suitable for the studies of distribution of viral antigens in plasma membrane, since both gp71 and glycosylated proteins of gag genome can be expressed on the surface.

The cells infected with AKR-L1 virus grown in the presence and absence of interferon (150 u/ml, 24 hrs) were selectively iodinated under conditions[15] where

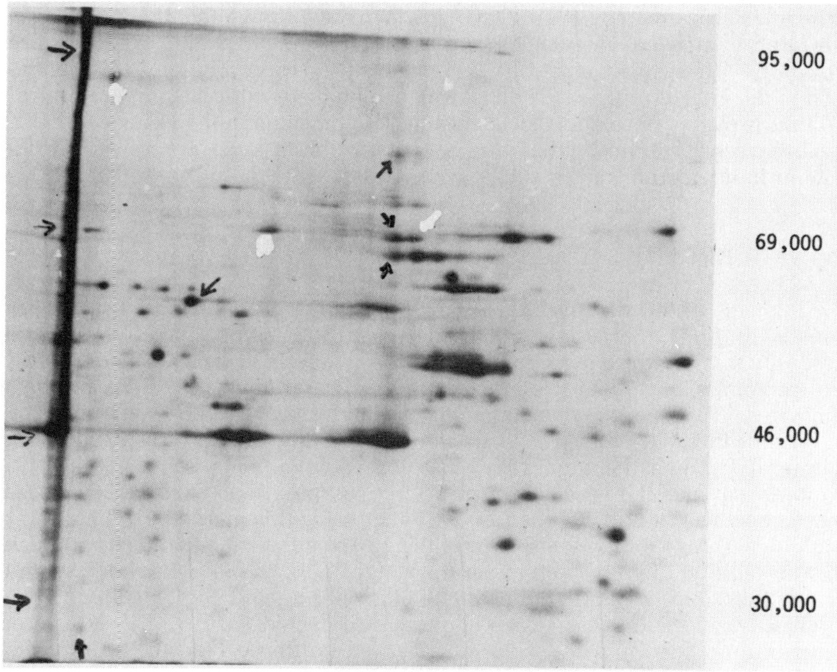
95,000
69,000
46,000
30,000

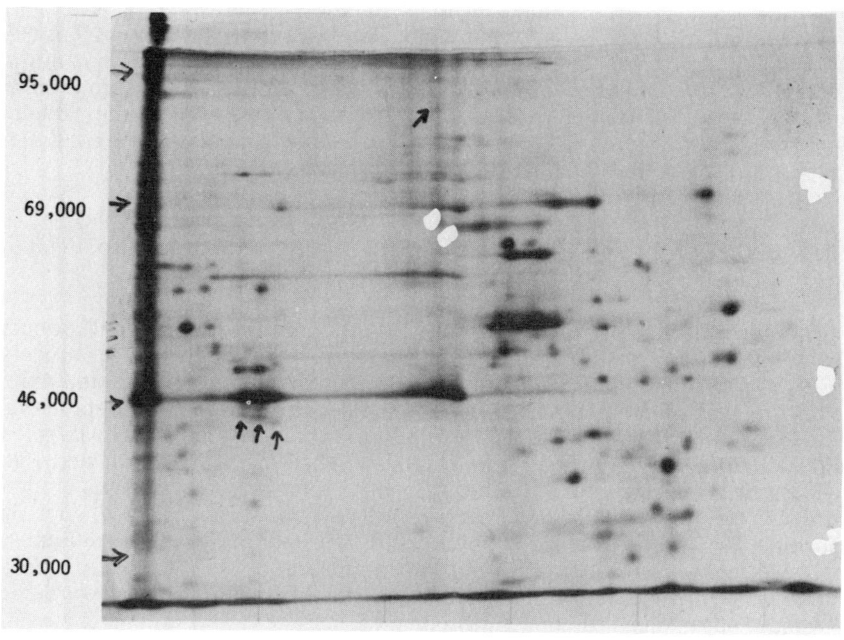
95,000
69,000
46,000
30,000

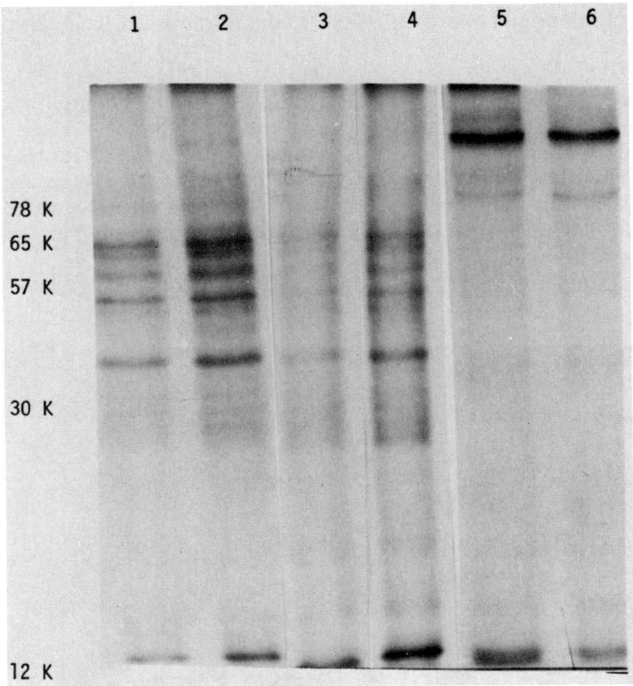

FIGURE 6. Surface labeling of proteins on the external and internal part of plasma membrane in mouse cells infected with AKR virus.

The external proteins of plasma membranes were labeled with ^{125}I, membranes were isolated, and the labeled proteins analyzed. Control cells (1,3) and interferon-treated cells (2,4). Two different methods of membrane isolation were used.[21,31] Iodination of the proteins in the cytoplasmic part of the membranes.[31] Control cells (5) and interferon-treated cells (6).

only the cell surface proteins are labeled, then plasma membranes were isolated and purified[29] and analyzed on a one-dimensional gel electrophoresis (FIGURE 6). It can be seen that interferon treatment did not cause any qualitative difference in the pattern of labeled proteins. Independently of the method of plasma membrane isolation the surface proteins of interferon-treated cells were always more labeled than the controls, suggesting perhaps (within the limits of the assay) that the cell surface proteins are more exposed for iodination in interferon-treated than in untreated cells. This observation may correlate with the observed

---

FIGURE 5. Polypeptides from mouse cells infected with AKR virus pulse-chase labeled in the presence and absence of interferon.

Cells treated with interferon (24 hr) and untreated controls were pulse labeled for 20 min with [^{35}S]methionine and chased for 3 hr. The labeled proteins were analyzed on two-dimensional gels. The sample origin is at the left side of this figure and electrofocusing was toward the positive electrode. *Top:* Control cells—the arrow indicates proteins not labeled in the interferon-treated cells. *Bottom:* Interferon-treated cells—arrow represents proteins absent in the controls.

enhancement of antigen expression that occurs in mouse cells in the presence of interferon.[30]

The cytoplasmic part of the plasma membranes of interferon-treated cells and controls were also labeled by iodination[31] and the proteins compared. However, in this case no qualitative or quantitative differences were observed.

Finally, we examined the possibility that the interferon treatment leads to a redistribution of the viral proteins in the plasma membrane, which may cause the erroneous assembly. The surface membrane proteins of the interferon-treated cells and controls were selectively labeled with ^{125}I, and viral proteins analyzed after precipitation with anti-gp71 serum. The results in FIGURE 7 indicate that both in interferon-treated and untreated cells the major protein labeled is gp71.

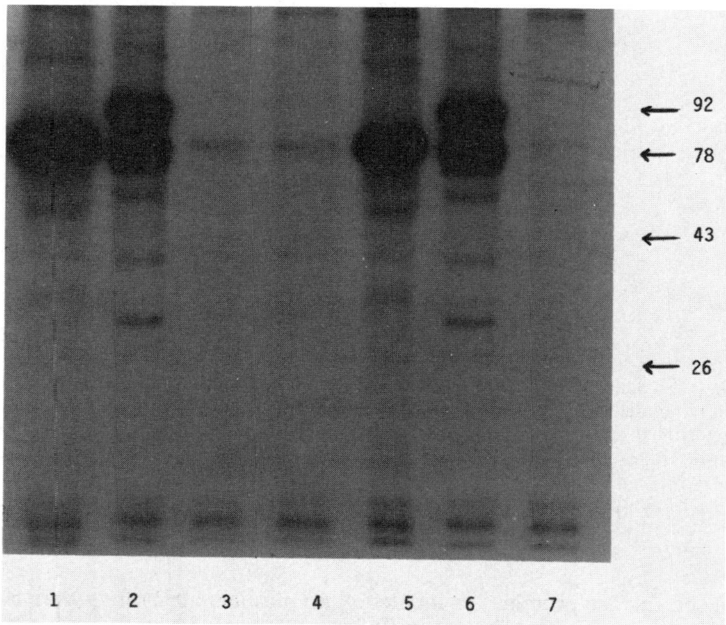

FIGURE 7. Surface labeling of infected cells grown in the presence and absence of interferon.

The isolated plasma membranes from interferon-treated cells (5,6,7) and controls (1,2,3) were iodinated and the ^{125}I-labeled viral proteins analyzed after precipitation with anti-gp71 serum (1,2,5,6) and anti-p30 serum (3,7); nonimmunized serum (4). Reducing (1,5) and nonreducing conditions (2,6). (Cells and virus identical to those in FIGURE 6.)

In cell membranes, as in virions, part of the gp71 is associated with p15E, and under nonreducing conditions the gp71-p15E complex is detected as gp90. However, unlike in the membrane of virions, the gp90 was detected both in the plasma membrane of interferon-treated and untreated cells. Both in interferon-treated cells and controls, the gp71 glycoprotein was the major viral surface protein detected.

These results indicate that either the interferon-induced changes in plasma membranes are too subtle, or transient (e.g. changes in antigen distribution or mobility) and therefore were not detected under the conditions used.

SUMMARY AND CONCLUSIONS

Highly purified mouse interferon inhibits the replication of MuLV in mouse cells. The inhibition is not due to the general inhibition of viral protein synthesis but occurs at the level of virus maturation and assembly, and the exact location of the interferon block seems to be determined by the host cell. In several cell lines interferon treatment does not prevent virus assembly but leads to a formation of noninfectious particles. The virions assembled in the presence of interferon do not differ in morphology and the content of virion 70S RNA from the control virions, but display a different polypeptide pattern when analyzed on SDS gel electrophoresis. The most striking difference is that they contain in addition to gp71 another glucosamine-containing glycoprotein of 90,000 MW. It remains to be determined whether the new glycoprotein present in the virions from interferon-treated cells is of cellular or viral origin since it is effectively recognized only by the antiserum to the disrupted virions but not by the anti gp71 or p30 serums.

The fact that in interferon-treated cells mature noninfectious particles accumulate on the cell surface indicates that the erroneous assembly leads both to the inhibition of virus release and to decrease in the infectivity of the virions.

The molecular basis for the lack of fidelity of virus maturation and assembly in interferon-treated cells remains unknown. Intracellular synthesis and processing of precursors of viral proteins do not seem to be affected by interferon treatment. Although there are several lines of evidence indicating that interferon affects the properties of cellular membranes, the interferon-induced changes are difficult to detect on the biochemical level. No qualitative differences were detected in the distribution of cellular and viral proteins in the plasma membranes of mouse lymphocytes infected with AKR virus grown in the presence and absence of interferon.

The two dimensional gel analysis of the total cellular proteins synthesized in mouse fibroblasts infected with AKR virus in the presence and absence of interferon shows that in cells treated with interferon four proteins were not detected in the pulse chase labeling when compared to the untreated controls. This raises the possibility of interferon-induced selective inhibition of (cellular or nonconstitutive viral) protein synthesis.

ACKNOWLEDGMENTS

The collaboration of Drs. D. P. Bolognesi, B. Fernie, H. P. Harper, M. N. Oxman, W. P. Rowe, S. P. Staal, N. A. Wivel, Mr. F. Maldarelli, and Miss E. Seigler during the course of these studies has been greatly appreciated.

REFERENCES

1. BILLIAU, A., H. HEREMANS, P. T. ALLENS, S. BARON & P. DESOMER. 1978. Interferon inhibits C-type virus at a posttranscriptional prerelease step. Arch. Virol. **57:** 205–220.

2. FRIEDMAN, R. M., E. H. CHANG, J. M. RAMSEUR & M. W. MEYERS. 1975. Interferon directed inhibition of chronic murine leukemic virus production in cell cultures; lack of effect on intracellular viral markers. J. Virol. **16:** 569–574.
3. FRIEDMAN, R. M. & J. M. RAMSEUR. 1974. Inhibition of murine leukemia virus production in chronically infected AKR cells; a novel effect of interferon. Proc. Nat. Acad. Sci. USA **71:** 3542–3544.
4. CHANG, E. H., S. J. MIMS, T. J. TRICHE & R. M. FRIEDMAN. 1977. Interferon inhibits mouse leukemia virus release: An electron microscopic study. J. Gen. Virol. **34:** 363–367.
5. CHANG, E. H., M. W. MEYERS, P. K. WONG, *et al.* 1977. The inhibitory effect of interferon on a temperature-sensitive mutant of Moloney murine leukemia virus. Virology **77:** 625–635.
6. BILLIAU, A., H. SORBIS & P. DESOMER. 1973. Influence of interferon on virus particle formation in different oncornavirus carrier cell lines. Int. J. Cancer. **12:** 464–653.
7. BILLIAU, A., V. G. EDY, H. SORBIS & P. DESOMER. 1974. Influence of interferon on virus particle synthesis in oncornavirus carrier line: Evidence for a direct effect on particle release. Int. J. Cancer. **14:** 335–340.
8. BILLIAU, A., V. G. EDY, E. DECLERCQ, H. HEREMANS & P. DESOMER. 1975. Influence of interferon on the synthesis of virus particles in oncornavirus carrier cell lines. III. Survey of effects on A-, B-, and C-type oncornaviruses. Int. J. Cancer. **15:** 947–953.
9. BILLIAU, A., H. HEREMANS, P. T. ALLEN, J. DEMAEYER-GUIGNARD & P. DESOMER. 1976A. Trapping of oncornavirus particles at the surface of interferon-treated cells. Virology **73:** 537–542.
10. PITHA, P. M., W. P. ROWE & M. N. OXMAN. 1976. Effect of interferon on exogenous, endogenous and chronic murine leukemia virus infection. Virol. **70:** 324.
11. PITHA, P. M., S. P. STAAL, D. P. BOLOGNESI, T. P. DENNY & W. P. ROWE. 1977. Effect of interferon on murine leukemia virus infection. II. Synthesis of viral components in exogenous infection. Virology **79:** 1.
12. PITHA, P. M., N. A. WIVEL, B. F. FERNIE & H. P. HARPER. 1979. Effect of interferon on MuLV infection. IV. Formation of noninfectious virus in chronically infected cells. J. Gen. Virol. **42:** 467.
13. PITHA, P. M. & S. P. STAAL. 1978. Effect of interferon on murine leukemia virus infection. III. The effect of interferon on MSV induced transformation. Virology. **90:** 151.
14. PITHA, P. M., B. FERNIE, F. MALDARELLI & N. A. WIVEL. 1980. Effect of Interferon on MuLV infection. V. Abnormal structural proteins in virions of Rauscher MuLV produced in the presence of interferon. J. Gen. Virol. **46:** 97.
15. PITHA, P. M., B. FERNIE, F. MALDARELLI & N. A. WIVEL. 1979. The errors in assembly of MuLV in interferon treated cells. J. Supramol. Struct. **12:** 35.
16. DEMAEYER, J. D., M. G. TORVEY, I. GRESSER & E. DEMAEYER. 1978. Purification of mouse interferon by sequential affinity chromatography on poly(U)- and antibody-agarose columns. Nature **271:** 622–625.
17. KNIGHT, E., JR. 1976. Antiviral and cell growth inhibitory activities reside in the same glycoprotein of human fibroblast interferon. Nature **262:** 302–303.
18. STEWART, W. E., II., I. GRESSER, M. G. TOVEY, M. T. BANDU & S. LEGOFF. 1976. Identification of the cell multiplication inhibitory factors in interferon preparations as interferons. Nature **262:** 300.
19. PAUCKER, K., B. J. DALTON, C. A. OGBURN & E. TORMA. 1976. Multiple active sites on human interferons. Proc. Nat. Acad. Sci. USA **72:** 4587–4591.
20. TOVEY, M., D. BROUTY-BOYE & I. GRESSER. 1975. Early effect of interferon on mouse leukemia cells cultivated in a chemostat. Proc. Nat. Acad. Sci USA **72:** 2265–2269.
21. KOHN, L. D., R. M. FRIEDMAN, J. M. HOLMES & G. LEE. 1976. Use of thyrotropin to cholera toxin to probe the mechanism by which interferon initiates its antiviral activity. Proc. Nat. Acad. Sci. USA **73:** 3695–3699.
22. PITHA, P. M. & W. P. ROWE. 1977. Effect of interferon on exogenous, endogenous, and chronic murine leukemia virus infection. *In* Control of Neoplasia by Modulation of the Immune System. M. A. Chirigos, Ed.:361–367. Raven Press. New York.

23. ABOUD, M., R. SHOOR & S. SALZBERG. 1978. Effect of interferon action on exogenous murine leukemia virus infection. Virol. **84:** 134–141.
24. MCGRATH, M., O. WITTE, T. PINCUS & I. WEISSMAN. 1978. Retrovirus purification: Method that conserves envelope glycoprotein and maximizes infectivity. J. Virol. **25:** 923–927.
25. PINTER, A., & E. FLEISSNER. 1977. The presence of disulfide linked gp70-p15(E) complexes in AKR murine leukemia virus. Virol. **83:** 417.
26. FRIEDMAN, R. M. 1977. Antiviral activity of interferon. Bact. Rev. **41:** 543–567.
27. BAUER, H., *et al.* 1974. The role of cell surface changes in RNA tumor virus transformed cells. Cold Spring Harbor Symposia on Quant. Biol. **39** (Part II): 1181.
28. O'FARRELL, P. H. 1975. High resolution two-dimensional electrophoresis of proteins. J. Biol. Chem. **250:** 4007–4021.
29. EVANS, R. M., & L. M. FINK. 1977. Identification of transmembrane bridging proteins in the plasma membrane of cultured mouse L cells. Proc. Nat. Acad. Sci. USA **74:** 5341–5344.
30. LINDAHL, P., P. LEARY & I. GRESSER. 1973. Enhancement by interferon of the expression of surface antigens on mouse leukemia L1210 cells. Proc. Nat. Acad. Sci. USA **70:** 2785–2788.
31. KENNEL, S. J., & R. A. LERNER. 1973. Isolation and characterization of plasma membrane associated immunoglobulin from cultured human diploid lymphocytes. J. Mol. Biol. **76:** 485–502.

EFFECTS OF INTERFERON-INDUCING AGENTS ON HEPATIC CYTOCHROME P-450 DRUG METABOLIZING SYSTEMS*

Gilbert J. Mannering, Kenneth W. Renton,† Rokea el Azhary,‡, and Laurel B. Deloria.

Department of Pharmacology
University of Minnesota School of Medicine
Minneapolis, Minnesota 55455

In 1976 we made the unexpected observation that the interferon-inducing agent, tilorone ((2,7-bis(2-diethylamino)ethoxy) fluoren-9-one-HCl), caused a marked depression of hepatic cytochrome P-450-linked monooxygenase systems in rodents.[1] Most drugs and other foreign chemicals either induce or have no effect on the hepatic P-450 systems; when chemicals depress these systems, they usually produce gross morphological changes in the liver or they form an adjunct with the heme of cytochrome P-450, which leads to the appearance of a green bile pigment.[2] Since neither liver damage nor the green pigment were seen after tilorone administration, we suspected that tilorone caused the loss of P-450 systems by some mechanism that had not previously been associated with low molcular weight chemicals. Several other known inducers of interferon (IF) were tested for their abilities to depress P-450 systems: small molecules (tilorone derivatives, quinacrine), an RNA virus (Mengo), a fungal mycophage (statolon), liver RNA, a synthetic double-stranded nucleotide (poly rI · rC), a bacterial lipopolysaccharide (*E. coli* endotoxin) and an attenuated bacterium (pertussis vaccine).[3] All of these agents caused losses of hepatic P-450 and monooxygenase activities. We suggested that the depression of hepatic P-450 systems may be a general property of IF-inducing agents.

Because immunologists appear to be no better informed about drug metabolism than experts in drug metabolism are informed about immunology, it is appropriate that this presentation begin with a brief description of the hepatic cytochrome P-450-linked monooxygenase system. Mixed function oxidases[4] or monooxygenases[5] are enzymes that transfer one atom of molecular oxygen to the substrate to form hydroxylated products while the other oxygen atom undergoes two-equivalent reduction to water. Thus, the reaction requires both O_2 and a reducing agent such as NADPH. Hepatic P-450-systems are comprised of a flavin reductase (NADPH-cytochrome P-450 reductase) and any one of at least six molecular species of cytochrome P-450.[6,7] The overall reaction is diagrammed in FIGURE 1. The reaction is initiated when the substrate (XH) combines with and activates the ferric form of P-450 to form ferricytochrome P-450 (a), which accepts an electron from NADPH-cytochrome P-450 reductase to form the reduced P-450-substrate complex (b). This reduced complex combines with O_2 (c) and the oxygen becomes activated when it accepts an electron from the iron of the heme

*Supported by United States Public Health Service Grant GM 15477.

†*Present address:* Department of Pharmacology, Dalhousie University, Halifax NS B3H 4H7, Canada.

‡*Present address:* Pharmacology Department, Cairo University, Kasr el-Eini, Cairo, Egypt.

0077-8923/80/0350-0314 $01.75/0 © 1980, NYAS

of P-450 (d). A second electron from either NADPH-cytochrome P-450 reductase or cytochrome b_5 is then added to the oxygenated complex (e or f), which then decomposes to form water, hydroxylated substrate and ferricytochrome P-450 (g–j).

Hepatic cytochrome P-450 systems exhibit unusually broad substrate specificities. Hundreds of chemicals are known to be substrates for these systems; in

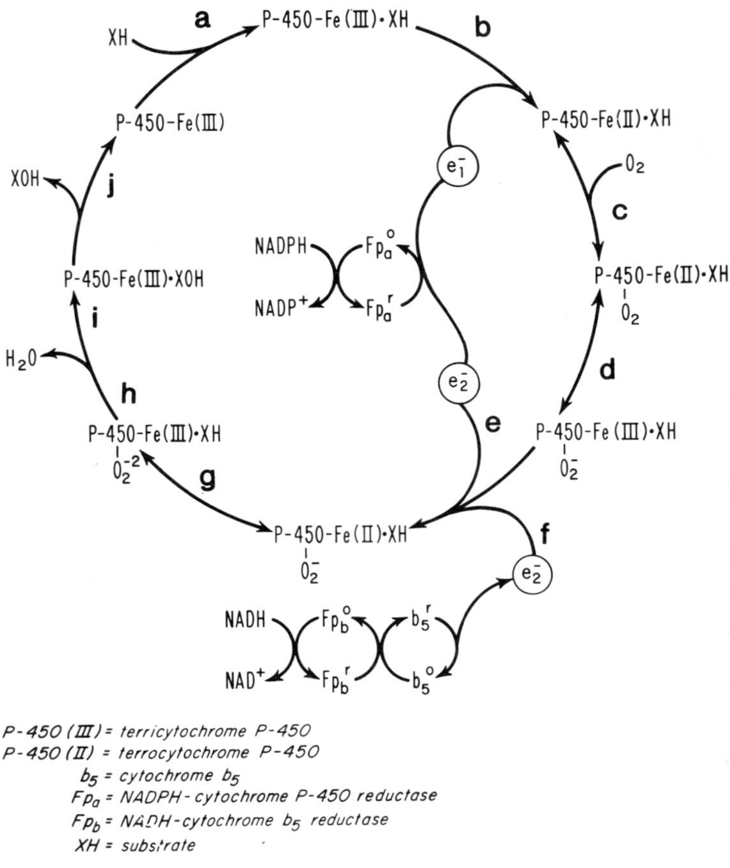

FIGURE 1. Cytochrome P-450-linked monooxygenase system of the hepatic endoplasmic reticulum.

fact, it seems likely that the great majority of lipophilic chemicals will be shown to react with P-450 systems. Moreover, these systems are highly inducible by many of these substrates. Because P-450 systems detoxify and occasionally activate drugs, pesticides, food additives and industrial wastes, they have attracted the interest of biologists in a variety of fields—pharmacologists, oncologists, toxicologists, environmentalists. Indeed, P-450 systems may be receiving more attention at this time than any other enzyme system.

The hepatic P-450 systems are of particular interest to pharmacologists and therapists. The oxidations, reductions, hydrolyses and conjugations that drugs undergo almost invariably result in products that are more polar than their parents; thus, they are more readily excreted by the kidney. Without these biotransformations the effects of some drugs would last for months, and even years,[8] and many could not be used because of their prolonged duration of action. The oxidative biotransformations catalyzed by the hepatic P-450 systems not only render drugs more polar, but in so doing, add functional groups that can participate in conjugation reactions (e.g., glucuronidation, acetylation) which further facilitate excretion. In short, P-450 systems largely determine the duration of action of drugs. They may also alter the intensity of drug action. When drugs are given repeatedly, they may accumulate and become toxic if P-450 systems are depressed; or conversely, if the P-450 systems are induced, the duration of action of the drug may be shortened to the extent that the drug loses much of its therapeutic effectiveness. In view of these considerations, it can be predicted that virus infections, vaccinations, endotoxins and other IF-inducing agents will be shown to have a profound effect on the toxicity and therapeutic activity of drugs.

Effect of the Administration of Interferon-Inducing Agents on the P-450 Systems of Hepatic Microsomes

Rats or mice were administered IF-inducing agents for one or more days. When multiple doses of the agents were given, hepatic microsomes were collected 24 hr after the last dose; when single doses were given, microsomes were obtained at various time intervals after administration of the agent. Microsomes were assayed for their cytochrome P-450,[9] cytochrome b_5[9] and protein[10] contents and for various monooxygenase activities.[1,3] Monooxygenase activities were determined by incubating these microsomes and various drug substrates with a buffered medium containing $NADP^+$ and an NADPH-generating system (e.g., glucose-6-phosphate + glucose-6-phosphate dehydrogenase) and measuring the rate of product formation (e.g., the rate of formaldehyde formation from the *N*-demethylation of ethylmorphine).

Dose response curves of the effects of tilorone on the cytochrome P-450 content and selected monooxygenase activities of hepatic microsomes are shown in FIGURE 2. Near maximal effects were observed in rats that had received 50 mg of tilorone/kg/day for 4 days. At this dose, the cytochrome P-450 content of microsomes was lowered by 40 percent. Ethylmorphine *N*-demethylase activity and aniline and benzo[a]pyrene hydroxylase activities were lowered by 50, 22 and 44%, respectively.

The time courses of loss and recovery of cytochrome P-450 and ethylmorphine *N*-demethylase activity after the single administrations of 50 mg/kg of tilorone and 10 mg/kg of poly rI · rC are shown in FIGURES 3 and 4. These doses of tilorone and poly rI · rC had been shown previously to produce near maximal responses. The time of onset of action of tilorone was considerably slower than that of poly rI · rC; the first statistically significant loss of cytochrome P-450 was observed 6 hr after the administration of poly rI · rC, but this did not occur until 16 hr after tilorone was given. The 10-hr delay in the onset of effects produced by tilorone may relate to the delayed induction of IF by this agent; tilorone induces IF 12–24 hr after its administration to mice,[11] whereas poly rI · rC causes one peak induction of IF at 2 hr after administration and another at 9–12 hr.[12] Disproportionate amounts of ethylmorphine *N*-demethylase activity and cytochrome P-450 were lost during the early stages of the depression of P-450 systems by poly rI · rC and tilorone. Four hours after the injection of poly rI · rC there was a 36% loss of ethylmorphine *N*-demethylase activity without a measurable loss of cytochrome P-450 (FIGURE 3). Similarly, 24 hr after the administration of tilorone, 45% of the ethylmorphine *N*-demethylase activity had been lost, but only 15% of the cytochrome P-450 had disappeared (FIGURE 4). This suggests that certain species of cytochrome P-450 are destroyed more rapidly than others by interferon-inducing agents.

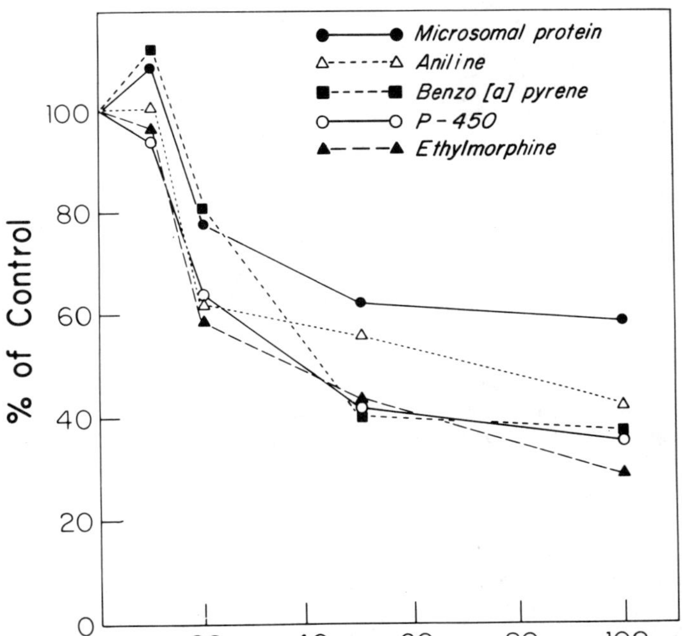

FIGURE 2. Effects of tilorone on the cytochrome P-450 content and monooxygenase activities of hepatic microsomes. Rats were administered (p.o.) the indicated daily doses of tilorone for 4 days. Aniline = aniline hydroxylation; Benzo[a]pyrene = benzo[a]pyrene hydroxylation; ethylmorphine = ethylmorphine *N*-demethylation.

The ability of animals to produce IF in response to inducing agents is rapidly lost when the agents are administered repeatedly at daily intervals. If the induction of IF is involved in the depressant effect of these agents on hepatic P-450 systems, it follows that the P-450 systems should recover during chronic administration of the agents. As can be seen in FIGURE 5, this was the case. The cytochrome P-450 levels of rat microsomes, which had fallen to about 55% of normal by 4 days, climbed slowly to about 90% of the normal value by 20 days. The recovery of ethylmorphine *N*-demethylase activity followed a similar time

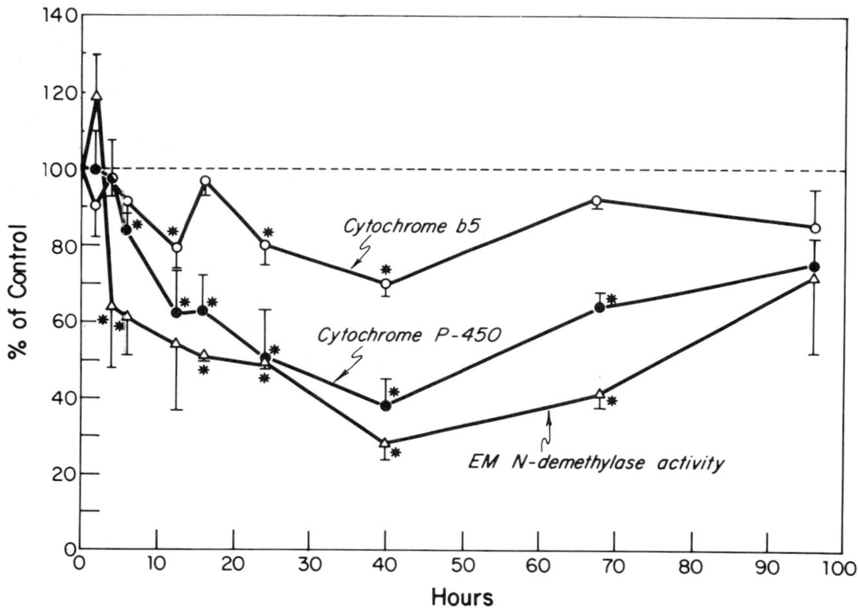

FIGURE 3. Time courses of loss and recovery of cytochromes P-450 and b_5 contents and ethylmorphine (EM) *N*-demethylase activity of hepatic microsomes from rats that had received a single i.p. dose of poly rI · rC (10 mg/kg).
*Significantly different from control value ($p < 0.05$).
(The figure is from el Azhary and Mannering.[13] Reproduced by permission of the publisher.)

course, but was not restored to as high a level. Similar results were obtained in mice injected chronically with poly rI · rC (data not shown).

TABLE 1 lists interferon-inducing agents that have been shown to depress hepatic P-450 systems. They represent the gamut of molecular sizes and structures and share only two features—the abilities to induce IF and to modulate the immune system. It is of interest that the inducers of both interferons I and II depress P-450 systems and that the times of interferon induction of each coincide with the times of depression of cytochrome P-450. Thus poly rI · rC, which induces IF within 1 or 2 hr of its administration, produces a measurable depression of the P-450 system 3 or 4 hr later (FIGURES 3 and 4), whereas *C. parvum*, which does not induce IF until 5 to 12 days after its administration, has a comparable delayed effect on the P-450 system.

Endotoxin is not a very good inducer of IF,[24] but of the IF inducers that have been tested, it is the most potent depressor of P-450 systems. As little as 1 μg per 20 g mouse caused a 30% loss of cytochrome P-450 or ethylmorphine *N*-demethylase activity (FIGURE 6).

Many drugs and other chemicals that induce hepatic P-450 systems also induce the biosynthesis of ascorbic acid in rats.[45,46] Poly rI · rC and tilorone suppressed the induction of ascorbate synthesis, cytochrome P-450, and monooxygenase activity (ethylmorphine *N*-demethylase and benzo[a]pyrene hydroxylase) by phenobarbital.[47] The induction of ascorbate synthesis by 3-

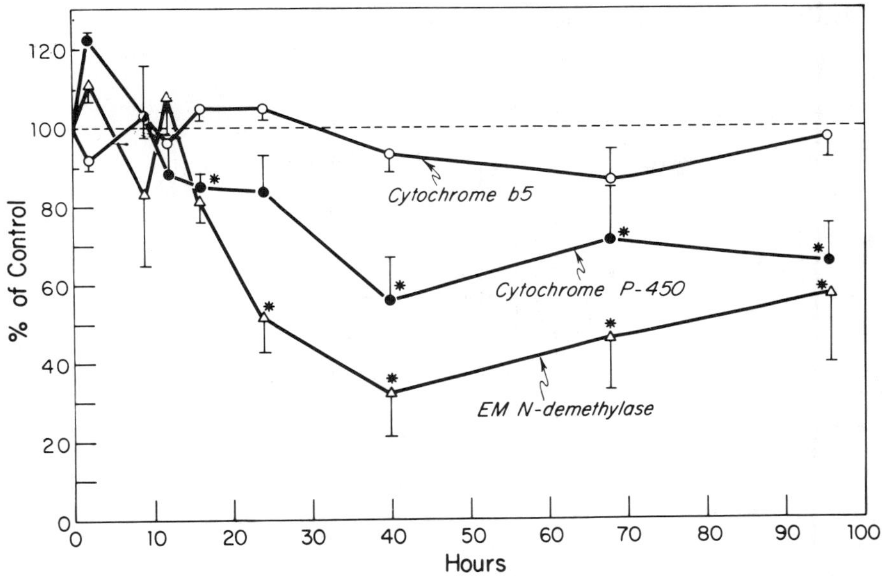

FIGURE 4. Time course of loss and recovery of cytochromes P-450 and b_5 contents and ethylmorphine (EM) N-demethylase activity of hepatic microsomes from rats that had received a single oral dose of tilorone (50 mg/kg).
*Significantly different from control value ($p < 0.05$).
(The figure is from el Azhary and Mannering.[13] Reproduced by permission of the publisher.)

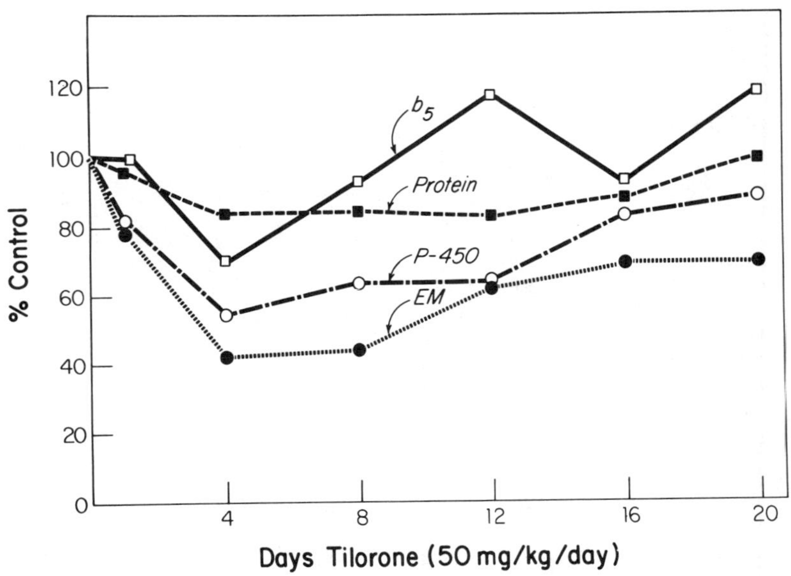

FIGURE 5. Effect of chronic tilorone administration on the cytochrome P-450 content and ethylmorphine *N*-demethylase activity of hepatic microsomes. Rats received 50 mg of tilorone daily, p.o.; microsomes were obtained from their livers at the indicated intervals. N = 4.

TABLE 1

INTERFERON-INDUCING AGENTS KNOWN TO DEPRESS HEPATIC CYTOCHROME P-450 SYSTEMS

		P-450				Interferon			
Name	Classification	Species	Substrate*	Time† (hr)	Ref.	Species‡	Type§	Time† (hr)	Ref.
Poly rI · rC	Double-stranded RNA	Rat	EM	6	13	Mouse	I	2	14
		Rat	AN, EM	(96)	3				
		Mouse	HX¶, AP, An	24	15				
		Mouse	HX¶	(15)	16				
Murine Hepatitis	Virus	Mice	AN	48	17	Mice	I	12	19
		Mice	HX, ST, PEN	72	18				
Mengo Virus	Double-stranded RNA virus	Rat	EM, AN	48	3	Mouse	I	15	20
Hepatic RNA	Single-stranded RNA	Rat	EM, AN	(96)	3	Mouse embryo cells	I	3	21
						(Rat cells)	I	4	22
Endotoxin	Lipopoly-saccharide	Rat	EM, AN	(96)	3	Mouse	I	2	24
		Rat	AN, BP	(24)	23				
		Mouse	EM	(96)	3				
		Mouse	HX¶	(15)	16				
Statolon	Fungal Mycophage	Rat	EM, AN	(96)	3	Mouse	I	12	25
		Mouse	EM	(24)	26				
B. Pertussis	Attenuated Bacteria	Rat	EM, AN	(96)	3	Mouse	I	2	27
		Rat	PH	(24)	28				
		Mouse	HX¶	(15)	16				
		Mouse	AP, EM, AN	(120)	29				

C. Parvum	Immunostimulator	Mouse	AP, AN, pNA, BP	24–168	30	Mouse	II	120–288	31
BCG‖	Immunoadjuvant	Rat	AN, DIC	72	32	Mouse	I,II	2	33
		Mouse	EM, AN	(24)	34				
		Human	AP	(1008)	35				
OK. 432**	Antitumor agent	Mouse	AN, AP, PEN¶	24	34	Mouse	II	24	36
Influenza A††	Virus	Human	TH	24	37	Human	II		38
Pyrans	Maleic Anhydride	Mouse	AP, AN	24	39	Mouse	I	24	40
	Divinyl Ethers	Mouse	AP, AN, HX¶	24	40				
Quinacrine	Small molecule	Rat	EM, AN	(96)	3	Mouse	I	18	41
Tilorone‡‡	Small molecule	Rat	EM, AN	(96)	3	Mouse	I	12–24	11
		Rat	HX¶, ZOX,¶ AP	24	42				
		Rat	EM	24	13				
		Rat	EM, AN, BP, HX¶	24	1				
		Rat	PEN¶	(120)	43				
CP 20, 901§§	Small molecule	Rat	EM, AN	(96)	3	Mouse	I	18	44

*EM = ethylmorphine N-Demethylase; AN = aniline hydroxylase; HX = hexobarbital; AP = aminopyrine N-demethylase; ZOX = zoxzolamine; PEN = pentobarbital; DIC = 5(3,3-dimethyl-1-triazeno)imidazole-4-carboxamide demethylase; PH = phenetoin; BP = benzo[a]pyrene hydroxylase; TH = theophylline; ST = strychnine. †Time in hours of maximal depression; ( ) only time reported. ‡*in vivo* assays except when in ( ). §Type II interferon has not always been looked for when an agent has been tested; therefore when type I only is indicated, the possibility is not excluded that type II may also be produced at a later time point, or in addition to type I. ¶Sleeping time or paralysis time. ‖Bacillus Calmette-Guerin. **Freeze dried material of penicillin-treated Streptococcus hemolyticus. ††Drug metabolism data obtained with Fluogen vaccine, lot #919961B, which is a mixture of Influenza A-USSR, Influenza A-Texas and Influenza B-Hong Kong. The interferon data were obtained with infants infected with Influenza A. ‡‡2,7-bis[(diethylamino)ethoxy]fluoren-9-one dihydrochloride. §§*N*-*N*-dioctadecyl-n^{1}n^1-bis(2-hydroxyethyl) propanediamine.

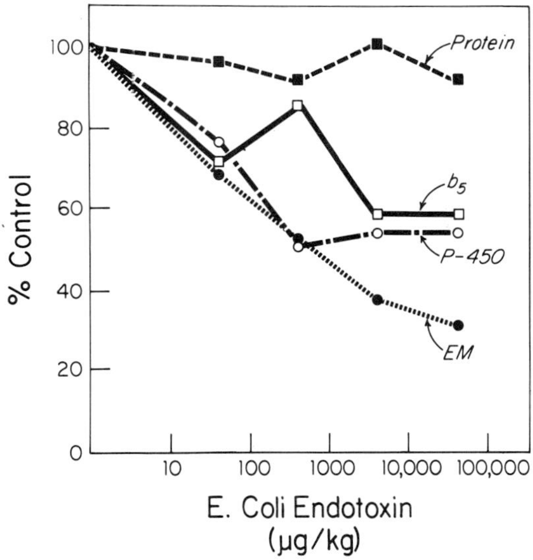

FIGURE 6. Effect of *E. coli* endotoxin (Sigma) on the cytochromes P-450 and b_5 content and ethylmorphine (EM) *N*-demethylase activity of hepatic microsomes. Mice received indicated doses of endotoxin, i.p., daily for 3 days. Each value is the mean of 3 mice.

methylcholanthrene was also suppressed by poly rI · rC. Induction of cytochrome P-450 by 3-methylcholanthrene was suppressed completely by poly rI · rC or tilorone, but that of benzo[a]pyrene was lowered by only 40%, again demonstrating the selective depressant action of IF-inducing agents on different species of cytochrome P-450.

EFFECT OF INTERFERON-INDUCING AGENTS ON *IN VIVO* DRUG METABOLISM

The length of time that an animal sleeps after receiving a hypnotic dose of a barbiturate has been used frequently as a measure of the rate of *in vivo* oxidation of these drugs by the hepatic P-450 system.[48] The daily oral administration of 20 mg of tilorone per kg for 4 days increased the mean hexobarbital sleeping time from 27 to 54 min.[1] Four of eight rats that received a 50 mg/kg dose of tilorone died; the remaining animals slept a mean of 114 min. The concentration of hexobarbital in the blood of control rats 30 min after they had received 100 mg of hexobarbital/kg, i.p., was 22 μg/ml; that of animals that had received 20 and 50 mg of tilorone/kg, p.o., daily for 4 days was 51 and 54 μg/kg, respectively. Similar increased pentobarbital sleeping times and blood barbiturate levels were also observed after tilorone administration.[43] Twenty-four hours after being vaccinated with influenza vaccine (TABLE 1), the serum half-life of theophylline of three patients in the recovery phase of chronic obstructive lung disease was increased 1.9-, 2.9- and 3.2-fold.[37] The patient whose metabolism of theophylline was depressed the most developed acute signs of theophylline toxicity. The mean half-life of serum theophylline of four healthy subjects rose from 3.3 hr to 7.3 hr within 24 hr after the administration of the same vaccine. These studies demonstrate that IF-inducing agents may have a profound effect on the toxicity and therapeutic efficacy of drugs.

Depression of Hepatic Catalase and Tryptophan 2,3-Dioxygenase by Interferon-inducing Agents

The possibility was considered that hepatic hemoproteins other than cytochrome P-450 might be depressed by IF-inducing agents. Accordingly, the effects of administered tilorone and poly rI · rC on levels of hepatic catalase, tryptophan 2,3-dioxygenase (tryptophan pyrrolase) and mitochondrial cytochromes were determined. The time courses of loss and recovery of catalase activity of homogenates of livers from rats that had received a single dose of tilorone or poly rI · rC are shown in FIGURE 7. Maximal depression of catalase activity occurred between 24 and 40 hr after the administration of poly rI · rC, but was delayed until about 48 hr after tilorone was given. Thus the delayed depressive effect of tilorone on catalase relative to that produced by poly rI · rC was consistent with that observed for the depression of cytochrome P-450 by these agents.

The effects of a single dose of poly rI · rC on tryptophan 2,3-dioxygenase activity (holoenzyme) and total enzyme activity (holoenzyme + apoenzyme) are shown in FIGURE 8. Three hours after administration of the agent there was a 40% rise in holoenzyme, but no change in the total enzyme. By 6 hr, both the total enzyme activity and the holoenzyme level were decreased to 58% and 66% of control values, respectively. Levels of the total enzyme returned to the control level by 15 hr, but the heme-saturated enzyme was still depressed by 68% at that time. However, the level returned to 90% of the control level by 24 hr. The significance of this sequence of events will be discussed in the next section. Tilorone, which was generally proved to be less active than poly rI · rC in most of

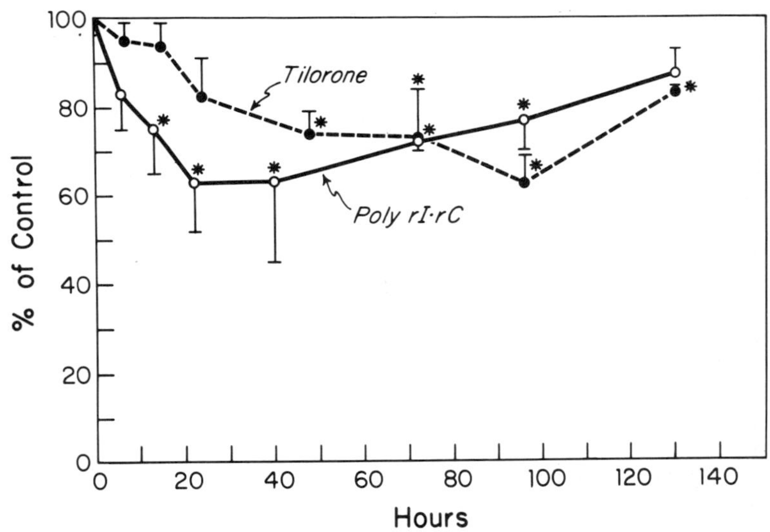

FIGURE 7. Time course of loss and recovery of catalase from liver homogenates of rats that had received a single dose of tilorone (50 mg/kg, p.o.) or poly rI · rC (10 mg/kg, i.p.). *Significantly different from control value ($p < 0.05$).
(The figure is from el Azhary and Mannering.[13] Reproduced by permission of the publisher.)

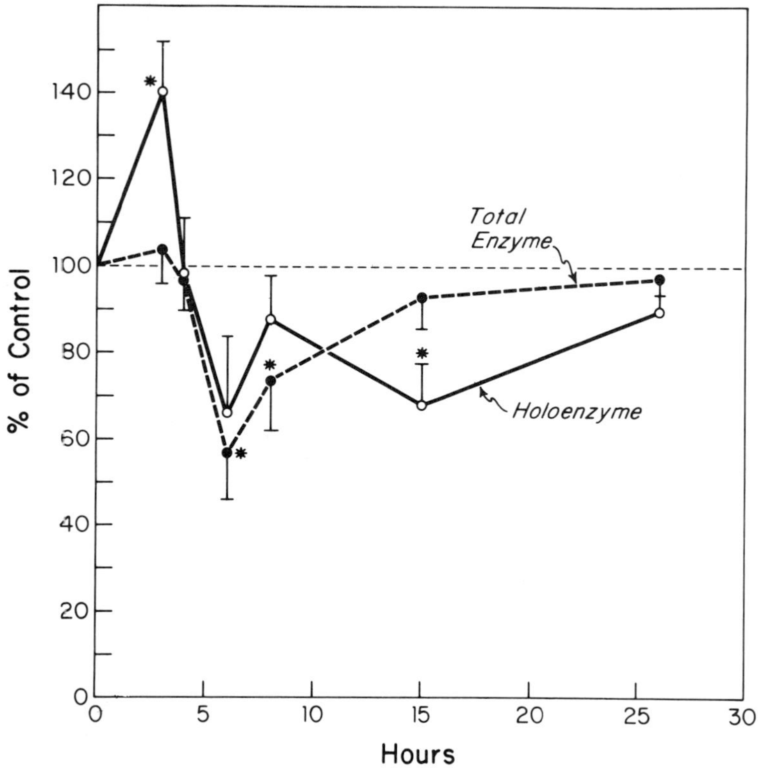

FIGURE 8. Time course of loss and recovery of tryptophan 2,3-dioxygenase from the 100,000 × g supernatant fraction of the livers of rats that had received a single injection of poly rI · rC (10 mg/kg, i.p.).
*Significantly different from control value ($p < 0.05$).
(The figure is from el Azhary and Mannering.[13] Reproduced by permission of the publisher.)

these studies, did not alter either total or holo tryptophan 2,3-dioxygenase activity when given as a single 50 mg/kg dose *per os*.

Hepatic mitochondrial cytochromes a, b and c were not depressed significantly after four daily doses of 10 mg of poly rI · rC/kg, i.p.; cytochrome c_1 was depressed about 20 percent. The cytochrome P-450 content and benzo[a]pyrene activity of intestinal mucosa and adrenal were not affected by four daily doses of poly rI · rC (10 mg/kg, i.p.); the cytochrome P-450 content of the kidney cortex was not altered, but the benzo[a]pyrene hydroxylase activity was lowered by 40 percent.

The time courses of the depression of hepatic hemoproteins after poly rI · rC or tilorone administration differ widely. This can be attributed to the turnover rates of the respective enzymes. The level of an enzyme in a cell is determined by its rate of synthesis and its rate of degradation, but the time required for an enzyme to change from one steady state to another is dependent solely on the rate of degradation.[49] Thus enzymes with rapid turnover rates reach new steady state levels faster than enzymes with slow turnover rates. Six hours after poly rI · rC treatment, the tryptophan 2,3-dioxygenase level was maximally depressed to 60% of the control value and returned to the control value within 24 hr. Catalase and cytochrome P-450 levels were maximally depressed to about 50% of the control values between 24 and 40 hr and were still below control values after 96 hr. The effect of poly rI · rC on the cytochrome b_5 level was less pronounced than for the other hemoproteins except those of the mitochondria, which were not affected appreciably. These differences in the time courses of loss and recovery of the hemoproteins are related to their half-lives. Tryptophan 2,3-dioxygenase has a half-life of 2.3 hr,[50] catalase, 30–36 hr,[51] cytochrome b_5, 4–5 days,[52] and mitochondrial cytochromes, 5–6 days.[53,54] The hepatic cytochrome P-450s can be grouped into two populations, one with a half-life of 7–8 hr and the other with a half-life of 42 hr.[55]

Effects of Interferon-inducing Agents on the Heme of Cytochrome P-450

Poly rI · rC and tilorone depressed hepatic δ-aminolevulinic acid synthetase (ALA-S), the rate-limiting enzyme in heme synthesis,[56] and induced heme oxygenase, the rate-limiting enzyme in heme breakdown.[57] Endotoxin has the same effects on these enzymes.[58,59] As was shown in Figure 8, poly rI · rC increases the ratio of holo:total tryptophan 2,3-dioxygenase. Figure 9 shows the temporal order of these events. The first event is a short-lived increase in the

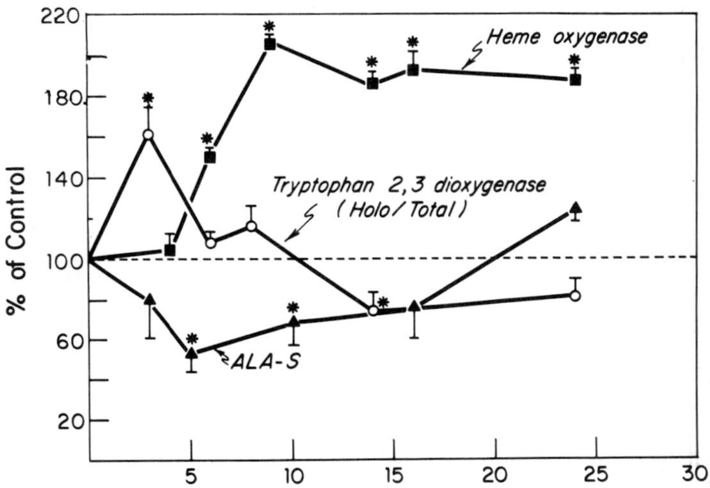

Figure 9. Temporal aspects of the effect of a single dose of poly rI · rC (10 mg/kg, i.p.) on the δ-aminolevulinic acid synthetase (ALA-S) and heme oxygenase and the relative heme saturation of tryptophan 2,3-dioxygenase activities of rat livers.
*Significantly different from control value ($p < 0.05$).
(The figure is from el Azhary and Mannering.[13] Reproduced by permission of the publisher.)

conversion of apotryptophan 2,3-dioxygenase to the active heme-saturated holoenzyme. This occurs within 3 hr of the administration of poly rI · rC. At this time ALA-S was partially depressed and heme oxygenase was not affected. At 5 hr the ratio of holo to total tryptophan 2,3-dioxygenase had returned to normal, and the depression of ALA-S was maximal. Induction of heme oxygenase activity began between 4 and 6 hr and reached a maximum at 8 hr. The induced level of heme oxygenase activity was maintained throughout the period during which ALA-S and the ratio of holo to total tryptophan dioxygenase levels were returning to normal. If one accepts the concept that heme synthesis is regulated by a heme pool,[2,59,60] the sequence of these events can be interpreted as follows: (1) Interferon-inducing agents cause an increase in the size of the regulatory heme pool. This could occur if these agents cause an increased dissociation of heme from cytochrome P-450 or other hepatic hemoproteins. It could also occur if the IF-inducing agents depress the synthesis of apocytochrome P-450 and the apoproteins of other hemoproteins, thereby decreasing the demand for heme from the heme pool; (2) The temporary increase in the ratio of holo to total tryptophan 2,3-dioxygenase is caused by the temporary increase in the size of the heme pool;[59] (3) the increase in the size of the heme pool depresses ALA-S synthesis; (4) Heme in excess of that necessary to depress ALA-S synthesis induces heme oxygenase, which relieves the inhibition of ALA-S by destroying heme.

Effect of Single-stranded Polynucleotides on Hepatic P-450 Systems

Single-stranded poly rI and single-stranded poly rC do not induce interferon[61-63] nor do they depress hepatic P-450 systems.[3] However, when injected consecutively, with the injection of poly rI preceding that of poly rC, both an antiviral effect[63] and a depression of the P-450 system are observed (Figure 10), even though no IF is produced.[62,63] The effects of poly rI plus poly rC are seen even when the injections of the two nucleotides are separated by 2 hr. It is essential that the poly rI be injected before the poly rC; when the order of the injections is reversed, no antiviral effect or depression of P-450 systems is observed.

Effect of Poly rI · rC on the P-450 Systems of Cultured Hepatocytes

With the expectation that the use of cultured hepatocytes would provide a more accessible means than intact animals of studying the mechanism by which IF-inducing agents depress P-450 systems, measurements were made of the effects of poly rI · rC on the cytochrome P-450 content and aminopyrine *N*-demethylase activity of primary, nonreplicating mouse hepatocytes maintained on floating collagen membranes.[64] During the first 24 hr of culture, hepatocytes lost about 80% of their cytochrome P-450, 97% of their aminopyrine *N*-demethylase and 90% of their benzo[a]pyrene hydroxylase activities. The specific activity of cytochrome P-450 relative to the *N*-demethylation of aminopyrine was lowered to as little as 10% of that of the freshly isolated, uncultured hepatocytes. Exposure of the cultures to poly rI · rC during the second 24 hr of culture caused a 55% increase in the cytochrome P-450 content of the hepatocytes (Figure 11), but did not restore the level to that of the original hepatocytes. However, the specific activity (nmoles aminopyrine metabolized/nmole of P-450) of the *de novo* cytochrome P-450 induced by poly rI · rC was restored to normal. Thus, paradoxical effects of poly rI · rC on the P-450 systems of *in situ* and *in vitro* hepatocytes were observed. Interferon was shown to be induced in cultured hepatocytes by poly rI · rC.[64]

Discussion

While there would appear to be little question that the depression of hepatic cytochrome-P-450-linked drug metabolizing systems is a general property of interferon-inducing agents, it is not known whether the effect is due to IF *per se*, to a process associated with the induction of IF, to a perturbation of one or more

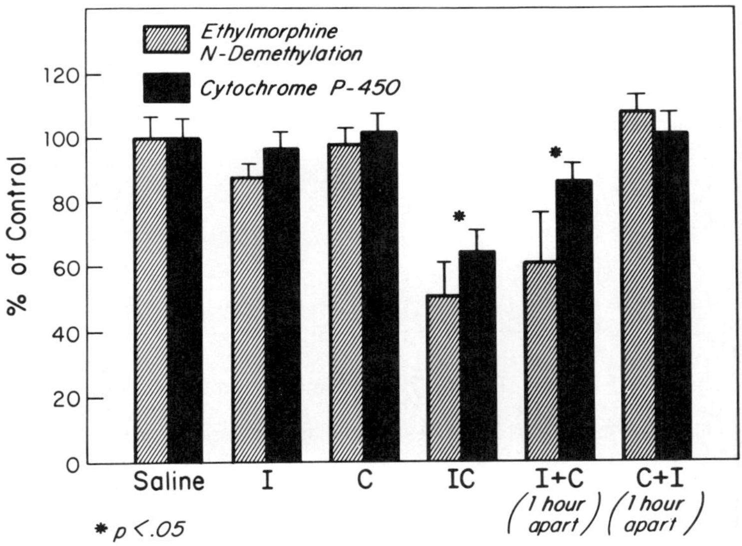

FIGURE 10. Effect of combined administration of single-stranded poly rI and poly rC on the cytochrome P-450 content and ethylmorphine *N*-demethylase activity of hepatic microsomes. Microsomes were collected 24 hr after the i.p. injection of 5 mg of poly rI (I), 5 mg of poly rC (C), 5 mg each of I + C or 10 mg of poly rI · rC (IC)/kg. N = 6 – 9. *Significantly different from values obtained with saline ($p < 0.05$).

components of the immune system, or to combinations of these processes. There is little to argue that IF *per se* is involved in the depression of hepatic P-450 systems other than the observations that apparently all IF-inducers cause the effect and that the different time courses of P-450 depression by poly rI · rC, tilorone and *C. parvum* agree with the time courses for IF induction by these agents. Other evidence suggests that IF may not be directly involved in the depression of hepatic P-450 systems: (1) There is a lack of parallelism between the extents of IF induction and depression of P-450 systems. For example, endotoxin (FIGURE 6) and maleic anhydride-divinyl ether (MVE) copolymers are poor inducers of interferon, but potent depressors of P-450 systems. However, it might be argued that the antiviral and P-450-depressant effects need not be parallel for all species of IF and that the IF induced by one agent may have a greater depressant effect on P-450 systems than that induced by another agent. The possibility should also be considered that the site of IF induction may be critical to its depressant effect on P-450 systems such that small amounts of IF induced by one agent at a suitable site may be more effective than a large amount of IF induced by another agent at a less suitable site. For example, IF induced in Kupffer cells might be expected to have a greater effect on the hepatocyte than IF induced elsewhere. It may even be necessary that the interferon be induced in

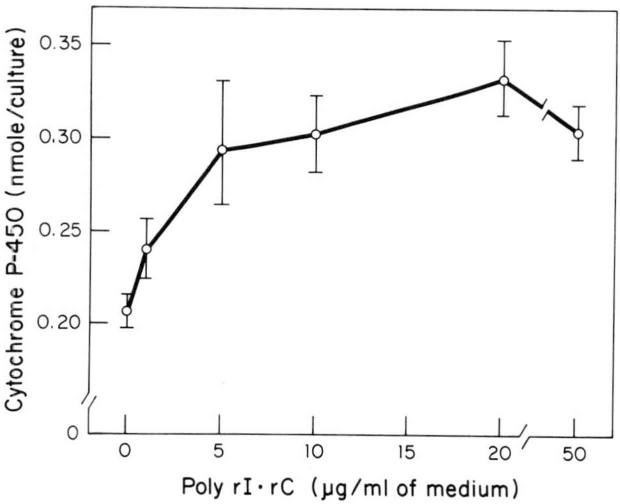

FIGURE 11. Induction of cytochrome P-450 in cultured mouse hepatocytes with poly rI · rC. Twenty-four-hour cultures were exposed to the indicated amounts of poly rI · rC and examined 24 hr later for their content of cytochrome P-450. Each point and bar represent the mean ± standard error of values obtained from three cultures; all cultures were obtained from the same mouse. The cytochrome P-450 content of the cells before culture was 1.58 nmoles/culture.
*Significantly different from the corresponding control ($p < 0.05$). The stimulatory effect of poly rI · rC (20 μg/ml) was demonstrated seven times in other experiments. (The figure is from Renton *et al.*[22] Reproduced by permission of the publisher.)

the hepatocyte for it to affect the P-450 system. We have shown that poly rI · rC induces IF in cultured hepatocytes.[64] (2) Administration of poly rI, followed by poly rC, depresses the P-450 system (FIGURE 10), but does not induce interferon.[61–63] (3) The subcutaneous injection of 75,000 units of mouse fibroblast (L cell) interferon (1.5×10^6 units/mg of protein),* followed 12 hr later with the same dose of interferon injected intraperitoneally, did not cause a depression of hepatic cytochrome P-450 or ethylmorphine *N*-demethylase activity that was significantly different than that produced by a mock IF preparation. This study is not conclusive for the same reasons given in (1), namely that the fibroblast IF

*Supplied by Dr. S. E. Grossberg, Medical College of Wisconsin, Milwaukee, Wisconsin.

used in this study may have a potent antiviral effect, but little effect on P-450 systems, or it may not have access to relevant internal components of hepatocytes. Interferon is rapidly destroyed by the liver. For IF to have an effect on P-450 systems it may be necessary that it be formed in the hepatocyte. Moreover, the amount of IF used in this study may not have been sufficient, or the time of assay may not have been appropriate.

Barnes and associates[39] have suggested that decreased hepatic monooxygenase activity may be a common property of all immunomodulators. In accordance with this concept, interferon would depress P-450 systems because it is an immunomodulator. This would explain why immunomodulators that are poor inducers of IF are still capable of depressing P-450 systems.

The observation that poly rI · rC induces P-450 systems in hepatocytes was unexpected in view of the observation that IF-inducing agents depress these systems in intact rats and mice. However, paradoxical results have been described for the activities of some other agents on P-450 systems. For example, biogenic amines depress P-450 systems *in vivo*, but induce aryl hydrocarbon hydroxylase activity markedly in cultures of fetal rat liver cells.[65] Dibutyryl cyclic AMP decreases P-450 systems in intact animals, perfused livers, and liver slices,[66-68] but induces aryl hydrocarbon hydroxylase activity in cultured mammalian cells.[69,70] Paradoxical results have also been described for the activities of IF on a variety of biological systems.[71]

That many nonspecific immunostimulators may produce changes in the maintenance or induction of the hepatic P-450 system may find an explanation in a concept proposed recently by Nebert,[72] who envisions a mechanism for the induction of multiple forms of P-450 which parallels the formation of antibodies by the immune system. At least six different cytochrome P-450s have been identified by isolation and immunochemical procedures.[6,7] Nebert suggests that this is only the tip of the iceberg, that in fact, hepatocytes may be capable of forming thousands of individual species of P-450 in response to exposure to an equal number of foreign chemicals. Each of these P-450s is designed to biotransform the chemical that induced it, although some other species of P-450 may also react with the chemical to a lesser extent. In accordance with this hypothesis, hepatocytes are capable of producing a great number of individual P-450s in much the same way that leukocytes produce individual antibodies by implementing a multitude of immunoglobulins that differ in their combinations of "heavy" and "light," "constant" and "variable" side chains. Nebert's concept would not only account for the broad substrate specificity of P-450 systems, but would also explain how the liver could "anticipate" the metabolism of a chemical before it had come into existence. The concept offers an exciting working hypothesis, but needs experimental support.

Summary

Duration and intensity of drug action are greatly influenced by the rates at which drugs are biotransformed by the cytochrome P-450-linked monooxygenase systems of the hepatic endoplasmic reticulum. Several interferon-inducing agents (poly rI · rC, tilorone, vaccines, viruses, endotoxin) are shown to markedly depress hepatic P-450 systems when administered to rodents. The interferon (IF) inducers that depress hepatic drug metabolism also modulate certain immune responses; it is therefore not known whether the depression of P-450 systems is due to IF *per se* or to the action of IF-inducing agents on one or more components of the immune system. The loss of cytochrome P-450 elicited by IF-inducing agents is accompanied by a perturbation of heme metabolism associated with the dissociation of heme from cytochrome P-450. The agents also cause losses of hepatic catalase and tryptophan 2,3-dioxygenase. These studies predict that viral infections, vaccinations, and treatment with IF-inducing agents will be shown to seriously impair the metabolism of drugs in humans.

References

1. Renton, K. W. & G. J. Mannering. 1976. Drug. Metab. Disp. **4:** 223–231.
2. De Matteis, F. 1978. *In* Heme and Hemoproteins. F. De Matteis & W. N. Aldridge, Eds.: 95–127. Springer-Verlag, New York.
3. Renton, K. W. & G. J. Mannering. 1976. Biochem. Biophys. Res. Commun. **73:** 343–348.
4. Mason, H. S., W. L. Fowlks & E. Peterson. 1955. J. Am. Chem. Soc. **77:** 2914–2915.
5. Hayaishi, O., M. Katagiri & S. Rothberg. 1955. J. Am. Chem. Soc. **77:** 5450–5451.
6. Guengerich, F. P. 1977. J. Biol. Chem. **252:** 3970–3979.
7. Thomas, P. E., A. Y. H. Lu, D. Ryan, S. B. West, J. Kawalek & W. Levin. 1976. Mol. Pharmacol. **12:** 746–758.
8. Brodie, B. B., G. J. Cosmides & D. P. Rall. 1965. Science **148:** 1547–1554.
9. Omura, T. & R. Sato. 1964. J. Biol. Chem. **239:** 2370–2378.
10. Lowry O. H., N. J. Rosebrough, A. L. Farr & R. J. Randall. 1951. J. Biol. Chem. **193:** 265–275.
11. De Clercq, E. & T. C. Merigan. 1971. J. Infect Diseases **123:** 190–199.
12. Campbell, J. B. & S. L. White. 1976. Can. J. Microbiol. **22:** 1595–1602.
13. El Azhary, R. & G. J. Mannering. 1979. Mol. Pharmacol. **15:** 698–707.
14. De Clercq, E., M. R. Nuwer & T. C. Merigan. 1970. J. Clin. Invest. **49:** 1565–1577.
15. Morahan, P. S., A. E. Munson, W. Regelson, S. L. Commerford & L. D. Hamilton. 1972. Proc. Nat. Acad. Sci. USA **69:** 842–846.
16. Floersheim, G. L. & J. J. Szeszat. 1971. Agents & Actions **2/3:** 150–155.
17. Budillon, G., M. Carrella & M. Coltorti. 1972. Experientia **28:** 1011–1012.
18. Kato, R., Y. Nakamura & E. Chiesara. 1963. Biochem. Pharmacol. **12:** 365–370.
19. Taguchi, F., N. Hirano, Y. Kiuchi & K. Fujiwara. 1976. Jap. J. Microbiol. **20:** 293–302.
20. Campbell, J. B. 1976. Can. J. Microbiol. **22:** 712–718.
21. Isaacs, A., R. A. Cox & Z. Rotem. 1963. Lancet, July 20: 113–116.
22. De Maeyer, E., J. De Maeyer-Guignard & L. Montagnier. 1971. Nature New Biol. **229:** 109–110.
23. Gorodischer, R., J. Krasner, J. J. McDevitt, J. P. Nolan & S. J. Yaffe. 1976. Biochem. Pharmacol. **25:** 351–353.
24. Youngner, J. S. & W. R. Stinebring. 1966. Virology **1:** 310–316.
25. Kleinschmidt, W. J. & E. B. Murphy. 1967. Bact. Rev. **31:** 132–137.
26. Deloria, L. B. & G. J. Mannering. Unpublished data.
27. Borecky, L. & V. Lackovic. 1966. Acta Virol. **10:** 271–272.
28. Renton, K. W. 1979. J. Pharmacol. Exp. Ther. **208:** 267–270.
29. Williams, J. F. & A. Szentivanyi. 1977. Eur. J. Pharmacol. **43:** 281–284.
30. Soyka, L. F., W. G. Hunt, S. E. Knight & R. S. Foster, Jr. 1976. Cancer Res. **36:** 4425–4428.
31. Kirchner, H., M. T. Scott, H. M. Hirt & K. Munk. 1978. J. Gen. Virol. **41:** 97–104.
32. Farquhar, D., T. L. Loo, J. U. Gutterman, E. M. Hersh & M. A. Luna. 1976. Biochem. Pharmacol. **25:** 1529–1535.
33. Nagano Y., K. Mizunoe, N. Maehara & Y. Kumazawa. 1971. Japan. J. Microbiol. **15:** 542–544.
34. Hojo, H. & Y. Hashimoto. 1977. Tox. Letters **1:** 89–93.
35. Lipton, A., G. W. Hepner, D. S. White & H. A. Harvey. 1978. Cancer **41:** 1680–1684.

36. MATSUBARA, S., F. SUZUKI & N. ISHIDA. 1974. Cancer Immunol. Immunother. **6:** 41–45.
37. RENTON, K. W., J. D. GRAY & R. HALL. Can. Med. Assoc. J. In press.
38. MCINTOSH, K. 1978. J. Pediatr. **93:** 33–36.
39. BARNES, D. W., P. S. MORAHAN, S. LOVELESS & A. E. MUNSON. 1979. J. Pharmacol. Exp. Ther. **208:** 392–398.
40. MORAHAN, P. S., W. REGELSON & A. E. MUNSON. 1972. Anti-Microb. Agents Chemother. **2:** 16–22.
41. GLAS, E. T., E. SZOLGAY, L. STOGER & M. TALAS. 1973. Anti-Microb. Agents Chemother. **3:** 537–541.
42. LEESON, G. A., S. A. BIEDENBACK, K. Y. CHAN, J. B. GIBSON & G. J. WRIGHT. 1976. Drug Metab. Disp. **4:** 232–238.
43. ABBOTT, V. & G. J. MANNERING. Unpublished results.
44. GLAS, E. T. & M. TALAS. 1978. Acta Microbiol. Acad. Sci. Hung. **25:** 87–96.
45. CONNEY, A. H., G. A. BRAY, C. EVANS & J. J. BURNS. 1961. Ann. N.Y. Acad. Sci. **92:** 115–127.
46. CONNEY, A. H. & J. J. BURNS. 1962. Adv. Pharmacol. **1:** 31–58.
47. RENTON, K. W., D. E. KEYLER & G. J. MANNERING. 1979. Biochem. Biophys. Res. Commun. **88:** 1017–1023.
48. CONNEY, A. H., C. DAVISON, R. GASTEL & J. J. BURNS. 1960. J. Pharmacol. Exp. Ther. **130:** 1–8.
49. SCHIMKE, R. T. 1973. Adv. Enzymol. Relat. Areas Mol. Biol. **37:** 135–187.
50. FEIGELSON, P., T. DASHMAN & F. MARGOLIS. 1959. Arch. Biochem. Biophys. **85:** 478–482.
51. PRICE, V. E., W. R. STERLING, V. A. TARANTOLA, R. W. HARTLY, Jr. & M. RECHCIGL. 1962. J. Biol. Chem. **237:** 3468–3475.
52. KURIYAMA, Y., T. OMURA, P. SIEKEVITZ & G. E. PALADE. 1969. J. Biol. Chem. **244:** 2017–2026.
53. ASCHENBRENNER, V., R. DRUYAN, R. ALBIN & M. RABINOWITZ. 1970. Biochem. J. **119:** 157–160.
54. DRUYAN, R., B. DEBERNARD & M. RABINOWITZ. 1969. J. Biol. Chem. **244:** 5874–5878.
55. LEVIN, W. & R. KUNTZMAN. 1969. J. Biol. Chem. **244:** 3671–3676.
56. GRANICK, S. & G. URATA. 1963. J. Biol. Chem. **238:** 821–827.
57. TENHUNEN, R., H. S. MARVER & R. SCHMID. 1969. J. Biol. Chem. **244:** 6388–6394.
58. BISSELL, D. M. & L. E. HAMMAKER. 1977. Biochem. J. **166:** 301–304.
59. BISSELL, D. M. & L. E. HAMMAKER. 1976. Biochem. J. **176:** 103-112.
60. TEPHLY, T. R., C. WEBB, P. TRUSSLER, E. KNIFFEN, A. HASEGAN & W. N. PIPER. 1973. Drug. Metab. Disp. **1:** 259–265.
61. DE CLERCQ, E. & P. DESOMER. 1971. Science **173:** 260–262.
62. DE CLERCQ, E., W. E. STEWART & P. DESOMER. 1973. Virol. **54:** 278–282.
63. STEBBING, N. & C. A. GRANTHAM. 1976. Arch. Virol. **51:** 199–215.
64. RENTON, K. W., L. B. DELORIA & G. J. MANNERING. 1978. Mol. Pharmacol. **14:** 672–681.
65. GIELEN, J. E. & D. W. NEBERT. 1972. J. Biol. Chem. **247:** 7591–7602.
66. WEINER, M., G. G. BUTERBAUGH & D. A. BLAKE. 1972. Res. Commun. Chem. Pathol. Pharmacol. **4:** 37–50.
67. ROSS, W. E., C. SIMRELL & W. W. OPPELT. 1973. Res. Commun. Chem. Pathol. Pharmacol. **5:** 321–328.
68. WEINER, M. 1973. Res. Commun. Chem. Pathol. Pharmacol. **6:** 551–564.
69. HUBERMAN, E., E. H. YAMASAKI & L. SACHS. 1974. Int. J. Cancer **14:** 789–798.
70. YAMASAKI, H., E. HUBERMAN & L. SACHS. 1975. J. Biol. Chem. **250:** 7766–7770.
71. GRESSER, I. 1977. *In* Cancer: Comprehensive Treatise. F. F. Becker, Ed. Vol. **5:** 521-571. Plenum Press, New York.
72. NEBERT, D. W. 1979. Mol. Cell. Biochem. **27:** 27–47.

ANTIGENIC PROPERTIES OF CROSSPROTECTING FACTORS IN HUMAN LEUKOCYTE AND MOUSE L CELL INTERFERONS*

Kurt Pauckert† and Barbara J. Dalton

Department of Microbiology
The Medical College of Pennsylvania
Philadelphia, Pennsylvania 19129

Human leukocyte interferons (IFs) were previously shown to possess some antiviral activity in mouse cells,[1,2] and mouse interferons some antiviral activity in human cells.[3] Human leukocyte IFs are also active in cells from many other species, as exhaustively reviewed by Stewart II.[4] The antigenic properties of crossprotecting factors in human IFs have been studied only in the rabbit system. The activity of human IFs in rabbit cells was antigenically unrelated to rabbit IF, and even the rabbit cell-protective action of human leukocyte and fibroblast IFs could be neutralized only by their respective antisera.[5] However, in the case of mouse IF, a recent report describes the finding that the heterologous antiviral protection of human cells is antigenically related to human leukocyte IF.[6] These divergent observations would seem to indicate that the protective action of IFs in cells from another species may or may not display the antigenic characteristics of the IF endogenously produced in that species.

Immunization of animals with interferon represents an amplification mechanism whereby minor constituents in an IF preparation, which escape detection by direct methods, can express themselves as antigens.[7,8] Therefore, we have reexamined the antigenic principle in human leukocyte IF which protects mouse cells, and that of mouse IF which is active in human cells, by means of antisera prepared against either of these IFs in sheep.

MATERIALS AND METHODS

Interferons

Human leukocyte interferon in crude form, prepared in buffy coats by stimulation with Sendai virus[9,10] and used for the initial series of immunizations of a sheep, was obtained from Dr.Kari Cantell, Helsinki, Finland. Leukocyte IF, which had been partially purified from acid ethanol[11,12] to a specific activity of 1.6×10^6 units per mg protein, was employed for booster inoculations, crossprotection and neutralization tests. That preparation was acquired from the Finnish Red Cross Blood Transfusion Service, Helsinki, Finland. Human fibroblast IF prepared in diploid embryonic skin muscle cells by priming and superinduction with poly rI:rC[13,14] and purified by controlled pore glass chromatography to a specific activity exceeding 1×10^6 [15] was obtained from Dr. Alphonse Billiau, Leuven, Belgium. Mouse L cell IF, stimulated by Newcastle disease virus,[16]

*This study was supported by Public Health Service Grant RO1 AI 13649 and Contract NO1 AI 82568 from the National Institute of Allergy and Infectious Diseases.

†Deceased.

0077-8923/80/0350-0332 $01.75/0 © 1980, NYAS

followed by precipitation with ammonium sulfate at acid pH[17] and chromatography on bovine plasma albumin-Sepharose[18] to a specific activity of 1×10^6, was utilized for the beginning series of injections of another sheep. For booster inoculations and all other tests, the ammonium sulfate-precipitated L cell IF was either chromatographed on Blue Sepharose CL-6B (Pharmacia Fine Chemicals, Piscataway, NJ), as modified from DeMaeyer-Guignard *et al.*[19,20] to a specific activity of 1×10^7, or subjected to antibody affinity chromatography[15] to a specific activity of 3×10^7.

Immunizations

Antibodies to human leukocyte and mouse L cell IFs were produced in female yearling sheep of Suffolk stock. The protocols followed and the quality of the IF antigens used for primary and booster inoculations are described in the legends of FIGURES 1 and 2. A goat antiserum against human fibroblast IF was received from Dr. Alphonse Billiau, Leuven, Belgium.

Assays

Titrations of human and mouse IFs were carried out in microplates essentially as described for the human system by Havell and Vilček,[13] except for minor modifications and the use of encephalomyocarditis virus, at a m.o.i. of 0.25 for challenge. Antiviral activity was expressed in terms of units per milliliter and the values were not corrected for international IF reference standards, since the nature of the factor responsible for antiviral activity in heterologous cells is unknown. In our FS-4 cell system, one unit of human leukocyte IF reference reagent G-023-901-527 and fibroblast IF reference standard G-023-902-527 registered as eight and four units of antiviral activity, respectively. One unit of mouse IF standard G-002-904-511 was recorded as two units in L929 cells. The standard reagents were obtained from the Research Resources Branch of the National Institute of Allergy and Infectious Diseases, Bethesda, MD.

Neutralization of human and mouse IFs in both human and mouse cells was measured by an adaptation of the microplate assay for IF.[5] This consisted of preincubating for 1 hr at room temperature serial twofold dilutions of antiserum with serial twofold dilutions of IF, covering the range from 1 to 32 units. Cells and virus were dispensed in the usual manner. The titer of the serum was expressed as the highest dilution corrected for one milliliter volume, neutralizing 8 units of antiviral activity by partially restoring viral cytopathogenicity.

RESULTS AND DISCUSSION

The Extent of Crossprotection

In order to determine the degree of antiviral activity expressed in heterologous cultures, human leukocyte and fibroblast IFs were assayed in parallel in mouse L cells and human fibroblasts. Mouse L cell IF was similarly titrated in both types of cells. The preparations were either crude or partially purified by a variety of methods to specific activities in the range of $1–3 \times 10^7$ units per mg protein. The results are shown in TABLE 1. Human leukocyte IF was on the average 350 times more active in homologous human than in heterologous mouse cells (Activities ratio R = 350:1). Human fibroblast IF was about 3,500 times more active in human than in mouse cells and paralleled the degree of crossprotection observed with mouse L cell IF in human fibroblasts (R = 2,500:1). This observation differs somewhat from previous findings that human fibroblast IF was inactive in mouse cells.[4] The discrepancy between those earlier reports and the present data is probably due to the difference in potency of the IF preparations used then and now.

Antibody Responses to Homologous and Heterologous Interferons

Hyperimmunization may allow for the antigenic expression of minor constituents in IF preparations which cannot be directly identified by other means. Inasmuch as recent evidence indicated that the antiviral activity expressed in a heterologous cell may bear an antigenic resemblance to the IF produced in that cell,[6] we looked for the serological evidence that would substantiate such findings. Accordingly, we examined the sera of two sheep that had been receiving massive injections of either partially purified human leukocyte or mouse L cell IF, for the development of antibodies to human leukocyte and fibroblast as well as mouse L cell IF antigens. In the case of the animal inoculated with leukocyte IF (FIGURE 1), neutralizing antibodies against leukocyte and fibroblast IF rose almost simultaneously about 20 weeks after start of the injections, except that the titers against the fibroblast IF antigen were more than 100-fold lower than those directed against the leukocyte IF antigen. There was no evidence of antibodies against mouse L cell IF. This would indicate that human leukocyte IF, though protective to some degree for mouse L cells, does not contain directly or indirectly measurable amounts of a component that antigenically resembles mouse L cell IF. *Ergo*, the antiviral effect of leukocyte IF in mouse L cells is antigenically unrelated to mouse L cell IF.

In contrast, immunization with L cell IF resulted in the formation of antibodies against both mouse L and human leukocyte IF (FIGURE 2). However, neutralizing antibody titers against the latter remained at a low level but rose with each booster inoculation in parallel with the antibodies against L cell IF. No antibodies neutralizing human fibroblast IF were found. These results indicate that mouse L cell IF harbors indeed a minor fraction that is antigenically related to or identical

TABLE 1

CROSSPROTECTION OF MOUSE CELLS BY HUMAN INTERFERONS AND OF HUMAN CELLS BY MOUSE INTERFERON

Source of Interferon	Number of Determinations	Ratio of Antiviral Activities* in Homologous/ Heterologous Cells†	
Human leukocytes	5	350/1	(250–600)
Human fibroblasts	2	3,500/1	
Mouse L cells	7	2,500/1	(500–6,000)

*Uncorrected for human and mouse interferon reference standards.

†Average based on number of tests indicated. Figures in parentheses denote range of values.

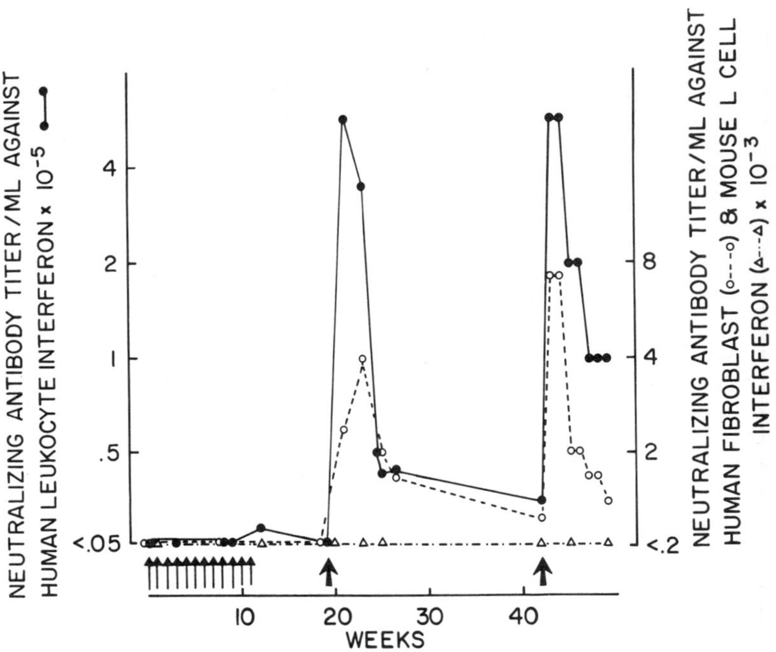

FIGURE 1. Formation of neutralizing antibodies to human and mouse IFs in a sheep immunized with human leukocyte IF. Small arrows indicate weekly injections of 2.5×10^6 units each of crude leukocyte IF. Large arrows indicate booster inoculations of 2.5×10^7 units each of acid ethanol-extracted leukocyte IF admixed with Freund's complete adjuvant. All injections were given intramuscularly.

with the foreign human leukocyte IF antigen. This fraction may well be responsible for the antiviral protection of mouse IF observed in human cells.

Neutralization of Human and Mouse Interferons in Homologous and Heterologous Cells

In order to show more convincingly that crossprotection of human cells by mouse IF was due to a component in the IF bearing the human leukocyte IF antigenic marker, whereas crossprotection of mouse cells by human leukocyte IF was caused by a factor unrelated to L cell IF, we performed neutralization tests against each IF in the homologous and heterologous cell systems. This was based on the expectation that the antiserum against human leukocyte IF (which lacks antibodies to L cell IF) would neutralize mouse and human IFs in human cells at about the same titer. On the other hand, antiserum against mouse L cell IF (which harbors antibodies to human leukocyte IF) was expected to neutralize leukocyte IF activity in L cells at a titer commensurate with the greater amount (350-fold) of that IF needed for the protection of heterologous L cells. The results presented in TABLE 2 show that neither assumption proved to be correct.

The anti-human leukocyte IF serum neutralized mouse L cell IF to an approximately 80-fold lower titer (1:20,000) than anticipated on the basis of its known antibodies against human leukocyte IF (1:1,600,000). This suggests that the dominant portion of antiviral activity of L cell IF in human cells is unlikely to be due to the component bearing the human leukocyte IF specific (Le) antigen. The antibody titer of the same serum against its homologous IF in L cells (1:12,000) corresponded closely to the expected level based on the ratio of activities of that IF in human and mouse cells (R = 250:1) exhibited in this test. As mentioned before, the antiserum had a low titer against fibroblast IF and contained no detectable antibodies against L cell IF when measured in L cells.

The anti-mouse L cell IF serum neutralized human leukocyte IF in L cells to a far greater titer (1:1,500) than anticipated (1:16) on the basis of its known anti-human leukocyte IF titer (1:4,000, R = 250/1) in this test. This strongly implies that the activity of leukocyte IF in mouse cells may also be caused by a constituent that does not bear the Le antigen of leukocyte IF. Moreover, this antiserum neutralized L cell IF in FS-4 cells to a considerably higher titer (1:40,000) than expected (1:100) if neutralization were due exclusively to a component carrying the mouse L IF antigen (R = 12,000:1) in this test. Antibodies against human fibroblast IF were absent. In other words, these serological relationships suggest to us that both cross-species activities may be due to a

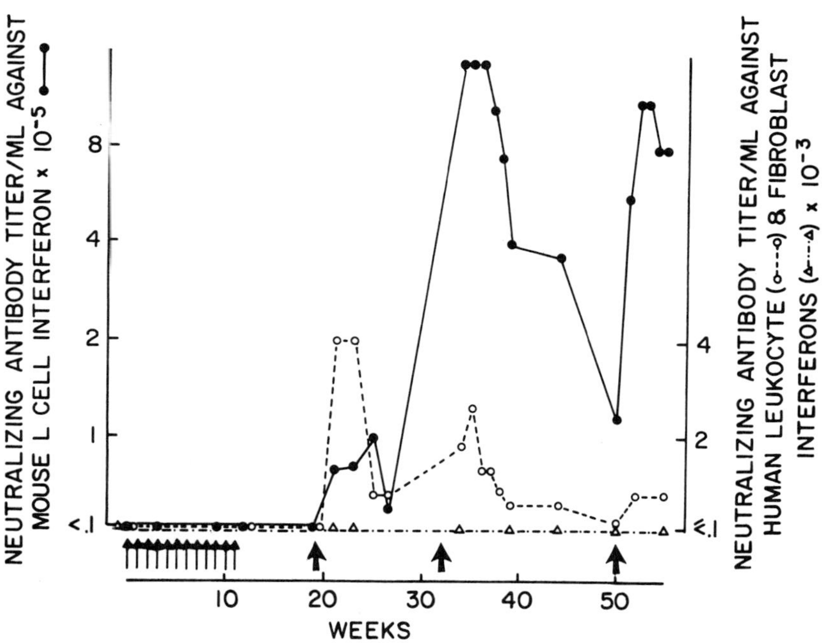

FIGURE 2. Formation of neutralizing antibodies to mouse and human interferons (IFs) in a sheep immunized with mouse L cell IF. Small arrows indicate weekly injections of 1.3×10^7 units each of L cell IF that had been chromatographed on bovine plasma albumin-Sepharose. Large arrows indicate booster inoculations of 2.5×10^7 units each of L cell IF admixed with Freund's Complete Adjuvant. The IF for this step was partially purified on Blue Sepharose CL-6B or by antibody affinity chromatography. All injections were given intramuscularly.

TABLE 2

NEUTRALIZATION OF THE CROSSPROTECTING ACTIVITIES OF HUMAN AND MOUSE INTERFERONS BY ANTI-INTERFERON SERA

Source of Interferon	Cell Used for Assay	Neutralizing Antibody Titer/ml* of the Following Anti-Interferon Sera		
		Anti-Leukocyte	Anti-Fibroblast	Anti-L Cell
Human leukocytes	FS-4	1,600,000	≤100	4,000
	L†	12,000	≤100	1,500
Human fibroblasts	FS-4	12,000	85,000	≤100
	L	ND‡	ND	ND
Mouse L cells	FS-4§	20,000	≤100	40,000
	L	≤40	≤40	1,200,000

*Determined against 8 units of antiviral activity in each system and recorded as reciprocal of endpoint dilution.

†Eight antiviral leukocyte interferon units correspond to 2,000 units in homologous FS-4 cells (R = 250/1 in this test).

‡Not done.

§Eight antiviral mouse interferon units correspond to 96,000 units in homologous L cells (R = 12,000/1 in this test).

component in each IF preparation which either lacks the main IF antigen characteristic of that IF (Le or L), or it contains so little of it that its neutralization is overshadowed by that of a distinct antigenic determinant that appears to be shared by the crossprotecting components of human leukocyte and mouse L cell IF.

The results also suggest that the mouse cell-protecting factor in human fibroblast IF is antigenically distinct from that in human leukocyte and mouse L cell IF, because the antiserum against fibroblast IF proved to be entirely monospecific, neutralizing only that IF and none of the other in either human or mouse cells. The relatively low activity of fibroblast IF in L cells (R = 4,400 in this instance) precluded conducting neutralization tests in mouse cells. The distinct antigenic character of the mouse cell protective effect of human fibroblast IF from that of leukocyte IF, parallels observations made earlier with these same IFs in heterologous rabbit cells.[5]

It should also be noted that control antisera prepared in sheep against IF-free fractions of human leukoctye and mouse L cell IFs that had been rejected from antibody affinity columns, failed to neutralize the crossprotecting effects of either IF (data not shown). This indicates that the crossprotecting principle was copurified with the IF during the affinity chromatography step and that insufficient amounts were left in the control material to elicit an immune response.

CONCLUSIONS

The interpretation of the results presented in this paper rests on the assumption that the known neutralizing titer of anti-IF sera can be used to identify the antigenic nature of the factor responsible for crossprotection of a heterologous cell. If the crossprotecting factor resembles antigenically the IF which is endogenously produced in that cell, it should be neutralized at a comparable titer by antibody against the endogenous IF. This was not the case in the present experiments. Anti-human leukocyte IF serum neutralized mouse L cell IF at a significantly (80-fold) lower titer than expected from its antibody titer against leukocyte IF in human cells. Anti-mouse L cell IF serum neutralized human leukocyte IF in mouse cells at a much higher titer (90-fold) than would be expected on the basis of its known neutralization of leukocyte IF in human cells. For the present, these results can best be explained as follows: (1) Crossprotection of mouse cells by leukocyte IF and of human cells by L cell IF is mostly due to a factor that is antigenically unrelated to the IF which is endogenously produced in the crossprotected cell. (2) Leukocyte If is devoid of a mouse L cell IF antigen, but L IF contains a minor fraction that bears the human leukocyte IF antigen. This fraction contributes to the antiviral protection expressed in heterologous human cells, but is not its sole cause. (3) The crossprotecting factors in leukocyte and L cell IFs share common antigens.

REFERENCES

1. LEVY-KOENIG, R. E., R. R. GOLGHER & K. PAUCKER. 1970. J. Immunol. **104**(4): 791–797.
2. BORECKÝ, L., N. FUCHSBERGER & V. HAJNICKÁ. 1974. Intervirol. **3:** 369–377.
3. BODO, G., P. PALESE & J. LINDNER. 1971. Proc. Soc. Exp. Biol. Med. **137:** 1392–1395.
4. STEWART II, W. E. 1979. The Interferon System.: 136–138. Springer-Verlag. Vienna, New York.
5. PAUCKER, K., B. J. DALTON, C. A. OGBURN & E. TÖRMÄ. 1975. Proc. Nat. Acad. Sci. USA **72**(11): 4587–4591.
6. HAVELL. E. A. 1979. Virol. **92:** 324–330.
7. PAUCKER, K., C. A. OGBURN & K. BERG. 1975 *In* Proceeding First Intersectional Congress of I.A.M.S. T. Hasegawa, Ed. Vol. **4:** 76–84. Science Council of Japan.
8. BERG, K., C. A. OGBURN, K. PAUCKER, K. E. MOGENSEN & K. CANTELL. 1975. J. Immunol. **114**(2): 640–644.
9. STRANDER, H. & K. CANTELL. 1966. *In* Annals Medicinae Experimentalis Et Biologiae Fenniae. K. O. Renkonen & T. U. Kosunen, Eds. Vol. **44:** 265–273. Finnish Medical Society. Helsinki.
10. CANTELL, K. 1970. *In* Immunobiological Standardization. International Symposium on Interferon and Interferon Inducers. F. T. Perkins & R. H. Regamey, Eds. Vol. **14:** 6–8. S. Karger. Basel, New York.
11. FANTES. K. H. 1970. Ann. N.Y. Acad. Sci. **173:** 118–125.
12. CANTELL, K., S. HIRVONEN, K. E. MOGENSEN & L. PYHÄLÄ. 1974. *In* In Vitro Monograph **3:** 35–38. C. Waymouth, Ed. The Tissue Culture Association. Rockville, MD.
13. HAVELL, E. A. & J. VILČEK. 1972. Antimicrob. Agents Chemother. **2:** 476–484.
14. BILLIAU, A., M. JONIAU & P. DE SOMER. 1973. J. Gen Virol. **19:** 1–8.
15. EDY V. G., I. A. BRAUDE, E. DE CLERCQ, A. BILLIAU & P. DE SOMER. 1976. J. Gen. Virol. **33:** 517–521.
16. OGBURN, C. A., K. BERG & K. PAUCKER. 1973. J. Immunol. **111**(4): 1206–1218.
17. KNIGHT. E., JR. 1975. J. Biol. Chem. **250:** 4139–4144.
18. DAVEY, M. W., E. SULKOWSKI & W. A. CARTER. 1976. J. Virol. **17**(2): 439–445.
19. DE MAEYER-GUIGNARD, J. & E. DE MAEYER. 1976. C. R. Acad. Sci. Paris. **283:** 709–711.
20. DE MAEYER-GUIGNARD, J., M. N. THANG & E. DE MAEYER. 1977. Proc. Nat. Acad. Sci USA. **74**(9): 3787–3790.

HYDROPHOBIC PROPERTIES OF INTERFERONS

Eugene Sulkowski, Kathleen Vastola, and Hung V. Le

Department of Viral Oncology
Roswell Park Memorial Institute
Buffalo, New York 14263

Hydrophobic amino acids are buried inside a protein molecule as a consequence of its folding in an aqueous environment.[1] However, it is now generally accepted that some hydrophobic residues may be localized near or at, the surface of many proteins.[2,3] As a result, those proteins may enter into hydrophobic interactions.

It may be useful, for the sake of this presentation, to distinguish between apparent and intrinsic hydrophobicities of proteins. *The apparent hydrophobicity* of a protein molecule will be defined as being due to the surface localization of hydrophobic residues. *The intrinsic hydrophobicity* will be directly related to the relative abundance of hydrophobic residues, regardless of their localization.

The surface localization of some hydrophobic residues could be due to their abundance in the polypeptide: as a result not all can be sequestered away from contact with water. This seems to be the case with some integral membrane proteins,[4] although the majority of these proteins have amino acid compositions similar to those of water-soluble proteins.[5] However, integral membrane proteins are amphipathic: they have both hydrophobic and hydrophilic domains.[6] The size of hydrophobic domains may vary from large to small as exemplified by insulin receptor[7] and adenylate cyclase,[8] respectively. Therefore, it is more appropriate to refer to the high intrinsic hydrophobicity of a protein domain rather than to the intrinsic hydrophobicity of the whole protein molecule, which may be quite average.

Some proteins, although neither particularly enriched in hydrophobic amino acids nor having discrete hydrophobic domains, display a propensity to enter into hydrophobic interactions. Serum albumin is a classical example: although a typically water-soluble protein, it is a physiological carrier for many hydrophobic molecules.[9-11] However, the hydrophobic binding sites on serum albumin are of very limited size.[12-14] The hydrophobicity of serum albumin is more apparent than intrinsic.

The majority of water-soluble proteins will not even display such an apparent hydrophobicity in their interactions with other hydrophobic molecules (ligands) unless the solvent conditions are artifically favorable (structure-forming ions, high ionic strength).[15]

Interferons (IFs) display high apparent hydrophobicity in their interactions with macro- and microligands. Bovine serum albumin, immobilized directly or via a molecular leash, was utilized as a ligand for the chromatography of human fibroblast interferon,[16,17] human leukocyte interferon,[18] mouse L-cell interferon,[19] mouse immune interferon,[20] and rabbit interferon.[21] The binding of human fibroblast interferon to immobilized concanavalin A was found to be due, in part, to a hydrophobic effect.[22,23] A similar phenomenon was recently reported for the nonspecific binding of human leukocyte interferon to an immobilized immunoglobulin.[24]

Hydrophobic interactions of several mammalian interferons were also

0077-8923/80/0350-0339 $01.75/0 © 1980, NYAS

observed on ω-carboxypentyl-agarose,[25] Affi-Gel 202,[19] alkyl-agaroses,[26] immobilized aromatic amino acids and their dipeptides,[27] phenyl-agarose[28-31] and Cibacron Blue F3GA-agarose.[32-36] Recently, the propensity of human leukocyte interferon for hydrophobic interactions was exploited for its purification to homogeneity by HPLC on Lichrosorb RP-8 (octyl groups bound to porous silica microparticles).[37]

Apparent Hydrophobicity of Interferons

Apparent hydrophobicity of several mammalian interferons was explored by studying their interactions with immobilized linear hydrocarbons (alkyl-agaroses) and aromatic hydrocarbons (phenyl-agarose).

Alkyl-agaroses

The hydrophobic interactions of human fibroblast interferon (HF-IF), human leukocyte interferon (HL-IF), mouse interferon (M-IF) and golden hamster interferon (Ha-IF) with immobilized straight chain hydrocarbons under physiological saline (PBS) solvent conditions are illustrated in Figure 1. All interferons are hydrophobically retained on decyl-agarose (C_{10}); HF-IF and HL-IF are still retained on hexyl-agarose (C_6) while M-IF and Ha-IF are not. By comparison, bovine serum albumin is not retained on hexyl-agarose under the same experimental conditions (PBS). The persistent binding of HF-IF to ethyl-agarose (C_2) and even to the unsubstituted agarose (not illustrated) cannot be readily

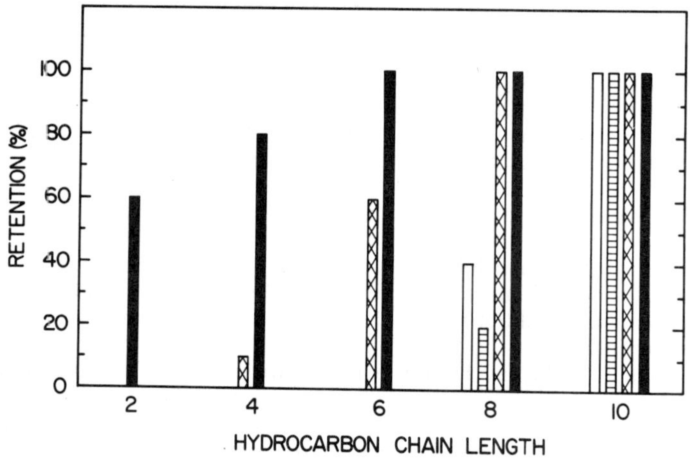

Figure 1. Binding of interferons to immobilized straight chain hydrocarbons. All interferon preparations were applied on alkyl-agaroses (Miles) columns in 0.02 M sodium phosphate, 0.15 M NaCl, pH 7.4 (PBS). The columns were washed with the equilibrating buffer and developed with (a) sodium chloride (1 M) in phosphate buffer and (b) ethylene glycol (50%) in the preceding eluant. Retention (%) is defined as this portion of activity which is recovered with ethylene glycol. HF-IF, solid bars; HL-IF, hatched bars; Ha-IF, open bars; M-IF, striped bars.

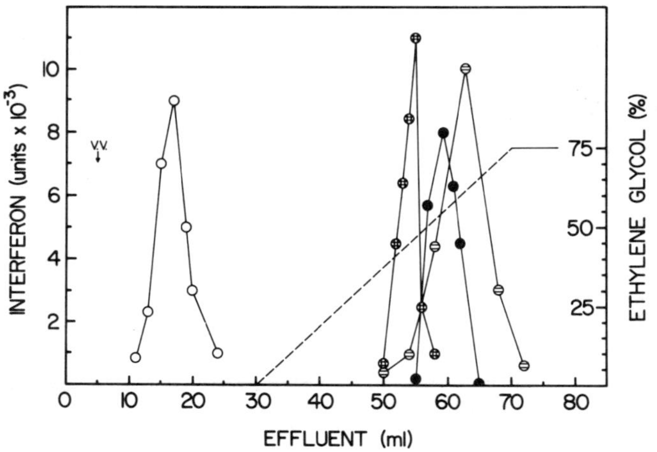

FIGURE 2. Binding of interferons to phenyl-agarose. All interferon preparations were applied in PBS on Phenyl-Sepharose CL-4B (Pharmacia) columns. After an initial wash with 0.02 M phosphate buffer (pH 7.4) a linear concentration gradient of ethylene glycol was developed. Ha-IF, open circles; HL-IF, hatched circles; HF-IF, closed circles; M-IF, striped circles.

explained in terms of hydrophobic interactions. It is quite plausible that HF-IF is retained as a result of charge-transfer phenomena.[38-40]

The hydrophobic interactions of mammalian interferons with alkyl-agaroses under low ionic strength of the solvent, are considerable by comparison with those of other water soluble proteins.* It is particularly noteworthy that mammalian interferons display significant variation in the strength of those interactions. It is, therefore, reasonable to anticipate that interferons will be shown to possess somewhat different surface topography. *A priori*, one can postulate that the difference in the apparent hydrophobicity of mammalian interferons may stem from (1) somewhat different tertiary structures of interferons or (2) from modifying influence of the varying extent of glycosylation, indirect (due to altered folding of the nascent interferon polypeptide) or direct (shielding of hydrophobic amino acid residues by hydrophilic sugar residues).

Phenyl-agarose

Chromatography of Ha-IF, HL-IF, HF-IF and M-IF is shown in FIGURE 2. All interferons were applied in physiological saline (PBS). Ha-IF interacted with phenyl-agarose weakly and as a result its elution from the column was merely retarded. HL-IF, HF-IF, and M-IF were retained and their desorption required ethylene glycol, a solute which weakens hydrophobic interactions.[44] A growing list of other interferons displaying high affinity for phenyl-agarose includes now:

*Some proteins can be induced to interact with alkyl- or aryl-agaroses but the ionic strength of the solvent has to be very high.[41-42] It has been also suggested that under those solvent conditions hydrogen bonding may occur as well.[43]

TABLE 1
AFFINITY OF SOME SOLUBLE PROTEINS FOR PHENYL-SEPHAROSE CL-4B

Protein	MW	$H\Phi_{ave}$	Interaction
Pancreatic trypsin inhibitor	6,520	1,270	—
Cytochrome *c* (horse)	11,700	1,170	—
Pancreatic ribonuclease	13,690	960	—
Lysozyme (egg)	14,310	1,070	weak
Micrococcal nuclease	16,790	1,140	—
Soybean trypsin inhibitor	20,100	1,200	—
α-Chymotrypsin*	25,670	1,080	weak
Concanavalin A	25,570	1,110	—
Ovalbumin (chicken)	45,000	1,170	—
α-1 Trypsin inhibitor	54,200	1,220	—
Serum albumin (bovine)	66,300	1,180	—

*MW and $H\Phi_{ave}$ calculated for chymotrypsinogen A.

human fibroblastoid interferon,[45] monkey interferon,[29] mouse immune interferon,[31] rabbit interferon[30] and mouse serum interferon[46] induced by Brucella.† It seems, thus, that mammalian interferons display a peculiar affinity for phenyl-agarose, which can almost serve as a group-specific sorbent for those proteins.

In order to evaluate the uniqueness of this affinity, we have selected several water-soluble proteins of diverse origin, biological function and molecular size.

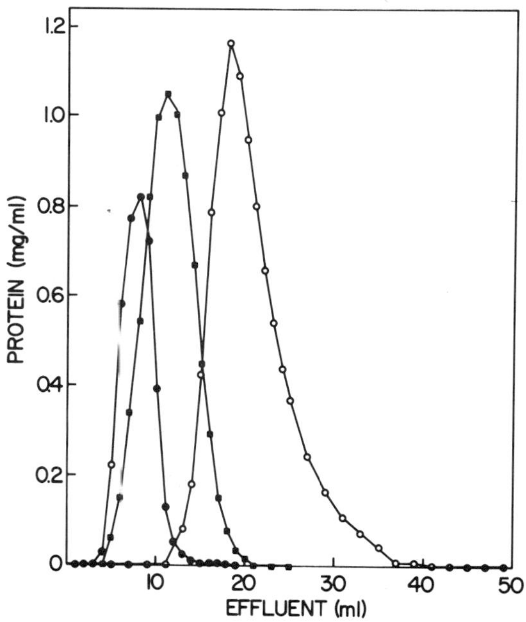

FIGURE 3. Weak interaction of α-chymotrypsin and lysozyme with Phenyl-Sepharose CL-4B. Protein samples were applied on columns in PBS. The columns were then developed with the same solvent. α-Chymotrypsin, solid squares; lysozyme, open circles. The elution profile of pancreatic trypsin inhibitor, closed circles, indicates an absence of any interaction.

†This interferon was not retained on phenyl-agarose when applied in a crude preparation; it was strongly retained after a partial purification.

The interactions of those proteins with phenyl-agarose, under the same conditions, are given in TABLE 1, and illustrated, in part, in FIGURE 3. By and large, all those proteins displayed little or no affinity for phenyl-agarose. By constrast, 5′ nucleotidase, an integral membrane protein, is retained on a phenyl-agarose column and can be displaced only with ethylene glycol at the concentration used for elution of interferons (L. J. Skrzeczkowski, personal communication). The high affinity of other integral membrane proteins, adenylate cyclase[47] and cytochrome *c* oxidase,[48] for aromatic ligands has been also reported.

TABLE 2

CALCULATION OF THE AVERAGE HYDROPHOBICITY ($H\Phi_{ave}$) OF HUMAN FIBROBLAST INTERFERON

AA	Residues	HΦ (cal/res)	HΦ (cal)
Asx	19		
Thr	7		
Ser	11		
Glx	27		
Pro	3	2,770	8,310
Gly	8		
Ala	10	870	8,700
Cys	2	1,520	3,040
Val	6	1,870	11,220
Met	3	1,670	5,010
Ile	9	3,150	28,350
Leu	20	2,170	43,400
Tyr	8	2,670	21,360
Phe	9	2,870	25,830
His	5	870	4,350
Lys	12	1,640	19,680
Arg	11	850	9,350
Trp	1	3,770	3,770
Total	171		192,370

$H\Phi_{ave} = 192{,}370 \div 171 = 1{,}125$

The apparent hydrophobicity of mammalian interferons, as probed by their interactions with immobilized hydrocarbons, aliphatic and aromatic, is quite conspicuous by comparison to the other water-soluble proteins. Is this remarkable propensity of interferons to enter into hydrophobic interactions, unlike other soluble proteins and quite like integral cell membrane proteins, a direct reflection of their intrinsic hydrophobicity?

INTRINSIC HYDROPHOBICITY OF INTERFERONS

A perusal of amino acid composition of a protein may indicate relative abundance or shortage of particular polar or hydrophobic residues. However, a more objective evaluation requires a quantitative parameter of the proportion of both. In order to calculate and compare the intrinsic hydrophobicities of interferons we have utilized such a parameter, an average hydrophobicity ($H\Phi_{ave}$), introduced by Bigelow.[49] A protocol for the calculation‡ of $H\Phi_{ave}$ for HF-IF is shown in TABLE 2. $H\Phi_{ave}$ values for HF-IF, HL-IF, HLy-IF and M-IF are shown in TABLE 3. Amino acid compositions used in calculations were taken from Knight *et al.*[51] for HF–IF; Rubinstein *et al.*[37] for HL-IF; Zoon *et al.*[52] for HLy-IF; and Cabrer *et al.*[53] for M-IF. A comparison of the $H\Phi_{ave}$ values for interferons with those for several other proteins (TABLE 1) reveals that the intrinsic hydrophobicities of interferons, in general, are not significantly different in contrast to their apparent hydrophobicities (FIGURES 1 and 2). Of course, the validity of this conclusion rests entirely on the amino acid compositions utilized in our calculations.

Among interferons themselves, HL-IF seems to have the highest intrinsic hydrophobicity, significantly higher than that of HF-IF. This is an unexpected result in view of a much more pronounced apparent hydrophobicity of HF-IF (FIGURES 1 and 2). Although one cannot treat apparent hydrophobicity as a direct reflection of intrinsic hydrophobicity, an opposite result would seem to be more plausible. Clearly, only further refinement of the amino acid compositions of HF-IF and HL-IF will provide the definitive answer. However, it is our expectation that HF-IF will be eventually found to have a higher average hydrophobicity value than that of HL-IF. Moreover, in view of our previous findings,[27] we also anticipate significantly higher contents of aromatic amino acids in HF-IF by comparison to that of HL-IF and, in particular, their more pronounced surface localization.

TABLE 3

AVERAGE HYDROPHOBICITIES ($H\Phi_{ave}$) OF INTERFERONS

Interferons	HF-IF	HL-IF	HLy-IF	M-IF
Number of residues	171	158	166	164
Total $H\Phi$ (cal)	192,370	197,060	183,690	172,600
$H\Phi_{ave}$	1,125	1,247	1,107	1,052

SURFACE TOPOGRAPHY OF INTERFERONS

The high and rather selective affinity of mammalian interferons for phenyl-agarose is the most conspicuous finding of this report. The existence of a specific binding site with a good steric fit on an interferon molecule could underlie this affinity. In such a case the lining of the binding site may not involve aromatic residues as well exemplified by the architecture of the specificity binding site of α-chymotrypsin.[54] However, an attractive alternate interpretation which we favor, is an occurrence of π-π interactions between phenyl residues of the ligand and aromatic amino acid site chain(s) localized on the surface of an interferon molecule.[30,35] The notion of the presence of some aromatic residues on the surface of interferon molecules was advanced by us in order to rationalize the nature of interactions between human interferons, HF-IF and HL-IF, and immobilized

‡The modifications introduced into the calculations include, (1) updating the values for amino acids' hydrophobicities ($H\Phi$, cal/res)[50] and (2) introduction of the hydrophobicity for histidine and omission of that for threonine.

aromatic amino acids and dipeptides.[27] That hypothesis would account for inordinately strong binding of interferons to aromatic *vis à vis* aliphatic ligands. One must bear in mind that the hydrophobicity of the phenyl-residue is equivalent to less than four methylene units.[55,56] However, an aromatic effect (π-π interaction) in addition to hydrophobicity inherent in aromatic ligands (lyotropic effect) may have a synergistic influence on the strength of binding.[42,57]

A report by Berthold *et al.*[58] on the accessibility of tyrosine residues for iodination and nitration is consistent with our hypothesis. Moreover, the chemical modification of tyrosine residue(s) abolished the antiviral activity of human fibroblast interferon.[58] It will be of interest to extend this observation to other interferons. Perhaps, the aromatic residues present on the surface of interferons are intimately involved in their binding to cell membrane receptors and in the triggering of biological effects.

Conclusions

Mammalian interferons display a propensity to enter into hydrophobic interactions with immobilized ligands. The avid binding of interferons to aromatic ligands, in particular, may result from a synergistic effect of hydrophobic and π-π interactions. The aromatic residues localized on the surface of interferons may participate in their interactions with cell membrane receptors.

References

1. Tanford, C. 1962. J. Am. Chem. Soc. **84:** 4240.
2. Klotz, I. M. 1970. Arch. Biochem. Biophys. **138:** 704.
3. Lee, B. & F. M. Richards. 1971. J. Mol. Biol. **55:** 379.
4. Barrantes, F. J. 1973. Biochem. Biophys. Res. Commun. **54:** 395.
5. Tanford, C. & J. A. Reynolds. 1976. Biochim. Biophys. Acta **457:** 133.
6. Singer, S. J. 1974. Annu. Rev. Biochem. **45:** 805.
7. Cuatrecasas, P. 1972. J. Biol. Chem. **247:** 1980.
8. Neer, E. J. 1974. J. Biol. Chem. **249:** 6527.
9. McMenamy, R. H. & J. L. Oncley. 1958. J. Biol. Chem. **233:** 1436.
10. Jacobsen, J. 1969. FEBS Lett. **5:** 112.
11. Spector, A. A., K. John & J. E. Fletcher. 1969. J. Lipid. Res. **10:** 56.
12. Cunningham, V. J., L. Hay & H. B. Stoner. 1975. Biochem. J. **146:** 653.
13. Pande, C. S. & R. H. McMenamy. 1974. Biochim. Biophys. Acta **342:** 60.
14. Bruderlein, H. & J. Bernstein. 1979. J. Biol. Chem. **254:** 11570.
15. Hofstee, B. H. J. 1979. Pure Appl. Chem. **51:** 1537.
16. Huang, J. W., M. W. Davey, C. J. Hejna, W. von Muenchhausen, E. Sulkowski & W. A. Carter. 1974. J. Biol. Chem. **294:** 4665.
17. Huang, J. W., C. J. Hejna, E. Sulkowski, W. A. Carter, G. H. Silver, H. Munayyer & P. Came. 1975. Virology **65:** 268.
18. Chen, J. K., W. J. Jankowski, J. A. O'Malley, E. Sulkowski & W. A. Carter. 1976. J. Virol. **19:** 425.
19. Davey, M. W., E. Sulkowski & W. A. Carter. 1976. J. Virol. **17:** 439.
20. Osborne, L. C., J. A. Georgiades & H. M. Johnson. 1979. Infect. Immun. **23:** 80.
21. Jeng, D. K. H. 1977. Proc. Soc. Exp. Biol. Med. **154:** 534.
22. Davey, M. W., J. W. Huang, E. Sulkowski & W. A. Carter. 1974. J. Biol. Chem. **249:** 6354.
23. Davey, M. W., E. Sulkowski & W. A. Carter. 1976. Biochemistry **15:** 704.

24. MOGENSEN, K. E., K. CANTELL. 1979. J. Gen. Virol. **45:** 171.
25. DAVEY, M. W., J. W. HUANG, E. SULKOWSKI & W. A. CARTER. 1975. J. Biol. Chem. **250:** 348.
26. DAVEY, M. W., E. SULKOWSKI & W. A. CARTER. 1976. J. Biol. Chem. **251:** 7620.
27. SULKOWSKI, E., M. W. DAVEY & W. A. CARTER. 1976. J. Biol. Chem. **251:** 5381.
28. MIKULSKI, A. J., J. S. HOROSZEWICZ, E. SULKOWSKI & W. A. CARTER. 1976. Int. Sci. Mem., October, I-A335/1.
29. YAKOBSON, E., M. REVEL & D. GURARI-ROTMAN. 1979. Arch. Virol. **59:** 251.
30. BOLLIN, E., JR & E. SULKOWSKI. 1979. Prep. Biochem. **9:** 339.
31. WIETZERBIN, J., S. STEFANOS, M. LUCERO, E. FALCOFF, J. A. O'MALLEY & E. SULKOWSKI. 1979. J. Gen. Virol. **44:** 773.
32. JANKOWSKI, W., W. VON MUENCHHAUSEN, E. SULKOWSKI & W. A. CARTER. 1976. Int. Sci. Mem., April. I-A268/1.
33. JANKOWSKI, W. J., M. W. DAVEY, J. A. O'MALLEY, L. R. DAVIS, JR., E. SULKOWSKI & W. A. CARTER. 1976. ASM, 76th Annual Meeting, May, Atlantic City, Abstracts: 253.
34. BOLLIN, E., JR., K. VASTOLA, M. ITO, E. SULKOWSKI & W. A. CARTER. 1976. Int. Sci. Mem., July, I-A295/1.
35. JANKOWSKI, W. J., W. VON MUENCHHAUSEN, E. SULKOWSKI & W. A. CARTER. 1976. Biochemistry **15:** 5182.
36. BOLLIN, E., JR., K. VASTOLA, D. OLESZEK & E. SULKOWSKI. 1978. Prep. Biochem. **8:** 259.
37. RUBINSTEIN, M., S. RUBINSTEIN, P. C. FAMILLETTI, R. S. MILLER, A. A. WALDMAN & S. PESTKA. 1979. Proc. Nat. Acad. Sci. USA **76:** 640.
38. PORATH. J. & B. LARSSON. 1978. J. Chromat. **155:** 47.
39. EGLY, J.-M. & J. PORATH. 1979. J. Chromat. **168:** 35.
40. VIJAYALAKSHMI, M. A. & J. PORATH. 1979. J. Chromat. **177:** 201.
41. HOFSTEE, B. H. J. 1976. J. Macromol. Sci.-Chem. A10:111.
42. HOFSTEE, B. H. J. & N. F. OTILLIO. 1978. J. Chromat. **161:** 153.
43. FUJITA, T., Y. SUZUKI, J. YAMAUTI, I. TAKAGAHARA, K. FUJII, J. YAMASHITA & T. HORIO. 1980. J. Biochem. **87:** 89.
44. HOFSTEE, B. H. J. 1973. Anal. Biochem. **52:** 430.
45. BERTHOLD, W., C. TAN & Y. H. TAN. 1978. J. Biol. Chem. **253:** 5206.
46. BOUSQUET-VELA, C., J. WIETZERBIN & E. FALCOFF. 1980. Arch. Virol. **63:** 57.
47. HOMCY, C. J., S. M. WRENN & E. HABER. 1977. J. Biol. Chem. **252:** 8957.
48. NAGASAWA, T., H. NAGASAWA-FUJIMORI & P. C. HEINRICH. 1979. Eur. J. Biochem. **94:** 31.
49. BIGELOW, C. C. 1967. J. Theoret. Biol. **16:** 187.
50. NOZAKI, Y. & C. TANFORD. 1971. J. Biol. Chem. **246:** 2211.
51. KNIGHT, E., JR., M. W. HUNKAPILLER, B. D. KORANT R. W. F. HARDY & L. E. HOOD. 1980. Science **207:** 525.
52. ZOON, K. C., M. E. SMITH, P. J. BRIDGEN, C. B. ANFINSEN, M. W. HUNKAPILLER & L. E. HOOD. 1980. Science **207:** 527.
53. CABRER, B., H. TAIRA, R. J. BROEZE, T. D. KEMPE, K. WILLIAMS, E. SLATTERY, W. H. KONIGSBERG & P. LENGYEL. 1979. J. Biol. Chem. **254:** 3681.
54. STEITZ, T. A., R. HENDERSON & D. M. BLOW. 1969. J. Mol. Biol. **46:** 337.
55. JENCKS, W. P. 1969. Catalysis in Chemistry and Enzymology. McGraw-Hill, Inc. pp. 393–436.
56. TANFORD, C. 1973. Hydrophobic Effect. John Wiley & Sons, Inc. pp. 49–53.
57. HOFSTEE, B. H. J. 1979. Biochem. Biophys. Res. Commun. **91:** 312.
58. BERTHOLD, W., C. TAN & Y. H. TAN. 1978. Eur. J. Biochem. **87:** 367.

ELECTROPHORETICALLY PURE MOUSE INTERFERON EXERTS MULTIPLE BIOLOGICAL EFFECTS*

Jaqueline De Maeyer-Guignard and Edward De Maeyer

Institut Curie-Biologie
Université de Paris-Sud, Bât. 110
91405 Orsay, France

Michael G. Tovey and Ion Gresser

Institut de Recherches sur le Cancer
94800 Villejuif, France

INTRODUCTION

Interferon (IF), preparations exert multiple effects on cells, *in vitro* and in the organism. The most extensively investigated of these "non-antiviral" effects are the cell-multiplication inhibitory effect,[1-4] the antitumor effect,[5-7] and various effects on humoral and cellular immunity.[8-20] Moreover, effects of IF preparations on the synthesis of IF itself, such as priming and blocking, have also been described.[21-25]

Except for studies on the cell-multiplication inhibitory activity,[26-27] none of this work has been carried out using pure IF, and in many preparations that were used for these studies IF represented only 0.1 or 0.01% of the protein; in the best preparations IF protein constituted at most only 1% of the total protein content. Most investigators however have been careful enough to use IF preparations of different cellular origins and of varying degrees of purity, all of which had comparable effects. In addition, mock IF and IF derived from different species were usually devoid of effect. Nevertheless, and in spite of these precautions, there remained some legitimate doubt as to whether all these non-antiviral effects were due to the same molecules responsible for the antiviral activity.

We have recently succeeded in preparing electrophoretically pure (EP) mouse interferon,[27] and present herein results which show that a number of the biological effects previously observed with crude or partially purified preparations are also observed with this EP interferon. These results provide the most direct evidence to date that IF not only inhibits viral multiplication, but that it also exerts a variety of important biological effects on cells.

PURIFICATION OF MOUSE INTERFERON USED IN OUR EXPERIMENTS

The interferon used in our studies was induced with Newcastle disease virus (NDV) in the high interferon-producing C-243 cell line.[28] Purification was achieved by two-step affinity chromatography, first on a poly U-agarose column[29] and then on a column of sheep anti-mouse interferon globulin coupled to

*This work was supported in part by the D.R.E.T. (78-34-210), D.G.R.S.T. (79-7-205/206), I.N.S.E.R.M. (ATP 78-90), C.N.R.S. (AI 0031858), the Lique Nationale Française contre le Cancer, and the Fondation pour la Recherche Médicale Française.

0077-8923/80/0350-0347 $01.75/0 © 1980, NYAS

affigel.[30] The purity of the eluted material was assessed by electrophoresis on 15% polyacrylamide slab gels in the presence of sodium dodecyl sulfate (SDS).[27] When enough IF is electrophoresed (i.e. at least 6×10^6 mouse interferon reference units per slot in a volume of 20 or 30 μl) two bands are seen after staining with Coomassie brilliant blue. Elution of two mm gel slices showed that antiviral activity was associated with these two bands, which had molecular weights of 35,000 and 22,000. Electrophoretic analysis of three purified IF preparations revealed each time only these two bands in the absence of any other stainable bands. The activity at a MW of 35,000 is in contrast to the MW of 38,000 described by Stewart *et al.*[31] The difference in results is due to our use of a discontinuous tris-glycine buffer system described by Laemmli[32] whereas Stewart *et al.* used a phosphate buffer. When electrophoresed in 0.01 M phosphate buffer, our IF preparations also exhibited peak of activity at a MW of 38,000. The difference in migration rates in different buffers obtained with the higher MW component can be attributed to its greater sugar content (as determined by P.A.S. staining[27] compared to the 22,000 MW component whose migration is identical in tris-glycine and phosphate buffer).

The specific activities of three different EP interferon preparations used in these studies were 9.9×10^8, 1.2×10^9, and 1.5×10^9 reference units per mg of protein as determined by the method of Böhlen *et al.*[33] These values are in accord with our previously published value of 2.4×10^9 reference units/mg protein.[27] To reduce loss of activity of highly purified interferon, bovine serum albumin (BSA), 100 μg/ml in PBS was added to the EP interferon. For purposes of comparison it was at times also added to the partially purified IF used as a comparative control in several experiments.

RESULTS

Effects of EP Interferon on the Immune System

Antibody Formation[11-13]

C3H mouse spleen cells (6×10^6 cells in 1 ml) where stimulated *in vitro* with sheep erythrocytes (SRBC)[34] and incubated with 0.1 ml of BSA (100 μg/ml) or 0.1 ml of partially purified or EP interferon (titer 1.2×10^5). After 5 days incubation the number of plaque-forming cells (PFC) was determined. A 94% inhibition in the generation of PFC was observed for cultures treated with both IF preparations in contrast to 11% inhibition for cultures incubated with BSA alone.

Cell-mediated Immunity

Enhancement of Natural Killer Cell Activity in Vivo *and* in Vitro.[35-37] Six-week-old male BALB/c mice were inoculated i.p. with 0.2 ml of either BSA (100 μg/ml), 0.2 ml of partially purified interferon (titering 9.6×10^5) or EP interferon (titer 6.4×10^5) or were left untreated. Twenty-four hours later the spleens of the two mice per group were tested individually for cytotoxicity on YAC target cells.[35] A significant enhancement in cytotoxicity was observed for spleen cells from interferon-treated mice.

Likewise incubation *in vitro* of splenic lymphoctyes for 2½ hours with partially purified or EP interferon (titer 1.2×10^4) enhanced their cytotoxicity for ^{51}Cr-labeled YAC target cells from the baseline value of 29% specific ^{51}Cr release to 55% and 44%, respectively (effector : target cell ratio of 100:1).

Delayed Hypersensitivity in Vivo. Interferon can affect both afferent and efferent pathways of DH in the mouse.

—*Sensitization.*[19] Eight-week-old female BALB/c mice were sensitized intravenously with 10^6 SRBC. One group was injected with 5×10^6 units of EP interferon i.p., 24 hours prior to sensitization, whereas the control group was injected with PBS. Four days after sensitization, 10^8 SRBC were injected into the left footpad of mice of both groups and footpad swelling was recorded 24 and 48 hr later. Footpad swelling was significantly inhibited in the IF-treated group.

If, however, EP interferon is administered 2 hours after sensitization, footpad swelling is significantly enhanced; however, for this stimulatory effect to occur, a suboptimal amount (10^5) of SRBC has to be used for sensitization.

Thus, EP interferon can either decrease or enhance sensitization, depending on the timing of its administration.

—*Expression.*[20] For this experiment mice were sensitized with 10^6 SRBC and the interferon was administered 4½ hours before footpad challenge, 4 days after sensitization. Footpad swelling, measured 24 and 48 hours after challenge, was reduced in IF-treated mice.

For both the experiments on sensitization and expression a mixture of the 35,000 and 22,000 MW was used. In another experiment, described elsewhere,[38] an effect on sensitization and expression was also obtained using only the 35,000 MW form, eluted from a PAGE gel. In one experiment, inhibition of sensitization was also observed when mice were treated 24 hours before sensitization with the 22,000 MW form.

Antitumor Effect in Vivo[5-6]

The antitumor activity was determined in BALB/c mice injected intraperitoneally (i.p.) with Ehrlich ascites (EA) cells.[6] Six-week-old female BALB/c mice were injected i.p. with 1.6×10^4 EA cells. Two hours later, and daily thereafter, for the next 9 days, mice were inoculated i.p. with 0.25 ml of either BSA (100 μg/ml), partially purified or EP mouse IF preparations. The titers of the partially purified or EP preparations were 1.28×10^{-6} and 3.2×10^{-5}, respectively. BSA (100 μg/ml) was added to the EP interferon. Daily injection of both partially purified and EP mouse IF preparations resulted in an inhibition of the multiplication of EA cells in the peritoneal cavity and an increase in mouse survival time.

Effects on Interferon Synthesis: Priming and Blocking

Interferon can influence its own synthesis, and pretreatment of cells with relatively low amounts often results in increased production upon subsequent induction, a phenomenon called "priming."[21,22] There is also evidence for an opposite effect in that treatment of cells with higher doses results in subsequent inhibition of interferon synthesis, and this has been called "blocking."[23-25]

Both effects were reexamined with EP interferon.

Results in MEF Cultures

Secondary cultures of mouse embryo fibroblasts were incubated for 18 hr with varying concentrations or partially purified and EP interferon prior to addition of 30 μg of poly I.poly C, in the presence of DEAE dextran (100 μg/ml). After 1 hour at 37°C, the inducer was removed, the cell sheet washed, medium replaced and harvested 24 hours later for determination of interferon content. Pretreatment of cells with 18 or more units of partially purified or EP interferon resulted in an increase in the mean interferon titer from 1:960 to 1:7680. Blocking was not observed, even at the highest concentrations (50,000 units/ml) of EP interferon used to preincubate the cells.

Results Obtained in C-243 Cells

Pretreatment of C-243 cells with EP interferon, at all concentrations tested, up to 160,000 units/0.15 ml, did not block subsequent IF induction by poly(I.C) (100 μg - DEAE dextran 500 μg/ml) but had significant priming effect; the optimal priming effect consisting in a 30-fold increase of IF yield, was obtained using 6000 units. The unpurified material also has priming effect at a low concentration (400 units), but this priming effect did not increase with increasing concentrations. This suggests that there are factors present in the crude preparation inhibiting the priming effect of interferon.

When IF production is induced with NDV instead of poly(I.C), pretreatment of C-243 cells or MEF with pure IF results in significant inhibition of subsequent IF synthesis. We ascribe this effect to the antiviral action of IF, inhibiting formation of NDV-dependent ds RNA, and not to a direct effect on IF synthesis.

Discussion

The interferon used in these studies was derived from one large batch of crude interferon, made in C-243 cells, but was purified on three separate occasions. We want to emphasize that the endproduct of each of the three purification runs was analyzed by PAGE, and only the two IF bands previously described were visualized after staining with Coomassie brilliant blue. The definition of purity is clearly relative and depends on the sensitivity of the methods used to measure possible contaminants. The lower limit of detection of this method in our hands is 0.07 μg of protein per band, using either bovine serum albumin or ovalbumin as reference proteins. Although we can of course not exclude that some minor contaminants, undetectable by staining of the gels, were present in our EP interferon preparations, we believe our results show that the same molecules are responsible for the antiviral and for the other biological effects.

In view of the relatively large amount of IF needed for some *in vivo* experiments—e.g. the antitumor effect— a mixture of the 35,000 and the 22,000 MW form was used in many experiments. When the two bands were eluted from a gel, and tested separately, such as for the inhibitory effect on sensitization to SRBC, both were found to have activity, and this activity correlated well with the antiviral titer of each preparation. It is however entirely possible that for some of the effects described in this paper, if both MW forms are examined separately, one form will be found to be more efficient than the other, since a different degree of glycosylation may conceivably influence clearance rates and uptake of IF molecules by various cells of the organism. This is a subject for further investigation.

Our results confirm the broad biological significance of interferon, and remove any reasonable doubt concerning the various effects of interferon on antibody formation and cell-mediated immunity.

When the effects of EP interferon on poly(I.C.)-induced IF synthesis were examined, only a stimulation of synthesis (priming) was observed, and no inhibition (blocking). In fact, priming was much more efficient when pure IF was used to preincubate the cells, suggesting that inhibitors of priming are present in our unpurified starting material. Priming was observed both when poly(I.C) and NDV were used as inducer, indicating that the biochemical changes occurring in the cell as a result of the IF-induced antiviral state are favoring IF synthesis. In poly(I.C)-induced cells, blocking of IF synthesis was not observed after pretreatment with EP interferon, even with the very high dose of 160,000 units. This shows that IF is not capable of inhibiting its own synthesis, which rules out negative feedback as a mechanism for the arrest of IF synthesis but indirectly lends weight to the repressor hypothesis, first advanced by Vilček and Ng.[39] When a viral inducer is involved, necessitating viral RNA synthesis, as is the case for NDV, pure IF when given in sufficient amounts can block IF synthesis; this effect, in all likelihood is indirect, through inhibition of ds RNA synthesis.

In addition to their theoretical interest, our results are also pertinent to the clinical usefulness of IF. Relatively crude and partially purified human leukocyte interferon preparations are currently being used in the treatment of patients with different neoplasms and some of the preliminary results are most encouraging.[40-44] The results presented above show that in one mouse transplantable tumor system, IF itself is responsible for an antitumor effect. Likewise, since IF interacts with the immune system, and affects the division and function of normal cells, therapeutic uses may now be envisaged for interferon that have not been heretofore considered.

Summary

Electrophoretically pure (EP) mouse interferon (IF), was examined for a number of biological effects previously ascribed to crude or partially purified interferon preparations. The following effects were observed: inhibition of antibody formation *in vitro;* inhibition or enhancement of sensitization to sheep erythrocytes in the mouse, depending on time of administration of IF, and dosage of antigen; inhibition of the expression of delayed type hypersensitivity *in vivo;* enhancement of natural killer cell activity *in vitro* and *in vivo;* inhibition of mouse tumor cells multiplication *in vitro;* inhibition of the growth of a transplantable tumor in mice. EP mouse IF had a very pronounced priming effect but had no blocking activity.

Acknowledgments

We are grateful to Drs. H. Fridman and A. Senik for their generous help in the experiments on the *in vitro* antibody response, and the cytotoxicity of NK cells respectively. We are indebted to Mrs. M.T. Bandu, J. Buywid and Miss A. Cachard for excellent technical assistance.

References

1. Paucker, K., K. Cantell & W. Henle. 1962. Virology **17:** 324–334.
2. Gresser, I., D. Brouty-Boyé, M. T. Thomas & A. Macieira-Coelho. 1970. Proc. Nat. Acad. Sci. USA **66:** 1052–1058.
3. Lindahl-Magnusson, P., P. Leary & I. Gresser. 1971. Proc. Soc. Exp. Biol. Med. **138:** 1044–1050.
4. Gresser, I., M. T. Bandu & D. Brouty-Boyé. 1974. J. Nat. Cancer Inst. **52:** 553–559.
5. Gresser, I., C. Bourali, J. P. Levy, D. Fontaine-Brouty-Boyé & M. T. Thomas. 1969. Proc. Nat. Acad. Sci. USA **63:** 51–57.
6. Gresser, I. & C. Bourali. 1970. J. Nat. Cancer Inst. **45:** 365–374.
7. Gresser, I. 1977. *In* Cancer: A Comprehensive Treatise. F. Becker, Ed. Vol. **5:** 521–571. Plenum. New York.
8. Braun, W. & H. B. Levy. 1972. Proc Soc. Exp. Biol. Med. **141:** 769–773.
9. Chester, T., K. Paucker & T. C. Merigan. 1973. Nature (London) **246:** 92–94.
10. Brodeur, B. R. & T. C. Merigan. 1974. J. Immunol. **113:** 1319–1325.
11. Gisler, R. H., P. Lindahl & I. Gresser. 1974. J. Immunol. **113:** 438–444.
12. Johnson, H., B. G. Smith & S. Baron. 1975. J. Immunol. **114:** 403–409.
13. Booth, R. J., J. Booth & J. Marbrook. 1976. Eur. J. Immunol. **6:** 769–772.
14. Lindahl-Magnusson, P., P. Leary & I. Gresser. 1972. Nature (London) New Biol. **273:** 120–121.
15. Lindahl, P., P. Leary & I. Gresser. 1972. Proc. Nat. Acad. Sci. USA **69:** 721–725.
16. De Maeyer, E., L. Mobraaten & J. De Maeyer-Guignard. 1973. C.R. Hebd. Séances Acad. Sci. **277:** 2101–2103.
17. Mobraaten, L., E. De Maeyer & J. De Maeyer-Guignard. 1973. Transplantation **16:** 415–420.
18. Hirsch, M. S., D. A. Ellis, P. H. Black, A. P. Monaco & M. L. Wood. 1973. Transplantation **17:** 234–236.
19. De Maeyer-Guignard, J., A. Cachard & E. De Maeyer. 1975. Science **190:** 574–576.
20. De Maeyer, E., J. De Maeyer-Guignard & M. Vandeputte. 1975. Proc. Nat. Acad. Sci. USA **72:** 1753–1757.
21. Isaacs, A. & D. C. Burke. 1958. Nature (London) **182:** 1073–1074.
22. Stewart, W. E. II, L. B. Gosser & R. Z. Lockart, Jr. 1971. J. Virol. 792–801.
23. Vilček, J. & B. Rada. 1962. Acta Virol. **6:** 9–16.
24. Paucker, K. & M. Boxaca. 1967. Bacteriol. Rev. **31:** 145–156.
25. Youngner, J. S. & J. V. Hallum. 1969. Virology **37:** 473–475.
26. Knight, E. 1976. Nature (London) **262:** 302–303.
27. De Maeyer-Guignard, J., M. G. Tovey, I. Gresser & E. De Maeyer. 1978. Nature (London) **271:** 622–625.
28. Oie, H. K., A. F. Gazdar, C. E. Buckler & S. Baron. 1972. J. Gen. Virol. **17:** 107–109.
29. De Maeyer-Guignard, J., M. N. Thang & E. De Maeyer. 1977. Proc. Nat. Acad. Sci. USA **74:** 3787–3790.
30. Sipe, J. D., J. De Maeyer-Guignard, B. Fauconnier & E. De Maeyer. 1973. Proc. Nat. Acad. Sci. USA **70:** 1037–1040.
31. Stewart, W. E. II, I. Gresser, M. G. Tovey, M. T. Bandu & S. Le Goff. 1976. Nature (London) **262:** 300–302.
32. Laemmli, U. K. 1970. Nature (London) **227:** 680–685.
33. Böhlen, P., S. Stein, W. Dairman & S. Udenfriend. 1973. Arch. Biochem. Biophys. **155:** 213–220.
34. Mishell, R. I. & R. W. Dutton. 1967. J. Exp. Med. **126:** 423–442.
35. Gidlund, M., A. Orn, H. Wigzell, A. Senik & I. Gresser. 1978. Nature (London) **273:** 759–761.
36. Welsh, R. M., Jr. 1978. J. Exp. Med. **148:** 163-181.

37. DJEU, K. Y., J. A. HEINBAUGH, H. T. HOLDEN & R. B. HERBERMAN. 1979. J. Immunol. **122:** 175–178.
38. DE MAEYER, E. & J. DE MAEYER-GUIGNARD. 1980. *In* Biochemical Characterization of Lymhokines. Proceedings of the Second International Lymphokine Workshop. A. De Weck, F. Kristensen & M. Landy, Eds.: 383–391.
39. VILČEK, J. & M. H. NG. 1971. J. Virol. **7:** 588–594.
40. STRANDER, H., K. CANTELL, G. CARLSTRÖM & P. A. JAKOBSSON. 1973. J. Nat. Cancer Inst. **51:** 733–742.
41. BLOMGREN, H., K. CANTELL, B. JOHANSSON, C. LAGERGREN, U. RINGBORG & H. STRANDER. 1976. Acta Med. Scand. **199:** 527–532.
42. STRANDER, H. 1977. Blut **35:** 277–288.
43. MERIGAN, T. C., K. SIKORA, H. H. BREEDEN, R. LEVY & S. A. ROSENBERG. 1978. N. Engl. J. Med. **299:** 1449–1453.
44. MELLSTEDT, H., M. BJÖRKHOLM, B. JOHANSSON, A. AHRE, G. HOLM & H. STRANDER. 1979. Lancet **i:** 245–247.

PURIFICATION AND PROPERTIES OF NATIVE AND MODIFIED INTERFERONS*

Lulu A. Pickering, Irwin A. Braude, Leo S. Lin, and William E. Stewart II

Interferon Laboratories
Memorial Sloan-Kettering Cancer Center
New York, New York 10021

INTRODUCTION

The variety in the interferon forms produced by cells of a given animal species is likely to be meaningful to the organisms producing these molecules, but this heterogeneity of interferon molecules reveals itself to us only as a curious phenomenon. To date the only functional distinction apparent in these diverse interferon forms is their pharmacological properties.[1] The heterogeneity of mouse type I interferons exhibited as size components of 38,000 and 22,000 daltons in SDS-polyacrylamide gels[2,3] appears to arise from glycosylation of precursor polypeptide, the 16,000 dalton "interferoid."[4] As yet we have been unable to discern any functional differences in these apparently extensively glycosylated, partially glycosylated, or nonglycosylated mouse interferon forms, as each appears equally able to induce antiviral, priming, toxicity-enhancing, and cell-multiplication-inhibitory activities.[5]

Similar studies with human leukocyte interferon have suggested that the size heterogeneities of these molecules, revealed as 21,000 and 15,000 dalton components in SDS-polyacrylamide gels,[6] is also carbohydrate-contributed. Thus, periodate oxidation eliminates the size and charge heterogeneity of human leukocyte interferons, apparently converting the larger forms to the smaller molecules,[7] and human leukocyte interferon preparations produced in the presence of glycosylation inhibitors contain only the smaller interferon forms.[8]

Our recent studies have been directed toward identification of the origins of the heterogeneities of human leukocyte interferons, by attempting conversion of one form to another, either by glycolytic or proteolytic processing, and by identification of the primary translation product of the interferon messenger RNAs obtained from different lymphoid cell populations producing distinct forms of human leukocyte interferons.

PROTEOLYTIC MODIFICATION OF HUMAN LEUKOCYTE INTERFERONS: ALTERED MOLECULAR HETEROGENEITIES AND CROSS-SPECIES ACTIVITY RATIOS

The antiviral activity of human leukocyte interferon preparations can be efficiently assayed on either human, lupine, feline, porcine or bovine cells,[9-11]

*This work was supported by Grant RO1-CA-20863 awarded by the National Cancer Institute and Institutional Core Grant NCI-CA-08748-13. I.A.B. was supported by a National Institutes of Health training grant (#T32-CA-09193-01A1). W.E.S.II is the recipient of United States Public Health Service Research Career Development Award #AI-00219 from the National Institutes of Allergy and Infectious Diseases.

0077-8923/80/0350-0354 $01.75/0 © 1980, NYAS

and certain of the molecular weight species of human leukocyte interferon have been shown to be significantly more cross-reactive on feline and bovine cells than other human leukocyte interferon forms.[11,12]

When a human leukocyte interferon preparation with similar ratios of human: bovine cell activities was treated with α-chymotrypsin at an enzyme-substrate ratio of 1:10 at 4°C, the activity on human cells was rapidly lost while the activity on bovine cells was retained.[13] We have observed this same phenom-

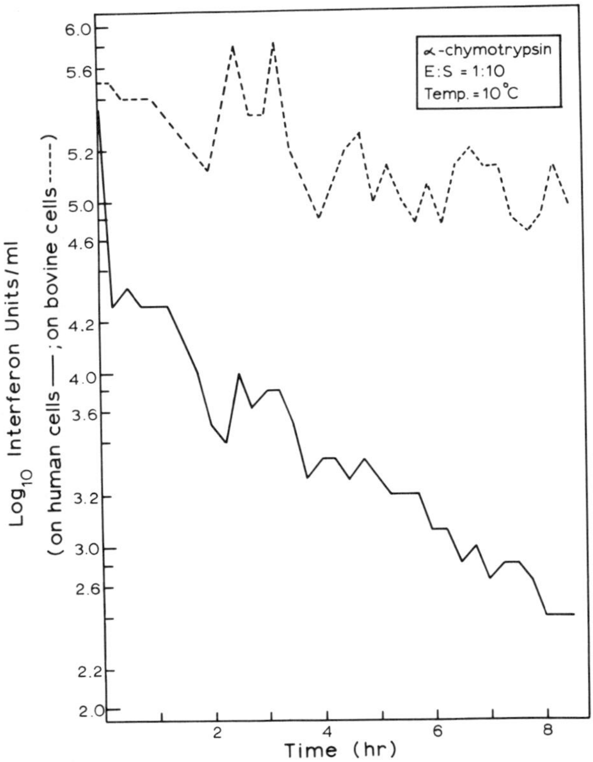

FIGURE 1. α-chymotrypsin treatment of human leukocyte interferon at 4°C. Human leukocyte interferon (HuLeIF), with a specific activity of 4.6×10^5 units/mg, was dialyzed against 20mM sodium-phosphate buffer, pH 7.6, and treated with α-chymotrypsin at an enzyme-substrate (E:S) ratio of 1:10. Samples were removed at 15-min intervals and the reaction inhibited with lima bean trypsin inhibitor (enzyme inhibitor, E:I, ratio ≥ 1:10). The pH was maintained at 7.6 with a Radiometer pH-Stat and the temperature maintained at 4°C with a Haake F2-C circulating water bath.

enon with several proteolytic enzymes under conditions of limited digestion (FIGURES 1–3), in each case heterologous cell activity being retained while homologous activity was lost. Thus, as each of these proteases cleaves with different specificities, this loss of homologous activity appears to be a general phenomenon. It should be noted, however, that although the activity of the

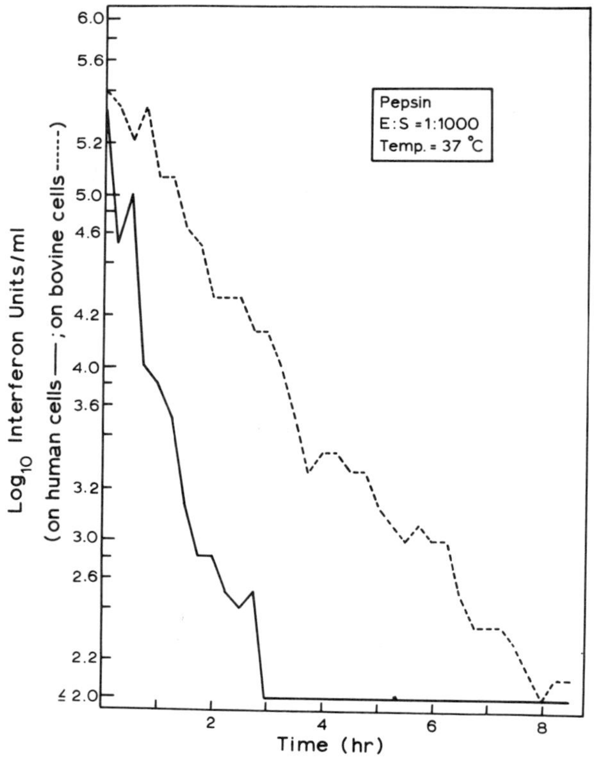

FIGURE 2. Pepsin treatment of human leukocyte interferon. HLeIF dialyzed against 10mM sodium-acetate buffer, pH 3.1, was treated with pepsin at an E:S of 1:1000. A pH of 3.1 and a temperature of 37°C was maintained as described in the legend to FIGURE 1. Samples were removed at 15-min intervals and the enzyme inhibited by increasing the pH to between 7–8 with 1N NaOh.

interferon for heterologous cells was less sensitive to proteolytic digestion than was the homologous activity, under more drastic conditions (e.g. α-chymotrypsin at 37°C, FIGURE 4) the enzymes rapidly inactivated both homologous and heterologous activities.

When analyzed by electrophoresis on SDS-polyacrylamide gels, the digestion with α-chymotrypsin reveals that the faster migrating components with more pronounced activity on bovine cells[12] are retained while those at the higher molecular weight with the more pronounced human cell activity are rapidly inactivated.[13] These data might suggest that the more heavily glycosylated interferon forms were contorted such that residues sensitive to the enzyme were exposed, while those on the smaller (less-glycosylated) molecules were shielded. However, when human leukocyte interferon preparations that had been treated with acidic periodate buffer, to remove carbohydate moeities,[7] were exposed to α-chymotrypsin, the same divergence of human and bovine activities was observed (FIGURE 5). These data suggest that even within the same size molecules of human leukocyte interferons there are those active on bovine cells and resistant to the protease and those active on human cells and sensitive to the enzyme. This is in agreement with our previous observation that two-dimensional gel electrophoresis of periodate-treated human leukocyte interferon resolves two spots of interferon protein, one active on both human and bovine cells and one active only on bovine cells.[14]

Properties of Native Human Interferons Derived from Different Lymphoblastoid Cell Lines

Rather than trying to convert one interferon form to another, an alternative approach to determining the origins of interferon heterogeneities is to study their sources. We have attempted this by trying to identify cell populations making distinct interferon forms and to study the products of translations of their interferon messenger RNAs. Human interferon preparations obtained from primary leukocyte buffy coat suspensions induced by viruses consistently distribute into two major size components at about 2,100 and 15,000 daltons when analyzed by SDS-polyacrylamide gels.[6,8,15] Human lymphoblastoid cell interferon derived from virus-induced Namalva cells migrates as predominantly the lower molecular weight form of leukocyte interferon in SDS-polyacrylamide gels,[15] and the product of Namalva cell interferon messenger RNA translated in *Xenopus laevis* oocytes has also been reported to migrate as a single peak at about 16,000 daltons in these gels.[16] Thus, either human peripheral blood leukocytes are better

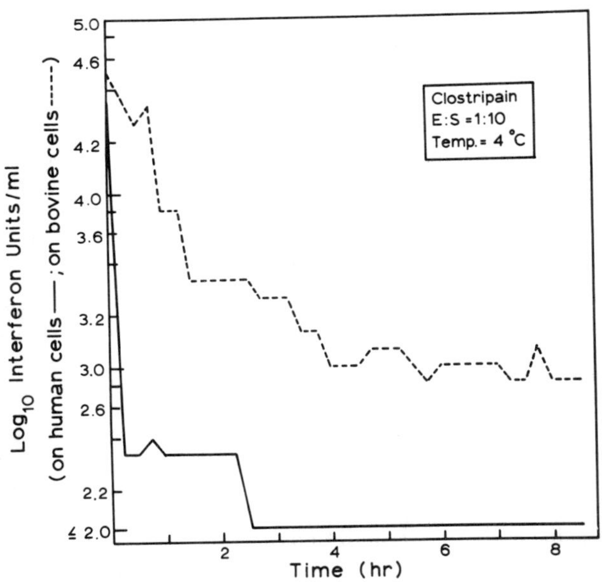

FIGURE 3. Clostripain treatment of human leukocyte interferon. HLeIF, dialyzed against 10mM sodium-phosphate buffer, pH 7.6, and 2.5 mM dithiothreitol, was treated with clostripain (which was first activated with 1.0 mM calcium acetate and 2.5 mM dithiothreitol) at an E:S of 1:10. A pH of 7.6, and a temperature of 4°C was maintained. Samples were removed at 15 minute intervals and the enzyme inhibited (E:I ≥ 1:1) with *p*-hydroxymercuribenzonae.

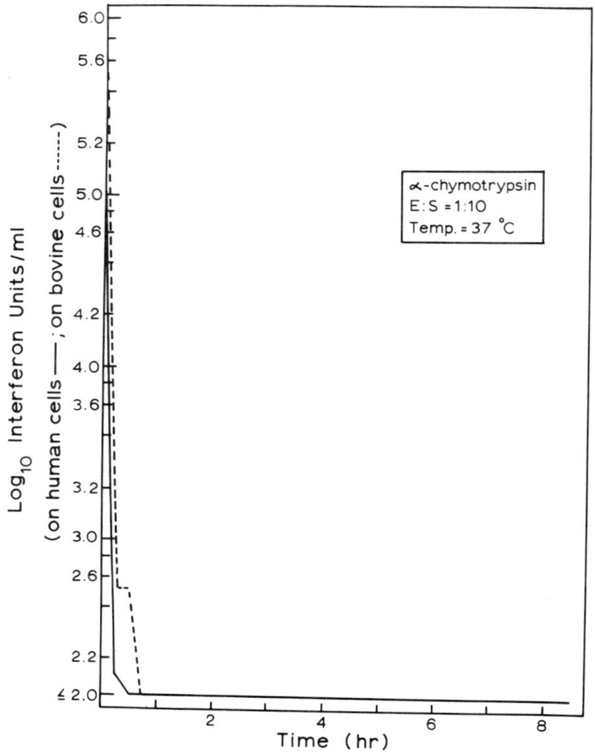

FIGURE 4. α-chymotrypsin treatment of human leukocyte interferon at 37°C. HLeIF was treated with α-chymotrypsin essentially as described in FIGURE 1. The reaction temperature in this experiment was maintained at 37°C.

able to glycosylate part the of interferon they produce than are Namalva cells or there are different cell populations in the peripheral blood that can produce different interferon forms, these in turn resulting either from different abilities of the producing cells to glycosylate them or from differences in their messenger RNAs.

To our knowledge, no one has yet determined the molecular weights of the interferon made from any lymphoblastoid cells other than that induced in Namalva cells. As there might be different types of lymphoid cells producing the different leukocyte-type interferon forms (and which thus might be sources of different messenger RNAs) we undertook to examine the interferons produced by different lymphoblast cells. Our first effort in this direction was a screening of several lines of lymphoblastoid cells for ability to produce interferon; several representatives of this search are listed in TABLE 1. These lymphoblastoid cell-types can be divided into those that produced interferon when induced with Sendai virus, those that did not produce any detectable interferon when induced with Sendai virus, and those that produced interferon even without being induced. Surprisingly, in our hands the best interferon-producing cells were those that did so spontaneously. Thus, an EB virus-transformed cell line designated EP 2 spontaneously produced between 30 to 100 reference units of interferon/ml, a myeloma cell line spontaneously produced just detectable levels of interferon, and a particular clone of the acute myelogenous leukemia cell line 8866 spontaneously released several hundred interferon reference units/ml into the growth medium. None of the cell lines that spontaneously produce interferon made any higher levels of interferon when they were induced with Sendai or Newcastle disease virus.

The spontaneously produced interferons (spIFs) were compared to poly I · poly C-induced human fibroblast interferon, to virus-induced human buffy coat leukocyte interferon, and to Namalva cell interferon for activity on bovine cells. Like the leukocyte and Namalva interferons, the spIFs were highly active on bovine cells, whereas the human fibroblast interferon, as is well documented,[17] was not significantly active on these cells (TABLE 2). It is noteworthy that the spIFs were somewhat less cross-reactive on the bovine cells than were the virus-induced interferons derived from Namalva cells or from peripheral blood leukocytes, as it has been reported that the larger molecular species of

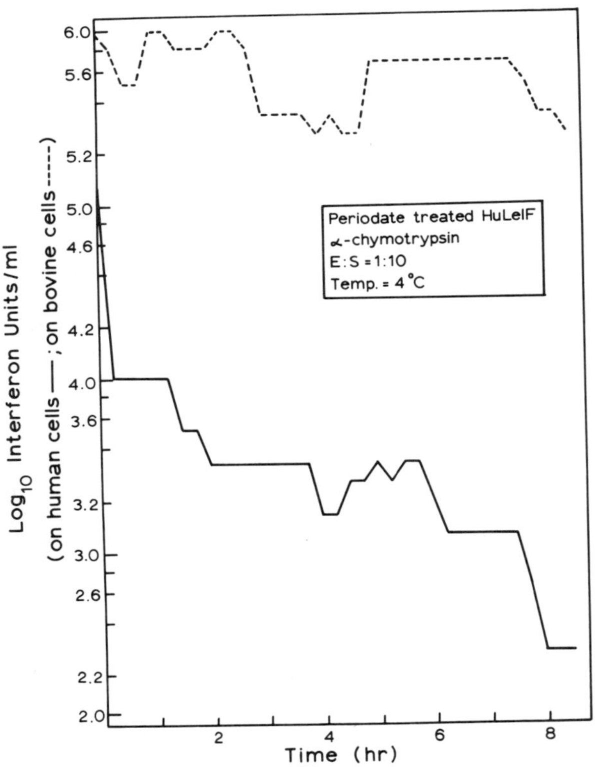

FIGURE 5. α-chymotrypsin treatment of periodate-oxidized human leukocyte interferon. Periodate-oxidized HLeIF was treated with α-chymotrypsin essentially as described in FIGURE 1.

TABLE 1

INDUCED AND SPONTANEOUS INTERFERON PRODUCTION BY HUMAN LYMPHOBLASTOID CELLS

Cell Type	Interferon Production (units/ml)	
	Spontaneous	Induced
Burkitt's lymphoma		
Namalva	<1	100–300
Daudi	<1	<1
Raji	<1	30–100
Myeloma		
BM	10	*
Plasmocytoma		
Sultan	<1	<1
Unknown derivations		
Platz (SKW-4)	<1	<1
Manca	<1	<1
EBV-transformed peripheral blood lymphocytes		
EP2	30–100	*
Acute myelogenous leukemia		
8866 · 7	100–600	*

*No increased production when induced.

human leukocyte interferon is slightly less active on bovine cells than on human cells, while the smaller molecular species is slightly more active on bovine cells than on human cells.

The spIFs were also characterized as to antigenic type by neutralizations using antisera prepared against human leukocyte interferon (a gift from Dr. Kari Cantell, Helsinki) antiserum to Namalva interferon (a gift from Dr. Karl Fantes, Wellcome Laboratories), antiserum to human fibroblast interferon (a gift from Dr. Jan Vilček, New York), and two different antisera to mouse interferon (one a gift from Dr. Anna Inglot, Wroclaw, Poland and one produced by I.A. Braude).

The spIFs were both antigenically leukocyte-type interferons as they were neutralized by the anti-human leukocyte and the anti-Namalva interferon antisera, but not by the anti-human fibroblast interferon antiserum (TABLE 3). Surprisingly, spIFs were also neutralized by each of the anti-mouse interferon antisera, whereas neither Namalva lymphoblastoid interferon nor human leukocyte interferon was neutralized by the anti-mouse interferon antisera. Thus, a form of human interferon has been identified that is neutralized by antiserum

TABLE 2

CROSS-REACTIVITY OF HUMAN INTERFERONS ON BOVINE CELLS

Interferon	Percent of Homologous Antiviral Activity on Bovine Cells
Fibroblast	≤1%
Leukocyte	100–200%
Namalva	100–200%
Spontaneous	30–50%

against mouse interferon. This is particularly intriguing as a mouse interferon has also recently been identified which is neutralized by anti-human leukocyte antiserum.[8] This mouse interferon form that is antigenically related to human leukocyte interferon, migrates at about 21,000 daltons in SDS-polyacrylamide gels.[19]

These data on cross-species activity levels on bovine cells and neutralizations by heterologous antisera suggested that spIF might be a human lymphoblastoid interferon form physically distinct from the Namalva lymphoblastoid interferon. Therefore, a batch of spIF was concentrated and purified by ammonium sulfate precipitation at pH 2.0 and was analyzed by SDS-polyacrylamide gel electrophoresis in simultaneously run parallel gels with Namalva interferon and human leukocyte interferon. As usual, the virus-induced "buffy-coat" leukocyte interferon was heterogeneously distributed into 21,000 and 15,000 dalton activity peaks (FIGURE 6a), while the virus-induced lymphoblastoid interferon from Namalva cells migrated predominantly as the lower molecular weight species (FIGURE 6b). The spIF activity, in contrast, migrated as a homologeneous band of activity with a peak at 20,000 daltons (FIGURE 6c).

TABLE 3

NEUTRALIZATION OF HUMAN LYMPHOID INTERFERONS BY VARIOUS ANTI-INTERFERON ANTISERA

	Neutralizing Activity Against			
	Spontaneous		Induced	
Antiserum	EP-2	8866 · 7	Namalva	Leukocyte
Anti-leukocyte	+	+	+	+
Anti-Namalva	+	+	+	+
Anti-fibroblast	–	–	–	–
Anti-mouse (Inglot)	+	+	–	–
Anti-mouse (Braude)	+	+	–	–

Thus, the spIF is a molecular form of lymphoblastoid interferon distinct from lymphoblastoid interferon derived from Namalva cells in the relative degrees of cross-species activities on bovine cells, in antigenic relation to mouse interferon, and in size. This interferon form should provide new approaches for determining the contribution of carbohydrate moieties to the heterogeneities of the lymphoid interferons. Translations of the interferon messenger RNA from these cells and from Namalva cells in *Xenopus laevis* oocytes should allow us to determine whether the biological, antigenic and physical distinctions between these two lymphoid interferon forms are gene-derived or arise from secondary embellishments. The availability of these two lymphoblastoid interferons with these several dissimilarities, one representing the larger leukocyte interferon form and the other the smaller leukocyte interferon form, affords an opportunity to evaluate the pharmacokinetic properties of the distinct molecular species of interferons present in native human leukocyte interferon preparations.

Further studies with these interferon-generating cells should provide interesting new information concerning the mechanisms regulating induction and production of interferons. Finally, the availability of lymphoblastoid cells able to

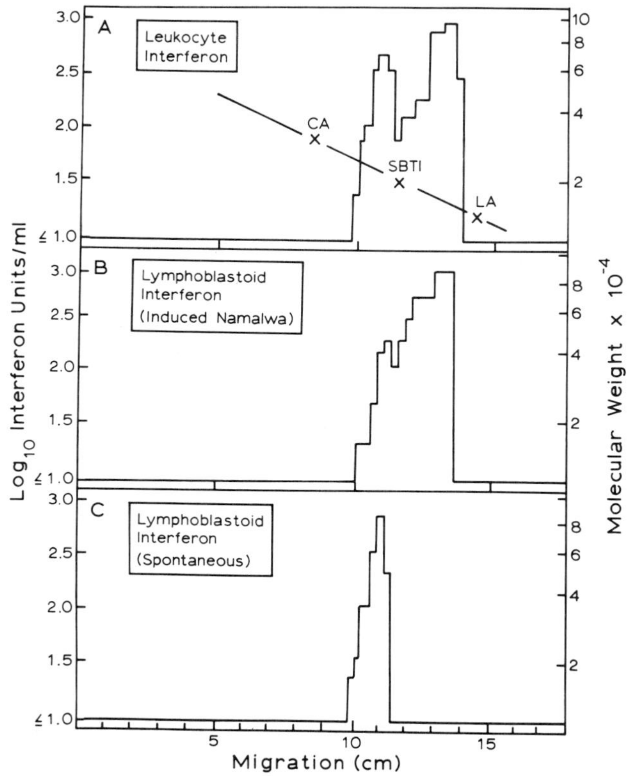

FIGURE 6. SDS-polyacrylamide gel electrophoresis of human lymphoid cell interferons. Gels were loaded with: A, Human leukocyte interferon; B, Human lymphoblastoid cell interferon induced in Namalva cells by Sendai virus; C, Spontaneously produced human lymphoblastoid cell interferon. Molecular weight markers: CA, carbonic anhydrase; SBTI, soy bean trypsin inhibitor; LA, α-lactalbumin.

spontaneously produce significant levels of human leukocyte-type interferon should make it possible for everyone who can grow cells to become involved in studies of the interferon system.

References

1. Hanley, D. F., M. Wiranowska-Stewart & W. E. Stewart II. 1979. Pharmacology of interferons. I. Pharmacologic distinctions between human leukocyte and fibroblast interferons. Int. J. Immunopharm. **1:** 219–226.
2. Stewart II, W. E. 1974. Distinct molecular species of interferons. Virology **61:** 80–86.
3. De Maeyer-Guignard, J., M. G. Tovey, I. Gresser & E. De Maeyer. 1978. Purification of mouse interferon by sequential affinity chromatography on poly(U)- and antibody-agarose columns. Nature **271:** 622–625.
4. Stewart II, W. E., T. Chudzio, L. S. Lin & M. Wiranowska-Stewart. 1978. Interferoids: *In vitro* and *in vivo* production of modified interferons. Proc. Nat. Acad. Sci. USA **75:** 4814–4818.

5. STEWART II, W. E., L. S. LIN & M. WIRANOWSKA-STEWART. 1978. Antiviral and other activities of pure interferons and interferoids. Proc. IVth Int. Cong. Virol. The Hague.
6. STEWART II, W. E. & J. DESMYTER. 1975. Molecular heterogeneity of human leukocyte interferon: Two populations differing in molecular weights, requirements for renaturation and cross-species antiviral activity. Virology **67:** 68–78.
7. STEWART II, W. E., L. S. LIN, M. WIRANOWSKA-STEWART & K. CANTELL. 1977. Elimination of size and charge heterogeneities of human leukocyte interferons by chemical cleavage. Proc. Nat. Acad. Sci. USA **74:** 4200–4204.
8. STEWART II, W. E., M. WIRANOWSKA-STEWART, V. KOISTINEN & K. CANTELL. 1979. Effects of glycosylation inhibitors of the production and properties of human leukocyte interferon. Virology **97:** 473–478.
9. DESMYTER, J., W. E. RAWLS & J. L. MELNICK. 1968. A human interferon that crosses the species line. Proc. Nat. Acad. Sci. USA **59:** 69–76.
10. GRESSER, I., M. T. BANDU, D. BROUTY-BOYE & M. TOVEY. 1974. Pronounced antiviral activity of human interferon on bovine and porcine cells. Nature **251:** 543–545.
11. DESMYTER, J. & W. E. STEWART II. 1976. Molecular modification of interferon: Attainment of human interferon in a conformation active on cat cells but inactive on human cells. Virology **70:** 451–458.
12. LIN, L. S., M. WIRANOWSKA-STEWART, T. CHUDZIO & W. E. STEWART II. 1978. Characterization of the heterogeneous molecules of human interferons: Differences in the cross-species antiviral activities of various molecular populations in human leukocyte interferons. J. Gen. Virol. **39:** 125–130.
13. BRAUDE, I. A., L. S. LIN & W. E. STEWART II. 1979. Differential inactivation and separation of homologous and heterologous antiviral activity of human leukocyte interferon by a proteolytic enzyme. Biochem. Biophys. Res. Commun. **89:** 612–619.
14. STEWART II, W. E., L. S. LIN & M. WIRANOWSKA-STEWART. 1979. Purification of interferons. Proc. 2nd International Workshop on Interferon. Rockefeller University Press. In press.
15. HAVELL, E. A., Y. K. YIP & J. VILČEK. 1978. Characteristics of human lymphoblastoid (Namalva) interferon. J. Gen. Virol **38:** 51–60.
16. CAVALIERI, R. L. , E. A. HAVELL, J. VILČEK & S. PESTKA. 1977. Synthesis of human interferon by *Xenopus laevis* oocytes: Two structural genes for interferons in human cells. Proc. Nat. Acad. Sci. USA **74:** 3287–3291.
17. STEWART II, W. E. 1979. The Interferon System. Springer-Verlag, Vienna, New York.
18. HAVELL, E. A. 1979. Isolation of a subspecies of murine interferon antigenically related to human leukocyte interferon. Virology **92:** 324–330.
19. STEWART II, W. E. & E. A. HAVELL. 1980. Characterization of a subspecies of mouse interferon cross-reactive on human cells and antigenically related to human leukocyte interferon. Virology **101:** 315–318.

HUMAN FIBROBLAST INTERFERON PURIFIED TO HOMOGENEITY BY A TWO-STEP PROCEDURE

J.W. Heine, M. De Ley, J. Van Damme,
A. Billiau, and P. De Somer

Rega Institute
University of Leuven
B-3000 Leuven, Belgium

Introduction

Although interferon of various animal species have been studied extensively for many years, pure interferons have only fairly recently been obtained.[2,3,6,10,12,17] The techniques that have been described have allowed the preparation of sufficient quantities of pure interferon to determine the specific activities (units/mg protein) of mouse interferon,[6,10,12] human fibroblast interferon,[2,11-13] and human leukocyte interferon.[12,17] Studies involving pure mouse interferon have also allowed assignment of some nonantiviral activities to the interferon molecules.[10]

Larger quantities of pure interferon are needed for elucidating its chemical structure. Also, for the determination of clinical potential of interferon the ultimate goal should be to perform trials with completely pure interferon rather than with semipurified preparations, which contain pharmacologically active substances, some of which may be responsible for the effect as well as the side-effects seen in current clinical trials.

One of the main difficulties to be overcome in achieving this goal is the great loss of interferon activity during multistep purification procedures described until now. In the present paper, we describe a two-step method for the purification of human fibroblast interferon (HF-IF) to a specific activity of 2×10^9 units/mg protein, with an over-all recovery of $> 50\%$ of the original crude activity.

Materials and Methods

Production and Purification

Human fibroblast interferon was produced by human diploid fibroblast cells from human embryos upon superinduction with poly-I:C as described earlier.[3,9] It was concentrated and partially purified by a method involving adsorption of the interferon on CPG beads at neutral pH and its desorption under acid conditions. The chromatographic procedure, originally described by Edy *et al.*,[8] was adapted into a batch procedure for processing large volumes.[3] This method was used as a first step in the complete purification of HF-IF, as outlined in Figure 1. The second step consisted of a modified and large-scale adaptation of the Zn^{++} chelate chromatographic purification method originally designed by Edy *et al.*[7] as a first step in the purification of crude HF-IF. The column was prepared by chelating zinc to iminodiacetate (Aldrich-Europe, Beerse, Belgium) immobilized on epoxy-activated Sepharose 6B (Pharmacia Fine Chemicals, Uppsala, Swe-

0077-8923/80/0350-0364 $01.75/0 © 1980, NYAS

I. Controlled pore glass (CPG) purification

Mix 1 volume of CPG beads with 30 volumes of crude HF-IF and stir for 2 hr.

↓

Wash 2x

1 Volume of CPG with 10 volumes of PBS.

↓

Wash 1x

1 Volume of CPG with 10 volumes of 0.01M glycine-HCl buffer, pH 3.5.

↓

Elute 2x

Stir 1 volume of CPG with 1 volume of 0.3M glycine-HCL buffer, pH 2.0, containing 0.09 mg/ml of plasma protein fraction, for 5 min.

↓

Elute 2x

Stir 1 volume of CPG with 1 volume of above buffer for 30 min.

↓

Dialyse

Pool eluates and dialyse aginst 0.02 PB, 1M NaCl, pH 7.4, to reduce 0.3M glycine concentration to 0.1 micromolar.

↓

II. Zn^{++} chelate chromatography

Apply sample at 15-20 ml/hr

Sample	Column
5-50 ml	0.9 x 8 cm (K9/15, Pharmacia)
100-400 ml	1.5 x 16 cm (K15/30, Fine Chemicals)

↓

Wash

With 1 1/2 bed volumes of 0.02M PB, 1M NaCl, pH 7.4.

↓

Wash

With 5 bed volumes of 0.1M sodium acetate, 1M NaCl, pH 5.9.

↓

Elute

Initially with 1 bed volume of 0.1M sodium acetate, 1M NaCl, pH 4.2, followed by 2 bed volumes of same buffer, pH 4.0.

Collect 1 ml fraction and determine pH.

Pool pH range 5.6 to 4.2 containing 98 % of purified HF-IF.

FIGURE 1. Purification procedure for human fibroblast interferon at 4°C.

den), as described by Porath *et al.*[16] HF-IF eluted from CPG was dialyzed extensively against 0.02M phosphate buffer (PB) at pH 7.4 containing 1M sodium chloride (NaCl) prior to application to Zn^{++} chelate chromatography (FIGURE 1). All buffers used in this purification procedure were made up with pyrogen-free water, containing 1M NaCl and is indicated by buffer-NaCl to prevent nonspecific binding of proteins with the zinc and were sterilized by filtration.

After sample application, the column was washed with PB-NaCl to remove the remaining unbound proteins. This was followed by a wash with 0.1M sodium acetate-NaCl (pH 5.9) which removed other contaminating proteins. Occasionally a small fraction (<10%) of the HF-IF was also removed with this treatment.

For large scale purification the interferon was then eluted with 0.1M sodium acetate-NaCl (pH 4.2), while for experimental purpose a pH 6–4 gradient of the same buffer was employed. With this final elution 1 ml fractions were collected and 98% of the HF-IF eluting from the column was contained in the fractions having a pH from 5.6–4.2. From each fraction 0.1 ml was removed for protein determination by the fluorometric method.[4] Then, 0.1 ml of 4.5% human plasma protein fraction (HPPF, Belgian Red Cross National Blood Transfusion Service) was added for stabilization of the IF during handling and storage.

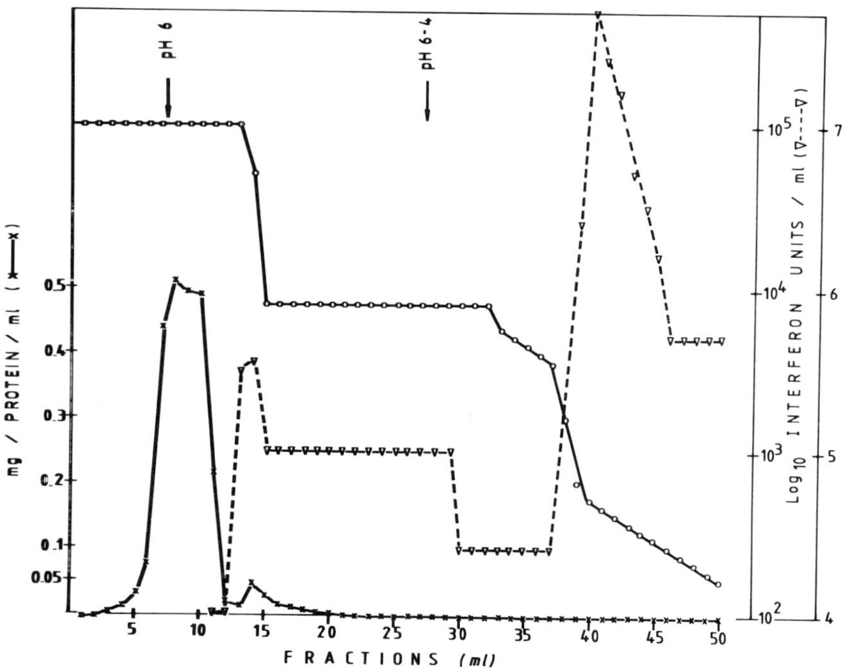

FIGURE 2. Chromatography of human fibroblast interferon on Zn^{++} chelate-agarose. Five ml of CPG-purified HF-IF with a titer of 10^5 reference units/ml were dialyzed against PB-NaCl (pH 7.4) and applied to a 0.9 × 8 cm column (K 9/15, Pharmacia Fine Chemicals) at 4°C (15–20 ml/hr). The column was washed with 0.1M sodium acetate-NaCl (pH 6, 25 ml) followed by the pH gradient. The gradient was developed by mixing 20 ml of each 0.1M sodium acetate-NaCl at pH 6 and pH 4.

TABLE 1

LARGE SCALE PURIFICATION OF HUMAN FIBROBLAST INTERFERON IN TWO STEPS: BY CPG AND Zn^{++} CHELATE CHROMATOGRAPHY

Designation	Volume (ml)	Total Protein (mg)	Total Activity (units)	Specific Activity (units/mg)
CPG Purification				
Crude	3200	1075.2	6.4×10^7	5.9×10^4
Unadsorbed	3200	—	—	—
Wash	1500	—	—	—
Eluate I	140	124.6	3.68×10^7	2.96×10^5
Eluate II	140			
Recovery			57.5%	
Zinc Chelate Purification				
Dialyzed fraction of eluate pool	100	44.46	1.32×10^7	2.96×10^5
Void + pH 7.4 wash	130	42.51	<200	—
pH 5.9 wash	150	1.60	0.76×10^6	0.47×10^6
Purified HF-IF	6	~0.007	12.02×10^6	$\sim 1.7 \times 10^9$
Recovery			91.4%	
Overall Recovery			52.6%	

The column was regenerated by the following procedure. First, it was stripped by washing with five bed volumes of 0.05M ethylenediaminetetraacetic acid (EDTA) in PB-NaCl (pH 7.4). The EDTA was removed by washing with an equal volume of PB-NaCl (pH 7.4). The column was then equilibrated with 0.1M sodium acetate-NaCl (pH 4.0). Zinc was then reintroduced by washing with 0.1M sodium acetate-NaCl (pH 4.0) containing 1 mM zinc chloride ($ZnCl_2$). The saturation point was determined by the formation of a precipitate when a drop of the column eluate was mixed with a test quantity of sodium carbonate solution. The excess zinc was removed by washing with five bed volumes of the pH 4.0 acetate-NaCl buffer. Then the column was equilibrated to pH 7.4 for sample application by washing with five bed volumes of PB-NaCl buffer. All washings as well as sample application were done by gravity flow with an operating pressure of 60 cm, resulting in a flow rate of about 15–20 ml/hr.

Radiolabeling

For the ^{125}I-iodination of interferon the procedure of Knight,[11] employing the ^{125}I-Bolton-Hunter reagent (New England Nuclear Chemicals GmbH, Dreieichenhain, W. Germany) was used. An aliquot (33 λ) taken from the pooled pH (5.6–4.2) range immediately after elution from the Zn^{++} chelate column and prior to addition of a stabilizing agent was mixed in a microtest tube (1.5 ml, Eppendorf 3810 Hamburg, W. Germany) with 20 λ of 0.2M sodium borate resulting in a final pH of 8.5. This mixture was transferred to a microtest tube in which 30 λ of the ^{125}I-Bolton-Hunter reagent (2000 Ci/mmole) had been evaporated to dryness. This mixture was incubated at RT for 30 min, whereupon 0.3 ml of 0.2M glycine was added. After incubation of 10 min, 0.2 ml of phosphate-buffered saline (PBS) containing 0.05% sodium dodecyl sulfate (SDS) and 100 μg/ml of HPPF or ovalbumin (OVA) (Serva GmbH & Co., Heidelberg, W. Germany) was added. The sample was then processed as described by Knight.[11]

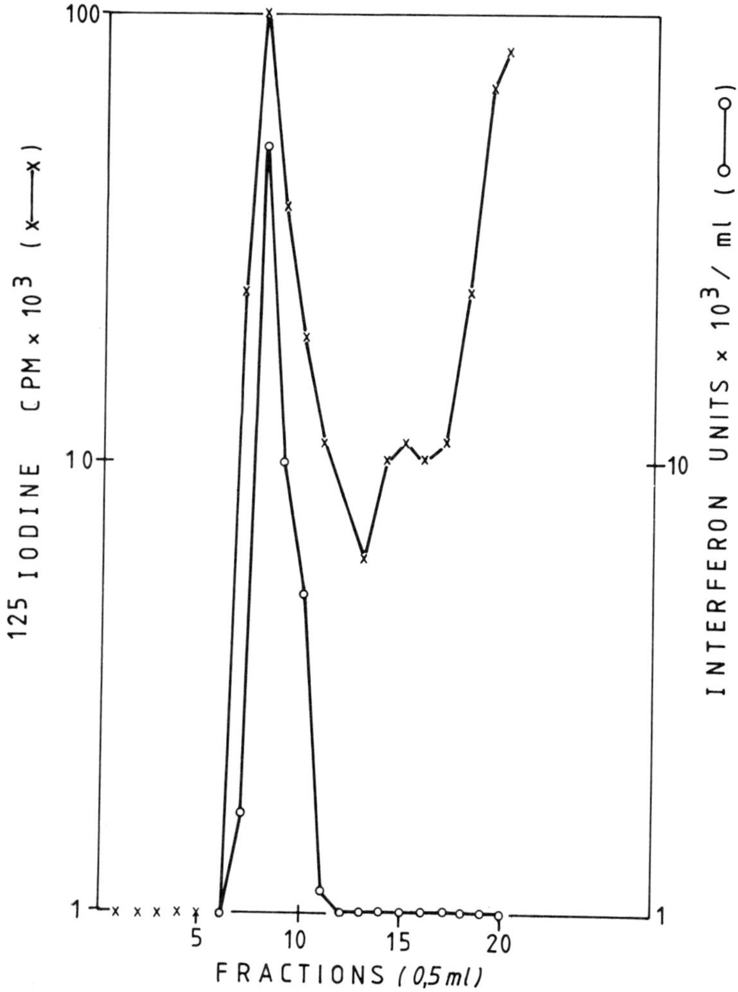

FIGURE 3. Gel filtration of ^{125}I-iodinated CPG-Zn^{++} chelated purified human fibroblast interferon employing Biogel P-30 (100–200 mesh, 0.8 × 20 cm) column which was equilibrated with PBS containing 0.05% SDS and 100 μg/ml of HPPF. The ^{125}I-interferon reaction mixture (0.5 ml) was loaded onto the column, fractions (0.5 ml) were collected at a flow rate of 12 ml/hr at 25°C. This procedure is essentially that of Knight.[11] The gel filtration of ^{125}I-interferon stabilized with OVA was indistinguishable from the above and thus is not presented.

For *in vivo* labeling of HF-IF, one roller bottle containing a monolayer of 50 × 10^6 primed fibroblast cells were induced in Eagle's minimum essential medium (EMEM) containing 0.75% of normal concentration of amino acids and at time of addition of media with HPPF (for details of priming and induction schedule, see ref. 3), 250 μCi of ^{14}C-protein hydrolysate (CFB 25, Amersham Radiochemicals, Buckinghamshire, England) in 30 ml of above medium containing 0.09 mg/ml of HPPF was added. The supernatant was harvested 20–24 hr later, centrifuged at

1000 × g for 15 min and purified by CPG-Zn^{++} chelate chromatography (FIGURE 1).

After purification, the HF-IF fraction was placed in dialyse tubing and concentrated by submersion in viscous PBS-ficol solution, upon concentration to about 50 λ, the sample was dialyzed against PBS to lower the salt concentration and then analyzed by discontinuous SDS-PAGE[14] employing a 8–24% polyacrylamide gel cross-linked with *N-N'*-diallyltartardiamide (DATD)[1] and a 3% stacking gel.[5] The gels were prepared for fluorography and exposed to x-ray films (Curix RP_2, Agfa Gevaert, Mortsel, Belgium) at −70°C.[5]

RESULTS

In an attempt to determine the possible use of Zn^{++} chelate chromatography in conjunction with CPG chromatography for the purification of HF-IF to a greater purity, 5–10 ml of CPG-purified material was chromatographed. FIGURE 2, illustrates a typical elution profile with 95% of the protein being recovered in the combined void and pH 6 wash and >90% of the HF-IF starting to elute at pH 5.2

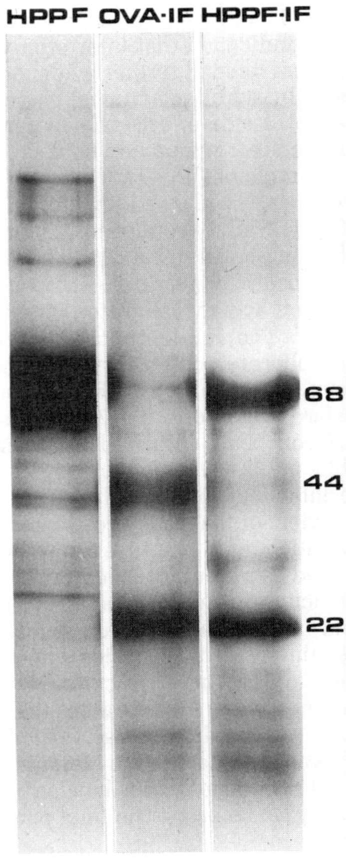

FIGURE 4. Autoradiogram of SDS-PAGE of ^{125}I-HPPF and ^{125}I-interferon stabilized after iodination neutralization reaction with HPPF (main component human serum albumin – 68,000 daltons) or OVA (main component – 44,000 daltons). Daltons × 10^3.

TABLE 2

Zn^{++} CHELATE CHROMATOGRAPHY OF CPG-PURIFIED *IN VIVO* ^{14}C-AMINO ACID-LABELED HF-IF

	Total ^{14}C		Total Protein		Total Activity	
Fractions	cpm	%	mg	%	units	%
Eluate of CPG (dialyzed)	765,320	100	0.406	100	0.3×10^6	100
Void + pH 7.4 wash	672,540	87.87	0.345	84.97	<200	
pH 5.9 wash	49,500	6.47	0.033	8.13	<200	
Pooled eluate	2,080	0.27	Not detectable		0.28×10^6	93.3
Total recovery		94.6		93.1		93.3

with completion of elution at pH 4.2. A small percentage of interferon together with a small fraction of protein eluted at pH 6. As no protein was detectable under the HF-IF peak, the Zn^{++} chelate chromatography was scaled up. In TABLE 1 the results of the combined large scale purification of CPG and Zn^{++} chelate are presented. The purification yielded a product purified with a specific activity of 1.5 to 3.1×10^9 reference units/mg, averaging at 2×10^9 reference units/mg protein. The over-all recovery was 50% of the original crude activity.

The indication that interferon was purified to homogeneity by this two-step procedure needed further evidence and this was sought by radiolabeling experiments. In addition, clinical experiments were initiated to demonstrate the absence of side-effects known for CPG-purified material. These data will be presented in a companion note.

A sample of CPG-Zn^{++} chelate purified HF-IF was ^{125}I-iodinated and subsequently stabilized by addition of HPPF. It was then chromatographed on a Biogel P-30 (Bio-Rad Laboratories, Richmond, CA, USA) column; this gel filtration profile is shown in FIGURE 3. The interferon activity eluted with the first ^{125}I-radioactivity peak. ^{125}I-Radioactivity eluting in a second broad peak had no interferon activity associated with it. These data are in agreement with those of Knight.[11] The HF-IF-containing fractions (7, 8, 9, and 10) were individually electrophoresed on an acrylamide gel slab to verify homogeneity of the labeled protein. ^{125}I-Labeled HPPF was also chromatographed for comparison. All four interferon fractions delivered similar profiles. As shown in FIGURE 4, the interferon band, localized by determination of biological activity, was clearly visible at 22,000 daltons. However, in addition, a number of bands were detectable that corresponded to the major components of radio-iodinated HPPF.

In view of the small protein content of the iodinated interferon fraction prior to addition of a stabilizer, it seemed likely that the extensive labeling had occurred as a result of label transfer to the stabilizer added after the radiolabeling reaction was completed and neutralized. If this is so, this type of experiment would not be suitable for detecting small amounts of proteins present as contaminants of the purified interferon. That extensive label transfer to added protein did occur after completion of the reaction was demonstrated in an experiment where OVA rather than HPPF was used as stabilizer. It can be seen in FIGURE 4 that, in this case, OVA components become labeled.

It was then decided to attempt an *in vivo* labeling of HF-IF with ^{14}C-amino acids. In order to obtain labeled interferon, a large dose of radioactive amino acids had to be used. The final pooled purified product contained only 0.04% of the labeled protein present in the original crude interferon or 0.3% of that present in the CPG-purified preparation. TABLE 2 shows the recoveries of the protein radioactivity and biological activity from the Zn^{++} chelate chromatography, which are all better than 90 percent. In FIGURE 5, the purity of the interferon preparation is demonstrated by the presence of only one band with a molecular weight of 22,000.

DISCUSSION

A two-step procedure for the purification of HF-IF to homogeneity is described. Earlier reports showed the independent purification capacity of CPG and Zn^{++} chelate chromatography.[2,7,8,18] Initial studies on the purification of HF-IF by the combination of the CPG and Zn^{++} chelate methods showed that it was an advantage to follow the CPG by the Zn^{++} chelate method, rather than the reverse. Further, if lyophilized CPG-purified material was utilized for purification on Zn^{++} chelate columns, a large amount of protein was found to co-purify with the interferon. This was also observed in combinations with other purifica-

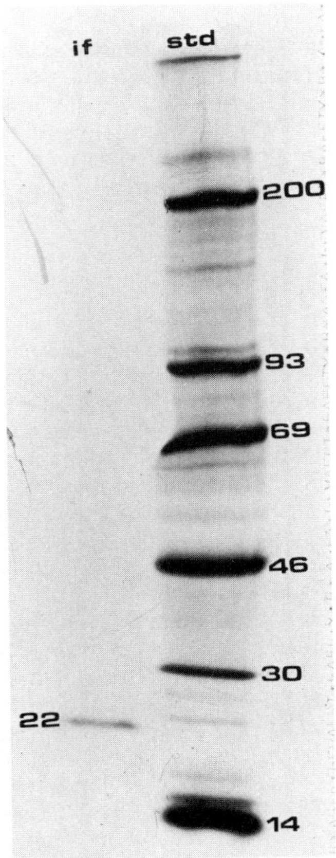

FIGURE 5. Autoradiogram of SDS-PAGE of *in vivo* ^{14}C-amino acid-labeled HF-IF purified by CPG-Zn^{++} chelate chromatography. A ^{14}C-labeled molecular weight mixture (14,000–200,000 daltons, Amersham Radiochemicals, Buckinghamshire, England) was co-electrophorized for molecular weight determination. Daltons $\times 10^3$.

tion procedures (unpublished observations). However, when the HF-IF was employed as a fresh eluate from the CPG beads, no protein could be detected with the sensitive fluorometric protein assay. Upon purification of larger quantities of HF-IF by the combined CPG-Zn^{++} chelate method, an average specific activity in the end-products of 2×10^9 reference units/mg protein was observed. This value is in agreement with the theoretical estimation of Ng *et al.*[15] and is slightly higher than that reported by Berthold *et al.*[2] and Knight.[13] In view of the low recoveries found by these workers,[2,13] it is possible that the specific activity was lower because of the presence of inactivated interferon. Furthermore, our value reported here is more realistic in view of the specific activity of $10^{8.3}$ units/mg of partially purified material reported by Edy *et al.*[7]

Radio-iodination of the purified interferon allowed to demonstrate the presence of a major radiolabeled protein of 22,000 daltons corresponding to the biological activity. By using different proteins (HPPF and OVA) as stabilizers, it was found that extensive transfer of label to stabilizers occurred after completion and neutralization of the radio-iodination reaction. Therefore, the complete purity of the interferon preparation prior to addition of stabilizer could not be demonstrated with this technique. However, the purity of the interferon was clearly demonstrated by the presence of only one band (at 22,000 daltons) in the autoradiogram prepared from the purified interferon labeled *in vivo* with ^{14}C-amino acids.

The purification method described here has several advantages over those available until now. Firstly, the method is simple in that it involves only two steps, one of which is a batch procedure. Secondly, it is inexpensive in that the reagents can be regenerated indefinitely, and thirdly, the method yields a homogeneous end-product with an average recovery of over 50% of the original biological activity.

Summary

Human fibroblast interferon, produced by superinduction of diploid skin fibroblasts, was concentrated and partially purified by adsorption to controlled pore glass (CPG) beads. Further purification to a specific activity of $\sim 10^9$ units/mg, was achieved by zinc chelate affinity chromatography. The over-all recovery of this two-step procedure was ~50 percent. Complete homogeneity of the final preparation was demonstrated by radiolabeling followed by gel electrophoresis and autoradiography.

Acknowledgments

This investigation was supported by a grant from the Cancer Research Foundation of the Belgian General Savings and Retirement Fund (A.S.L.K.C.G.E.R.). The production of interferon was made possible by a research contract (No. 76/81-10) obtained from the "Geconcerteerde Onderzoeksacties." The work has profited from the experience gained by the senior author (J.W.H.) in the laboratories of Dr. E. Sulkowski (Roswell Park Memorial Institute, Buffalo, New York, USA). The technical assistance of Francine Cornette, Chris Neuckermans-Dillen, Isabelle Claes-Ronsse, R. Conings, W. Put, and J.P. Lenaerts is acknowledged. The authors thank Jane Putzeys for excellent editorial help.

References

1. Anker, H.S. 1970. A solubilizable acrylamide gel for electrophoresis. FEBS Letters **7:** 293.
2. Berthold, W., C. Tan & Y.H. Tan. 1978. Purification and *in vitro* labeling of interferon from human fibroblastoid cell lines. J. Biol. Chem. **253:** 5206–5212.
3. Billiau, A., J. Van Damme, F. Van Leuven, V.G. Edy, M. De Ley, J.J. Cassiman, H. Van den Berghe & P. De Somer. 1979. Human fibroblast interferon for clinical trials: Production, partial purification and characterization. Antimicrob. Agents Chemother. **16:** 49–55.
4. Böhlen, P., J. Stein, W. Dairman & S. Udenfriend. 1973. Fluorometric assay of proteins in the nanogram range. Arch. Biochem. Biophys. **155:** 213–220.
5. De Ley, M., A. Billiau & P. De Somer. 1979. Interferon-induced synthesis of a 63, 000 dalton protein in mouse cells. Biochem. Biophys. Res. Commun. **89:** 701–705.
6. De Maeyer-Guignard, J., M.G. Tovey, I. Gresser & E. De Maeyer. 1978. Purification of mouse interferon by sequential affinity chromatography on poly(U)- and antibody-agarose columns. Nature **271:** 622–625.
7. Edy, V.G., A. Billiau & P. De Somer. 1977. Purification of human fibroblast interferon by zinc chelate affinity chromatography. J. Biol. Chem. **252:** 5934–5935.
8. Edy, V.G., I.A. Braude, E. De Clercq, A. Billiau & P. De Somer. 1976. Purification of interferon by adsorption chromatography on controlled pore glass. J. Gen. Virol. **33:** 517–521.
9. Havell, E.A. & J. Vilček. 1972. Production of high titered interferon in cultures of human diploid cells. Antimicrob. Agents Chemother. **2:** 476–484.
10. Iwahura, Y., S. Yonehara & Y. Kawade. 1978. Purification of mouse L cell interferon. J. Biol. Chem. **253:** 5074–5079.
11. Knight, E. Jr. 1978. Preparation of ^{125}iodine-labelled human fibroblast interferon. J. Gen. Virol. **40:** 681–684.
12. Knight, E., Jr. 1978. Purification of interferons. Pharmacol. Therap. A **2:** 439–446.
13. Knight, E., Jr. 1976. Interferon: Purification characterization from human diploid cells. Proc. Nat. Acad. Sci. USA **73:** 520–523.
14. Laemli, U.K. 1970. Cleavage of structural proteins during the assembly of the head of bacteriophage T4. Nature **227:** 680–684.
15. Ng, M.H. & J. Vilček, 1972. Interferon: Physicochemical properties and control of cellular synthesis. Adv. Protein Chem. **26:** 179–241.
16. Porath, J., J. Carlsson, I. Olsson & G. Belfson. 1975. Metal chelate affinity chromatography, a new approach to protein fractionation. Nature **258:** 598–599.
17. Rubinstein, M., S. Rubinstein, P.G. Familletti, R.S. Miller, A.A. Waldman & S. Pestka. 1979. Human leukocyte interferon: Production, purification to homogeneity, and initial characterization. Proc. Nat. Acad. Sci. USA **76:** 640–644.
18. Sulkowski, E. 1978. Personal communication.

TOLERABILITY OF PURE FIBROBLAST INTERFERON IN MAN

A. Billiau, J. W. Heine, J. Van Damme,
H. Heremans, and P. De Somer

Rega Institute
University of Leuven
B-3000 Leuven, Belgium

Partially purified human fibroblast interferon (IF) has been shown to evoke a febrile response after intramuscular injection in man.[1] Also, intracutaneous injection of partially pure fibroblast IF elicits inflammatory skin reactions.[1,2] Until recently it was impossible to determine to what extent these effects were due to biological activity of the IF molecule itself rather than to the impurities present. We here describe results obtained with fibroblast IF purified to homogeneity by the method described in the accompanying paper.[4]

Skin reactivity towards partially and completely pure IF was tested by injecting 100,000 units/0.1 ml intracutaneously on the ventral side of the fore-arm of patients or volunteers.

A first type of reaction occurred only in patients who had already received several intramuscular doses of partially pure interferon; it consisted of a wheel and flare reaction appearing within minutes after intracutaneous challenge with partially pure interferon. Most probably it represented an atopic (type I) reaction to calf serum components which were present in the IF preparations used for intramuscular as well as intracutaneous injections.[1-3] When such sensitized patients were given an intracutaneous challenge with 100,000 units/0.1 ml of completely pure IF, no immediate type reaction did occur, indicating that all immunogenic material had been removed by the purification procedure.

A second type of skin reaction occurred in all patients or volunteers at about 6 to 16 hr after intracutaneous injection of partially pure interferon. It consisted of an infiltration with mononuclear cells resembling a delayed type (type II) allergic response. With completely pure IF preparations no such reactions were seen; instead, the skin reactivity was recovered in the void volume of the second purification step (Zn^{++} chelate chromatography).

The pyrogenicity of partially and completely pure interferons was tested by measuring body temperature in rabbits injected intravenously or in patients injected intramuscularly or intraveneously. The results of these tests are shown in TABLE 1. As described in a previous paper[1] fibroblast IF purified only by controlled pore glass (CPG) absorption contained variable but small amounts of material that activated the Limulus amoebocyte lysate (LAL) test. In contrast, the IF that underwent additional purification by Zn^{++} chelate chromatography was always LAL-negative. In rabbits, injected intravenously, partially pure IF was either not or marginally pyrogenic. The pure IF, in contrast, was always devoid of any pyrogenic activity in rabbits. Purification by the Zn^{++} chelate chromatography eliminated the pyrogenicity seen in man after intramuscular injection. Unexpectedly, however, completely pure interferon, when injected by intravenous infusion, still evoked a distinct febrile response in man. Thus we have until now been able to separate all pyrogenic activity from the fibroblast interferon molecules, indicating that this molecule may be a pyrogen itself.

TABLE 1

PYROGENICITY OF FIBROBLAST INTERFERON

	Dose		Purification Method (Specific Activity)		
	U/kg	U/kg/hr	CPG (10^6 U/mg)	Zn-chelate (10^8 U/mg)	CPG + Zn (>10^9 U/mg)
Limulus Assay			pos/neg (<50 ng/30,000 U)		neg (10^6 U/ml)
Pyrogenicity					
rabbits, i.v.	30,000		0.05–0.55*		
	200,000		0.63		0.02
man, i.m.	40,000		1.2	0.4	
	160,000		1.8		
	111,000		0.6	−0.1	
	350,000		1.2		
	50,000		1.0		0.0
man, i.v.		20,000	3.2		
		4,000			2.0
		10,000			1.8

*Temperature rise (Δ°C).

ACKNOWLEDGMENTS

The authors thank their colleagues Prof. Dr. R. Verwilghen and Prof. Dr. J. Vossen for collaboration received.

REFERENCES

1. BILLIAU, A., P. DE SOMER, V. G. EDY, E. DE CLERCQ & H. HEREMANS. 1979. Human fibroblast interferon for clinical trials: Pharmacokinetics and tolerability in experimental animals and humans. Antimicrob. Agents Chemother. **16:** 56–63.
2. DE SOMER, P., V. G. EDY & A. BILLIAU. 1977. Interferon-induced skin reactivity in man. Lancet **2:** 47–48.
3. BILLIAU, A., J. VAN DAMME, F. VAN LEUVEN, V. G. EDY, M. DE LEY, J. J. CASSIMAN, H. VAN DEN BERGHE & P. DE SOMER. 1979. Human fibroblast interferon for clinical trials: Production, partial purification and characterization. Antimicrob. Agents Chemother. **16:** 49–55.
4. HEINE, J. W., M. DE LEY, J. VAN DAMME, A. BILLIAU & P. DE SOMER. 1980. Human fibroblast interferon purified to homogeneity by a two-step procedure. Ann. N.Y. Acad. Sci. **350:** 364–373. This volume.

ISOLATION OF HUMAN FIBROBLASTOID INTERFERON FOR STRUCTURE AND FUNCTION ANALYSES

Y. H. Tan, H. Smith-Johannsen, and H. Okamura

Division of Medical Biochemistry, Faculty of Medicine
The University of Calgary
Calgary, Alberta T2N 1N4 Canada

W. Berthold

Tumor Biology
Karolinska Institute
Stockholm, Sweden

INTRODUCTION

Several biological activities have been attributed to interferon (IF) preparations. They include the well known antiviral, cell multiplication inhibitory, and immunoregulatory effects.[1-3] Recently IFs have also been shown to enhance the natural killer activity of lymphocytes.[4] What the underlying mechanism is for these pleiotropic effects poses an interesting question. A knowledge of the interferon molecule's structure and function relationship should shed some light on this problem. Toward this end we are working to isolate enough pure IF protein for such analyses, including amino acid sequence determination.

PURIFICATION OF HUMAN FIBROBLASTOID INTERFERON

Interferon was produced from cultures of human fibroblastoid cells and purified by two different procedures. Enough purified IF was produced by a conventional procedure to develop the second procedure, which utilized an immunosorbent column.[5,6] The purity of the IF isolated by the first procedure is indicated in FIGURE 1. Purified IF was then used to inoculate a rabbit. Neutralizing activity was observed in the serum of the rabbit after 3 months of weekly interferon (1–2 μg) inoculations. This neutralizing activity was extremely specific for human fibroblastoid IF, indicating some differences in the antigenic sites on the different types of human IF as well as on mouse IF (TABLE 1).

The rabbit antiserum was cross-linked to activated Sepharose and the resulting immunosorbent column tested in the purification of human fibroblastoid interferon. Before this step, however, crude IF was partially purified by chromatography on controlled-pore glass, as described previously,[6] and then on carboxymethyl cellulose (CM-cellulose). When such a preparation was applied at neutral pH to the immunosorbent column, IF activity was bound tightly. The 100 mM acetic acid elute contained most of the antiviral activity, but analysis revealed the presence of numerous other proteins besides interferon. The source of these contaminants is unlikely to be antibodies directed specifically against these proteins. Furthermore, experiments in which a column with bound IF was treated with mild detergent before acid elution indicated that the extraneous proteins are probably not bound to IF via hydrophobic interactions. On the other hand, there is some evidence to suggest that some of the non-IF proteins are

0077-8923/80/0350-0376 $01.75/0 © 1980, NYAS

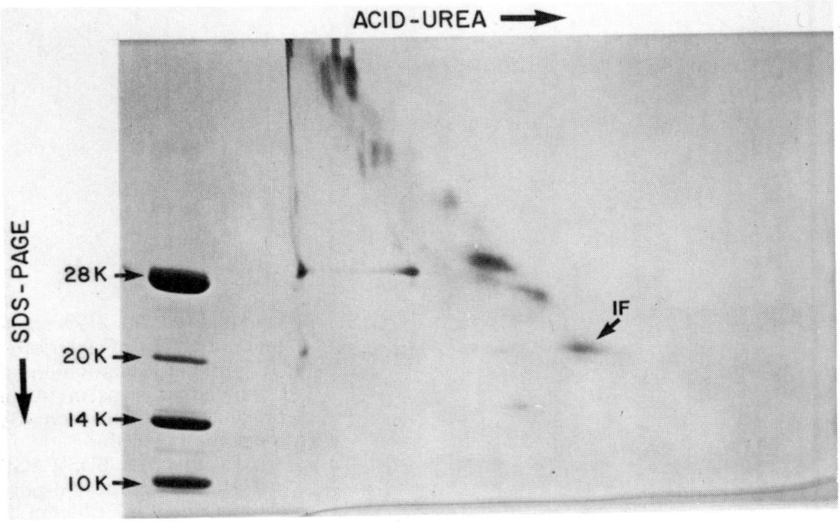

FIGURE 1. Two-dimensional gel electrophoresis of human fibroblastoid interferon. The arrow indicates interferon protein (IF) and molecular weight markers of 28,000, 20,000, 14,000 and 10,000 are given in the second dimensional gel.

immunoglobulins which "leak" from the column and others are proteins from the CM-cellulose-purified preparation which are bound nonspecifically to the column. To obtain pure IF, the immunosorbent column-purified material was subjected to sodium dodecyl sulfate-polyacrylamide gel electrophoresis (SDS-PAGE), and the region of the gel containing antiviral activity cut out and eluted. The products of the two purification procedures described here are compared in FIGURE 2. Both methods yield a single molecular weight species of about 20,000.

PURITY AND RECOVERY

The identity of the product of the first purification procedure as interferon and its purity by various criteria has already been established.[6] Moreover, the amino acid composition of this protein has been determined. Having this information at hand, we felt that the criteria for the purity of IF derived from the procedure utilizing the immunosorbent column were (1) the amino acid composi-

TABLE 1

SPECIFICITY OF NEUTRALIZATION OF ANTIVIRAL ACTIVITY BY RABBIT ANTISERUM

Type of Interferon	Neutralizing Activity (units/ml)
Human leukocyte interferon (partially pure)	0
Human fibroblastoid interferon (partially pure)	1.72×10^6
Mouse L cell interferon (crude)	0
Human fibroblastoid interferon (crude)	7.2×10^6

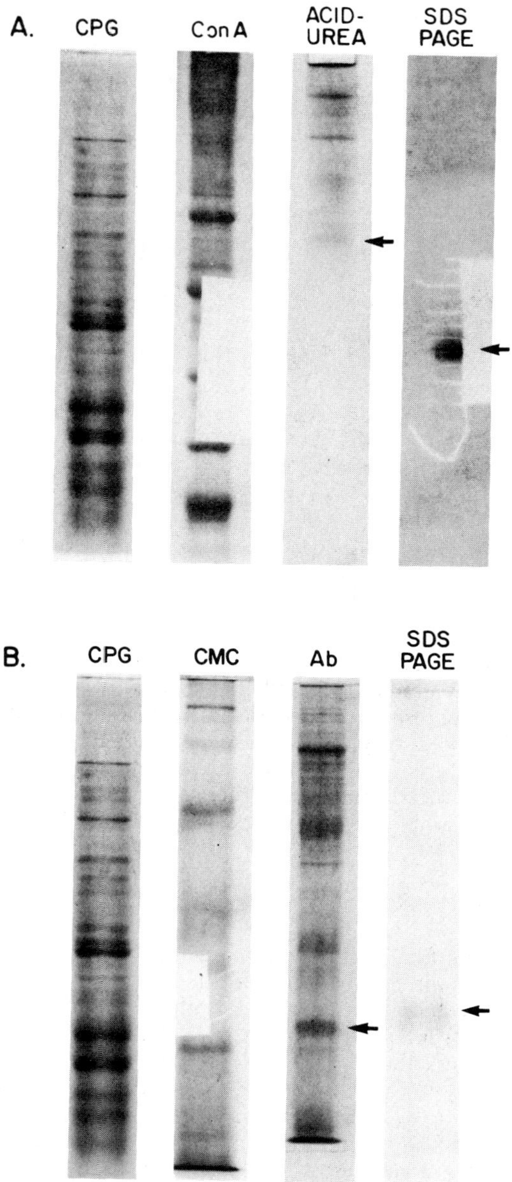

FIGURE 2. Gel electrophoretic analyses of interferon (IF) preparations obtained from various steps in (A), a previous procedure and (B), the present procedure.

(A) *Column 1:* SDS-PAGE analysis of controlled-pore glass-purified IF. *Column 2:* SDS-PAGE analysis of Con A-purified IF. *Column 3:* Acid-urea gel electrophoresis of Con A-purified IF. *Column 4:* SDS-PAGE analysis of the final purified product.

(B) *Column 1:* Same as column 1 in (A). *Column 2:* SDS-PAGE analysis of CM-cellulose-purified material. *Column 3:* SDS-PAGE analysis of immunosorbent-purified material. *Column 4:* SDS-PAGE analysis of the final purified product.

Arrows indicate IF protein.

tion and (2) the R_f of the stained protein in an acid-urea gel. This value was found to be 0.45 as previously reported for interferon.[6] Both analyses confirm the purity of the immunosorbent column-purified IF by these criteria.[8]

Although the first procedure allowed purification of interferon to homogeneity, the recovery was low, 50 nmols of crude IF yielding 0.25 to 1 nmol pure material. With the immunosorbent column, however, one can reproducibly obtain 5.0 to 7.5 nmols pure IF. Clearly, this represents a significant improvement in the efficiency of IF purification.

PROBLEMS

Once the immunosorbent column has been made, it can be used more than once, since the agarose matrix is relatively resistant to the conditions required for elution of the IF. Such a column has been used up to three times without reduction in the recovery of IF. However, it is possible that with increasing use the column may lose some of its efficiency through loss or modification of the bound immunoglobulins.

Since pure interferon is isolated from the immunosorbent column-purified preparation by SDS-PAGE, it is subject to contamination by acrylamide. Therefore, in order to remove acrylamide, IF eluted from the polyacrylamide gel was first centrifuged at high speed and then dialyzed extensively.

PHYSIOCHEMICAL PROPERTIES OF FIBROBLASTOID IINTERFERON

Detergents, especially SDS, have been widely used in an effort to stabilize IF activity. However, depending on the conditions, detergent treatment of IF can result in either stabilization, partial inactivation or severe loss of its biological activity. This appears to be related to a number of factors including the kind and concentration of detergent used, the detergent:protein ratio and the purity of the IF (TABLE 2). Paradoxically, lower concentrations of detergent inactivate all partially purified IF preparations to a greater degree than do higher concentrations, which either partially inactivate or stabilize biological activity. At these higher concentrations, detergent molecules are known to aggregate into micelles. It is conceivable that these micelles may be responsible for the stabilization of biological activity, but the exact mechanism is not yet known. Thus, in view of the complexity of detergent and protein interactions, it is not surprising that conflicting results have been reported concerning the stabilizing effect of detergent on IF activity. For example, we have observed that SDS at all concentrations, in the presence or absence of urea and reducing agents, can inactivate purified IF from 50 to 99 percent. Consequently, the notion that SDS treatment stabilizes IF activity is not a universally accepted phenomenon and certainly requires critical reevaluation.

Crude IF preparations from fibroblastoid cells are labile in neutral and alkaline pH. However, on partial purification IF becomes more stable at these pH values. This suggests that the lability could reflect the presence of some endogenous enzymes. However, at all levels of purity, IF activity is susceptible to both reducing and strong oxidative conditions. This has been attributed to the presence of tyrosyl residues as well as disulfide bridges, which are involved in maintaining the active conformation.[6,7] Although a small amount of methionyl residue is present, cyanogen bromide treatment does not generate detectable peptide fragments suggesting the methionyl residue(s) are at the end(s) of the polypeptide. It is also possible that the polypeptide must be extensively unfolded in order to expose the otherwise inaccessible methionyl residue(s).

TABLE 2

EFFECTS OF DETERGENT ON HUMAN FIBROBLASTOID INTERFERON PREPARATIONS OF DIFFERENT PURITY*

Detergent and Concentration (%)	Purity (specific activity in units/mg protein)	% Loss of Activity
IONIC		
Sodium dodecyl sulfate		
1	1×10^5	0, 80
1	1×10^8	0, 72
0.001	1×10^5	0, 40
0.001	1×10^8	99, 98
Dodecylamine		
0.1	1×10^8	35, 0
0.01	1×10^8	65, 40
Decyltrimethyl ammonium bromide		
0.1	1×10^8	35, 0
0.01	1×10^8	65, 65
Octylamine		
0.1	1×10^8	35, 0
0.01	1×10^8	65, 80
Decylsulfate		
0.1	1×10^8	35, 0
0.01	1×10^8	65, 94
Octylsulfate		
0.1	1×10^8	55, 90
0.01	1×10^8	65, 90
NONIONIC		
Triton X-100		
0.1	1×10^8	0, 0
0.001	1×10^8	65, 66
Tween 20		
0.001	1×10^8	50, 0
0.1	1×10^8	65, 0

*All experiments were performed in 10 mM acetic acid.

INTERFERON PEPTIDE FRAGMENTS

Many attempts have been made to chemically and enzymatically degrade the IF peptide to obtain an active fragment. However, a fragment possessing biological activity has not yet been found. One might expect some difficulties in obtaining such a fragment, since the induction of the antiviral state by IF involves at least two different events. First, IF must bind to the cell surface and then it initiates the cascade of biochemical reactions culminating in the antiviral state. The failure to include either one of the sites responsible for the binding or catalytic activity in the interferon fragment could result in a biologically inert peptide. The probability of a polypeptide considerably smaller than the intact molecule, yet possessing both binding and catalytic sites, is correspondingly limited. Nevertheless, the desirability of an active fragment of IF with its considerable therapeutic potential and its amenability to chemical synthesis explains the continued interest in this area.

Regardless of their biological activity, peptide fragments of IF are useful for determining the protein's complete amino acid sequence. For this purpose, ^{125}I-labeled pure IF was used to establish optimal conditions for the production and recovery of peptide fragments. Preliminary experiments involving a series of enzymatic treatments indicate that tryptic digestion of IF produces a peptide of about 10,000 molecular weight (FIGURE 3). Such a radioactive fragment can serve as a marker for the identification and recovery of unlabeled peptides produced when nanomoles of pure IF are subjected to tryptic digestion.

CHEMICAL CLEAVAGE BY CYANOGEN BROMIDE

Human fibroblastoid IF was purified to homogeneity as described above and radiolabeled under reducing conditions. When the pure material was exposed to 25 mg/ml CNBr under different conditions, a number of fragments were reproducibly generated. Maximal cleavage resulted in roughly 50% of the IF being converted to lower molecular weight material. The effect of increasing concentrations of acid on the pattern of fragmentation is shown in FIGURE 4. In "weaker acid" conditions (75–88% formic acid, 1:1 formic acid and HFBA,

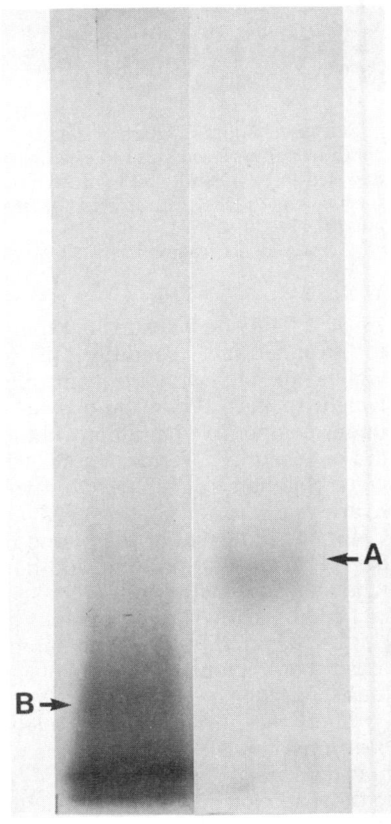

FIGURE 3. Autoradiography of SDS-PAGE analyzed ^{125}I-labeled interferon (A), and the 10,000 MW interferon fragment (B) derived from a tryptic digest.

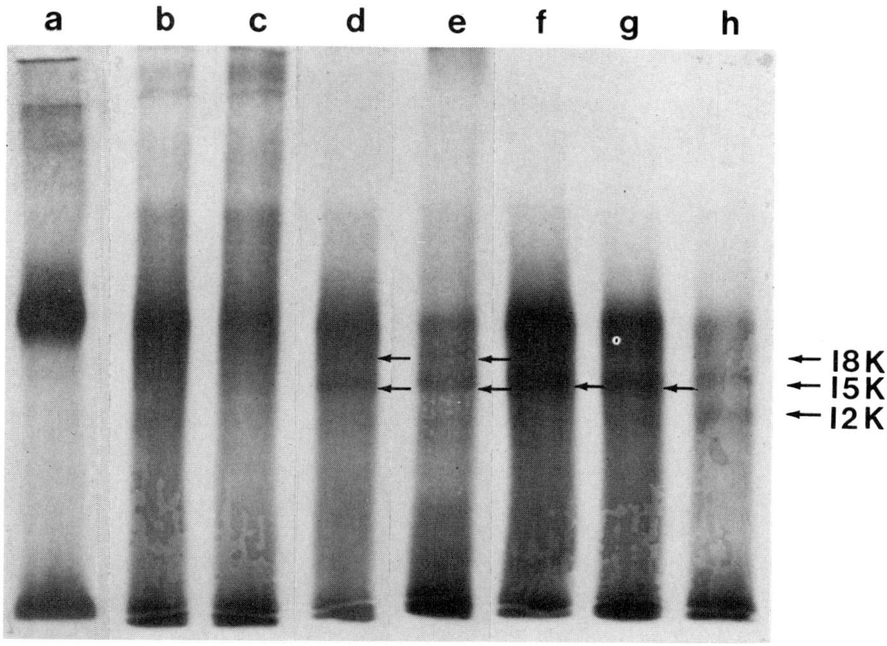

FIGURE 4. Autoradiogram of human fibroblastoid IF cleaved by CNBr under various acid conditions. Interferon was radio-iodinated, treated to reduce and block disulfide bonds, and exposed to 25 mg/ml CNBr for 24 h at 20°C in (a) no acid; (b) 75% formic acid; (c) 80% formic acid; (d) 88% formic acid; (e) 1:1 88% formic acid:HFBA; (f) 75% TFA; (g) 80% TFA; and (h) 85% TFA.

Arrows locate fragments of 18,000, 15,000 or 12,000 molecular weight.

75–80% TFA), 18,000 and 15,000 molecular weight species were observed, while in "stronger acid" conditions (85% TFA) a third fragment of 12,000 molecular weight appears with the concomitant disappearance of the 18,000 molecular weight species. When the protein was exposed to these concentrations of acid under comparable conditions but in the absence of CNBr, a similar breakdown did not occur. Therefore, the 18,000, 15,000, and 12,000 molecular weight species were obtained from specific cleavage at methionine residues and not from acid hydrolysis of other peptide or glycosidic bonds. Increasing the concentration of CNBr to 125 mg/ml or the period of exposure of interferon to CNBr to 48 hr in 85% TFA did not produce additional fragments, although cleavage was somewhat more extensive under these conditions. Cleavage by CNBr was also carried out in 8 M urea. Three fragments of 18,000, 15,000 and 12,000 molecular weight can be liberated by CNBr treatment in the presence of this denaturant. In some experiments a fourth fragment of 8,000 molecular weight was also detected under these conditions.

Until recently, attempts to cleave human fibroblastoid IF with CNBr have been unsuccessful. The presence of at least three methionines in this protein is now confirmed[8]; thus, the previous lack of reactivity with CNBr can be attributed to the oxidation of methionyl residues in IF during purification. To avoid this, the isolation and labeling of IF were performed under reducing conditions and is now possible to obtain four fragments of 18,000, 15,000, 12,000 and 8,000 molecular weight using CNBr. The number and sizes of these fragments, the conditions required to produce them and partial sequence data[8] allow certain predictions to be made regarding the number and location of methionyl residues in human fibroblastoid IF. These predictions are summarized in FIGURE 5. To construct this model, we considered interferon to consist of about 150 amino acids. The model shows that there are four methionines in fibroblastoid IF, which is more than indicated by composition studies. The low methionine value from amino acid analysis is probably related to the lability of methionine. The location of one of the methionyl residues [i] is already known to be at the N-terminal.[8] The positions of two other methionines are calculated to be at or near amino acids 36 [iii] and 128 [ii] (see FIGURE 5). The location of the fourth methionyl residue is likely to be in the region of either amino acid 71 or amino acid 93. Thus, cleavage of IF by CNBr at site [ii] and [iii] would liberate fragments of approximately molecular weights of 18,000 and 15,000, respectively. If cleavage occurred at both sites in the same molecule, a 12,000 molecular weight species would be produced. If the residue at site [iv] were exposed to CNBr, an 8,000 molecular weight fragment would appear. Theoretically, scission at [ii] and [iii] should also release smaller fragments of 2,000 and 5,000 molecular weight from the C-terminal and N-terminal, respectively. Similarly, cleavage at site [iv] and [ii] should produce a 4,000 molecular weight species. However, such fragments were not observed

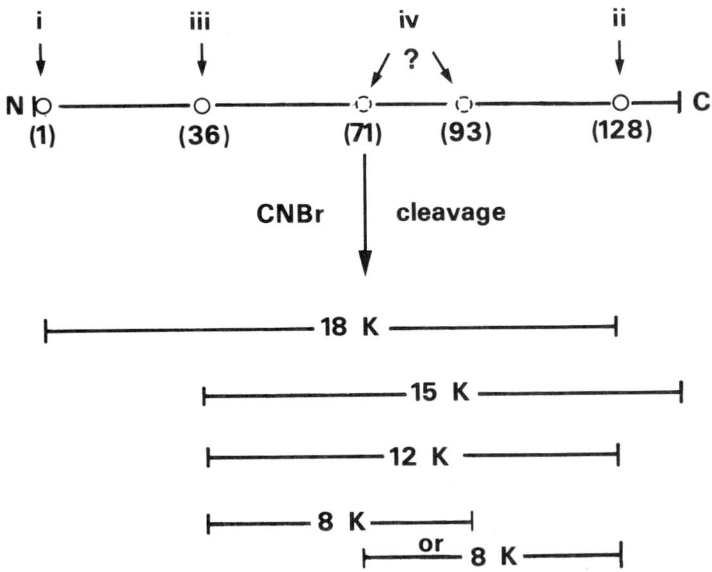

FIGURE 5. Location of methionine residues in human fibroblastoid IF. Methionyl residues are indicated by circles. Cleavage at sites [ii] and [iii] would produce fragments of 18,000 and 15,000 molecular weight, respectively. Cleavage at both sites in the same molecule would liberate a 12,000 molecular weight species. The position of methionine [iv] could be at either one of two sites, and cleavage would produce an 8,000 molecular weight fragment.

possibly because the 5,000 molecular weight species does not bear the radioactive label. These possibilities also apply to the smaller fragments, which in addition may have migrated too quickly to allow their resolution by SDS-PAGE.

One of the unanswered questions in this study is the location of disulfide bridge(s) with respect to the fragments produced by CNBr; namely, are some or all of the cleavage products held together by disulfide bonds?[5] The reducing conditions used in this study, however, do not permit the testing of IF with intact disulfides. Another concerns whether any of the CNBr-generated fragments contain biological activity. Unfortunately, the strong denaturing conditions required for rendering the IF susceptible to cleavage abolish biological activity.

SUMMARY

An efficient procedure for purifying interferon has enabled the preparation of nanomole amounts of pure interferon, permitting the partial amino acid sequence of this scarce protein to be determined. Also, experiments indicate the feasibility of preparing peptide fragments which would facilitate the complete analysis of interferon's primary structure.

REFERENCES

1. FINTER N. B. 1973. Interferons and Interferon Inducers. 2nd Edition. Elsevier Press. N.Y. 598 pp.
2. HO M. & J. A. ARMSTRONG. 1975. Ann. Rev. Microbiol. **29:** 131–161.
3. HUANG K. 1977. Tex. Rep. Biol. Med. **35:** 350–357.
4. SANTOLI D., G. TRINCHIERI & H. KOPROWSKI. 1978. J. Immunol. **121:** 532–538.
5. TAN Y. H., F. BARAKAT, W. BERTHOLD, H. SMITH-JOHANNSEN & C. TAN. 1979. J. Biol. Chem. **254:** 8067–8073.
6. BERTHOLD W., C. TAN & Y. H. TAN. 1978. J. Biol. Chem. **253:** 5206–5212.
7. BERTHOLD W., C. TAN & Y. H. TAN. 1978. Eur. J. Biochem. **253:** 5206–5212.
8. OKAMURA H., W. BERTHOLD, L. HOOD, M. HUNKAPILLER, M. INOUE, H. SMITH-JOHANNSEN & Y. H. TAN. 1980. Biochemistry. In press.

PURIFICATION, AMINO ACID COMPOSITION, AND N-TERMINAL AMINO ACID SEQUENCE OF HUMAN FIBROBLAST INTERFERON

Ernest Knight, Jr.

Central Research and Development Department
E. I. du Pont de Nemours & Co.,
Wilmington, Delaware 19898

Michael Hunkapiller

Division of Biology
California Institute of Technology
Pasadena, California 91125

The chemical characterization of interferons is necessary in order to understand its actions at the molecular level. Characterization has been slow since only microgram quantities have been available of any interferon. Interferons from human fibroblast cells,[1,2] human lymphoblastoid cells,[3] human leukocytes,[4] and mouse cells[5-8] have recently been purified to homogeneity and some limited structural information has been reported.[9,10] A major goal of the structural studies in interferons is the determination and comparison of amino acid sequences.

We report in this paper an improved procedure for the purification of human fibroblast interferon (HF-IF) that has been used to provide interferon for amino acid sequencing. Using an automated protein microsequencing technique previously described,[11,12] we have determined the sequence of the 13 amino acid residues at the N-terminus of the HF-IF prepared by this method. We also report an amino acid composition.

Human diploid fibroblast cells (FS-4) were cultured and HF-IF was produced as previously described.[1] Interferon was assayed by a microassay technique,[13] with vesicular stomatitis virus as the challenge virus. Interferon units are given in National Institutes of Health human fibroblast interferon units.

The crude HF-IF, 10–15 liters produced in the absence of serum, is made 1 M in NaCl and passed at room temperature through a column (4 × 10 cm) of Blue Sepharose (Pharmacia, Inc.) equilibrated with 0.02 sodium phosphate buffer, pH 7.2, containing 1 M NaCl. The HF-IF is retained while greater than 95% of the total protein passes through the column. The interferon is eluted with a 1:1 mixture of the column buffer and ethylene glycol, and each fraction is diluted immediately with 0.5 volume of the buffer (FIGURE 1a). Fractions containing interferon activity are pooled, diluted with two volumes of the column buffer, and passed through a small (1 × 6 cm) Blue Sepharose column for concentration. The interferon is eluted as described above (FIGURE 1b).

Fractions containing HF-IF are pooled, dialyzed against 1 mM Tris·HCl, pH 6.8, containing 0.02% sodium dodecyl sulfate (SDS, BioRad electrophoresis grade), and concentrated to dryness in a vacuum centrifuge. The HF-IF is then subjected to electrophoresis on a SDS-polyacrylamide slab gel and the HF-IF eluted as previously described[1] (FIGURE 2a). Fractions eluted from the gel are assayed for interferon activity (FIGURE 2a). Approximately 0.2 μg of HF-IF from the peak activity fraction is subjected to electrophoresis in this system again, and the gel is stained with Coomassie Blue (FIGURE 2b).

0077-8923/80/0350-0385 $01.75/0 © 1980, NYAS

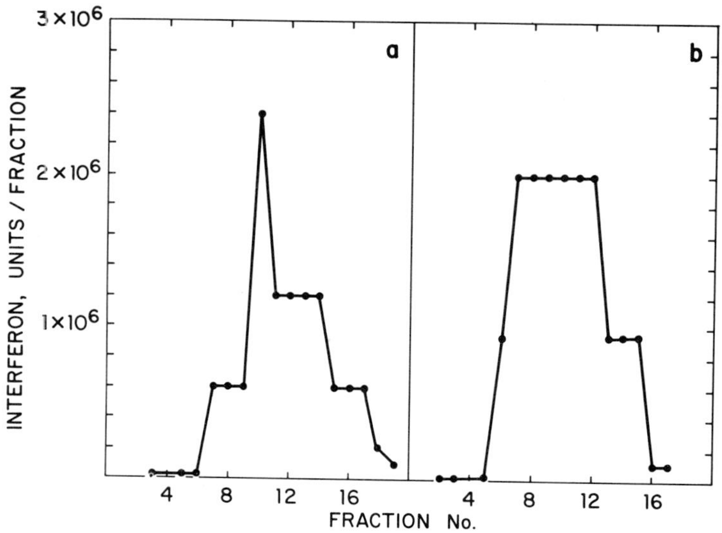

FIGURE 1 (a) Fractionation of crude interferon on a large column of Blue Sepharose. Elution of interferon with 50% ethylene glycol in column buffer begins at fraction 1. (b) Small Blue Sepharose column. Fractions 7–17 in (a) were pooled, passed through the small column, and eluted with 50% ethylene glycol in column buffer (fractions 1–20).

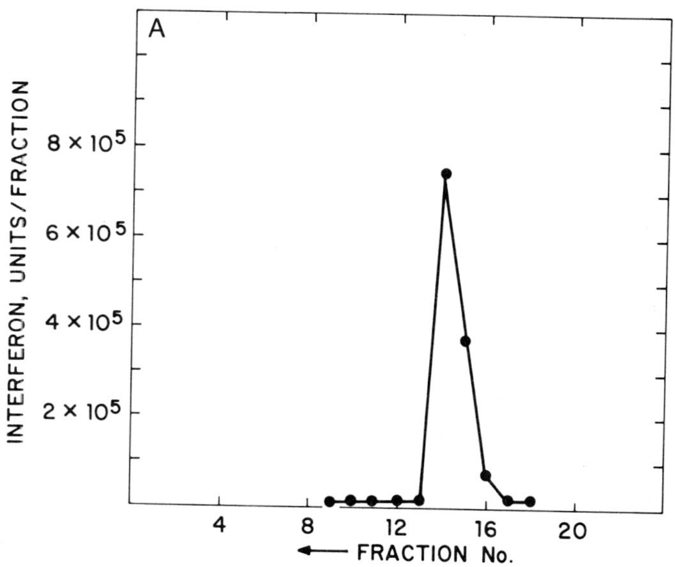

FIGURE 2a. Preparative electrophoresis of interferon, activity profile. Fractions 6–15 in FIGURE 1b were pooled, concentrated, and subjected to electrophoresis in a polyacrylamide slab gel, 0.75 mm thick. Fractions 14 and 15 (FIGURE 2a) were pooled and processed for amino acid sequencing.

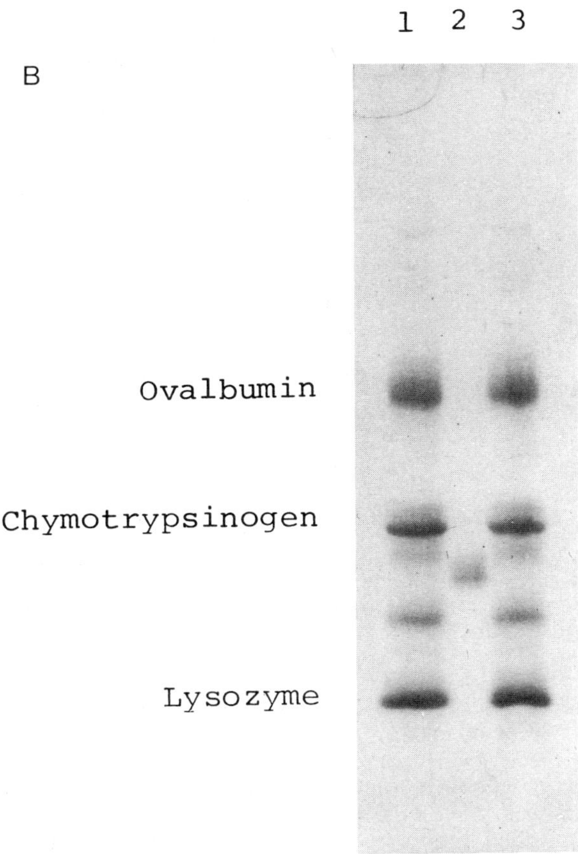

FIGURE 2b. Polyacrylamide slab gel, staining of proteins eluted from preparative gel in FIGURE 2a. Approximately 2% of the protein in fractions 14 and 15 (FIGURE 2a) was subjected to electrophoresis and stained.

The preparative electrophoresis fractions containing HF-IF are pooled and centrifuged for 30 min at 30,000 rpm, 4°C, to remove polyacrylamide gel particles. The interferon solution is dialyzed first against 0.15 M NaCl containing 0.1% SDS and then against 0.02% SDS, and it is concentrated to dryness in a vacuum centrifuge.

This purification procedure is simpler and shorter than that described previously.[1] Recoveries from the large Blue Sepharose column have ranged from 50–100%, and those from the small column approach 100%. The interferon (5×10^7 units/mg) eluted from these columns is stable for at least four weeks at 4°C in 1 M NaCl, 35% ethylene glycol, pH 7.2. Recoveries of activity from the SDS gels have ranged from 5–20%, and specific activities of this protein have ranged from 2-9 $\times 10^8$ units/mg. Accurate specific activities are difficult to determine, and two- to fourfold differences above 1×10^8 units/mg are probably

TABLE 1

AMINO ACID COMPOSITION OF HUMAN FIBROBLAST INTERFERON

	Mol %	Residues per 20,000 Daltons
Asp	11.1	18.9
Thr	4.0	6.8
Ser	6.2	10.5
Glu	15.9	27.0
Pro	1.6	2.7
Gly*	4.6	7.8
Ala	5.9	10.0
Cys†	1.0	1.7
Val	3.5	6.0
Met	1.7	2.9
Ile	5.3	9.0
Leu	12.0	20.4
Tyr	4.4	7.5
Phe	5.5	9.4
His	2.9	4.9
Lys	6.8	11.6
Arg	6.4	10.9
Trp‡	0.6	1.0

*Includes correction for free glycine present in unhydrolyzed protein.
†Determined after performic acid oxidation.
‡Determined after hydrolysis with mercaptoethane-sulfonic acid.

not meaningful. Overall yields of purified HF-IF from 10–15 liter batches of crude material ($5–7 \times 10^7$ total units, 8×10^4 units/mg) have averaged around 10 percent. This gives 5–20 μg of homogeneous interferon.

Amino acid analysis on 1–2 μg aliquots was performed on a Durrum D-500 amino acid analyzer (TABLE 1). Automated Edman degradation on 0.4–2 μg aliquots of the purified interferon was performed in a spinning cup sequentator as previously described.[11,12] Phenylthiohydantoin (Pth) amino acids were identified by high performance liquid chromatography on a Du Pont Zorbax CN column.[14]

The sequence of the N-terminal 13 amino acid residues of human fibroblast interferon determined by this microsequencing technique is given in FIGURE 3. Yields of Pth-Met at cycle 1 for three sequenator runs ranged from 60–100% (based upon protein quantitation by amino acid analysis), and the sequenator repetitive cycle yields were 92–95 percent. Any unblocked minor peptide sequence present at >5% of the reported sequence could have been detected by the methods used, but none has been observed. This result, coupled with the high initial Pth yields, confirms the homogeneity of the HF-IF polypeptide preparation.

1				5						11		
Met	Ser	Tyr	Asn	Leu	Leu	Gly	Phe	Leu	Gln	Arg	Ser	Ser

FIGURE 3. The N-terminal amino acid sequence of human fibroblast interferon.

This paper reports the amino acid composition and the N-terminal sequence of 13 amino acid residues of human fibroblast interferon.[15] It is essential to determine the amino acid sequences of the interferons in order to identify an active site and to understand at the molecular level its mechanism of action. Moreover, determination of the amino acid sequences will allow comparison of structural features of interferons from different sources. This is an interesting possibility since interferons from different species and even from different cell types within an animal are thought to be different proteins.

References

1. Knight, E., Jr. 1976. Proc. Nat. Acad. Sci. USA **73:** 520.
2. Berthold, W., C. Tan & Y. H. Tan. 1978. J. Biol. Chem. **253:** 5206.
3. Zoon, K. C., M. E. Smith, P. J. Bridgen, D. zur Nedden & C. B. Anfinsen. 1980. Proc. Nat. Acad. Sci. USA. **76:** 5601.
4. Rubinstein, M., S. Rubinstein, P. C. Familletti, R. S. Miller, A. A. Walman & S. Pestka. 1979. Proc. Nat. Acad. Sci. USA **76:** 640.
5. Knight, E., Jr. 1975. J. Biol. Chem. **250:** 4139.
6. Yamamoto, Y. & Y. Kawade. 1976. J. Gen. Virol. **33:** 225.
7. Kawakita, M., B. Cabrer, H. Taira, M. Rebello, E. Slattery, H. Weideli & P. Lengyel. 1978. J. Biol. Chem. **254:** 598.
8. DeMaeyer-Guignard, J., M. G. Tovey, I. Gresser & E. DeMaeyer. 1978. Nature **271:** 622.
9. Cabrer, B., H. Taira, R. J. Broeze, T. D. Kemple, K. Williams, E. Slattery, W. H. Konigsberg & P. Lengyel. 1979. J. Biol. Chem. **254:** 3681.
10. Tan, Y. H., F. Barakat, W. Berthold, H. Smith-Johannsen & C. Tan. 1979. J. Biol. Chem. **254:** 8067.
11. Hunkapiller, M. W. & L. E. Hood. 1978. Biochemistry **17:** 2124.
12. Bell, J. R., M. W. Hunkapiller, L. E. Hood & J. H. Strauss. 1978. Proc. Nat. Acad. Sci. USA **75:** 2722.
13. Armstrong, J. A. 1971. Appl. Microbiol. **21:** 723.
14. Johnson, N. J., M. W. Hunkapiller & L. E. Hood. 1979. Anal. Biochem. **100:** 335.
15. Knight, E., Jr., M. W. Hunkapiller, B. D. Korant, R. W. F. Hardy & L. E. Hood. 1980. Science **207:** 525.

HUMAN LYMPHOBLASTOID INTERFERON: PURIFICATION, AMINO ACID COMPOSITION, AND AMINO-TERMINAL SEQUENCE

Kathryn C. Zoon, Mark E. Smith, Pamela J. Bridgen, Dorothy zur Nedden, Dorothea M. Miller, and Christian B. Anfinsen

Laboratory of Chemical Biology
National Institute of Arthritis, Metabolism and Digestive Diseases
National Institutes of Health
Bethesda, Maryland 20205

Michael W. Hunkapiller and Leroy E. Hood

Division of Biology
California Institute of Technology
Pasadena, California 91125

Introduction

The purification and characterization of human interferons (IFs), type I and type II (immune), are currently under investigation because of the clinical potential of these molecules as antiviral, antitumor, and immunomodulatory agents.[1] Recently, the purification and initial characterization of several mouse[2,3] and human[4-7] IFs have been described. Major advances in the large-scale production of IFs[7-12] and improvements in the detection and analysis of picomole quantities of amino acids, peptides, and proteins[4,13-15] have contributed to this success. In spite of developments in production, only minute quantities of these purified interferons are currently available for sequencing studies.

Purified human lymphoblastoid interferon has been obtained in nanomole quantities from Namalwa cells induced with Newcastle disease virus (NDV).[16] The major component, with an apparent molecular weight of 18,500, has been purified to homogeneity.[16] This report describes the isolation of two components of human lymphoblastoid IF with the apparent molecular weights of 21,500 and 18,500 by sodium dodecyl sulfate polyacrylamide gel electrophoresis. The amino acid composition and the amino-terminal sequence of the 18,500 dalton component is presented.

Materials and Methods

Production and Concentration of Crude Interferon

Human lymphoblastoid interferon was obtained from Namalwa cultures induced with NDV, strain B1, as previously described.[10] The crude IF was concentrated by precipitation with 5% (wt/vol) trichloroacetic acid (TCA).[11] A major portion of the IF was supplied by Litton Bionetics under National Cancer Institute contract NO1-CO-75380 as the redissolved TCA precipitate. Newcastle disease virus was prepared by Jack Campbell, National Institute of Arthritis, Metabolism, and Digestive Diseases, National Institutes of Health, Bethesda, MD.[10]

0077-8923/80/0350-0390 $01.75/0 © 1980, NYAS

Interferon Assay

IF was assayed on low passage human foreskin fibroblast cells (HSF-4) with vesicular stomatitis virus as the challenge virus, using a modification of the semi-micro method described by Armstrong.[17] All IF titers are expressed as reference units based on the human leukocyte standard G-023-901-527 obtained from the Research Resources Branch, National Institute of Allergy and Infectious Diseases, National Institutes of Health, Bethesda, MD.

Protein Determination and Amino Acid Analyses

Protein concentrations were determined by the method of Lowry *et al.*[18] with bovine serum albumin as a standard, or by amino acid analyses. The latter analyses were done in the laboratory of P. E. Hare, Geophysical Laboratory, Carnegie Institute of Washington, D.C., using high-performance liquid chromatography (HPLC), and fluorescence detection of o-phthalaldehyde amino acid derivatives.[13,14] Samples were analyzed directly or were dialyzed prior to analysis twice against 6-liter volumes of phosphate buffered saline, pH 7.4, 0.05% NaN_3 (PBS) containing 0.1% sodium dodecyl sulfate (SDS) and then twice against 1-liter volumes of 0.01% SDS prepared with Baker HPLC reagent water (J. T. Baker Chemical Co., Phillipsburg, NJ) at 25°C over a 24-hr period. The analyses were done with samples containing 1–3 μg protein. Contaminating amino acids were monitored by analyzing duplicate unhydrolyzed samples. The quantity of each residue in the unhydrolyzed sample was less than 5% of that found in the hydrolyzed sample for all the amino acids with the exception of Ser and Gly, which were less than 10 percent. These values were subtracted from the values observed with the hydrolyzed samples. Proline was measured by gas chromatography as described,[19] except that trifluoroacetic anhydride was used rather than pentafluoropropionic anhydride to form the derivative. Cysteic acid and methionine sulfone were measured after performic acid oxidation.[20–21] Tryptophan was determined after hydrolysis in 6 N HCl/4% (vol/vol) thioglycolic acid.[22]

Immunoabsorbant Affinity Chromatography

Sheep anti-lymphoblastoid IF was prepared, purified, and coupled to Sepharose 4B as described.[16] Columns were successively eluted with PBS, McIlvaine's citrate/phosphate buffer, pH 5.0, McIlvaine's citrate/phosphate buffer, pH 2.4–2.6, PBS, PBS containing 4M Guanidine · HCl and PBS, respectively.[16] Components of lymphoblastoid IF, antigenically identical to human leukocyte IF, were eluted by the pH 2.6 buffer and were stored at −70°C until a sufficient quantity ($2–5 \times 10^8$ units) was accumulated for the next purification step.

Sephadex G-150 Chromatography

The pH 2.6 eluates from the immunoabsorbant affinity columns were thawed and concentrated on a Pellicon cassette ultrafiltration system (Millipore) PT series, (Millipore, Bedford, MA) to a volume of 75–100 ml.[16] The concentrate was adjusted to pH 3.5 with 1N NaOH and applied to a Sephadex G-150 column (46.5

cm in height, 6200 ml in volume) and developed with McIlvaine's citrate/phosphate buffer pH 3.5 containing 0.05% NaN_3 at 4–6°C. Interferon was eluted, at a flow rate of 60 ml/hr, between the effluent volumes 3800–5000 ml.

SP-Sephadex Chromatography and Treatment of Interferon with Glycosidase Mixture

The Sephadex G-150 fractions containing the major antiviral activity peak were concentrated by ultrafiltration to 300–450 ml and applied to an SP-Sephadex C-25 column (1.5 cm in diameter, 5 cm in height) and equilibrated with McIlvaine's citrate/phosphate buffer pH 3.5. The column was developed with a step pH gradient at a flow rate of 1.3 ml/min as previously described.[16] An average of 90% of the recovered IF was eluted at pH 5.5. This fraction was adjusted to pH 6.0 with 1N NaOH and incubated at 37°C for 4–5 hr with a mixture of glycosidases from *Streptococcus pneumoniae*, Type 1, prepared by S. Bose,[23] which was shown to remove most of the carbohydrate moiety of the leukocyte IF.[23]

L-Tryptophyl-L-Tryptophan-Affi-Gel 10 Chromatography

After the glycosidase mixture treatment, the IF preparation was applied to an L-tryptophyl-L-tryptophan-Affi-Gel 10 column (11.3 cm in height, 22.7 ml in volume) at a flow rate of 1.3 ml/min. It was developed with PBS, PBS containing 1.0 M NaCl, and then PBS containing 1.0 M NaCl and 75% (vol/vol) ethylene glycol as described.[16] Interferon was eluted with the buffer containing 75% ethylene glycol and collected in an equal volume of 0.1% SDS. The eluate was then dialyzed three times against 6-liter volumes of 0.05% SDS over a 24-hr period at 23°C.

Preparative and Analytical SDS Polyacrylamide Gel Electrophoresis

After dialysis, the ethylene glycol eluate was concentrated by ultrafiltration to 0.5–1.0 ml.[16] The samples were adjusted to 0.05 M Tris HCl pH 6.8, 10% (vol/vol) glycerol, 1.0% SDS, and 0.002% bromophenol blue, and incubated 2–3 hr at 25°C. Polyacrylamide gel electrophoresis was performed using a modification of the Laemmli system.[24-25] Preparative gels were 1.5 mm in thickness and 24–27 cm in length. Analytical gels were 0.75 mm in thickness and 9 cm in length. A 3.7% acrylamide stacking gel and a 16% acrylamide separating gel were used in both preparative and analytical procedures. Details of the electrophoresis, staining and destaining of the slab gels, and excision and elution of the IF components from the gels have been reported.[16]

Amino-terminal Sequence Determination

Samples to be sequenced were dialyzed twice against 6-liter volumes of PBS containing 0.1% SDS and then three times against 1-liter volumes of 0.01% SDS prepared with Baker HPLC reagent water at 25°C. The SDS was purchased from

Bio-Rad Laboratories, Inc., Richmond, CA. The amino-terminal sequence was primarily determined using a Caltech spinning cup sequencer, the nonprotein carrier Polybrene, and slight modification of the Edman Quadrol program as previously described.[15] A portion of the amino-terminal sequence was also obtained using a LKB solid phase sequencer as described by Bridgen.[26] The amino acid phenylthiohydantoins (PTHs) from the spinning cup sequencer were identified by high-performance liquid chromatography using a Du Pont Zorbax CN column developed by gradient elution employing methanol/acetonitrile (17:3) in sodium acetate buffer, pH 5.4.[27] Radioactive PTHs from the solid-phase sequencer were identified by adding a mixture of unlabeled standards, running on HPLC on a Zorbax ODS column, and collecting and counting each peak.

TABLE 1

PURIFICATION OF HUMAN LYMPHOBLASTOID INTERFERON

Step	Interferon Units $\times 10^{-6}$	Protein (mg)	Specific Activity (interferon units $\times 10^{-6}$/mg protein)	Cumulative Recovery (%)
Trichloroacetic Acid precipitation	800			
Sephadex G-25	690	334,756	.0021	86
Anti-lymphoblastoid interferon-Sepharose 4B	640	878	.73	80
Storage at −70°C	400			50
Ultrafiltration	220	700		28
Sephadex G-150	190	61.9	3.1	24
Ultrafiltration	140			18
SP-Sephadex*	110	31.9	3.4	14
Glycosidase treatment	101	32.3	3.1	13
L-tryptophyl-L-tryptophan Affi-gel 10	83	7.6	11	10
Dialysis and ultrafiltration	48			6
SDS PAGE				
Total†	48			6
A	5	.065	77	0.6
B	23	.104	220	3
C	9	.101	89	1

*pH 5.5 eluate only.
†The total quantity of interferon eluted from the gels.

Solvent A was 21mM sodium acetate pH 4.5, solvent B was acetonitrile. A step gradient of 19% B for 4 min followed by 34% B at a flow rate of 2 ml/min was used.

RESULTS

A summary of the purification of human lymphoblastoid interferon is shown in TABLE 1. As previously described, the IF present in the redissolved trichloroacetic acid precipitate was chromatographed on Sephadex G-25 to remove the trichloroacetate ions and to equilibrate the sample in PBS prior to immunoabsorbant affinity chromatography.[11] The eluate of the Sephadex G-25 column containing 35.2–88.2 g protein and 0.5–2 × 10^8 units of IF was then applied to a sheep anti-lymphoblastoid interferon-Sepharose 4B column. In this preparation an average of 93% of the antiviral activity was eluted by McIlvaine's citrate/phosphate buffer pH 2.6. This step yielded the largest purification, a 350-fold increase in the specific activity over the Sephadex G-25 eluate. The pH 2.6 fractions were then stored at −70°C until sufficient IF (1–5 × 10^8 units) was accumulated for the next purification step. As shown in TABLE 1, a 37% loss in the antiviral activity was observed after the pH 2.6 fractions were stored at −70°C for 2 months and thawed. Recent studies in this laboratory have indicated that partially purified IF having protein concentrations below 100 μg/ml lose up to 60% of their antiviral activity after brief storage at 6°C or −70°C in plastic bottles and tubes. Collection in siliconized glass bottles and concentration of the dilute protein solutions by ultrafiltration prior to storage have reduced losses. The next step in the purification is the concentration of the partially purified IF by the Pellicon cassette ultrafiltration system. In this preparation, 55% of the antiviral activity was recovered in the concentrate; less than 1% was found in the filtrate. Two previous preparations did not exhibit this loss (i.e. 44% of the antiviral activity); 90% of the antiviral activity was recovered in the concentrates. Gel filtration on Sephadex G-150 followed. Approximately 5% of the antiviral activity eluted at the void volume and 86% eluted between 3800–5000 ml. The major peak of antiviral activity obtained from Sephadex G-150 column was then purified by an SP-Sephadex column. Approximately 90% of the applied IF was eluted with pH 5.5 buffer and 10% with pH 7.0 buffer. Although the increase in specific activity of the IF preparation appears slight, as shown in TABLE 1, analysis by analytical SDS gel electrophoresis showed that several polypeptide species migrating in the region of the antiviral activity were removed by this step. The pH 5.5 eluate was then incubated with a mixture of glycosidases, which removes a major portion of the carbohydrate moiety.[23] Examination of the glycosidase preparation by analytical SDS polyacrylamide gel electrophoresis showed that no detectable Coomassie brilliant blue R-250 staining components were present in the region of the antiviral activity.

Amino acids and dipeptides bound to solid phase supports have been used previously to purify a variety of IFs.[28] The dipeptide, L-tryptophyl-L-tryptophan coupled to Affi-gel 10 was effective in the purification of human lymphoblastoid IF. A 75% (vol/vol) ethylene glycol solution was required to elute the IF. Extended exposure of lymphoblastoid IF to this high concentration of ethylene glycol resulted in large losses of antiviral activity. These losses were virtually eliminated by collecting the eluate in an equal volume of 0.1% SDS. This procedure immediately reduced the concentration of ethylene glycol and added SDS which stabilizes the interferon. This stabilization by low concentration of SDS has been shown with several other IFs.[6,29,30] FIGURE 1 shows a typical preparative SDS gel. The Coomassie brilliant blue R-250-stained components, A and B, with the apparent molecular weights of 21,500 and 18,500 respectively, comigrated with the peaks of antiviral activities recovered from the gel. As shown in TABLE 1 and FIGURE 1, B is the major IF species. A third component migrating slightly faster than the major 18,500 dalton species (C) is also observed and appears as a shoulder on B. Recovery of the IF activity from the stained gels ranges from 50 to 100 percent. The B component was then analyzed by analytical gel electrophoresis as shown in FIGURE 2. Only one Coomassie brilliant blue R-250-stained polypeptide was detected. The amino acid composition of B is shown in TABLE 2. The combination of Leu, Ile, Val, Ala, and Phe accounted for 31% of the amino acid residues; Leu alone was present at a level of 11%. The high content of these residues is consistent with the hydrophobicity of IF. Approximately 12% of the molecule consisted of the basic amino acids, Arg and

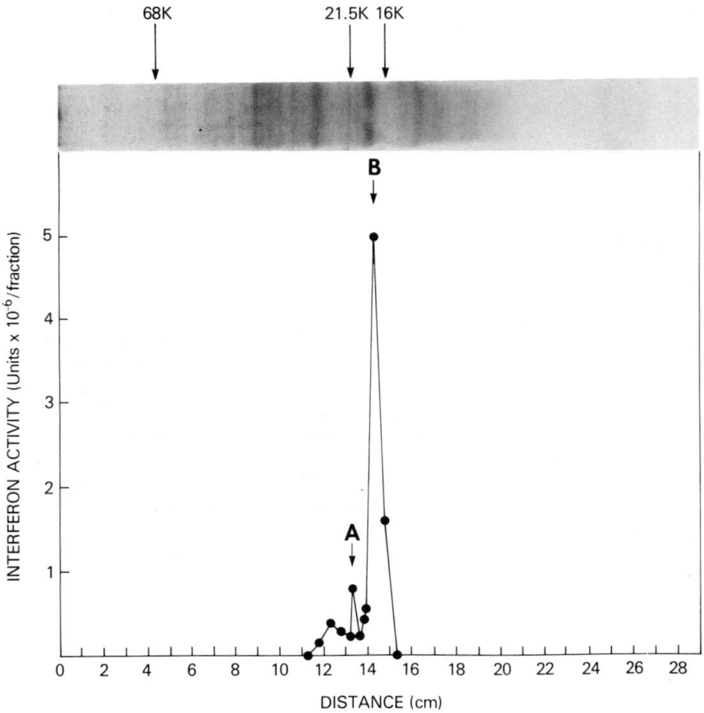

FIGURE 1. Preparative SDS polyacrylamide gel electrophoresis of human lymphoblastoid interferon (IF). Partially purified IF (1.9×10^7 units, 1.2 mg protein) was applied to the gel. Total IF recovered was 9.7×10^6 units; 8×10^5 units comigrated with the 21,500 dalton species (A); 5.0×10^6 units comigrated with the 18,500 dalton species (B); 1.6×10^6 units comigrated with C (defined in text). The Coomassie brilliant blue R-250 polypeptide pattern shown at the top of the figure represents one lane of the preparative gel. In this experiment the total recovery of antiviral activity was 51 percent.

Lys. The value obtained for met, shown in TABLE 2, represents a minimum value because of losses incurred during the oxidation.[21]

The amino acid sequence of the amino-terminal 20 residues of B is presented in FIGURE 3. Multiple analyses (6 determinations) using the spinning cup sequencer on three independent preparations of interferon (20–500 pmol protein) yielded the sequence shown in FIGURE 3. A portion of the amino-terminal sequence, to residue 10, was obtained with the solid-phase sequencer (500 pmol protein, one determination). These results were in essential agreement with those obtained with the spinning cup sequencer. A second sequence (approximately 10%) was found in an earlier preparation of B. Fraction C had equal amounts of both sequences and one-half the specific activity of B (TABLE 1), indicating that the second sequence is probably a contaminant. Improved fractionation of B from the preparative SDS polyacrylamide gels essentially eliminated this sequence. Two recent preparations have yielded the sequence shown in FIGURE 3 with undetectable quantities (<3%) of the contaminant.

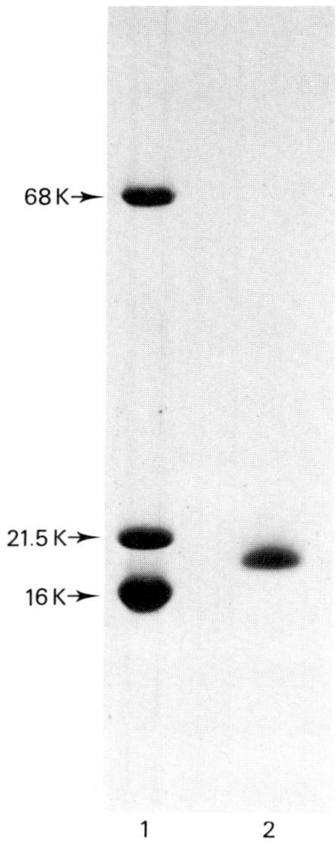

FIGURE 2. Analytical SDS polyacrylamide gel electrophoresis of the purified 18,500 dalton component of human lymphoblastoid interferon. *Lane 1*, molecular weight standards: 2.5 μg bovine serum albumin (68,000) and 5.0 μg each of soybean trypsin inhibitor (21,500) and myoglobin (16,000). *Lane 2*, 2.2 μg B from the preparative SDS polyacrylamide gel shown in FIGURE 1.

DISCUSSION

A human lymphoblastoid interferon with an apparent molecular weight of 18,500[8] has been purified to homogeneity and has a specific activity of $2.2–2.5 \times 10^8$ units/mg protein. Major advances in the large scale production of lymphoblastoid IF[10-12] coupled with improvements in amino acid analysis[13,14] and microsequencing[15] have permitted the purification and initial characterization of this IF species.

A preparation of IF from uninduced Namalwa cells, which produce low levels of IF constitutively,[16,31] was purified by the steps described in TABLE 1. Analysis of

TABLE 2

AMINO ACID COMPOSITION OF THE MAJOR 18,500 DALTON COMPONENT OF HUMAN LYMPHOBLASTOID INTERFERON

Amino Acid	Residues*
Asx	14.9
Thr	8.0
Ser	10.7
Glx	27.3
Pro	10.9
Gly	10.7
Ala	11.0
Cys	1.8
Val	7.7
Met	1.2
Ile	6.9
Leu	17.8
Tyr	3.8
Phe	7.1
His	4.4
Lys	10.4
Arg	9.6
Trp	0.6

*The number of amino acid residues is 165, based on the apparent molecular weight of 18,500 determined by SDS polyacrylamide gel electrophoresis.

the ethylene glycol eluate from the L-tryptophyl-L-tryptophan-Affi-gel 10 column by SDS polyacrylamide gel electrophoresis showed A and B in greatly diminished amounts.[16] This provides additional evidence that we are indeed purifying proteins produced during the induction of IF.

The amino acid composition of B showed an abundance of hydrophobic amino acid residues. Similarly, several human[4,7] and mouse[32] interferons have been characterized as being enriched in hydrophobic amino acids by amino acid analysis. In addition, 8 of the first 20 amino acid residues of B consisted of Leu, Ile, and Ala, and contribute a very hydrophobic character to the amino-terminal portion of the IF molecule.

Preliminary sequencing of the amino-terminus of B to approximately residue 40 is currently being reexamined using larger quantities (0.5–2 nmol) of protein. Fragment production using cyanogen bromide and trypsin, and subsequent peptide purification and sequence determination are in progress.

Amino-terminal sequencing studies of A and C yielded one sequence similar to B (the major 18,500 dalton component) plus a second sequence (preliminary

Ser^{1}-Asp-Leu-Pro-Gln^{5}-Thr-His-Ser-Leu-Gly^{10}-

Asn-Arg-Arg-Ala-Leu^{15}-Ile-Leu-Leu-Ala-Gln^{20}

FIGURE 3. The sequence of the 20 amino-terminal residues of the 18,500 dalton component of human lymphoblastoid interferon.

amino-terminal sequence data are available on the second protein). It is of interest that the second amino-terminal sequence observed in A appears to be the same as that observed in C. At this point it is not clear whether this second protein is a modification of B or if it is a contaminant of the IF preparation. The observation that the specific activities of A and C are approximately twofold less than that of B and that both A and C contain 25–50% of the second protein suggests that the second sequence is a contaminant. Purification of this other protein and the determination of its antiviral activity should distinguish between these two possibilities.

References

1. Baron, S. & F. Dianzani, Ed. 1977. Tex. Rep. Biol. Med. **35:** 394–541.
2. Kawakita, M., B. Cabrer, H. Taira, M. Rebello, E. Slattery, H. Weideli & P. Lengyel. 1978. J. Biol. Chem. **253:** 598–602.
3. Iwakura, Y., S. Yonehara & Y. Kawade. 1978. J. Biol. Chem. **253:** 5074–5079.
4. Rubenstein, M., S. Rubinstein, P. Familletti, R. Miller, A. Waldman & S. Pestka. 1979. Proc. Nat. Acad. Sci. USA **76:** 640–644.
5. Lin, L. S. & W. E. Stewart II. 1978. Fed. Proc. Fed. Am. Soc. Exp. Biol. **37:** 1441.
6. Knight, E., Jr. 1976. Proc. Nat. Acad. Sci. USA **73:** 520–523.
7. Tan, Y. H., F. Barakat, W. Berthold, H. Smith-Johannsen & C. Tan. 1979. **254:** 8067–8073.
8. Cantell, K. & S. Hirvonen. 1978. J. Gen. Virol. **39:** 541–543.
9. Edy, V. G. 1977. Tex. Rep. Biol. Med. **35:** 132–137.
10. Zoon, K. C., C. E. Buckler, P. J. Bridgen & D. Gurari-Rotman. 1978. J. Clin. Microbiol. **7:** 44–51.
11. Bridgen, P. J., C. B. Anfinsen, L. Corley, S. Bose, K. C. Zoon, U. T. Rüegg & C. E. Buckler. 1977. J. Biol. Chem. **252:** 6585–6587.
12. Klein, F., R. T. Ricketts, W. I. Jones, I. A. De Armon, M. J. Temple, K. C. Zoon & P. J. Bridgen. 1979. Antimicrob. Agents Chemother. **15:** 420–427.
13. Hare, P. E. 1977. Methods. Enzymol. **47:** 3–18.
14. Benson, J. R. & P. E. Hare. 1975. Proc. Nat. Acad. Sci. USA **72:** 619–622.
15. Hunkapiller, M. W. & L. E. Hood. 1978. Biochemistry **17:** 2124–2133.
16. Zoon, K. C., M. E. Smith, P. J. Bridgen, D. zur Nedden & C. B. Anfinsen. 1979. Proc. Nat. Acad. Sci. USA **76:** 5601–5605.
17. Armstrong, J. A. 1971. Appl. Microbiol. **21:** 723–725.
18. Lowry, O. H., N. J. Rosebrough, A. L. Farr & R. J. Randall. 1951. J. Biol. Chem. **193:** 265–275.
19. Frank. H., G. J. Nicholson & E. Bayer. 1977. J. Chromatogr. Sci. **15:** 174–176.
20. Hirs, C. H. W. 1967. Methods. Enzymol. **11:** 197–199.
21. Moore, S. 1963. J. Biol. Chem. **238:** 235–237.
22. Matsubara, H. & R. M. Sasaki. 1969. Biochem. Biophys. Res. Commun. **35:** 175–181.
23. Bose, S., D. Gurari-Rotman, U. T. Rüegg, L. Corley & C. B. Anfinsen. 1976. J. Biol. Chem. **251:** 1659–1662.
24. Laemmli, U. K. 1970. Nature (London) **227:** 680–685.
25. Weintraub, H., K. Palter & F. Van Lente. 1975. Cell **6:** 85–110.
26. Bridgen, J. 1976. Biochemistry. **15:** 3600–3604.
27. Johnson, N. D., M. W. Hunkapiller & L. E. Hood. 1979. Anal. Biochem. **100:** 335–338.
28. Sulkowski, E., M. W. Davey & W. A. Carter. 1976. J. Biol. Chem. **251:** 5381–5385.
29. Törma, E. T. & K. Paucker. 1976. J. Biol. Chem. **251:** 4810–4186.
30. Stewart, W. E., II, P. DeSomer, V. G. Edy, K. Paucker, K. Berg & C. A. Ogburn. 1975. J. Gen. Virol. **26:** 327–331.
31. Adams, A., B. Lidin, H. Strander & K. Cantell. 1975. J. Gen. Virol. **28:** 219–223.
32. Cabrer, B., H. Taira, R. J. Broeze, T. D. Kempe, K. Williams, E. Slattery, W. H. Konigsberg & P. Lengyel. 1979. J. Biol. Chem. **254:** 3681–3684.

GROWTH-INHIBITORY AND ANTIVIRAL ACTIVITY OF PURIFIED LEUKOCYTE INTERFERON

Marian Evinger, Menachem Rubinstein, and Sidney Pestka

Roche Institute of Molecular Biology
Nutley, New Jersey 07110

Numerous cell-regulatory properties have been attributed to interferon (IF). The ability to inhibit viral growth was the first recognized biological activity of interferon and was the property for which the protein was named. Later the ability to inhibit cell multiplication, i.e., the antiproliferative activity, was detected not only with murine IF but also with human leukocyte and fibroblast IF.[1-3] Interferon has also been reported to exert antitumor effects with virus-induced, transplantable, and spontaneous tumors.[4] Immunomodulatory activities of IF may include suppression of the immune response to T-dependent and -independent antigens in the mouse (for review of this and other activities, see Johnson and Baron[5]). Additional responses of the cell to IF involve activation of natural killer T-cells and a corresponding increase in the phagocytic activity of macrophages.[6] Furthermore, cell-mediated immunity and graft-versus-host rejections are diminished after treatment with interferon.

Effective administration of IF as a therapeutic agent requires a thorough knowledge of its biological properties. The most direct method of obtaining this information involves testing each of the potential biological activities separately with homogeneous IF. However, such studies have been hampered by the lack of homogeneous IF. The purification of human leukocyte IF was accomplished recently in this laboratory with the use of high performance liquid chromatography.[7] Therefore, the availability of leukocyte interferon (with specific activities of 2–4 × 10^8 units/ml) has enabled us to probe several of the biological activities attributed to IF. In these studies, we report that the growth-inhibitory activity of leukoctye IF purifies with antiviral activity. Enhancement of natural killer cell activity as a property of homogeneous IF is also described by Herberman *et al.*[6]

The antiproliferative effects of IF may be examined by measuring the amount of inhibition the IF exerts on cell multiplication. A growth assay analogous to that described by Stewart *et al.*[2] measures the growth-inhibitory activity of IF on the sensitive human lymphoid Daudi cell line. As shown in FIGURE 1, this assay is performed by adding interferon to 1–2 × 10^5 cells/ml. After 3 days, the number of cells is determined and the amount of growth inhibition is expressed as the percent change in cell number in IF-treated cultures relative to that in untreated control cultures.

The amount of growth-inhibitory activity can be compared to the amount of antiviral activity in each sample. The antiviral activity is measured as the amount of interferon (in international reference units/ml) necessary to reduce the cytopathic effects of vesicular stomatitis virus by 50 percent. In these studies, the antiviral activity of IF was measured on human AG-1732 fibroblast and on bovine MDBK endothelial cells. Leukocyte IF exerted maximal growth-inhibitory activity on the Daudi cells at concentrations of ≥10 units/ml. Fifty percent of maximal growth inhibition was produced by 3–5 units/ml of interferon. In all experiments, data are expressed as the average of triplicate determinations with a standard error of ±5 percent.

0077-8923/80/0350-0399 $01.75/0 © 1980, NYAS

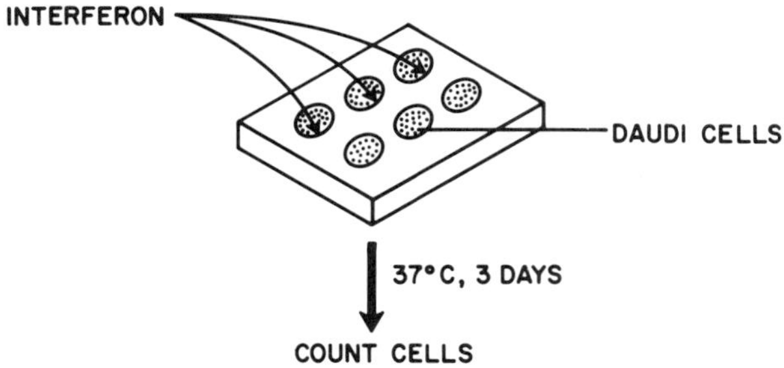

FIGURE 1. Growth-inhibitory activity. The amount of growth inhibition was determined by comparing the cell number in interferon-treated cultures to that in nontreated control cultures. Human lymphoid Daudi cells were incubated 1–2 × 10^5 cells/ml in the presence or absence of IF at 37°C for 3 days.

Partition chromatography on Sephadex G-150 in the presence of 4M urea is the initial step in fractionation of leukocyte IF (for details of leukocyte IF purification, see Rubinstein *et al.*[7]). Each of the fractions eluting from this column was tested for growth-inhibitory activity and antiviral activity as shown in FIGURE 2. Growth-inhibitory activity occurs as a broad distribution in fractions 65–87,

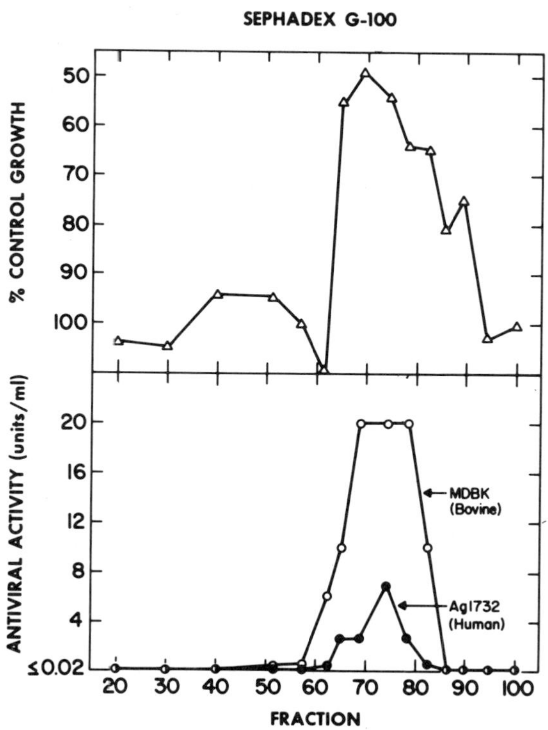

FIGURE 2. Fractionation of crude human leukocyte interferon on Sephadex G-100 in 4M urea. The growth-inhibitory activity (*upper panel*) is expressed as the percent control growth of the Daudi cells as described in the text. The antiviral activity (*lower panel*) in reference units/ml was measured on human AG-1732 and bovine MDBK cells.

which is also the only region of the elution profile exhibiting antiviral activity. The material in some fractions, e.g., fraction 62, appears to stimulate Daudi cell growth; and it is therefore represented as greater than 100% of control growth. In addition, there is inhibition of cell growth in certain other fractions; however, these fractions do not possess corresponding antiviral activity and conceivably may represent other growth-inhibitory factors.

Further purification of the material in the peak fractions from the Sephadex column with high performance liquid chromatography is shown in FIGURE 3. An increase in the antiviral specific activity of the IF profile is observed when the

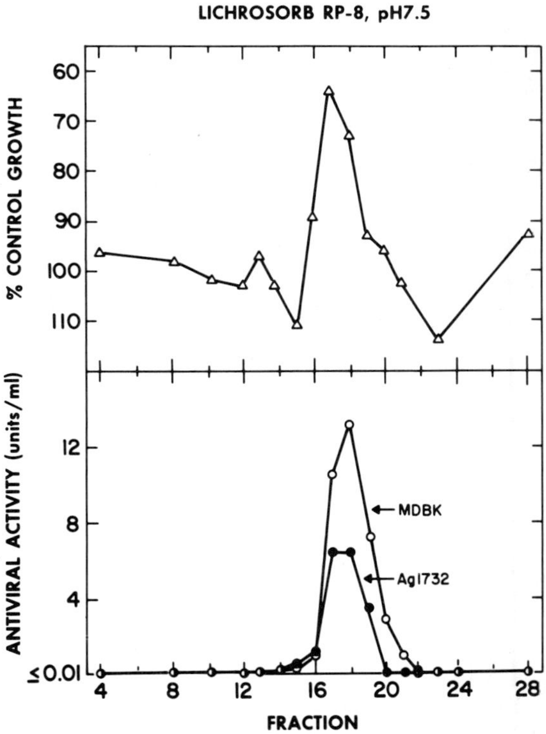

FIGURE 3. Chromatography of interferon on Lichrosorb RP-8 at pH 7.5. Growth-inhibitory activity (*upper panel*) and antiviral activity (*lower panel*) were measured as described in the text.

fractions from the Sephadex G-100 column are partitioned on Lichrosorb RP-8 at pH 7.5. It can be seen that growth-inhibitory activity elutes in a narrow region of the profile which corresponds to the region of antiviral activity.

Although the biological activity of IF is confined to a relatively narrow area in the elution profile from Lichrosorb RP-8, three distinct peaks of leukocyte IF are resolved by chromatography on Lichrosorb Diol. As shown in FIGURE 4, three peaks of antiviral activity have been designated α, β, and γ in the order of their elution from Lichrosorb Diol. It is significant that each of these exhibits substantial growth-inhibitory activity. Although the reason is not known, the relative proportion of antiviral activity in each of these peaks differs according to the cell

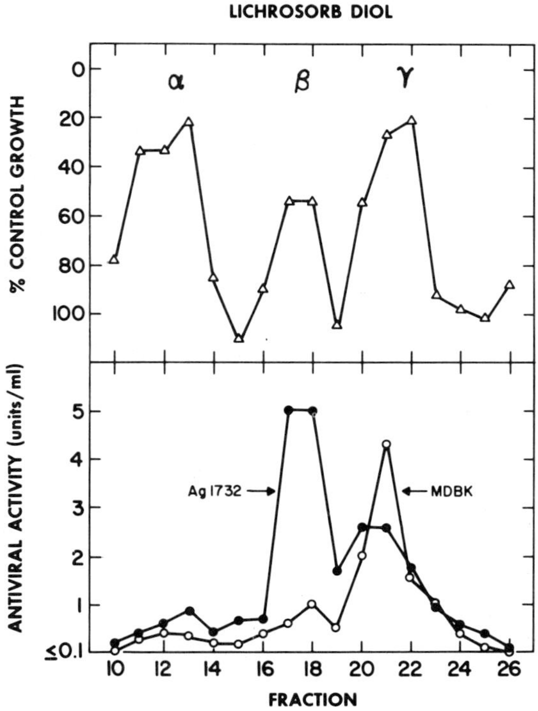

FIGURE 4. Chromatography of interferon on Lichrosorb Diol. Growth-inhibitory activity (*upper panel*) and antiviral activity (*lower panel*) were measured as described in the text.

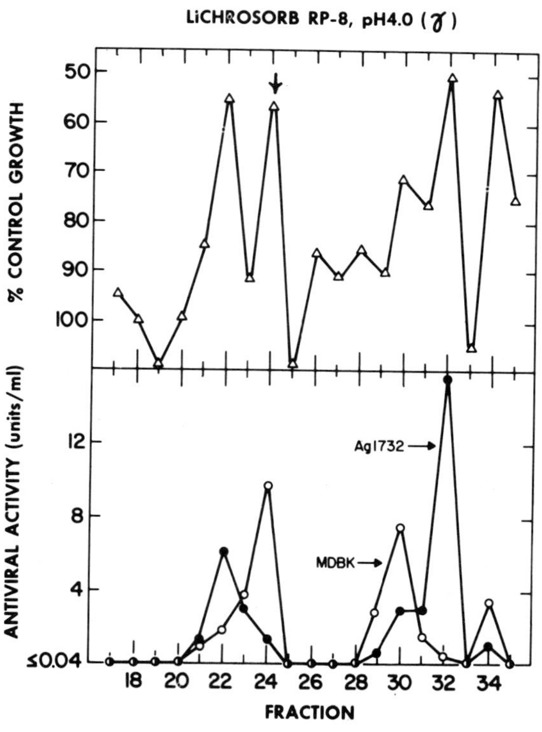

FIGURE 5. Chromatography of interferon on Lichrosorb RP-8 at pH 4. Growth-inhibitory activity (*upper panel*) and antiviral activity (*lower panel*) were measured as described in the text.

species used to titer the antiviral activity. In addition, the relative fraction of antiviral activity in the α peak is observed to be small in comparison to that in the β and γ peaks. This appears to be a characteristic for leukocyte IF which has been prepared from cells of patients with chronic myelogenous leukemia.[8] Nevertheless, the α peak exhibits substantial growth-inhibitory activity.

The γ peak of the Diol column, which possesses considerable amounts of both growth-inhibitory and antiviral activities, was selected for closer study. Chromatography of the material in the γ peak on Lichrosorb RP-8 at pH 4 further resolves the interferon into numerous species (FIGURE 5). As shown in FIGURE 5, the presence of growth-inhibitory activity corresponds precisely with the occurrence of antiviral activity. When the protein in fraction 24 was subjected to electropho-

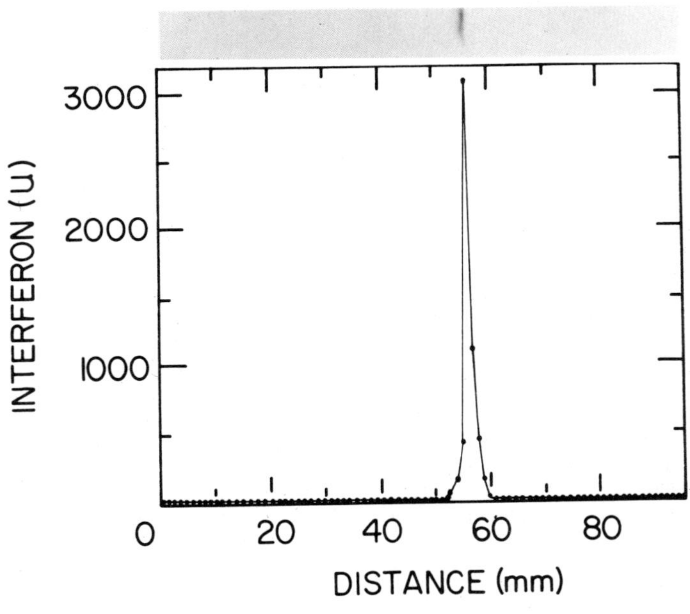

FIGURE 6. Sodium dodecyl sulfate-polyacrylamide gel electrophoresis and antiviral activity of the interferon in fraction 24 from the Lichrosorb RP-8, pH 4, column (FIGURE 5). After electrophoresis, the gel was sliced into 1-mm segments and assayed for antiviral activity on bovine MDBK cells as described by Rubinstein et al.[9]

resis on sodium dodecyl sulfate-polyacrylamide gels, a single band was detected by staining with Coomassie blue (FIGURE 6). When 1-mm segments corresponding to the electrophoretic profile were assayed, all the antiviral activity corresponded to the stained protein band. Furthermore, amino acid analyses of this material and achievement of constant specific activity upon rechromatography established the homogeneity of the IF in this fraction. As is evident in FIGURE 5, this material exerts substantial growth-inhibitory activity. Therefore, the presence of both activities in this fraction demonstrate that human leukocyte IF possesses growth-inhibitory activity in addition to antiviral activity.

Copurification of the antiviral and antigrowth activities indicates that each of these activities is an intrinsic property of leukoctye interferon. In all cases where antiviral activity was detected, growth-inhibitory activity was always present. The significance of diverse ratios of antiviral to growth-inhibitory activity and of antiviral activity on human and bovine cells in various fractions remains to be determined. Such differences may represent structural heterogeneities in the IF protein. The existence of such differences, however, suggests that there may be some distinct mechanisms for antiviral and antiproliferative activities.

As presented by Herberman *et al.*,[6] it has been demonstrated that pure leukocyte IF can enhance the activity of natural killer cells. The availability of homogeneous IF will enable us to determine whether the IF protein possesses additional biological activities. It is clear, however, that antiproliferative activity and enhancement of cytolytic activities are intrinsic properties of leukocyte interferon.

References

1. Paucker, K., K. Cantell & W. Henle. 1962. Quantitative studies of viral interference in suspended L-cells. Effect of interfering viruses and interferon on the growth rate of cells. Virology **17:** 324–334.
2. Stewart, W. E. II., I. Gresser, M. G. Tovey, M.-T. Bandu & S. Le Goff. 1976. Identification of the cell multiplication inhibitory factors in interferon preparations as interferons. Nature **262:** 300–302.
3. Knight, E. Jr. 1976. Antiviral and cell growth inhibitory activities reside in the same glycoprotein of human fibroblast interferon. Nature **262:** 302–303.
4. Gresser, I. 1977. On the mechanisms of the antitumor effects of interferon. *In* The Interferon System: A Current Review to 1978. S. Baron and F. Dianzani, Eds. Vol. **35:** 394–398. University of Texas Medical Branch, Galveston, TX.
5. Johnson H. M., & S. Baron. 1977. Evaluation of effects of interferon and interferon inducers on the immune response. Pharmacol. Ther.[A] **1:** 349–367.
6. Herberman, R. B., J. R. Ortaldo, J. Y. Djeu, H. T. Holden, J. Jett, N. P. Lang, M. Rubinstein & S. Pestka. 1980. Role of interferon in regulation of cytotoxicity by natural killer cells and macrophages. Ann. N.Y. Acad. Sci. **350:** 63–71.
7. Rubinstein, M., S. Rubinstein, P. C. Familletti, R. S. Miller, A. A. Waldman & S. Pestka. 1979. Human leukocyte interferon: Production, purification to homogeneity, and initial characterization. Proc. Natl. Acad. Sci. USA **76:** 640–644.
8. Rubinstein, M., S. Rubinstein, P. C., Familletti, R. D. Hershberg, L. D. Brink, J. Gutterman, J. Hester & S. Pestka. 1980. Human leukocyte interferon. Production and purification to homogeneity by HPLC. *In* Proteins: Structure and Biological Function. E. Gross & J. Meienhofer, Eds.: 99–103. Pierce Chemical Company. Rockford, IL.
9. Rubinstein, M., S. Rubinstein, P. C. Familletti, M. S. Gross, R. S. Miller, A. A. Waldman & S. Pestka. 1978. Human leukocyte interferon purified to homogeneity. Science **202:** 1289–1290.

SYNTHESIS, STRUCTURE, AND FUNCTION OF POLY(I) · POLY(C)-INDUCED HUMAN FIBROBLAST INTERFERON mRNA*

Pravinkumar B. Sehgal and Igor Tamm

The Rockefeller University
New York, New York 10021

We have investigated various aspects of the synthesis, structure, and regulated function of interferon mRNA induced by poly(I) · poly(C) in FS-4 human fibroblasts. The kinetics of interferon (IF) synthesis by oocytes of *Xenopus laevis* microinjected with IF mRNA preparations were reevaluated.[1-3] Evidence was obtained to suggest that the size of the transcription unit for human fibroblast IF mRNA is several times larger than that of the mature mRNA species.[4] In collaboration with Dr. Hermona Soreq, it was found that approximately 200 residues at the 3′ end of IF mRNA internal to the poly(A) junction are not necessary for translation of this molecule in oocytes.[5] That the post-transcriptional mechanism which inactivates or degrades IF mRNA during the shutoff phase of poly(I) · poly(C) induction does not affect bulk cellular mRNA was also documented.[6] Finally, in collaboration with Dr. Sohan Lal Gupta, evidence was obtained which strongly suggests that the 2′,5′-oligo(A)-dependent nuclease system is not involved in the post-transcriptional shutoff mechanism.[6]

Kinetics of Synthesis of Interferon by Oocytes of *Xenopus laevis*

We used the oocyte assay for interferon mRNA, first described by Reynolds, Premkumar, and Pitha in 1975[7] as the basic tool in our investigations. This is a fairly reliable and sensitive assay for quantitation of IF mRNA and is now in wide use for this purpose. Figure 1 depicts the kinetics of accumulation of biologically active IF in oocytes microinjected with mRNA preparations from superinduced human fibroblast cultures as determined in our laboratory.[1,2] It should be emphasized first, that groups of oocytes were homogenized in the same aliquot of Barth's medium in which they had been incubated,[1,2] and that the IF titers in oocyte homogenates therefore reflect the total amount of IF present in the system. Second, the ordinate in this figure is logarithmic whereas the abscissa is not. On the basis of data of this kind we concluded that the half-life of IF mRNA microinjected into oocytes is in the 6–8-hr range.[2] This conclusion was called into question in a recent paper.[8] Colman and Morser[8] observed an apparently linear total accumulation of biologically active IF following microinjection into oocytes of lymphoblastoid interferon mRNA preparations, and suggested that IF mRNA was essentially stable within the oocyte.

The appearance of interferon in the incubation medium outside the oocytes has been described recently in several laboratories. Colman and Morser[8] suggest that this represents an active secretory process.

*Research in the authors' laboratory was supported by Grants AI-16262, CA-18608, and CA-18213 from the National Institutes of Health, Department of Health, Education, and Welfare.

0077-8923/80/0350-0405 $01.75/0 © 1980, NYAS

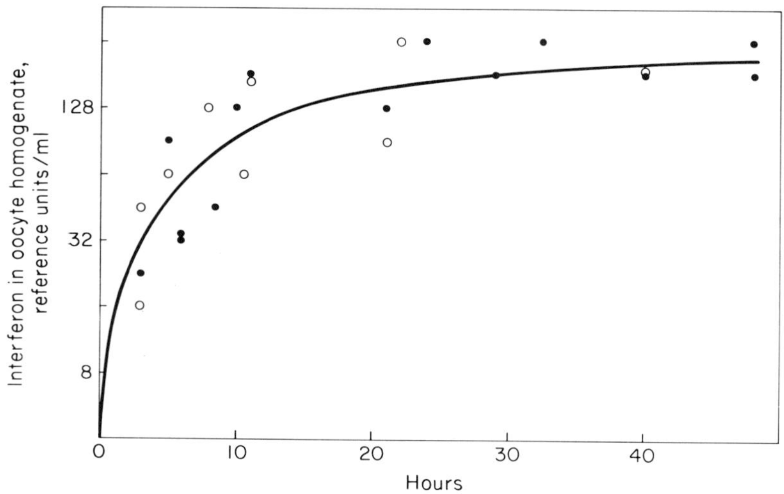

FIGURE 1. Synthesis of interferon in oocytes of *Xenopus laevis* microinjected with poly(A)-containing (●) and deadenylated (○) human fibroblast IF mRNA preparations. Oocytes were homogenized in the same aliquot of modified Barth's medium in which they were incubated. From Sehgal *et al.*[2]

In view of the widespread use of the oocyte assay in the interferon mRNA field we have reevaluated these issues.[3] We have injected ^{3}H-labeled mRNA preparations, derived from superinduced FS-4 cultures, into oocytes and have monitored the following: the degradation of ^{3}H-labeled injected mRNA, the total accumulation of interferon, and the amounts and concentrations of interferon inside and outside the oocytes over a period of 4 days. We have also injected partially purified human fibroblast IF into oocytes and monitored the total amount of IF in the system as well as the amount and concentration inside and outside of the oocytes over a period of 24 hr. The injected oocytes appeared normal even 4 days after microinjection. The main observations and conclusions were as follows: (A) Maximal rates of IF synthesis were observed within one hour of microinjection of mRNA. After 48 hr, there was no detectable increase in the accumulated amount of IF in the system. In some experiments the accumulation was apparently linear up to 48 hr. However, there was always a slow decay of IF titers thereafter. Trichloroacetic acid (10%)-precipitable radioactivity in mRNA inside the oocytes decayed rapidly such that it was 10–15% of the original level at ~24 hr. These results support our earlier conclusion that the half-life of human fibroblast IF mRNA injected into oocytes is 6–8 hr. (B) The *concentration* of IF, outside of the oocytes never exceeded 10–25% of that inside the oocyte cytoplasm. This further justifies our view that we did not grossly damage or kill the oocytes during microinjection. (C) Partially purified human fibroblast IF injected into oocytes decayed minimally (at most twofold) over a period of 24 hr, but leaked out into the surrounding medium such that the *concentration* of interferon inside and outside the oocytes was the same at 24 hr after injection. At this time, because the volume of the outside incubation medium was large compared to the oocyte volume, the total amount of IF outside was 10–20-fold higher than that inside. These data prevent us from excluding leakage as a basis for the appearance of fibroblast IF outside of oocytes after injection of its mRNA. However, we are also unable to rule out secretion at the present time.

SIZE OF THE TRANSCRIPTION UNIT FOR HUMAN FIBROBLAST INTERFERON

Fifteen years ago, Jaqueline and Ed DeMaeyer[9] showed that interferon synthesis could be inhibited by ultraviolet irradiation of induced cells. We have used ultraviolet irradiation to inhibit IF mRNA synthesis and have obtained evidence which suggests that the transcription unit for human fibroblast IF mRNA is severalfold larger than the mature mRNA.[4] The design of these experiments allows us to be reasonably certain that we are dealing with the target size of the transcription unit for the interferon gene *per se* and not with that of an aggregate of genes that might be involved in IF induction.

FIGURE 2 summarizes the result of the experiments carried out in FS-4 cultures. The inactivation characteristics of 18S and 28S ribosomal RNA synthesis are representative of DNA targets of 4000 and 11,000 base-pairs, respectively. The inactivation of interferon mRNA in confluent FS-4 cultures was carried out in one of two ways. FS-4 cultures were first irradiated for varying periods and then incubated for 90 min with poly(I) · poly(C) in the presence of cycloheximide. Alternatively, cultures were first induced with poly(I) · poly(C) and cycloheximide for 30 min, and then irradiated and incubated for a further period of 90 min in the continued presence of cycloheximide. Cycloheximide was included in the culture medium to obtain maximal "superinduction" of IF mRNA synthesis

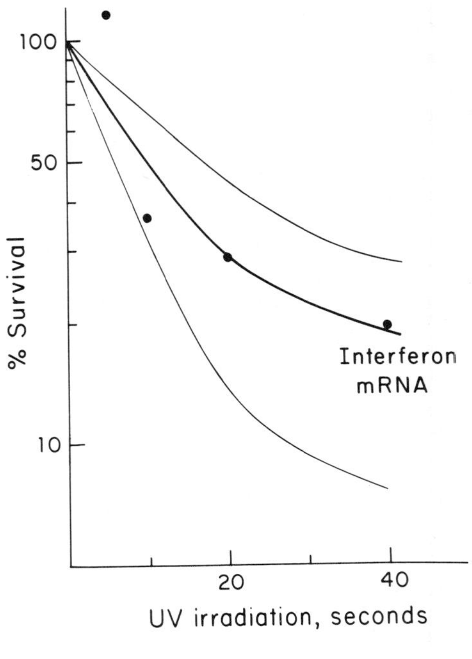

FIGURE 2. Inactivation of the synthesis of poly(I) · poly(C)-induced human fibroblast interferon mRNA (●) by UV-irradiation. The 100% value for interferon mRNA corresponds to an interferon titer of 60 ref. U/ml in the oocyte homogenate. The upper and lower fine lines correspond to the inactivation of the synthesis of 18 S and 28 S ribosomal RNA, respectively.

and thus to prevent the superinducing effect of UV irradiation on IF synthesis from masking the inhibitory effect of UV irradiation on IF mRNA synthesis. Nevertheless, the slight leakiness of the effects of cycloheximide may explain why UV irradiation for 5 sec consistently gave a slightly higher level of IF mRNA than unirradiated controls. Since the [^{3}H]uridine-labeled cultures used in the calibration experiment were incubated for 90 min after UV irradiation,[4] the IF experiments were also terminated at 90 min after irradiation. Polyadenylated RNA was prepared from induced, irradiated cells and assayed for interferon mRNA content using the *Xenopus laevis* oocyte translation assay.

The assumption that the UV sensitivity of interferon mRNA induction is directly proportional to the size of the transcriptional unit for the interferon gene was tested by carrying out the inactivation experiment in the two different ways mentioned. The possibility existed that the RNA product of one or more inducible genes might be necessary for the derepression of the IF gene. If several different genes were functionally linked *in series*, the UV sensitivity of IF induction would not be directly proportional to the size of the transcriptional unit of the IF gene itself. Since exposure of FS-4 cells to poly(I) · poly(C) for 30 min at 37°C is known to be sufficient for full derepression of the interferon gene,[10] we reasoned that all intermediate steps that may be responsible for derepression of the IF gene must be virtually complete within 30 min. If transcription of multiple genes in series were necessary during IF derepression, the UV target size for inactivation of IF induction estimated by irradiating FS-4 cultures prior to induction would be much larger than that estimated by irradiating cultures subsequent to complete induction. However, the results of the two kinds of experiments were closely similar and have been pooled in FIGURE 2.[4] We conclude that the assumption that the UV sensitivity of interferon induction reflects the size of the transcription unit for the interferon gene(s) *per se* is reasonable.

Human fibroblast interferon mRNA appears to be transcribed from a DNA segment of a size within the range from 4 to 11 kb whereas the mature mRNA is approximately 850–900 residues long. Thus, human fibroblast IF mRNA appears to be processed from a precursor RNA roughly 10 times longer than the mature mRNA. These results raise the possibility that human fibroblast (F) and human leukocyte (Le) interferon mRNA species may represent the end products of alternative pathways of processing and splicing of a long precursor RNA, depending upon the phenotype of the induced cell and on the nature of the IF inducer.[4] A precedent for this phenomenon has been established by the work of Segal and colleagues,[11] who described alterations in splicing of SV-40 transcripts depending upon the state of differentiation of host murine teratocarcinoma cells.

STRUCTURE OF HUMAN FIBROBLAST INTERFERON mRNA

TABLE 1 summarizes current information about the structure of human fibroblast interferon mRNA.[5,12] The size of the molecule was estimated by sedimentation of denatured mRNA through a sucrose gradient. The poly(A) length was estimated by determining the concentration of formamide required to elute the mRNA from poly(U)-Sepharose columns. The size of the coding region was derived from data of other investigators, which suggest that the apparent molecular weight of the polypeptide for human fibroblast IF is approximately

15,000–16,000. The assignment of 50–60 residues for an NH_2-terminal signal sequence was based on an assumption that may or may not be true. A signal sequence may be internal and not NH_2-terminal. The extent of the noncoding region was originally arrived at by subtraction. We have now, in collaboration with Dr. Hermona Soreq, obtained evidence indicating that the IF mRNA molecule does indeed contain 200–250 noncoding residues located at the 3′ end internal to the poly(A) junction.[5]

In 1974, Dr. Soreq and coworkers described an elegant procedure for trimming RNA molecules in a controlled and synchronous manner from the 3′ end.[13] The *E. coli* enzyme polynucleotide phosphorylase, abbreviated PNPase, under appropriate ionic conditions binds to the 3′ end of RNA molecules. At 0°C, this enzyme behaves as a 3′ exonuclease and degrades poly(A) in a processive manner, but digests mixed sequence RNA extremely slowly. At 37°C, digestion extends fairly rapidly and includes residues internal to the poly(A). Synchrony is preserved for several minutes at 37°C corresponding to a digestion of up to approximately 600 residues per chain (reviewed in references 14 and 15).

About a year ago we published experiments describing the removal of poly(A) from fibroblast interferon mRNA preparations using PNPase at 4°C, and observed no alteration in the functional stability of the mRNA in oocytes.[2] We have reconfirmed this observation and have since extended this experiment to sequences internal to the poly(A).[5]

TABLE 1

STRUCTURE OF HUMAN FIBROBLAST INTERFERON mRNA

	Residues
Size (12 S)	850–900
Poly(A)	>100
Coding	450–500
Signal (?)	50–60
3′ Terminal noncoding	~200

[^{3}H]Uridine-labeled polyadenylated mRNA preparations from superinduced FS-4 cultures were first trimmed for 20 min on ice with a molar excess of PNPase to remove the poly(A). The temperature was then raised to 37°C and the progress of the reaction monitored in various ways by following ^{3}H radioactivity. We obtained a linear rate of digestion of the RNA. By 120 sec approximately 450 residues had been trimmed from the RNA chains. The residual IF mRNA activity (assayed in oocytes) and the residual cellular mRNA activity (assayed by stimulation of cell-free incorporation of [^{3}H]leucine in a reticulocyte lysate) were determined in mRNA samples digested for 30, 60, 90 and 120 sec at 37°C with PNPase.[5] It was found that the activities both of IF mRNA and cellular mRNA were undiminished for up to 60 sec of incubation with PNPase at 37°C, but decreased thereafter. This corresponds to a loss of approximately 200–300 residues per RNA chain. The data suggest that there may exist a rather large, 3′ noncoding segment in IF mRNA if we assume that the average rate of digestion of mRNAs in a mixture is applicable to interferon mRNA *per se*. Most pure mRNA preparations that have been analyzed by Dr. Soreq and colleagues[14,15] are digested at the same rate as mixtures of RNA. Nevertheless, the crucial experiment will be to document that IF mRNA trimmed for 60 sec at 37°C is shorter than the native molecule by 200–300 residues. Preliminary experiments using sucrose gradient sedimentation suggest that this is likely; however, the resolution is too poor for reliable quantitation. We are in the process of carrying out gel analyses of native and trimmed interferon mRNA molecules in order to substantiate our conclusions about the 3′ end of interferon mRNA.

INTERFERON SUPERINDUCTION AND THE SPECIFICITY OF THE POST-TRANSCRIPTIONAL SHUTOFF MECHANISM

The central effort in our research program relates to the mechanism of interferon superinduction (reviewed in references 16–18). Exposure of confluent FS-4 cultures to poly(I) · poly(C) leads to rapid induction of IF production. The rate of IF secretion peaks within 3 hr and production is then rapidly shut off by 6–8 hr. The transcription of IF mRNA is largely complete in the first 3 hr. However, the *rapid* shutoff of IF production does not appear to be due to the cessation of mRNA transcription but is mediated through a post-transcriptional mechanism which specifically inactivates or degrades IF mRNA. The major basis for this hypothesis is the phenomenon of IF superinduction, first discovered by Youngner and colleagues in 1965 in mice,[19] and subsequently reproduced in cell culture by Vilček and colleagues in 1969[20] and Tan and coworkers in 1970.[21] Judicious exposure of induced cultures to inhibitors of RNA and protein synthesis dramatically increases IF yields.

The main mechanism underlying superinduction is a 15-fold increase in the half-life of interferon mRNA.[1,12,22] We, and others, hypothesize that the rapid shutoff of IF production reflects the existence of a post-transcriptional repressor mechanism which degrades or inactivates IF mRNA and that in the presence of inhibitors of RNA and protein synthesis this mechanism is not activated and thus IF mRNA remains functional for extended periods of time. This markedly increases cumulative interferon yields. We have extensively investigated this phenomenon and are currently engaged in an attempt to unravel the biochemical basis of the shutoff mechanism. We have recently made the basic observation that the shutoff mechanism does not affect bulk cellular mRNA.[3]

Thus, while the rate of IF secretion in FS-4 cultures declines rapidly after reaching a peak subsequent to induction of cells with poly(I) · poly(C), the rate of cellular protein synthesis remains constant.[6] The rate of cellular protein synthesis was monitored by pulsing cultures with [^{3}H]leucine for 10 min at different times during the first 6 hr of induction. Likewise, while the level of fibroblast IF mRNA assayed in oocytes decreases during the shutoff phase, the level of cellular mRNA assayed in reticulocyte lysates remains constant.

The possibility that the level of bulk cellular mRNA remains constant because of continuous synthesis while interferon mRNA level decreases because synthesis is terminated by 3 hr after induction has been eliminated by following the survival of a cohort of cellular mRNA species synthesized during the first 2.5 hr of induction. This was done by labeling cultures with [^{3}H]uridine for 2.5 hours and monitoring the survival of ^{3}H in polyadenylated mRNA during the shutoff phase.[6] The data clearly indicate that the shutoff mechanism does not affect bulk cellular mRNA, but that it inactivates or degrades interferon mRNA in a rather specific manner.

Lack of Involvement of the 2′,5′-Oligo(A)-dependent Nuclease System in the Shutoff Mechanism

Is the 2′,5′ oligo(A)-dependent nuclease involved in the shutoff of IF production? The issue arises because the fibroblast cultures are treated with dsRNA to induce IF production and are then in contact with IF that they have themselves synthesized. Some suggestive evidence that the 2′,5′-oligo(A) system is not involved in the shutoff process is already available in the literature. First, the shutoff mechanism is remarkably specific, whereas the 2′,5′-oligo(A)-dependent nuclease appears to be nonspecific.[6,23,24] Second, numerous descriptions of IF priming[10] suggest that the 2′,5′-oligo(A) system is not involved in the shutoff process. In order to settle this issue, we have, in collaboration with Dr. Sohan Gupta, estimated directly the level of 2′,5′-oligo(A) synthetase in poly(I) · poly(C)-induced FS-4 cultures.[6] There is a low basal level of synthetase activity in confluent FS-4 cultures. Five hours after the start of poly(I) · poly(C) induction this level is virtually unchanged.

We have increased the level of 2′,5′-oligo(A) synthetase by greater than 200-fold in fibroblasts and asked whether this accelerates the decay of interferon mRNA. The increase was achieved by exposing FS-4 cultures to human fibroblast IF (250 reference units/ml, for 17 hr). These cultures were then induced with poly(I) · poly(C) alone as well as in combination with a cycloheximide-actinomycin D superinduction regime. The elevation in synthetase level at 5 hr after induction was simultaneously documented. The data obtained showed that despite a documented 200-fold increase in 2′,5′-oligo(A) synthetase level there was little change in the apparent half-life of IF mRNA in IF-treated cultures as compared to untreated controls during ordinary induction and superinduction. There was however an 8-fold higher level of interferon synthesis at all times in IF-treated cultures, which is evidence of the well-known priming effect of IF.[10]

We conclude that it is very unlikely that the 2′,5′-oligo(A)-dependent mechanism is involved in regulating the half-life of IF mRNA.

References

1. Sehgal, P. B., B. Dobberstein & I. Tamm. 1977. Proc. Nat. Acad. Sci. USA **74:** 3409–3414.
2. Sehgal, P. B., H. Soreq & I. Tamm. 1978. Proc. Nat. Acad. Sci. USA **75:** 5030–5033.
3. Sehgal, P. B. In preparation.
4. Sehgal, P. B. & I. Tamm. 1980. Virology **102:** 245–249.
5. Soreq, H., A. D. Sagar & P. B. Sehgal. In preparation.
6. Sehgal, P. B. & S. L. Gupta. 1980. Proc. Nat. Acad. Sci. USA. **77:** 3489–3493.
7. Reynolds, F. H., E. Premkumar & P. M. Pitha. 1975. Proc. Nat. Acad. Sci. USA **72:** 4881–4885.
8. Colman, A. & J. Morser. 1979. Cell **17:** 517–526.
9. De Maeyer-Guignard, J. & E. De Maeyer. 1965. Nature **205:** 985–987.
10. Stewart, W. E. II. 1979. The Interferon System. Springer-Verlag. Vienna and New York.
11. Segal, S., A. J. Levine & G. Khoury. 1979. Nature **280:** 335–338.
12. Sehgal, P. B., D. Lyles & I. Tamm. 1978. Virology **89:** 186–198.
13. Soreq, H., U. Nudel, R. Salomon, M. Revel & U. Z. Littauer. 1974. J. Mol. Biol. **88:** 233–245.
14. Littauer, U. Z., H. Soreq & P. Cornelis. 1979. *In* Proceedings of the special FEBS meeting on Enzymes. Pergamon Press. In press.

15. LITTAUER, U. Z. & H. SOREQ. 1980. Prog. Nuc. Acid Res. Mol. Biol. In press.
16. TAMM, I. & P. B. SEHGAL. 1978. Adv. Virus Res. **22:** 187–258.
17. SEHGAL, P. B. & I. TAMM. 1978. Biochem. Pharmacol. **27:** 2475–2485.
18. TAMM, I. & P. B. SEHGAL. 1979. *In* Specific Eukaryotic Genes, Alfred Benzon Symposium 13. J. Engberg, H. Klenow & V. Leick. Eds.:424–439. Munksgaard. Copenhagen.
19. YOUNGNER, J. S., W. R. STINEBRING & S. E. TAUBE. 1965. Virology **27:** 541–550.
20. VILČEK, J., T. A. ROSSMAN & F. VARACALLI. 1969. Nature **222:** 682–683.
21. TAN, Y. H., J. A. ARMSTRONG, Y. K. KE & M. HO. 1970. Proc. Nat. Acad. Sci. USA **67:** 464–471.
22. CAVALIERI, R. L., E. A. HAVELL, J. VILČEK & S. PESTKA. 1977. Proc. Nat. Acad. Sci. USA **74:** 4415–4419.
23. CLEMENS, M. J. & B. R. G. WILLIAMS. 1978. Cell **13:** 565–572.
24. HOVANESSIAN, A. G., J. WOOD, E. MEURS & L. MONTAGNIER. 1979. Proc. Nat. Acad. Sci. USA **76:** 3261–3265.

THE INDUCTION AND CHARACTERIZATION OF INTERFERON FROM PURE CULTURES OF MURINE MACROPHAGES*

Edward A. Havell and George L. Spitalny

Trudeau Institute, Inc.
Saranac Lake, New York 12983

Introduction

The macrophage is an integral element in both humoral and cell-mediated immunity. A number of studies have shown that either the *in vivo* or *in vitro* administration of either interferon (IF) or interferon-inducing agents can have a pronounced effect on macrophage morphology and function.[1-3] Interferon or agents that elicit interferon have been demonstrated to enhance both macrophage spreading[2] and the ingestion of IgG-coated erythrocytes.[4] Furthermore, IF has rendered macrophages cytotoxic for syngeneic tumor cells.[3] Macrophages have also been found to produce IF in response to a wide variety of agents, including viruses, double-stranded RNA, polysaccharides, bacteria, endotoxin, and polyanions.[5,6] Several studies have implicated the macrophage as the source of the early appearing serum IF after the intravenous administration of either endotoxin[7] or the synthetic polyribonucleotide Poly (I)·Poly (C).[8]

The studies on both IF induction and the effect of IF on macrophage functions have been carried out for the most part with freshly seeded adherent cell populations obtained from the peritoneal cavity. While attached cells have been considered to be macrophages, these cultures are known to consist of a heterogeneous array of other cell types, which includes lymphoid cells.[9] In this report, we have examined the ability of different agents to induce IF in pure murine macrophage cultures derived from bone marrow. These pure macrophage cultures were derived from bone marrow and were grown to confluency *in vitro*. The IF produced by these macrophage cultures has been compared to other murine IFs with regards to certain physical and antigenic properties.

Materials and Methods

Bone Marrow-derived Macrophage Cultures

Murine bone marrow macrophages were obtained by perfusing femurs and tibias from $AB6F_1$ mice (A × C57BL/6) with 1–2 ml of medium. Cell aggregates were dispersed by repeated pipetting and then centrifuged at 200 × g for 5 min. The cell pellets were then suspended at a concentration of 2×10^6 cells/ml and 35 × 10 mm dishes (Falcon Plastics) were seeded with 1 ml of the cell suspension in culture medium. A modified version of the growth medium originally used by Stewart *et al.*[10] to propagate murine macrophages was used in these studies. The

*This work was supported by United States Public Health Service Grants AI-15348 and CA-21360, and Contracts N00014-78-C-0610 from the Office of Naval Research, and RR05705 from the Division of Research Resources, National Institutes of Health

0077-8923/80/0350-0413 $01.75/0 © 1980, NYAS

modified growth medium consisted of RPMI 1640 (GIBCO) medium containing 10% fetal bovine serum (FBS), 5% horse serum, and supplemented with 10% of 0.22 μm filtered L-cell-conditioned medium that was originally used to grow murine L929B cells. The macrophage growth medium also contained penicillin (100 units/ml), streptomycin (100 μg/ml) and gentamycin (50 μg/ml). The cultures were incubated at 37°C in a 5% CO_2 atmosphere for 48 hr, after which the cultures were washed to remove nonadherent cells and reincubated with 3 ml of growth medium. The cultures were replenished with 3 ml of fresh growth medium 4 days later. The macrophages routinely reached confluency after 9 days in culture and were induced on the following day. The day before IF induction, the growth medium containing L-cell-conditioned medium was changed to RPMI 1640 containing 10% FBS and antibiotics, without conditioned L-cell medium, to stop proliferation.

Interferon-inducing Agents and Induction Procedures

Newcastle disease virus (Hickman strain) was propagated in 11-day-old fertile hen eggs and had a titer of 10^9 plaque-forming units/ml when assayed on chick embryo cells. The synthetic polyribonucleotide polyinosinic-polycytidylic acid, Poly (I)·Poly (C), was purchased from P-L Laboratories (Milwaukee, WI). *Salmonella enteritidis* (3105–25) endotoxin was purchased from Difco (Detroit, MI).

Triplicate cultures of macrophages were routinely induced for 2 hr, after which the cultures were washed 4X with Hanks' balanced salt solution (GIBCO) and 1 ml of RPMI 1640 containing 5% FBS was placed on the cultures and the cultures reincubated at 37°C in 5% CO_2. Interferon preparations obtained from virus-induced cultures were acidified to pH 2.0 for 5 days (to inactivate virus) and then returned to pH 7.4 by dialysis against phosphate buffered saline (pH 7.4).

The murine L-cell IF was made by inducing confluent 4-day-old L929B cultures with 20 μg/ml Poly (I)·Poly (C) and 400 μg/ml of diethylaminoethyl (DEAE)-dextran in Eagle's Minimal Essential Medium (MEM) for 6 hr. After the incubation period, the cultures were extensively washed, and replenished with MEM containing 0.1% FBS. Phytohemagglutinin (Burroughs Wellcome, Co.)-induced "immune" IF was obtained from spleen cell cultures established according to a method previously described.[12] Phytohemagglutinin was added to the spleen cultures at a concentration of 5 μg/ml for 48 hr.

Interferon Assays and Antibody Neutralizations

Interferon assays were done by the micromethod of Armstrong[12] as modified by Havell and Vilček[13] using murine L-929B cells. All IF assays included the murine IF standard (G-002-904-511) and all titers given are in international IF reference units.

The antiserum neutralization assays of IF activities on L929B cells were performed as previously described by Havell *et al.*[14] The rabbit anti-murine L-cell IF globulin (A-L Inf. No. 12, 3/17/72) was obtained from the Research Resources Branch of the National Institute of Allergy and Infectious Diseases (Bethesda, MD).

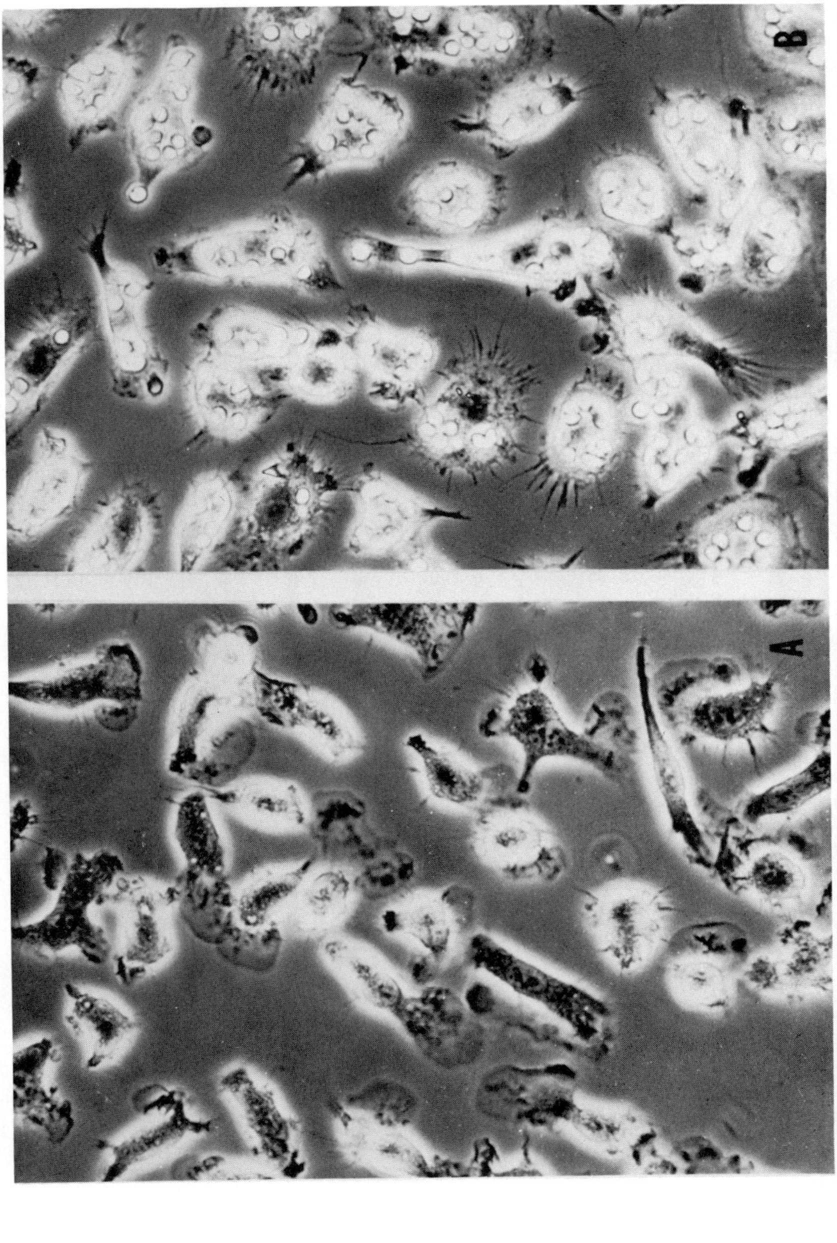

FIGURE 1. *Panel A* shows the morphological features of murine bone marrow-derived macrophages in culture. The evidence that these cells are macrophages is presented in *Panel B*, which shows the ability of these cultures to ingest IgG-coated sheep red cells.

Results

Ten-day-old bone marrow-derived macrophage cultures (FIGURE 1) were treated with different inducing agents in order to determine if the cultures could be stimulated to produce IF (TABLE 1). Newcastle disease virus (NDV) at high multiplicities of infection (MOI) induced high titers of IF and at the highest MOI (100) the yield per cell was equivalent to or exceeded the yields of IF produced by L-cells (Havell and Spitalny, unpublished observations). The synthetic polyribonucleic acid Poly (I)·Poly (C) at a concentration of 10 μg/ml with or without diethylaminoethyl-dextran (DEAE-dextran) did not induce IF. However, 100 μg/ml of Poly (I)·Poly (C) stimulated the macrophages to produce 128 units of IF. Exposure of macrophages to 50 μg/ml of endotoxin failed to elicit IF.

The rate of IF synthesis by macrophages was measured in cultures induced with either 100 μg/ml of Poly (I)·Poly (C) or NDV at a MOI of 10 (FIGURE 2). After a 2-hr induction period, the cultures were washed and reincubated with fresh medium and at the indicated intervals the culture fluids were collected and the cells washed and reincubated with fresh medium. The yields of IF are expressed as IF units synthesized/hr. The Poly (I)·Poly (C)-induced macrophage cultures produced peak levels of IF between 3–5 hr from the start of induction, whereas NDV-induced macrophages produced considerably more interferon with peak levels synthesized between 10–12 hr.

Incubation of cells with low doses of IF prior to induction has been reported to enhance or "prime" IF production in a number of different systems.[13,15] The effect of priming macrophage cultures with varying concentrations of L-cell IF for 18 hr prior to induction was examined (TABLE 2). Pretreatment of the macrophages with IF followed by induction with either Poly (I)·Poly (C) (100 μg/ml) or endotoxin (50 μg/ml) resulted in enhanced levels of IF activity. For both Poly (I)·Poly (C) and endotoxin inductions, there appeared to be a dose-dependent relationship between the amount of IF used to pretreat the macrophages and the resulting IF yield. The results also show that IF pretreatment of the macrophage cultures induced with NDV (MOI of 10) inhibited the production

TABLE 1

INTERFERON INDUCTION IN MURINE MACROPHAGES DERIVED FROM BONE MARROW

Interferon-inducing Agent*	24-Hour Interferon Titer (units/ml)
Newcastle disease virus	
0.1 (MOI)	32
1	384
10	1024
100	16,384
Poly (I) · Poly (C)	
10 μg/ml	<4
100 μg/ml	128
Poly (I) · Poly (C) 10 μg/ml	
+ DEAE dextran (100 μg/ml)	<4
Endotoxin 50 μg/ml	<4

*Newcastle disease virus was added to cultures in 0.4 ml of phosphate-buffered saline (pH 7.4) at the designated MOI. The cultures were then tilted every 15 min for the 2-hr induction period. Cultures induced with either Poly (I). Poly (C) or endotoxin received 1 ml of the agents in RPMI 1640.

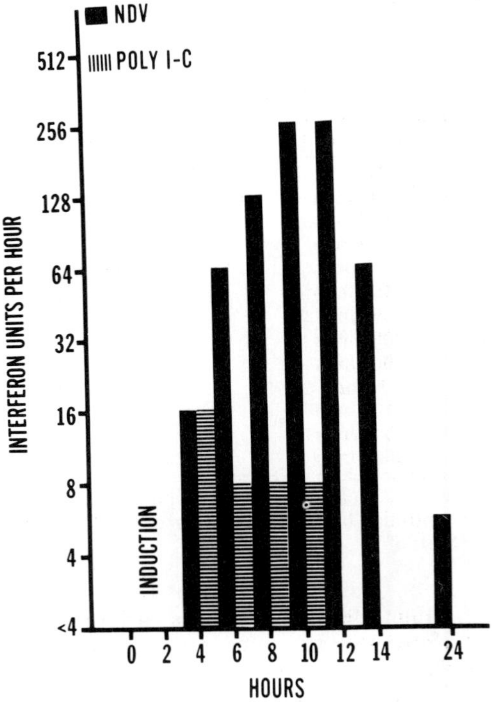

FIGURE 2. Kinetics of interferon released from macrophages after a 2-hr induction period with 100 μg/ml of Poly (I)·Poly (C) or with Newcastle disease virus (MOI of 10). The culture fluids were collected at the indicated hours and the cultures were reincubated with fresh medium, until the next collection time. The interferon yield per hour was calculated by dividing the units/ml present in a sample at the indicated hour of collection by the number of hours elapsed from the time the previous sample was collected.

of IF by the cultures. It was also noticed that exposure of the macrophages to IF resulted in a dramatic change in morphology and the cells exhibited increased spreading, ruffled plasma membranes, and vacuolization.

Studies were carried out to characterize several properties of macrophage IF. The macrophage IF, like L-cell or a serum interferon preparation obtained two hours after the intravenous injection of 20 μg of Poly (I)·Poly (C), was relatively stable at a low pH (2.0) for 5 days (TABLE 3). An "immune" serum interferon preparation obtained by injecting old tuberculin (OT) into mice, which 3 weeks earlier were infected with BCG, was totally inactivated by the acid treatment. Heating these same IFs at 56°C for 30 minutes abolished all of the macrophage IF activity and virtually all of the serum IF activity induced by Poly (I)·Poly (C). On the other hand, the L-cell IF and the OT-induced serum interferon activities were relatively more stable to heat. In a preliminary experiment, we have observed that both macrophage and Poly (I)·Poly (C)-induced serum IF expressed higher antiviral activities when assayed on both human and bovine cultures than did a Poly (I)·Poly (C) L-cell IF preparation. On the basis of these observations, macrophage IF appears to be very similar to the Poly (I)·Poly (C) serum IF preparation. Differences were also found between the molecular weights of L-cell and macrophage IFs when analyzed by sodium dodecyl sulfate-poly-acrylamide gel electrophoresis. The L-cell IF activity was found to migrate as two molecular weight components of 43,000 and 26,000, whereas the macrophage IF appeared to be composed of a single molecular weight component with an apparent molecular weight of 43,000 (results not shown).

TABLE 2

INTERFERON INDUCTION IN BONE MARROW MACROPHAGE CULTURES PRETREATED WITH INTERFERON

Interferon (units/ml) Pretreatment*	Interferon-inducing Agent	24-hr Interferon Titer (units/ml)
None	Poly (I) · Poly (C) (100 μg/ml)	128
10 Units	↓	256
50 Units		1056
100 Units		2048
None	Endotoxin (50 μg/ml)	<4
10 Units	↓	4
50 Units		8
100 Units		32
100 Units	None	<4
None	Newcastle disease virus†	768
10 Units	↓	<4
50 Units		<4
100 Units		<4

*Murine L-cell interferon was added directly to the culture medium to achieve the final concentration of interferon (units/ml) 18-hr prior to the interferon-inducing agents.

†MOI of 1.

A neutralization assay was performed on the antiviral activity of macrophage interferon using an antiserum prepared against murine L-cell IF (TABLE 4). The results show that the antiviral activities of macrophage, L-cell, and serum IF preparations were all neutralized to approximately the same degree by the antiserum. The antiviral activity of an IF produced by spleen cell cultures, which were induced by exposure to the T-cell mitogen phytohemagglutinin (PHA), was not neutralized by the antiserum. This PHA-induced spleen cell IF has been classified as "immune" or type II IF because of its inactivation by acid.

TABLE 3

THE EFFECT OF LOW pH ON THE ANTIVIRAL ACTIVITIES OF VARIOUS MURINE INTERFERON PREPARATIONS

Source of Interferon	Interferon-Inducing Agent	Interferon Treatment: Interferon Units pH 2.0‡ Before	After	Interferon Units 56°C/30″ Before	After
Serum	Poly (I) · Poly (C)*	8,192	8,192	1024	16
	Old tuberculin†	512	<8	192	48
L cells	Poly (I) · Poly (C)	12,288	16,384	2048	512
Macrophages	Poly (I) · Poly (C)	256	128	128	<4

*Serum interferon was collected 2 hr after the intravenous injection of either 20 μg of Poly (I) · Poly (C) or 10 mg protein of old tuberculin (OT).

†Mice receiving OT were immunized intravenously 3 weeks earlier with 10^7 BCG.

‡Samples were dialyzed against Sorensen's Glycine-HCl buffer (pH 2.0) for 5 days at 4°C. The samples were returned to pH 7.4 by dialysis against phosphate-buffered saline (pH 7.4) prior to assay.

DISCUSSION

Three distinct human interferons have been identified,[14,17] and there is growing evidence that other species are capable of producing multiple IFs.[16,18] The differences between IFs have been detected by physiochemical, biological, and antigenic analysis. Interferon has become a generic term used to describe a class of induced glycoproteins that are characterized by the common ability of rendering cells resistant to viral multiplication. In addition to this activity, there are a number of other biological activities attributed to IFs, which include inhibition of cell division[19] and immunoregulatory properties.[20] The existence of multiple IFs raises the fundamental question as to the exact function of each IF in the host's mechanism of defense against disease. Macrophages can act as effector cells in the response against infectious and neoplastic disease. Various lymphoid cells and macrophages are known to produce IF, and it is known that IF can alter macrophage morphology and certain functions.[1-3] Thus, it is essential that IFs derived from the different cells involved in the expression of immunity be characterized and analyzed to determine if they differ in abilities to exert different biological actions and influence other cellular components involved in immunity.

TABLE 4

ANTIGENIC NATURES OF DIFFERENT MURINE INTERFERON PREPARATIONS

Source of Interferon	Interferon-Inducing Agent	Degree of Neutralization* of Antiviral Activities by Anti-L-Cell Interferon Serum
Spleen cell	Phytohemagglutinin	< 10
L cells	Poly (I) · Poly (C)	900
Macrophages	Poly (I) · Poly (C)	1200
Serum	Poly (I) · Poly (C)	600

*The reciprocal of the dilution of rabbit anti-murine L-cell interferon which neutralizes the antiviral activity of 20 units/ml of interferon contained in an equal volume.

We have been examining the ability of pure populations of bone marrow macrophages to produce IF and have performed certain characterizations of this macrophage product. Our studies have demonstrated that under appropriate conditions macrophage cultures can be induced to produce IF with a variety of agents including endotoxin. Macrophages treated with NDV (MOI of 100) produce very high levels of IF, but treatment of these cultures with IF prior to NDV induction abolishes the IF-producing ability of these cells. On the other hand, IF "priming" of macrophages markedly enhanced the IF levels produced by induction with either Poly (I)·Poly (C) or endotoxin. Macrophage IF is clearly a type I IF in that it is relatively stable in acid (pH 2.0) and is neutralized by an antiserum raised against an L-cell IF preparation. However, unlike L-cell IF the antiviral activity is totally abolished by heating (56°C/30 min). A murine serum interferon preparation obtained 2 hr after intravenous injection of Poly (I)·Poly (C) was found to exhibit similar properties to macrophage-produced IF and it is conceivable that macrophages could be the source of the early appearing serum IF in response to certain inducing agents *in vivo*.

Interferons have been reported to be capable of modulating certain immune responses and our ultimate goal is to determine the possible function of IFs in the generation and expression of immunity. We have been able to induce IF in pure macrophage cultures and have partially characterized it with regards to certain properties. Eventually, we plan to compare the relative activity of different murine IFs on various macrophage functions such as phagocytosis, bactericidal, and tumoricidal activities. This approach may elucidate the possible functions of IFs in immunity.

REFERENCES

1. HUANG, K., R. M. DONAHOE, F. B. GORDON & H. R. DRESSLER. 1971. Enhancement of phagocytosis by interferon containing preparations. Infect. Immun. **4:** 581–588.
2. RABINOVITCH, M. R. E. MANEJIAS, M. RUSSO & E. E. ABBEY. 1977. Increased spreading of macrophages from mice treated with interferon inducers. Cell. Immunol. **29:** 86–95.
3. SCHULTZ, R. M., M. A. CHIRIGOS & U. I. HEINE. 1978. Functional and morphologic characteristics of interferon-treated macrophages. Cell. Immunol. **35:** 84–91.
4. HAMBURG, S. I., R. E. MANEJIAS & M. RABINOVITCH. 1978. Macrophage activation: Increased ingestion of IgG-coated erythrocytes after administration of interferon inducers to mice. J. Exp. Med. **147:** 593–598.
5. BORECKÝ, L., V. LACKOVIČ & N. FUCHSBERGER. 1970. Comparison of interferon production in mouse leukocytes by statolon and complexed polyribonucleotide (Poly (I)·Poly (C)). Acta Virol. **14:** 329–336.
6. SCHULTZ, R. M., J. D. PAPAMATHEAKIS & M. A. CHIRIGOS. 1977. Interferon: An inducer of macrophage activation by polyanions. Science **197:** 674–675.
7. ITO, Y., I. NAGATA & A. KUNII. 1973. Mechanism of endotoxin-type interferon production in mice. Virology **52:** 439–446.
8. TALAS, M., E. SZOLGAY, V. VARTERESZ & A. G. KOCZK. 1972. Influence of acute and fractional X-irradiation on induction *in vivo*. Arch. gesamte Virusforsch. **38:** 143–148.
9. NATHAN, C. F., R. ASOFSKY & W. D. TERRY. 1977. Characterization of the nonphagocytic adherent cell from the peritoneal cavity of normal and BCG-treated mice. J. Immunol. **118:** 1612–1621.
10. STEWART, C. C., H. S. LIN & C. ADLES. 1975. Proliferation and colony-forming ability of peritoneal exudate cells in liquid culture. J. Exp. Med. **141:** 1114–1132.
11. OSBORNE, L. C., J. A. GEORGIADES & H. M. JOHNSON. 1979. Large scale production and partial purification of mouse immune interferon. Infect. Immun. **23:** 80–86.
12. ARMSTRONG, J. A. 1971. Semi-micro, dye binding assay for rabbit interferon. Appl. Microbiol. **21:** 723–726.
13. HAVELL, E. A. & J. VILČEK. 1972. Production of high titered interferon in cultures of human diploid cells. Antimicrob. Agents Chemother. **2:** 476–484.
14. HAVELL, E. A., B. BERMAN, C. A. OGBURN, K. BERG, K. PAUCKER & J. VILČEK. 1975. Two antigenically distinct species of human interferon. Proc. Nat. Acad. Sci. USA **72:** 2185–2190.
15. BURKE, D. C. & A. ISAACS. 1958. Some factors affecting the production of interferon. Br. J. Exp. Pathol. **39:** 452–458.
16. HO, M. & J. A. ARMSTRONG. 1975. Interferon. Annu. Rev. Microbiol. **29:** 131–161.
17. VALLE, M. J., G. W. JORDAN, S. HAAHR & T. C. MERIGAN. 1975. Characteristics of immune interferon produced by human lymphocyte cultures compared to other human interferons. J. Immunol. **115:** 230–244.
18. MAEHARA, N., M. HO & J. A. ARMSTRONG. 1977. Differences in mouse interferons according to cell source and mode of induction. Infect. Immun. **17:** 572–579.

19. GRESSER, I., D. BROUTY-BOYE, M. T. THOMAS & A. MACIERIA-COELHO. 1970. Interferon and cell division. I. Inhibition of the multiplication of mouse leukemia L_{1210} cells *in vitro* by interferon preparations. Proc. Nat. Acad. Sci. USA **66:** 1052–1058.
20. JOHNSON, H. M. & S. BARON. 1976. Regulatory role of interferons in the immune response. Int. Res. Commun. Sys. Med. Sci. **4:** 50–52.

ANTIGENIC RELATIONSHIPS AMONG VARIOUS INTERFERON SPECIES

Y. Kawade, Y. Yamamoto, J. Fujisawa, and Y. Watanabe

Institute for Virus Research
Kyoto University
Kyoto 606, Japan

Multiple molecular forms of interferon (IF) are known to exist in various animal species, but the structural basis of the heterogeneity has remained largely unknown (see for review, Stewart[1]). The antigenicity of IF[2] has proved highly useful for analyzing the relationship of different interferons or the molecular composition of a given interferon preparation. Not only are IFs from different animal species antigenically different, but within a given species, type I (virus- or double-strand RNA-induced) and type II (immune) interferons are distinguishable. For human IFs, type I IF is further divided into two antigenically distinct species: leukocyte-type and fibroblast-type.[3]

Not much is known of the antigenicity of IFs from other animal species. Here we have summarized our studies on mouse IFs, which showed that various type I mouse IFs consist of two antigenically distinct species; the antigenicities of each of them from different sources are common, regardless of lymphoid or nonlymphoid origin. Furthermore, one of them was found to be neutralized by an antiserum against human leukocyte IF, suggesting a structural similarity between the important species of human and mouse IFs.

Distinct Antigenicity of the Two Species of L-Cell Interferon

L cells induced by Newcastle disease virus (NDV) are well known to produce two species of IF, which we call F (22-24K) and S (32-40K), differing in various properties.[4] They are both glycoproteins,[5] but their sugar moieties are different, as indicated by the binding of S, but not F, to a galactose-binding lectin from *Wistaria floribunda*.[6] On the other hand, their polypeptide moieties appeared to be partially common in the tryptic peptide analyses of the purified IFs.[7]

They were found to be distinct in antigenicity.[8] Antisera raised in rabbits against the isolated F and S IFs neutralized the respective IFs well, with titers (defined as the reciprocal of serum dilution that neutralizes 10 units of IF) of several thousands, but did not appreciably neutralize the heterologous IFs. The absence of cross-reactions was also indicated by affinity chromatographies using immobilized antibodies, as well as immobilized IFs. If a common structure is shared by the two IFs, it appears to be immunologically silent.

Interferons from poly C·poly I-induced L cells and from NDV-induced C243 cells were found also to consist of two species that are antigenically indistinguishable from F and S interferons, although S interferon was predominant in these preparations.

Interferon produced by NDV-induced L cells in the presence of tunicamycin, a glycosylation inhibitor, contains little F and S species, but consists of a nonglycosylated species with 18K,[5] termed here T. It was found to be F-type in antigenicity, with no measurable reactivity to anti-S antibody.[9] These findings are

0077-8923/80/0350-0422 $01.75/0 © 1980, NYAS

consistent with the idea that both F and S molecules are derived by glycosylation of the 18K species.[5,10] If this were true, however, one must assume a drastic change in antigenic specificity upon attachment of the sugar moiety to T to form S (but not F) molecules. This appears unlikely, since glycosidase treatment of S reduced its molecular weight by 5 to 10K without altering its antigenicity.[9] We tentatively favor the view that the protein moieties of F and S interferons are not identical, and anti-F and anti-S antibodies recognize the difference in their protein moieties, rather than the difference in the sugar or a change in protein structure that might occur upon glycosylation.

Mouse Interferons from Lymphocytes and Other Nonfibroblastic Origins

Type I IF from mouse lymphocytes was reported to be neutralizable by antibody against L-cell interferon,[11] in apparent contrast to human IFs. We examined various preparations of type I mouse interferons listed in Table 1 for their reactivity to anti-L cell interferon sera. All these were found to be

Table 1

Antigenicity of Type I Mouse Interferons of Nonfibroblastic Origins

			Antigenicity*		
Cell	Inducer	Reference	F-type	S-type	Other†
Spleen lymphocyte	Sendai virus	19	+	+	0
Spleen lymphocyte	UV-Sendai virus	19	+	+	0
Spleen lymphocyte	Influenza virus	20	+	+	0
Spleen macrophage	Influenza virus	20	+	+	0
L1210	NDV	21	0	+	0
M1‡	Poly C · poly I	22	+	+	0

*Presence of the designated species is indicated by +, and absence (less than 2%) by 0.
†Not neutralizable by anti-F and anti-S sera, or not retained by the antibody columns.
‡A line of myeloid leukemia cell.

efficiently neutralized by anti-L cell interferon or by a mixture of anti-F and anti-S antibodies. When analyzed for binding to the anti-F and anti-S antibody columns, they were found to consist of molecular species that are bound either to anti-F or anti-S antibody, and no significant fractions were found that were unreactive toward them.

The relative abundance of the two species varied in these IFs. Thus, F-type species generally predominated in virus-induced lymphocyte IFs, whereas S-type was the major species in macrophage and M1 interferons, and no F-type was found in L1210 interferon, although we do not know how variable the ratio is in independent preparations from the same sources.

We conclude that the two antigenic types we recognized in L-cell IF represent the two basic type I IF species in the mouse, regardless of the kind of producing cell.

This may appear at variance with human IFs, but recently it has become clear that human leukocytes[3] and lymphoblastoid cells,[12] as well as fibroblasts,[13] may produce both leukocyte- and fibroblast-type species. We may then speculate that

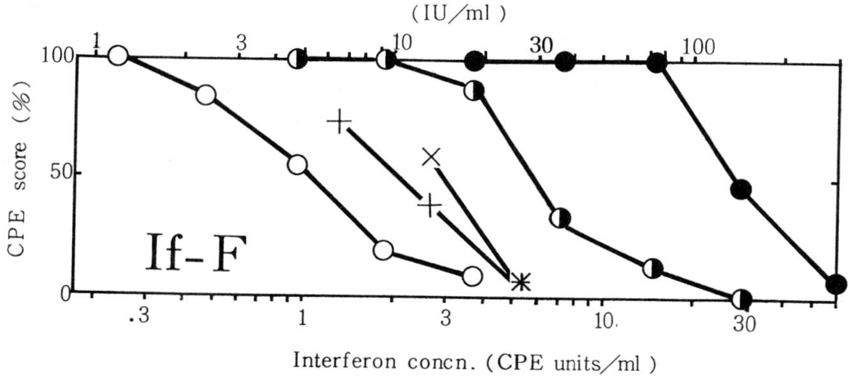

FIGURE 1. Neutralization of interferon F from L cell by anti-human leukocyte interferon sera. Interferon F was separated from S by polyacrylamide gel electrophoresis at pH 4.3 of partially purified L-cell interferon.[23] Interferon at indicated concentrations (lower scale in laboratory units, and upper scale in international reference units) and fixed concentrations of antiserum were added to L-cell cultures in microtiter plates. After 24 hr at 37°C, the cultures were challenged with vesicular stomatitis virus, and the cytopathic effect after 2 days was scored.[8] ○ Interferon without antibody. ◑,● Antiserum #1 from rabbit at dilutions of 1:200 and 1:50, respectively. +,x Antiserum #2 from sheep at 1:400 and 1:100.

the two species of mouse IF might be the mouse counterparts of human leukocyte- and fibroblast-type IFs. Broadly speaking, mouse F and human leukocyte IFs appear somewhat similar to each other in several respects, as do mouse S and human fibroblast IFs. Thus, compared to the latter two, the former two usually predominate in IFs of lymphoid origin, are more heat-stable at moderate temperatures, more susceptible to reducing agents upon heat denaturation in SDS,[14,15] and tend to have higher cross-species activities,[1,16,17] although the distinctions are not always clear-cut. In partial support of this notion, we found an antigenic relatedness between F and human leukocyte IFs, but not between the other pair.

ANTIGENIC CROSS-REACTION BETWEEN MOUSE AND HUMAN INTERFERONS

There has been no direct evidence indicating structural homology among IFs from different animal species, and few, if any, antigenic cross-reactions were observed. Recently, however, Havell[18] found that a small fraction of L-cell interferon (1 to 2%) reacted well with anti-human leukocyte IF antibody.

We examined the F and S species of L-cell IF individually for neutralization by antisera against human leukocyte and fibroblast IFs donated by Dr. J. Vilček of New York University. A rabbit antiserum against human leukocyte IF was found to neutralize F IF completely, as shown in FIGURE 1, although the neutralization titer was about one-tenth of that against human leukocyte interferon (8000). The F-type IF from mouse lymphocytes isolated by antibody affinity chromatography was similarly neutralized by the serum. Another antiserum from sheep with a titer of 5000 gave only marginal neutralization (FIGURE 1).

On the other hand, interferon F was not appreciably neutralized by anti-human fibroblast sera with homologous titers of 8000 and 2000, and interferon S likewise did not show clear signs of reaction with both antisera against human leukocyte and fibroblast IFs, as shown in FIGURE 2. The small decreases in virus resistance observed in these cases (FIG. 2) using high concentrations of the antisera (1:50) may not be regarded as significant.

The reverse situation, human IFs against anti-mouse IF antibodies, is now being investigated.

Our results thus strongly suggest a structural similarity, and hence an evolutionary relationship, between one of the two major species of type I mouse interferon, F, and human leukocyte interferon. Our results are qualitatively similar to Havell's,[18] but different in that the cross-reacting mouse IF represents one important species, rather than a small fraction. One of the reasons why this has escaped detection by other investigators may be that, when unfractionated mouse IFs are used, the other major species, S-type, will remain unreacted, and obscure the usual neutralization tests.

It seems worthwhile to further search for antigenic homologies of IFs from various animals, using fractionated IF species or antibody affinity column techniques.

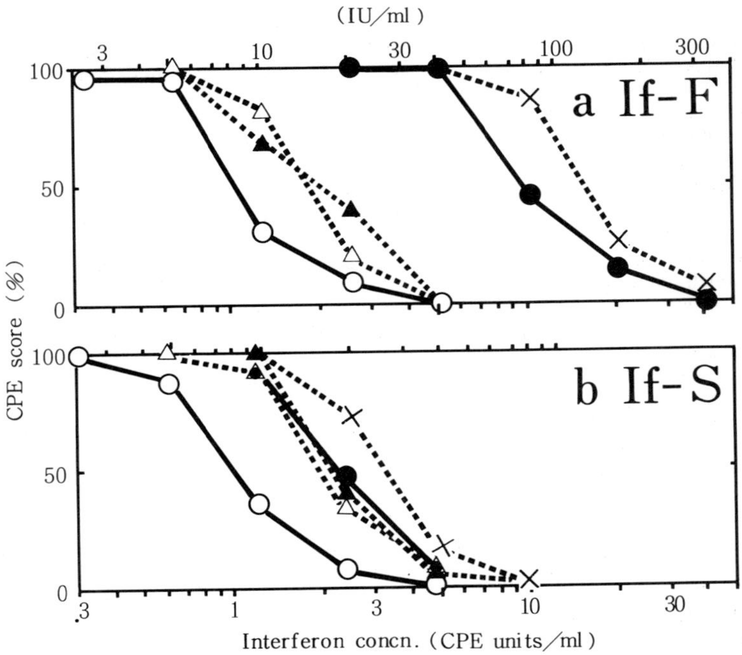

FIGURE 2. Lack of significant neutralization of (a) interferon F by anti-human fibroblast, and (b) interferon S by anti-human fibroblast and anti-human leukocyte sera. The experimental method was the same as that of Figure 1. —O— Interferon without antibody. ——△——,——▲—— Two batches of anti-fibroblast interferon sera, 1:50. —●— Anti-leukocyte interferon serum #1, 1:200 in (a) and 1:50 in (b). ——x—— Anti-fibroblast interferon, 1:50, plus anti-leukocyte interferon.

Summary

Mouse L-cell interferon consists of two antigenically distinct species, F (22 to 24K) and S (32 to 40K). Various type I mouse interferons, regardless of lymphoid or nonlymphoid origin, likewise consist of two species, whose antigenicities are indistinguishable from the two L-cell interferons. Interferon F was found to be completely neutralizable by an antiserum against human leukocyte interferon, suggesting a structural similarity between the important species of human and mouse interferons.

Acknowledgments

We thank Dr. J. Vilček of New York University for generous gifts of antisera, and Dr. Y. Ito of Nagoya University, Dr. K. Tsukui of the Red Cross Central Blood Center, Tokyo, and Dr. M. Tomida of the Saitama Cancer Center Research Institute for kindly providing interferons. This work was aided in part by a grant from the Japanese Ministry of Education.

References

1. Stewart II, W. E. 1979. The Interferon System. Springer Verlag. Vienna.
2. Paucker, K. 1977. Antigenic properties. *In* The Interferon System: A current review to 1978. S. Baron and F. Dianzani, Eds. Tex. Rep. Biol. Med. **35:** 23–28.
3. Havell, E. A., B. Berman, C. A. Ogburn, K. Paucker & J. Vilček. 1975. Two antigenically distinct species of human interferon. Proc. Nat. Acad. Sci. USA **72:** 2185–2187.
4. Kawade, Y. 1977. Purification of murine interferon. Tex. Rep. Biol. Med. **35:** 181–186.
5. Fujisawa, J., Y. Iwakura & Y. Kawade. 1978. Nonglycosylated mouse L cell interferon produced by the action of tunicamycin. J. Biol. Chem. **253:** 8677–8679.
6. Yamamoto, Y. 1979. Two molecular species of mouse L cell interferon differing in lectin binding. J. Gen. Virol. **42:** 533–539.
7. Iwakura, Y. Kawade & Y., S. Yonehara. 1978. Presence of a common structure in the two molecular species of mouse L cell interferon. Biochem. Biophys. Res. Commun. **84:** 557–563.
8. Yamamoto, Y. & Y. Kawade. 1980. Virology **103:** 80–88.
9. Fujisawa, J. & Y. Kawade. Unpublished results.
10. Stewart II, W. E., T. Chudzio, L. S. Lin & M. Wiranowska-Stewart. 1978. Interferoids: *In vitro* and *in vivo* conversion of native interferons to lower molecular weight forms. Proc. Nat. Acad. Sci. USA **75:** 4814–4818.
11. Maehara, N., M. Ho & J. A. Armstrong. 1977. Differences in mouse interferons according to cell source and mode of induction. Infect. Immun. **17:** 572–579.
12. Dalton, B. J. & K. Paucker. 1979. Antigenic properties of human lymphoblastoid interferons. Infect. Immun. **23:** 244–248.
13. Havell, E. A., T. G. Hayes & J. Vilček. 1978. Synthesis of two distinct interferons by human fibroblasts. Virology **89:** 330–334.
14. Stewart II, W. E. 1974. Distinct molecular species of interferons. Virology **61:** 80–86.
15. Mogensen, K. E. & K. Cantell. 1974. Human leukocyte interferon: Role for disulfide bond. J. Gen. Virol. **22:** 95–103.
16. Stewart II, W. E., S. LeGoff & M. Wiranowska-Stewart. 1977. Characterization of two distinct molecular populations of type I mouse interferons. J. Gen. Virol. **37:** 277–284.
17. Yamamoto, Y. & Y. Kawade. Unpublished results.

18. HAVELL, E. A. 1979. Isolation of a subspecies of murine interferon antigenically related to human leukocyte interferon. Virology **92:** 324–330.
19. ITO, Y., Y. NISHIYAMA, K. SHIMOKATA, I. NAGATA, H. TAKEYAMA & A. KUNII. 1978. The mechanism of interferon induction in mouse spleen cells stimulated with HVJ. Virology **88:** 128–137.
20. TSUKUI, K. 1977. Influenza virus-induced interferon production in mouse spleen cell culture: T cells as the main producer. Cell. Immunol. **32:** 243–251.
21. ITO, Y. Unpublished.
22. YAMAMOTO, Y., M. TOMIDA & M. HOZUMI. 1979. Stimulation of differentiation of mouse myeloid leukemic cells and induction of interferon in the cells by double-stranded polyribonucleotides. Cancer Research. **39:** 4170–4174.
23. YAMAMOTO, Y. & Y. KAWADE. 1976. Purification of two components of mouse L cell interferon: Electrophoretic demonstration of interferon proteins. J. Gen. Virol. **33:** 225–236.

AMINO TERMINAL SEQUENCE OF THE MOUSE INTERFERON SPECIES A FROM EHRLICH ASCITES TUMOR CELLS*

R. J. Broeze, H. Taira, B. M. Jayaram, and P. Lengyel

Department of Molecular Biophysics and Biochemistry
Yale University,
New Haven, Connecticut 06511

M. W. Hunkapiller and L. E. Hood

Division of Biology
California Institute of Technology
Pasadena, California 91125

There are several reports on the isolation and characterization of interferons (IFs) produced by cultured mouse cells upon infection with Newcastle disease virus.[1-9] The purified IFs are distributed over a broad size range. Those isolated from L929 cells and C243 cells were found to consist of two species, a larger one of 35,000 to 40,000 daltons and a smaller one of 22,000 to 28,000 daltons.[1-7] In a previous report[9] we described the purification of mouse IFs from Ehrlich ascites tumor (EAT) cells to a specific activity of about 2×10^9 NIH reference standard mouse interferon units/mg protein. The analysis of these by polyacrylamide gel electrophoresis in sodium dodecyl sulfate (SDS) revealed IFs of three size classes: A, 33,000 to 40,000 daltons, B, 26,000 to 30,000 daltons, and C, about 20,000 daltons. The amino acid compositions of IFs A, B, and C are similar. The tryptic peptide patterns of species A and B are similar; that of C is clearly different.[9]

Though pure IFs are available at present only in microgram quantities, the development of a highly sensitive amino acid sequencing technique[10] has made it possible to initiate a study of their amino acid sequences. A comparison of the sequences of different IFs should provide insights into the basis of species specificity of IFs, and the evolutionary relationship among different IFs. Furthermore, the knowledge of the sequences may facilitate the cloning of IF genes, e.g., by permitting the chemical synthesis of oligodeoxynucleotide primers for the enzymatic synthesis of cDNA to only partially purified interferon mRNA preparations.

Here we report the amino terminal sequence of the mouse IF species A from EAT cells.

The crude IFs were purified by a modification of our published procedure.[9] The initial steps, which involve chromatography on controlled pore glass, CM-Sephadex, and phosphocellulose result in fractions which are enriched in one of the three IF species. The fraction enriched in IF A was further purified by chromatography on octyl-sepharose and isoelectric focusing to a specific activity of 1.8×10^9 units/mg protein.[8,9] To remove from the interferon A small amounts of IFs B and C and ampholines (used in the isoelectric focusing) we fractionated the preparation further by polyacrylamide gel electrophoresis in the presence of

*Supported by Grants CA 16038 and AI-12320 from the National Institute of Health and by a grant from the Weingard Foundation, Los Angeles, California.

0077-8923/80/0350-0428 $0.175/0 © 1980, NYAS

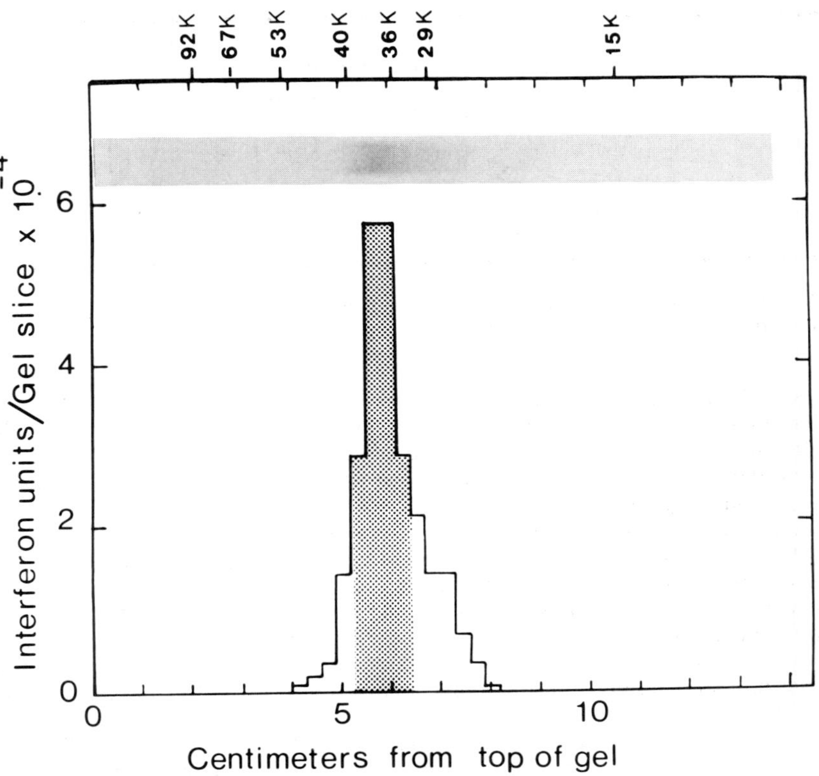

FIGURE 1. Polyacrylamide gel electrophoresis of mouse interferon A in the presence of SDS. Size distribution of interferon-active material and of protein.

A crude IF preparation from EAT cells induced with Newcastle disease virus was applied to a column of controlled pore glass (as described previously[9]) and eluted with 0.4 M glycine-Cl buffer (pH 3.5), 0.5%, (v/v) glycerol, 3.1 mM NaN_3, 10 μM phenymethylsulfonylfluoride (PMSF). The eluted material was fractionated by chromatography on CM-Sephadex and phosphocellulose.[8,9] The fraction eluted from phosphocellulose with 400 mM sodium phosphate buffer (pH 6.2) was further purified by chromatography on octyl-sepharose and by isoelectric focusing.[8,9] The interferon-active fractions were pooled, dialyzed against 2 mM sodium phosphate buffer (pH 6.2), 2% (v/v) glycerol, 10 μM PMSF and concentrated fivefold with Aquacide IIA (Calbiochem). The preparation (1.7×10^8 units of interferon) was dissolved in 0.7 ml of SDS sample buffer,[11] heated at 95°C for one minute and divided into five aliquots. Each of these was electrophoresed through a 15% polyacrylamide gel in the presence of SDS at 20 mA for 6 hours. To locate the protein, the gel was stained with Coomassie brilliant blue. To locate the IF, one gel track was cut into 3 mm wide slices and the proteins were extracted from them by soaking in 0.3 ml 137 mM NaCl, 2.7 mM KCl, 8.1 mM Na_2HPO_4, 1.5 mM KH_2PO_4, 0.1% (w/v) SDS, 10% (v/v) glycerol, 10 μM PMSF at room temperature overnight. Interferon activity in the eluate was detected by the cytopathic effect assay.[8] The IF-containing regions (shaded area in the figure) were eluted from the other gel tracks by electrophoresis according to Lazarides.[12] The eluate was dialyzed first against 150 mM NaCl, 0.1% (w/v) SDS, subsequently against 0.02% (w/v) SDS and was finally lyophilized. 40 to 50% of the protein was recovered. 400 pmoles of the eluted protein was used for amino terminal sequencing according to published procedure.[10] The location of protein size markers in the gel electropherograms are indicated.

1	5	10
H-Ile-Asn-Tyr-Lys-Gln-Leu-Gln-Leu-Gln-Glu-		
11	15	20
Arg-Thr-Asn-Ile-Arg-Lys-(?)-Gln-Glu-Leu-		
21		
Leu-Glu-Gln-Leu-		

FIGURE 2. Amino terminal sequence of mouse interferon A from EAT cells. The amino acid in position 17 has not been identified.

SDS.[11] The distributions of protein and of interferon activity in the gel electropherogram are shown in FIGURE 1: the protein (i.e., the Coomassie brilliant blue stainable substance, size range 35,000 to 40,000 daltons) and the IF-active material comigrate. The protein was recovered from the shaded region of the gel (see FIGURE 1) by electrophoresis.[12]

The amino terminal sequence of IF A was determined by automated Edman degradation involving the use of a spinning cup sequenator and high performance liquid chromatography for the analysis of amino acid phenylthiohydantoins. The sequence of the first 24 amino acids (except that in position 17 which has not been identified) is shown in FIGURE 2. Isoleucine[9] and smaller amounts of glycine and serine were detected in the first sequencing cycle. In all subsequent cycles only one amino acid was found, indicating that the IF A preparation is at least 95% pure.

Further studies will be needed to establish whether the broad size distribution of IF A (see FIGURE 1) is due to non-uniform glycosylation, non-uniform polypeptide cleavage, a difference in amino acid sequence of the molecules (in a region other than the amino terminus), or other phenomena. The sequencing of the amino terminal regions of mouse IFs B and C is underway.

ACKNOWLEDGMENTS

We thank E. Slattery for expert advice on interferon production and M. Gomez and T. Novicki for skillful assistance.

REFERENCES

1. OSBORN, C. A., K. BERG & K. PAUCKER. 1973. J. Immunol. **111:** 1206–1218.
2. STEWART II, W. E. 1974. Virology **61:** 80–86.
3. KNIGHT, E. 1975. J. Biol. Chem. **250:** 4139–4144.
4. IWAKURA, Y., S. YONEHARA & Y. KAWADE. 1978. J. Biol. Chem. **253:** 5074–5079.
5. DE MAEYER-GUIGNARD, J., M. G. TOVEY, I. GRESSER & E. DE MAEYER. 1978. Nature **271:** 622–625.
6. IWAKURA, Y. S. YONEHARA & Y. KAWADE. 1978. Biochem. Biophys. Res. Commun. **84:** 557–563.
7. FUJISAWA, J., Y. IWAKURA & Y. KAWADE. 1978. J. Biol. Chem. **253:** 8677–8679.

8. KAWAKITA, M. B. CABRER, H. TAIRA, M. REBELLO, E. SLATTERY, H. WEIDELI & P. LENGYEL. 1978. J. Biol. Chem. **253:** 598–602.
9. CABRER, B., H. TAIRA, R. J. BROEZE, T. D. KEMPE, K. WILLIAMS, E. SLATTERY, W. H. KONIGSBERG & P. LENGYEL. 1979. J. Biol. Chem. **254:** 3681–3684.
10. HUNKAPILLER, M. W. & L. E. HOOD. 1980. Science **207:** 528–530.
11. LAEMMLI, U. K. 1970. Nature **227:** 680–685.
12. LAZARIDES, E. 1976. J. Supramol. Structure **5:** 531–563.

THE MOLECULAR BASIS OF THE ANTIVIRAL ACTIVITY OF INTERFERONS

INTRODUCTORY REMARKS

Wolfgang K. Joklik

Department of Microbiology and Immunology
Duke University Medical Center
Durham, North Carolina 27710

Interferons (IFs) are powerful biological agents: first studied as inhibitors of the multiplication of almost all, if not all, animal viruses, they were subsequently found to be capable of affecting also a variety of cellular functions ranging from the ability to grow to the ability to synthesize specific proteins. The biological significance of the *anticellular* activity of IFs is still being explored, and there are hopes that it may be possible to utilize it in the fight against cancer; but there is no doubt at all about the biological importance of the *antiviral* activity of IFs. Several studies have clearly shown that virus-caused diseases are far more severe in animals to which antiserum to IF is administered than in control animals, thereby demonstrating that IFs are the first line of defence against viral infections.[1,2]

In this session we propose to examine in some detail the nature of the antiviral activity of IF*; and we have a variety of very interesting and thought-provoking papers that summarize the current state of the art. Most of these papers will focus on two approaches that are currently thought to provide an insight into the nature of the fundamental reactions by which IFs inhibit the multiplication of viruses; and it is my task as Session Chairman to place these experiments into perspective relative to the studies that have preceded them, as well as to the overall problem of how IFs interact with cells.

Let me start by listing three considerations basic to investigations of the mode of antiviral action of IF. First, the IF preparations used in this research should be as pure as possible. Ideally, of course, pure IFs should be used; in practice many studies have been carried out with IF preparations that contain less than 0.01% IF. It is conceivable that at least some of the more unusual biological effects of IFs that have been reported are caused by biologically active impurities in "interferon" preparations. Second, IF inhibits the replication of all animal viruses, both RNA-containing ones and DNA-containing ones, with both single-stranded and double-stranded nucleic acids, with both segmented and nonsegmented genomes. Therefore, it is likely that treatment of cells with IF elicits some specific reaction which is fundamental to the induction of the antiviral state. This is not to say that this fundamental reaction could not itself trigger a variety of subsequent events, thereby giving the impression that IF treatment induces a pleiotropic response. Third, it must always be kept in mind that IF is capable of inhibiting the multiplication of viruses under conditions when it fails to affect adversely the uninfected cell. Any proposed mechanism for the antiviral effect of IF must

*The mechanism by which IFs inhibit the multiplication of RNA tumor viruses differs from that by which they inhibit other viruses, and will not be discussed here.

0077-8923/80/0350-0432 $01.75/0 © 1980, NYAS

therefore include an explanation as to why some reaction basic to the multiplication of viruses is inhibited, while the analogous reaction in uninfected cells is not inhibited.

Reasoning along these lines suggested some 15 years ago that a possible target of IF action might be the ability of viral messenger RNAs to be translated;[3] and indeed it was found that in IF-treated cells infected with vaccinia virus protein synthesis was inhibited abruptly.[4] Under conditions of normal infection, vaccinia virus shuts down the translation of most host messenger RNA species rather rapidly, and most of the ribosomes that then cease translating host cell messenger RNAs begin to translate viral messenger RNAs. As a result, the overall rate of protein synthesis undergoes a minor depression which is followed by a rise as host messenger RNA translation gives way to viral messenger RNA translation.[5] In IF-treated infected cells host messenger RNA translation is also shut off, but ribosomes are not recruited to form polyribosomes with viral messenger RNA; as a result the amount of polyribosomes drops drastically, as does the overall rate of protein synthesis.[4] Similar observations were subsequently made with cells infected with reovirus,[6] mengovirus,[7] Semliki forest virus,[8] and others.

By 1972 it was generally agreed that one of the fundamental attributes of the antiviral state induced by IF is inhibition of the translation of early viral messenger RNAs. In most IF-treated cells, infection also shuts off the synthesis of host-specified proteins; but whereas this effect is irreversible in some cell systems, such as the vaccinia-infected L or HeLa cell,[4] it is reversible in others, such as the mengovirus-infected L or HeLa cell.[9] Interferon-treated infected cells may therefore die or survive; and since no viral progeny is formed in either case, uninfected cells in the population survive. Current work is very much concerned with defining, in molecular terms, the reasons why viral messenger RNAs are not translated in IF-treated cells. However, before examining these studies in some detail, let me digress briefly and point out that studies on two virus-cell systems have suggested that it is not always the translation, but rather sometimes the transcription of early viral messenger RNAs that is inhibited in IF-treated cells. These are VSV-infected and SV40-infected cell systems. The latter system was investigated in considerable detail; and there is no doubt that SV40-infected IF-treated cells contain far less early viral messenger RNA than infected cells not treated with IF. This was interpreted as signifying that in this particular system IF prevented the transcription, rather than the translation of virus-coded messenger RNAs.[10,11] However, two findings suggested that the real picture may be more complicated. First, it was found that in cells infected with SV40 DNA rather than with the whole virus, IF pretreatment did not reduce the amount of early viral messenger RNA;[12] and second, if SV40-infected cells were treated with IF after infection, the translation of viral messenger RNAs was drastically inhibited.[13] The latter finding showed that the translation of SV40 messenger RNAs is indeed inhibitable by interferon treatment, just like that of other viral messenger RNAs. The former result suggested that the lesion in the SV40 infection cycle in IF-treated cells may not be the transcription of viral messenger RNA, but rather some defect in the uncoating of parental genomes, or, in a more general sense, the delivery of transcribable parental DNA to that location in the cell where it is normally transcribed. The mechanism by which such a lesion might be induced could very well be via an effect of IF on the host cell membrane. Indeed, it is known that there are receptors for IFs on cells,[14] that IF must interact with these receptors in order to induce the antiviral state,[15] and that IF treatment alters a variety of membrane functions ranging from changes in cell morphology to changes in cellular electrophoretic mobility and changes in the antigenic composition of the cell surface.[16-19] As for the decreased amount of VSV messenger RNA in IF-treated cells,[20] a membrane-associated nuclease was detected in some (but not all) types of IF-treated infected cells;[21] and the suggestion was made that the reason why less viral messenger RNA appeared to accumulate in IF-treated cells and why less viral proteins were formed in such cells may be degradation of messenger RNA by such a nuclease. Attractive though this theory was, it did not explain why only viral, and not also host cell messenger RNAs, should be degraded.

1972 saw the first experiments designed to explore the nature of the antiviral effect of IF in cell extracts. It was found, and quickly confirmed in several laboratories, that whereas the ability to translate *endogenous* messenger RNAs or added poly(U) in cell-free extracts was unaffected by IF pretreatment, extracts of IF-treated cells were greatly inhibited with respect to their ability to translate added viral messenger RNAs.[22-24] Unfortunately, in many such extracts the translation of added host cell messenger RNAs was also inhibited;[25-28] but in one system the ability of IF-treated cells to discriminate between viral and host cell messenger RNAs was preserved in the cell-free state.[24] The reason for this discrepancy is not yet clear. However, all workers in the field agree that the reason for the inhibition is the presence of a factor associated with the ribosomes of IF-treated cells that can be solubilized in 0.5M KCl.[22,24,26,29]

For several years attention then focused on the findings that inability to translate messenger RNAs in extracts of IF-treated cells developed during the preincubation period normally employed to reduce levels of endogenous messenger RNA translation; and that this inability could be relieved, at least in part, by the addition of certain species of mammalian tRNA, in particular $tRNA_{leu}$.[30-35] It was also shown that the tRNA species that restored the translation of mengovirus RNA and of globin mRNA in IF-treated cell extracts were not the same,[31] which suggested a possible basis for the selective effect of IF on virus-versus-host protein synthesis, and that extracts of IF-treated cells inactivated added tRNA with respect to its ability to support protein synthesis much faster than extracts of untreated cells.[36] Further work to extend these interesting observations is temporarily suspended for two reasons. First, it was shown that tRNA isolated from untreated and from IF-treated mouse cells possessed the same number and relative amounts of $tRNA_{leu}$ isoacceptor species and have comparable stimulatory activity in reversing the IF-mediated inhibition of viral mRNA translation *in vitro*.[37] This suggests that the tRNA effect may be an artefact of cell-free extracts. Second, it has been found that the inhibition of translation caused by the presence of dsRNA, upon which attention is currently focused most intensely, is not relieved by the addition of tRNA and does not involve inactivation of tRNA species.[38] It is unlikely therefore that this line of research will be pursued before the role of dsRNA in IF-induced viral mRNA translation inhibition is resolved.

Attention was focused on dsRNA as an effector or amplifier of the antiviral state in 1974 when it was found that IF treatment renders cells very sensitive to the toxic effects of dsRNA and increases the sensitivity of viral protein synthesis to inhibition by dsRNA in cell extracts.[39] Interest in this effect was stimulated by concurrent work on globin synthesis in reticulocyte lysates. In such lysates either hemin deficiency[40,41] or addition of dsRNA[44,45] causes protein synthesis to be inhibited by activating a protein kinase that catalyzes the phosphorylation of the small subunit of the protein synthesis initiation factor eIF-2, thereby inactivating it.[42,43]

Work on the mechanism by which dsRNA activates the IF-induced inhibition of messenger RNA translation has proceeded along two avenues. First, it has been found that the combination of IF treatment and dsRNA addition greatly stimulates phosphorylation of the small subunit of eIF-2, thereby inactivating it.[46-52] It is also clear that the small subunit of eIF-2 is not the only protein the phosphorylation of which is stimulated in IF-treated cells, for increased phosphorylation of at least three other proteins, one of which has a molecular weight of about 67,000 and may itself be a protein kinase,[77] has also been reported.[47-51,55] Phosphorylation of some, but not of all, of these proteins is increased by dsRNA treatment. Second, it has been found that IF treatment induces the formation of an oligo(A) synthetase which in the presence of dsRNA polymerizes ATP into a family of 2′, 5′-linked oligoadenylates, the most prominent of which is usually the trinucleotide $ppp^{5'}A^{2'}p^{5'}A^{2'}p^{5'}A$.[56-69] The 2′5′ oligo(A) then activates a nuclease that is present in cells that have not been treated with IF.[58,60,62,64,70]

Just as in the case of studies of eIF-2 phosphorylation, which inactivates an initiation factor necessary for the translation not only of viral messenger RNAs but also of host cell messenger RNAs, it has not been demonstrated that this nuclease will hydrolize only viral, and not also host cell messenger RNAs. The selectivity for viral messenger RNAs is postulated to lie in the requirement for dsRNA for nuclease activation; in other words, the nuclease is postulated to be activated only in close proximity to the dsRNA of the replicative forms and intermediates which serve as primer-templates for viral RNA formation.[55,71] This is an ingenious *ad hoc* explanation the significance of which remains to be proved. In fact, these findings focus attention sharply on the general significance of the potentiation by dsRNA of IF-induced effects. It is known that in extracts of IF-treated cells viral messenger RNAs are degraded more rapidly, but not much more rapidly than in extracts of untreated cells[49]; that formation of the initial peptide bond is either not inhibited at all or only inhibited minimally, but that elongation is slowed[53]; that a factor that inhibits translation of viral messenger RNAs in extracts of untreated cells can be removed from ribosomes with 0.5 M KCl[22,24,26,29]; and that this inhibitory factor is not species-specific, that is, it will inhibit protein synthesis in extracts of cells of other species.[54] It is also known that if dsRNA is added to extracts of IF-treated cells, a nuclease present in untreated cells is strongly activated by 2′ 5′ oligo(A), and that eIF-2 is markedly inactivated by virtue of phosphorylation of its small subunit (see above). Does the functioning of the antiviral state then require the presence of dsRNA in infected cells? The answer to this question is not yet in. Certainly it is difficult to see how even the minute amounts of dsRNA that effect viral protein synthesis inhibition can be formed in cells infected with a dsDNA-containing virus such as vaccinia virus, even though it has been shown that dsRNA molecules can be isolated from vaccinia virus-infected cells[72]; but this is only after exposing such extracts to conditions conducive to annealing, conditions that are unlikely to occur in infected cells. Furthermore, similar treatment results in the isolation of dsRNA molecules even from uninfected cells.[73] Finally, it has been found that extracts of vaccinia virus-infected cells do not contain factors with dsRNA activity when tested in protein-synthesizing extracts of IF-treated cells.[39] In fact, it is questionable whether free dsRNA, that is, dsRNA recognizable as such by protein molecules, ever exists at all in cells infected with *any* virus. Thus the dsRNA in cells infected with reovirus is always coated by a protective shell. The same is probably true of replicative intermediates in cells infected with negative-stranded RNA viruses; certainly it is true of transcription complexes in such cells. Presumably the functional significance of the dsRNA-activated nuclease will only be revealed when careful studies are carried out on the formation and stability of virus-coded RNAs in IF-treated and untreated cells. Such studies are currently underway in my own laboratory. Perhaps we have here an indication that the antiviral state inhibits the multiplication of different viruses in different ways: that of certain RNA viruses via dsRNA activation, and that of other viruses via ribosome-associated factors the formation and activation of which is not dependent upon potentiation by dsRNA. This all leads back to the original question that I posed, namely whether the fundamental basis of these various mechanisms may not be a single IF-induced reaction. Recently several laboratories have taken the view that rather than search for such a needle in a haystack by multiple individual probings and testings, the problem may best be attacked frontally and one should ask simply whether there are specific protein species, or modifications (such as phosphorylation) of species, that are characteristic of IF-treated cells, using for this purpose the almost infinite resolving capacity of two-dimensional polyacrylamide gel electrophoresis. Such work is underway in several laboratories, including those of Lengyel, Knight, and my own. It has already yielded results: thus it has been found that IF-treated cells contain several polypeptide species that are not present in untreated cells.[74-76] No doubt it will require a major effort to isolate and characterize these proteins in molecular and functional terms, and no doubt some of them will turn out to have nothing to do with the antiviral activity of IF; but it may also be true that this approach represents our best chance of identifying the protein species that is fundamental to the induction of the antiviral state by IFs.

References

1. Gresser, I., M. G. Tovey, C. Maury & M.-T. Bandu. 1976. Role of interferon in the pathogenesis of virus diseases in mice as demonstrated by the use of anti-interferon serum. II. Studies with Herpes simplex, Moloney sarcoma, vesicular stomatitis, Newcastle disease, and influenza viruses. J. Exp. Med. **144:** 1316–1323.
2. Virelizier, J.-L. & I. Gresser. 1978. Role of interferon in the pathogenesis of viral diseases of mice as demonstrated by the use of anti-interferon Serum. V. Protective role in mouse hepatitis virus type 3 infection of susceptible and resistant strains of mice. J. Immunol. **120:** 1616–1619.
3. Joklik, W. K. 1965. The molecular basis of the viral eclipse phase. Progr. Med. Virol. **7:** 44–96.
4. Joklik, W. K. & T. C. Merigan. 1966. Concerning the mechanism of action of interferon. Proc. Nat. Acad. Sci. USA **56:** 558–565.
5. Joklik, W. K. 1966. The poxviruses. Bact. Rev. **30:** 33–66.
6. Wiebe, M. E. & W. K. Joklik, 1975. The mechanism of inhibition of reovirus replication by interferon. Virology **66:** 229–240.
7. Levy, H. B. & W. A. Carter. 1968. Molecular basis of the action of interferon. J. Mol. Biol. **31:** 561–577.
8. Friedman, R. M. 1968. Inhibition of arbovirus protein synthesis by interferon. J. Virol. **2:** 1081–1085.
9. Falcoff, R. & J. Sanceau. 1979. Mengovirus-induced inhibition of cell protein synthesis and subsequent recovery of cellular activity in interferon-pretreated cells. Virology **98:** 433–438.
10. Oxman, M. N. & M. J. Levine. 1971. Interferon and transcription of early virus-specific RNA in cells infected with simian virus 40. Proc. Nat. Acad. Sci. USA **68:** 299–302.
11. Metz, D. H., M. J. Levine & M. N. Oxman. 1976. Mechanism of interferon action: Further evidence for transcription at the primary site of action in Simian virus 40 infection. J. Gen. Virol. **32:** 227–240.
12. Yamamoto, K., N. Yamaguchi & K. Oda. 1975. Mechanism of interferon-induced inhibition of early simian virus 40 (SV40) functions. Virology **68:** 58–70.

13. YAKOBSON, E., M. REVEL & E. WINOCOUR. 1977. Inhibition of simian virus 40 replication by interferon treatment late in the lytic cycle. Virology **80:** 225–228.
14. CHANY, C., A. GRÉGOIRE, M. VIGNAL, J. LEMAITRE-MONCUTT, P. BROWN, F. BESANÇON, H. SUAREZ & R. CASSINGENA. 1973. Mechanism of interferon uptake in parental and somatic monkey-mouse hybrid cells. Proc. Nat. Acad. Sci. USA **70:** 557–561.
15. VENGRIS, V. E., B. D. STOLLAR & P. M. PITHA. 1975. Interferon externalization by producing cell before induction of antiviral state. Virology **65:** 410–417.
16. HUET, C., I. GRESSER, M. T. BANDU & P LINDAHL. 1974. Increased binding of concanavalin A to interferon-treated murine leukemia L1210 cells. Proc. Soc. Exp. Biol. Med. **147:** 52–57.
17. VIGNAUX, F. & I. GRESSER. 1977. Differential effect of interferon on the expression of H-2K, H-2D, and Ia antigens on mouse lymphocytes. J. Immunol. **118:** 721–723.
18. HERON, I., M. HOKLAND & K. BERG. 1978. Enhanced expresion of β_2-microglobulin and HLA antigens on human lymphoid cells by interferon. Proc. Nat. Acad. Sci. USA **75:** 6215–6219.
19. KNIGHT, E., JR. & B. D. KORANT. 1977. A cell surface alteration in mouse L cells induced by interferon. Biochem. Biophys. Res. Commun. **74:** 707–713.
20. MARCUS, P. I., D. L. ENGELHARDT, J. M. HUNT & M. J. SEKELLICK. 1971. Interferon action: Inhibition of vesicular stomatitis virus RNA synthesis induced by virion-bound polymerase. Science **174:** 593–598.
21. MARCUS, P. I., T. M. TERRY & S. LEVINE. Interferon action. II. Membrane-bound alkaline ribonuclease activity in chick embryo cells manifesting interferon-mediated interference. Proc. Nat. Acad. Sci. USA **72:** 182–186.
22. FRIEDMAN, R. M., D. H. METZ, R. M. ESTEBAN, D. R. TOVELL, L. A. BALL & I. M. KERR. 1972. Mechanism of Interferon Action: Inhibition of viral messenger ribonucleic acid translation in L-cell extracts. J Virol. **10:** 1184–1198.
23. FALCOFF, E., R. FALCOFF, B. LEBLEU & M. REVEL. 1973. Correlation between the antiviral effect of interferon treatment and the inhibition of in vitro mRNA translation in noninfected L cells. J. Virol. **12:** 421–430.
24. SAMUEL, C. E. & W. K. JOKLIK. 1974. A protein synthesizing system from interferon-treated cells that discriminates between cellular and viral messenger RNAs. Virology **58:** 476–491.
25. FALCOFF, E., R. FALCOFF, B. LEBLEU & M. REVEL. 1972. Interferon treatment inhibits mengo RNA and hemoglobin mRNA translation in cell-free extracts of L cells. Nature New Biology **240:** 145–147.
26. FALCOFF, E., R. FALCOFF, B. LEBLEU & M. REVEL. 1973. Correlation between the antiviral effect of interferon treatment and the inhibition of in vitro of messenger RNA translation in non-infected L cells. J. Virol. **12:** 421–430.
27. GUPTA, S. L., W. D. GRAZIADEI III, H. WIDELL, M. L. SOPORI & P. LENGYEL. 1974. Selective inhibition of viral protein accumulation in interferon-treated cells; non-discriminant inhibition of the translation of added viral and cellular messenger RNAs in their extracts. Virology **57:** 49–63.
28. HILLER G., I. WINKLER, G. VIEHHAUSER, C. JUNGWIRTH, G. BODO, S. DUBE & W. OSTERTAG. 1976. Failure of globin mRNA to stimulate globin synthesis in cell-free extracts of interferon-treated globin-synthesizing mouse erythroleukemic cells. Virology **69:** 360–363.
29. GUPTA, S. L., M. L. SOPORI & P. LENGYEL. 1973. Inhibition of protein synthesis directed by added viral and cellular messenger RNAs in extracts of interferon-treated Ehrlich ascites tumor cells. Location and dominance of the inhibitor(s). Biochem. Biophys. Res. Commun. **54:** 777–783.
30. GUPTA, S. L., M. L. SOPORI & P. LENGYEL. 1974. Release of the inhibition of messenger RNA translation in extracts of interferon-treated Ehrlich ascites tumor cells by added transfer RNA. Biochem. Biophys. Res. Commun. **57:** 763–770.
31. CONTENT, J., B. LEBLEU, A. ZILBERSTEIN, H. BERISSI & M. REVEL. 1974. Mechanism of the interferon-induced block of mRNA translation in mouse L cells: Reversal of the block by transfer RNA. FEBS Letters **41:** 125–130.
32. SAMUEL, C. E. 1976. Mechanism of interferon action. Studies on the mechanism of

interferon-mediated inhibition of reovirus messenger RNA translation in cell-free protein synthesis systems from mouse ascites tumor cells. Virology **75:** 166–176.

33. Zilberstein, A., B. Dudock, H. Berissi & M. Revel. 1976. Control of messenger RNA translation by minor species of leucyl-transfer RNA in extracts from interferon-treated L cells. J. Mol. Biol. **108:** 43–54.
34. Sen, G. C., S. L. Gupta, G. E. Brown, B. Lebleu, M. A. Rebello & P. Lengyel. 1976. Interferon treatment of Ehrlich ascites tumor cells: Effects of exogenous mRNA translation and tRNA inactivation in the cell extract. J. Virol. **17:** 191–203.
35. Falcoff, R., B. Lebleu, J. Sanceau, J. Weissenbach, G. Dirheimer, J. P. Ebel & E. Falcoff. 1976. The inhibition of translation of synthetic polyribonucleotides and mengo RNA in extracts from interferon-treated L cells and its reversion by tRNAs. Biochem. Biophys. Res. Commun. **68:** 1323–1331.
36. Falcoff, R., E. Falcoff, J. Sanceau & J. A. Lewis. 1978. Influence of preincubation on the development of the inhibition of protein synthesis in extracts from interferon-treated mouse L cells. Action on tRNA. Virology **86:** 507–515.
37. Colby, C., E. E. Penhoet, C. E. Samuel. 1976. A Comparison of transfer RNA from untreated and interferon-treated murine cells. Virology **74:** 262–264.
38. Lewis, J. A., E. Falcoff & R. Falcoff. 1978. Dual action of double-stranded RNA in inhibiting protein synthesis in extracts of interferon-treated mouse L cells. Translation is impaired at the level of initiation and by mRNA degradation. Eur. J. Biochem. **86:** 497–509.
39. Kerr, I. M., R. E. Brown & L. A. Ball. 1974. Increased sensitivity to double-stranded RNA of protein synthesis in cell-free systems from interferon-treated cells. Nature **250:** 57–59.
40. Levin, D. H., R. S. Ranu, V. Ernst & I. M. London. 1976. Regulation of protein synthesis in reticulocyte lysates: Phosphorylation of methionyl-tRNA binding factor by protein kinase activity of translational inhibitor isolated from heme-deficient lysates. Proc. Nat. Acad. Sci. USA **73:** 3112–3116.
41. Kramer, G., J. M. Cimadevilla & B. Hardesty. 1976. Specificity of the protein kinase activity associated with the hemin-controlled repressor of rabbit reticulocyte. Proc. Nat. Acad. Sci. USA **73:** 3078–3082.
42. De Haro, C. & S. Ochoa. 1978. Mode of action of the hemin-controlled inhibitor of protein synthesis: Studies with factors from rabbit reticulocyte lysates. Proc. Nat. Acad. Sci. USA **75:** 2713–2716.
43. Lenz, J. R. & C. Baglioni. 1978. Inhibition of protein synthesis by double-stranded RNA and phosphorylation of initiation factor eIF-2. J. Biol. Chem. **253:** 4219–4223.
44. Levin, D. & I. M. London. 1978. Regulation of protein synthesis: Activation by double-stranded RNA of a protein kinase that phosphorylates eukaryotic initiation factor 2. Proc. Nat. Acad. Sci. USA **75:** 1121–1125.
45. Farrell, P. J., K. Balkow, T. Hunt, R. J. Jackson & H. Trachsel. 1977. Phosphorylation of initiation factor eIF-2 and the control of reticulocyte protein synthesis. Cell **11:** 187–200.
46. Roberts, W. K., A. Hovanessian, R. E. Brown, M. J. Clemens & I. M. Kerr. 1976. Interferon-mediated protein kinase and low-molecular-weight inhibitor of protein synthesis. Nature **264:** 477–480.
47. Lebleu, B., G. C. Sen, S. Shaila, B. Cabrer & P. Lengyel. 1976. Interferon, double-stranded RNA, and protein phosphorylation. Proc. Nat. Acad. Sci. USA **73:** 3107–3111.
48. Zilberstein, A., J. P. Federman, L. Shulman & M. Revel. 1976. Specific phosphorylation in vitro of a protein associated with ribosomes of interferon-treated mouse cells. FEBS Letters **68:** 119–124.
49. Samuel, C. E., D. A. Farris & D. A. Eppstein. 1977. Mechanism of interferon action. Kinetics of interferon action in mouse L929 cells: Translation inhibition, protein phosphorylation, and messenger RNA methylation and degradation. Virology **83:** 56–71.
50. Samuel C. E. 1979. Mechanism of interferon action. Kinetics of interferon action in

mouse L929 cells: Phosphorylation of protein synthesis initiation factor eIF-2 and ribosome-associated protein P1. Virology **93:** 281–285.

51. SAMUEL C. E. 1979. Mechanism of interferon action. Phosphorylation of protein synthesis initiation factor eIF-2 in interferon-treated human cells by a ribosome-associated kinase possessing site-specificity similar to the hemin-regulated rabbit reticulocyte kinase. Proc. Nat. Acad. Sci. USA. **76:** 600–604.
52. KAEMPFER, R., R. ISRAELI, H. ROEN, S. KNOLLER, A. ZILBERSTEIN, A. SCHMIDT & M. REVEL. 1979. Reversal of the interferon-induced block of protein synthesis by purified preparations of eukaryotic initiation factor 2. Virology **99:** 170–173.
53. SAMUEL, C. E. 1976. Mechanism of interferon action. Studies on the mechanism of interferon-mediated inhibition of reovirus messenger RNA translation in cell-free protein synthesis systems from mouse ascites tumor cells. Virology **75:** 166–176.
54. SAMUEL, C. E. & D. A. FARRIS. 1977. Mechanism of interferon action. Species specificity of interferon and of the interferon-mediated inhibitor of translation from mouse, monkey, and human cells. Virology **77:** 556–565.
55. AUJEAN, O., J. SANCEAU, E. FALCOFF & R. FALCOFF. 1979. Location of enhanced ribonuclease activity and of a phosphoprotein kinase in interferon-treated mengovirus-infected cells. Virology **92:** 583–586.
56. HOVANESSIAN, A. G., R. E. BROWN & I. M. KERR. 1979. Synthesis of low molecular weight inhibitor of protein synthesis with enzyme from interferon treated cells. Nature **268:** 537–540.
57. KERR, I. M., R. E. BROWN & H. E. HOVANESSIAN. 1977. Nature of inhibitor of cell-free protein synthesis formed in response to interferon and double-stranded RNA. Nature **268:** 540–542.
58. RATNER, L., R. C. WIEGAND, P. J. FARRELL, G. C. SEN, B. CABRER & P. LENGYEL. 1978. Interferon, double-stranded RNA and RNA degradation. Fractionation of the endonuclease$_{INT}$ system into two macromolecular components; role of a small molecule in nuclease activation. Biochem. Biophys. Res. Commun. **81:** 947–954.
59. KERR, I. M. & R. E. BROWN. 1978. pppA$^{2'}$p$^{5'}$A$^{2'}$p$^{5'}$A: An inhibitor of protein synthesis synthesized with an enzyme fraction from interferon-treated cells. Proc. Nat. Acad. Sci. USA **75:** 256–260.
60. CLEMENS, M. J. & B. R. G. WILLIAMS. 1978. Inhibition of cell-free protein synthesis by pppA$^{2'}$p$^{5'}$A$^{2'}$p$^{5'}$A: A novel oligonucleotide synthesized by interferon-treated L-cell extracts. Cell **13:** 565–572.
61. BALL, L. A. & C. N. WHITE. 1978. Oligonucleotide inhibitor of protein synthesis made in extracts of interferon-treated chick embryo cells: Comparison with the mouse low molecular weight inhibitor. Proc. Nat. Acad. Sci. USA **75:** 1167–1171.
62. BAGLIONI, C., M. A. MINKS & P. A. MARONEY. 1978. Interferon action may be mediated by activation of a nuclease by pppA$^{2'}$p$^{5'}$A$^{2'}$p$^{5'}$A. Nature **273:** 684–687.
63. EPPSTEIN, D. A. & C. E. SAMUEL. 1978. Mechanism of interferon action. Properties of an interferon-mediated ribonucleolytic activity from mouse L929 cells. Virology **89:** 240–251.
64. EPPSTEIN, D. A., T. C. PETERSON & C. E. SAMUEL. 1979. Mechanism of interferon action: Synthesis and activity of the interferon-mediated low-molecular-weight oligonucleotide from murine and human cells. Virology **98:** 9–19.
65. MINKS, M. A., S. BENVIN, D. A. MARONEY & C. BAGLIONI. 1979. Synthesis of 2′5′-oligo(A) in extracts of interferon-treated Hela cells. J. Biol. Chem. **254:** 5058–5064.
66. KIMCHI, A., L. SHULMAN, A. SCHMIDT, Y. CHERNAJOVSKY, A. FRADIN & M. REVEL. 1979. Kinetics of the induction of three translation-regulatory enzymes by interferon. Proc. Nat. Acad. Sci. USA **75:** 3208–3212.
67. BAGLIONI, C., P. A. MARONEY & D. K. WEST. 1979. 2′5′ Oligo (A) polymerase activity and inhibition of viral RNA synthesis in interferon-treated Hela cells. Biochem. **18:** 1765–1770.
68. STARK, G. R., W. J. DOWER, R. T. SCHIMKE, R. E. BROWN & I. M. KERR. 1979. 2–5 A Synthetases: Assay, distribution and variation with growth or horomone status. Nature **278:** 471–473.

69. BALL, L. A. Induction of 2'5'-oligoadenylate synthetase activity and a new protein by chick interferon. Virology **94:** 282–296.
70. BALL, L. A. & C. N. WHITE. 1969. Nuclease activation by double-stranded RNA and by 2', 5'-oligoadenylate in extracts of interferon-treated chick cells. Virology **93:** 348–356.
71. NILSEN, T. W. & C. BAGLIONI. 1979. Mechanism for discrimination between viral and host mRNA in interferon-treated cells. Proc. Nat. Acad. Sci. USA **76:** 2600–2604.
72. COLBY, C. & P. H. DUESBERG. 1969. Double-stranded RNA in vaccinia virus-infected cells. Nature **222:** 940–944.
73. MONTAGNIER, L. 1968. Présence d'un acide ribonucléique en double chaîne dans des cellules animales. C. R. Acad. Sci. (Paris) **267:** 1417–1419.
74. DE LEY, M., A. BILLIAU & P. DE SOMER. 1979. Interferon-induced synthesis of a 63,000 dalton protein in mouse cells. Biochem. Biophys. Res. Commun. **89:** 701–705.
75. FARRELL, P. J., R. J. BROEZE & P. LENGYEL. 1979. Accumulation of an mRNA and protein in interferon-treated Ehrlich ascites tumour cells. Nature **279:** 523–525.
76. KNIGHT, E., JR. & B. D. KORANT. 1979. Fibroblast interferon induces synthesis of four proteins in human fibroblast cells. Proc. Nat. Acad. Sci. USA. **76:** 1824–1827.
77. KIMCHI, A., A. ZILBERSTEIN, A. SCHMIDT, L. SHULMAN & M. REVEL. 1979. The interferon-induced protein kinase PK-i from mouse L cells. J. Biol. Chem. **254:** 9846–9853.

DOUBLE-STRANDED RNA AND THE ENZYMOLOGY OF INTERFERON ACTION*

P. Lengyel, H. Samanta, J. Pichon, J. Dougherty, E. Slattery, and P. Farrell

Department of Molecular Biophysics and Biochemistry
Yale University
New Haven, Connecticut 06511

Interferons were discovered in 1957 as antiviral agents.[1] Investigations in the last 22 years, however, revealed their involvement in the regulation of a large variety of seemingly diverse physiological phenomena and processes. These include for example cell growth, delayed hypersensitivity, graft rejection, histocompatibility antigen expression, natural killer-cell recruitment and macrophage activation. It appears to be in line with this multiplicity of effects that the biochemistry of interferon (IF) action is also complex. Much of our knowledge of this biochemistry is based on the comparison of enzyme activities in extracts from IF-treated and control cells and has been gained in the last five years.[2-4]

In this communication we will summarize briefly our studies of two enzyme systems controlled by IF. The action of one results in the accelerated cleavage of single-stranded RNA, that of the other in the impairment of peptide chain initiation. The two enzyme systems are distinct, though both require double-stranded (ds) RNA for activation[5] (see also references 4 and 6–9). Our studies concerning other effects of IF treatment of cells on enzyme reactions (e.g., an impairment of mRNA cap methylation *in vitro* and *in vivo*[10-12] and the acceleration of tRNA inactivation *in vitro*[13]) have been summarized elsewhere.[14]

Interferon, Double-stranded RNA and Single-stranded RNA Cleavage

In the course of investigating the mechanism of inhibition of reovirus replication in mouse L cells by interferon we established that the early steps of replication e.g., virus binding to cells, penetration and partial uncoating are unaffected whereas viral protein and RNA accumulation are decreased.[15,16] These observations stimulated us to compare the rate of reovirus mRNA degradation in an extract prepared from cells treated with IF to that in an extract from untreated control cells. Reovirus mRNAs that had been prepared *in vitro* and were contaminated with the genomic dsRNAs of the virus were degraded faster in the extract from IF treated cells than in the extract from control cells when incubated under conditions of cell-free protein synthesis. Remarkably, the difference in the rate of degradation was not observed in experiments with purified reovirus mRNA preparations from which the contaminating ds reovirus RNA had been removed. However, added ds reovirus RNA (or poly(I) · poly(C)) greatly enhanced the rate of degradation of the purified reovirus mRNAs in the extract from IF-treated cells whereas it affected this rate in the extract from

*Research for this paper was supported by National Institutes of Health Research Grants AI 12320 and CA 16038.

0077-8923/80/0350-0441 $01.75/0 © 1980, NYAS

control cells barely if at all.[17] In addition to dsRNA, ATP was also required to accelerate reovirus mRNA degradation in the extract from IF-treated cells. Experiments involving the staggered additions and removals of dsRNA and ATP to and from extracts of IF-treated cells revealed that dsRNA and ATP are needed for the activation of an endonuclease activity but they do not have to be present during the actual cleavage of single-stranded RNA.[18] This dsRNA and ATP-dependent endonuclease activity in extracts from IF-treated cells was designated as endonuclease$_{INT}$.[17]

We fractionated the endonuclease$_{INT}$ system into two complementary enzyme fractions. One of these when incubated with dsRNA and ATP gives rise to a stable, low molecular weight substance. This substance activates the second enzyme fraction, a latent ribonuclease (designated as RNase L).[19] The substance is identical with a series of 2′–5′ oligoadenylates ((2′–5′)(A)$_n$)[19] (see also references 20 and 21). These were originally discovered by Kerr and coworkers as inhibitors of protein synthesis.[22]

(2′–5′)(A)$_n$ Synthetase

The treatment of Ehrlich ascites tumor cells (EAT) with IF increases the level of the enzyme synthesizing (2′–5′)(A)$_n$ (designated as (2′–5′)(A)$_n$ synthetase) 10- to 100-fold. We purified this enzyme to apparent homogeneity.[23] The starting material for the purification is obtained by washing with a salt solution ribosomes from IF-treated EAT cells. The purification consists of differential precipitation with ammonium sulfate, chromatography on DEAE cellulose and CM cellulose. The apparent molecular weight of the enzyme is 105,000 as determined by polyacrylamide gel electrophoresis in the presence of SDS and 85,000 as determined by centrifugation through a glycerol gradient. These results make it probable that, at least before activation, the enzyme occurs as a monomer. In the presence of dsRNA the purified enzyme catalyzes the synthesis from ATP of 2′–5′ linked oligoadenylates with 5′ terminal triphosphate residues. The size of the oligoadenylates extends from the dimer to the hexadecamer; the dimer, trimer and tetramer are predominant among the products.[23] Studies involving the use of α and γ ^{32}P ATP indicate that the stoichiometry of the formation of one molecule of (2′–5′)(A)$_n$ is the following

$$\text{nATP} \rightarrow \text{pppA}\,(2'\,\text{p5}'\text{A})_{n-1} + n - 1 \text{ pyrophosphate}$$

Pyrophosphate is not cleaved by the enzyme. It is remarkable that the extent of conversion of ATP to (2′–5′)(A)$_n$ is very high, 97% or above. It is in line with this observation that the extent of the reverse reaction i.e., the incorporation of [^{32}P]pyrophosphate into ATP (in the presence of unlabeled (2′–5′)(A)$_n$, dsRNA and enzyme) if any, is below 0.3 percent.

The rate of (2′–5′)(A)$_n$ synthesis in the absence of dsRNA is less than 4% of that in the presence of dsRNA. The affinity of (2′–5′)(A)$_n$ synthetase for ATP is remarkably low. Even 5 mM ATP does not saturate the enzyme; the rate of the reaction increases by about 10% if the concentration of ATP is increased to 10 mM (Samanta *et al.*, manuscript in preparation).

RNase L

We purified RNase L, the (2′–5′)(A)$_n$-activatable latent endonuclease several hundredfold.[24] The starting material for this purification is the high speed supernatant fraction from an extract of IF-treated EAT cells. The purification consists of differential precipitation with ammonium sulfate and chromatography on several ion exchange resins. RNase L is an acidic protein with an isoelectric point of 5.5 and a molecular weight of 185,000 as estimated by gel filtration. It cleaves RNA only in the presence of divalent cations but it is not known whether these are needed for the activation of the enzyme or its catalytic function or both. When assayed in reaction mixtures including 1 mM ATP RNase L is activated by $(2'-5')(A)_n$ of chain length 3, 4 and 5 at nanomolar concentrations.

Partially purified preparations of RNase L retain $[^{32}P]$-labeled $(2'-5')(A)_n$ on nitrocellulose filters. The following results are consistent with the possibility that the component of the partially purified enzyme preparation which retains $(2'-5')(A)_n$ is RNase L: (a) the agent retaining $(2'-5')(A)_n$ on nitrocellulose filters copurifies with RNase L both during ion exchange chromatography and gel filtration. (b) Treatment of the enzyme preparation with N-ethylmaleimide abolishes both its activatability by $(2'-5')(A)_n$ and its ability to retain $(2'-5')(A)_n$ on nitrocellulose filters.[25] It remains to be established whether or not affinity chromatography on immobilized $(2'-5')(A)_n$ is a good approach for isolating RNase L.

The activation of RNase L is reversible and is lost upon removal of $(2'-5')(A)_n$, as revealed by the following experiment:[24] Gel filtration of $(2'-5')(A)_n$-activated RNase L results in an inactive enzyme and the bulk of the $(2'-5')(A)_n$ is recovered from fractions eluting after the enzyme. The enzyme recovered from gel filtration can, however, be fully reactivated by re-addition of $(2'-5')(A)_n$.

Gel filtration of activated RNase L through Sephadex G-200 equilibrated with $(2'-5')(A)_n$ results in elution of activated RNase L in the same elution volume as that of the not activated RNase L passed through Sephadex G-200 in the absence of $(2'-5')(A)_n$. Thus it seems unlikely that the activation of RNase L should result in the multimerization of the enzyme, the binding of a large complementary protein or the release of a large regulatory subunit. Any one of these processes would probably cause a more pronounced change in elution volume. It remains possible, however, that the activation really does involve such a process and the elution volume still does not change because of a compensating change in the shape of the enzyme.

The activated RNase L which was passed through the Sephadex G-200 column in the presence of $(2'-5')(A)_n$ reverts to the latent state when $(2'-5')(A)_n$ is removed by ammonium sulfate precipitation and dialysis of the enzyme. The latent endonuclease can thereafter be reactivated by re-adding $(2'-5')(A)_n$. This makes it improbable that the activation should result in the release of a small regulatory subunit since this would have been separated from the enzyme during gel filtration in the presence of $(2'-5')(A)_n$. If such a hypothetical small subunit would have been involved in inhibiting activity then its absence would have kept the enzyme active even after removal of $(2'-5')(A)_n$. If conversely such a subunit were needed for activation then its removal would have impaired the repeated activation of the endonuclease by $(2'-5')(A)_n$.

The nonactivated enzyme recovered from gel filtration through Sephadex G-200 can be activated by addition of $(2'-5')(A)_n$. This makes it unlikely that a small complementary protein would be required for the activation by $(2'-5')(A)_n$. This would have been separated from the enzyme during gel filtration.

All the above observations are consistent with the possibility that the activation of the latent endonuclease may involve the binding of $(2'-5')(A)_n$ to RNase L and that this interaction elicits the activation of RNase L by some mechanism other than the release of a subunit or the binding of a complementary protein. The validity of this interpretation will have to be tested, however, when pure RNase L becomes available. The partially purified RNase L preparation if activated cleaves various single-stranded RNAs at widely different rates.[26]

The fact that reovirus mRNA is degraded much faster in IF-treated cells (half life 5.3 hr) than in control cells (half life 12.3 hr) is consistent with the involvement of activated RNase L in mediating at least some of the antiviral effects of interferon in the case of reovirus infection.[14]

Interferon, dsRNA and Protein Phosphorylation

The need for dsRNA and ATP for the regulation of the endonuclease$_{INT}$ system, the knowledge that several proteins are activated or inactivated by phosphorylation, and other considerations prompted us to examine the effect of dsRNA on protein phosphorylation in extracts of IF-treated and control cells. We found that the addition of dsRNA (reovirus dsRNA or poly(I)·poly(C)) to an extract from IF-treated EAT cells (but not or to a much lesser extent to an extract from control cells) results in the phosphorylation of at least two proteins, P1 (67,000 daltons) and P2 (37,000 daltons)[27] (see also references 28 and 29). It is in accord with this finding that dsRNA added to intact IF-treated cells (but not to control cells) also results in the phosphorylation of P1.[30] We purified the dsRNA-activatable protein kinase system several thousandfold from EAT cells treated with interferon.[31] This treatment increases the level of the system severalfold. The purified enzyme preparation is free of dsRNA-independent kinase activity,[31] and its phosphorylation site specificity is similar to that of a kinase in reticulocyte lysates.[32] (2′–5′)(A)$_n$ is not synthesized by the activated kinase and (2′–5′)(A)$_n$ does not substitute for dsRNA in activating the enzyme.

The P2 protein that can be phosphorylated by the kinase appears to be the small subunit of the peptide chain initiation factor eIF-2[5] (see also references 32 and 33). The identity of P1 has not been definitely established. However, P1 copurifies with the dsRNA-activatable protein kinase throughout a several thousandfold purification. The most highly purified kinase preparation we have at present consists of P1 as a major protein band and two minor bands (as tested by labeling with [^{125}I]) (Pichon *et al.*, unpublished data). Studies are underway to test whether or not P1 is identical with the protein kinase.

The addition of the activated protein kinase preparation to a cell-free protein synthesizing system from EAT cells or reticulocyte lysates results in the inhibition of peptide chain initiation. The inhibition can be overcome by the addition of further eIF-2 and is apparently the consequence of the phosphorylation of eIF-2.[5,34]

On the Two Distinct, Double-stranded RNA-Dependent Pathways for Controlling Protein Synthesis in Interferon-treated Cells

As discussed in the previous sections the treatment of cells with IF enhances the level of latent enzymes (e.g., of (2′–5′)(A)$_n$ synthetase and of a protein kinase). If activated by double-stranded RNA and ATP these inhibit protein synthesis by cleaving single-stranded RNA, and blocking peptide chain initiation apparently by phosphorylating the small subunit of the chain initiation factor eIF-2.

The RNase L that had been activated by (2′–5′)(A)$_n$ returns to the latent state upon release of (2′–5′)(A)$_n$.[24] (2′–5′)(A)$_n$ can be cleaved by several enzymes including a "(2′–5′)(A)$_n$ cleaving enzyme" which was reported to cleave 2′–5′ linkages preferentially.[35] The inhibition of peptide chain initiation can be reversed by the enzymatic dephosphorylation of phosphorylated eIF-2.[7]

The rationale for the multiple involvement of dsRNA in the functioning of the IF system remains to be established. It is conceivable that dsRNAs in some form (e.g., RNA molecules partially single-stranded and partially double-stranded, free or partially coated) are intermediates or side products in the replication of many viruses. (Such dsRNAs might arise in the case of RNA viruses, e.g., in the form of a replication complex,[36] and in the case of DNA viruses, e.g., in consequence of the symmetric transcription of parts of the genome[37,38] and the annealing of the complementary strands to form dsRNA.) If this is the case then dsRNAs might serve as signals revealing the presence of replicating viruses in cells. It should be noted, however, that at least one of the biochemical phenomena elicited by IF—i.e., the impairment of mRNA cap methylation *in vitro*, is manifested even in the absence of added dsRNA.[11]

The treatment of cells with IF induces the formation of new mRNAs[39,40] and new proteins.[39–42] It remains to be seen if the dsRNA-activatable (2′–5′)(A)$_n$ synthetase and protein kinase can be identified with some of the new proteins.

The finding of (2′–5′)(A)$_n$ in IF-treated virus-infected cells indicates that (2′–5′)(A)$_n$ formation is not only an artifact of the *in vitro* system.[6] However, the definite establishment of the role of the above enzymes in mediating interferon action will require studies with mutants (or conditional mutants) lacking one or the other of the above enzymes.

SUMMARY

Extracts from interferon-treated, not virus-infected Ehrlich ascites tumor cells differ in various biochemical characteristics from extracts of control cells. We studied three enzymes whose level is enhanced in cells upon treatment with IF and which are causing some of the differences. (2′–5′)(A)$_n$ synthetase, an enzyme converting ATP into a series of (2′–5′) linked oligoadenylates ((2′–5′)(A)$_n$) in the presence of dsRNA was purified to homogeneity and characterized. The second enzyme, RNase L, a latent endonuclease, which can be activated by (2′–5′)(A)$_n$ to cleave single-stranded RNAs, was purified several hundredfold. The activation of this enzyme is reversible and is lost upon removal of (2′–5′)(A)$_n$. The activation is not accompanied by a large change in shape or conformation of the enzyme. The third enzyme is a protein kinase which if activated by dsRNA can phosphorylate the peptide chain initiation factor eIF-2 and a protein designated P1 of 67,000 daltons. This enzyme was purified several thousandfold. The most highly purified preparation consists of three proteins with P1 as the most abundant component.

REFERENCES

1. ISAACS, A. & J. LINDENMANN. 1957. Virus interference I. The interferon. Proc. Roy. Soc. London B **147:** 258–267.
2. BARON, S. & F. DIANZANI, Eds. 1977. The Interferon System. Tex. Rep. Biol. Med. **35.**
3. STEWART II, W. E. 1979. The Interferon System. Springer Verlag. Vienna, New York.

4. BAGLIONI, C. 1979. Interferon induced enzymatic activities and their role in the antiviral state. Cell **17:** 255–264.
5. FARRELL, P. J. , G. C. SEN, M-F. DUBOIS, L. RATNER, E. SLATTERY & P. LENGYEL. 1978. Interferon action: Two distinct pathways for the inhibition of protein synthesis by double-stranded RNA. Proc. Nat. Acad. Sci. USA **75:** 5893–5897.
6. WILLIAMS, B. R. G., R. R. GOLGHER, R. E. BROWN, C. S. GILBERT & I. M. KERR. 1979. Natural occurrence of 2-5A in interferon-treated EMC virus-infected L cells. Nature **282:** 582–586.
7. ZILBERSTEIN, A., A. KIMCHI, A. SCHMIDT & M. REVEL. 1978. Isolation of two interferon-induced translational inhibitors: A protein kinase and an oligo-isoadenylate synthetase. Proc. Nat. Acad. Sci. USA **75:** 4734–4738.
8. LEWIS, J. A., E. FALCOFF & R. FALCOFF. 1978. Dual action of double-stranded RNA in inhibiting protein synthesis in extracts of interferon-treated mouse L cells. Translation is impaired at the level of initiation and by mRNA degradation. Eur. J. Biochem. **86:** 497–509.
9. EPPSTEIN, D. A., T. C. PETERSON & C. E. SAMUEL. 1979. Mechanism of interferon action: Synthesis and activity of the interferon-mediated low-molecular weight oligonucleotide from murine and human cells. Virology **98:** 9–19.
10. SEN, G. C., B. LEBLEU, G. E. BROWN, M. A. REBELLO, Y. FURUICHI, M. MORGAN, A. J. SHATKIN & P. LENGYEL. 1975. Inhibition of reovirus messenger RNA methylation in extracts of interferon-treated Ehrlich ascites tumor cells. Biochem. Biophys. Res. Commun. **65:** 427–434.
11. SEN, G. C., S. SHAILA, B. LEBLEU, G. E. BROWN, R. C. DESROSIERS & P. LENGYEL. 1977. Impairment of reovirus mRNA methylation in extracts of interferon-treated Ehrlich ascites tumor cells: Further characteristics of the phenomenon. J. Virol. **21:** 69–83.
12. DESROSIERS, R. C. & P. LENGYEL. 1979. Impairment of reovirus mRNA cap methylation in interferon-treated mouse L929 cells. Biochim. Biophys. Acta **562:** 471–480.
13. SEN, G. C., S. L. GUPTA, G. E. BROWN, B. LEBLEU, M. A. REBELLO & P. LENGYEL. 1976. Interferon treatment of Ehrlich ascites tumor cells: Effects on exogenous mRNA translation and tRNA inactivation in the cell extract. J. Virol. **17:** 191–203.
14. LENGYEL, P., R. DESROSIERS, R. BROEZE, E. SLATTERY, H. TAIRA, J. DOUGHERTY, H. SAMANTA, J. PICHON, P. FARRELL, L. RATNER & G. SEN. 1980. Bichemistry of the interferon system. *In* Microbiology 1980. D. Schlessinger, Ed p: 219–226. ASM Publications.
15. GUPTA, S. L., W. D. GRAZIADEI III, H. WEIDELI, M. L. SOPORI & P. LENGYEL. 1974. Selective inhibition of viral protein accumulation in interferon-treated cells: Nondiscriminate inhibition of the translation of added viral and cellular messenger RNAs in their extracts. Virology **57:** 49–63.
16. GALSTER, R. L. & P. LENGYEL. 1976. Formation and characteristics of reovirus subviral particles in interferon-treated mouse L cells. Nucleic Acids Res. **3:** 581–598.
17. BROWN, G. E., B. LEBLEU, M. KAWAKITA, S. SHAILA, G. C. SEN & P. LENGYEL. 1976. Increased endonuclease activity in an extract from mouse Ehrlich ascites tumor cells which had been treated with a partially purified interferon preparation: Dependence on double-stranded RNA. Biochem. Biophys. Res. Commun. **69:** 114–122.
18. SEN, G. C., B. LEBLEU, G. E. BROWN, M. KAWAKITA, E. SLATTERY & P. LENGYEL. 1976. Interferon, double-stranded RNA and mRNA degradation. Nature **264:** 370–373.
19. RATNER, L., R. WEIGAND, P. FARRELL, G. C. SEN, B. CABRER & P. LENGYEL. 1978. Interferon, double-stranded RNA and RNA degradation. Fractionation of the endonuclease$_{INT}$ system into two macromolecular components: Role of a small molecule in nuclease activation. Biochem. Biophys. Res Commun. **81:** 947–954.
20. BAGLIONI, C., M. A. MINKS & P. A. MARONEY. 1978. Interferon action may be mediated by activation of a nuclease by pppA2′p5′A2′p5′A. Nature **273:** 684–687.
21. CLEMENS, M. J. & B. R. G. WILLIAMS. 1978. Inhibition of cell-free protein synthesis by pppA2′p5′A2′p5′A: A novel oligonucleotide synthesized by interferon-treated L-cell extracts. Cell **13:** 565–572.
22. KERR, I. M. & R. E. BROWN. 1978. pppA2′p5′A2′p5′A: An inhibitor of protein synthesis synthesized with an enzyme fraction from interferon-treated cells. Proc. Nat. Acad. Sci. USA **75:** 256–260.

23. DOUGHERTY, J. P., H. SAMANTA, P. J. FARRELL & P. LENGYEL. 1980. Interferon, double-stranded RNA and RNA degradation: Isolation of homogeneous (2′–5′)$(A)_n$ synthetase from Ehrlich ascites tumor cells. J. Biol. Chem. **255:** 3813–3816.
24. SLATTERY, E., N. GHOSH, H. SAMANTA & P. LENGYEL. 1979. Interferon, double-stranded RNA and RNA degradation: Activation of an endonuclease by (2′–5′)$(A)_n$. Proc. Nat. Acad. Sci. USA **76:** 4778–4782.
25. SLATTERY, E., N. GHOSH, H. SAMANTA & P. LENGYEL. 1979. Mediators of interferon action: On the activation of an endonuclease by (2′–5′)$(A)_n$. *In* Interferon: Properties and Clinical Uses. A Khan, N. O. Hill & G. L. Dorn, Eds. Wadley Institutes of Molecular Medicine.
26. RATNER, L., G. C. SEN, G. E. BROWN, B. LEBLEU, M. KAWAKITA, B. CABRER, E. SLATTERY & P. LENGYEL. 1977. Interferon, double-stranded RNA and RNA degradation: Characteristics of an endonuclease activity. Eur. J. Biochem. **79:** 565–577.
27. LEBLEU, B., G. C. SEN, S. SHAILA, B. CABRER & P. LENGYEL. 1976. Interferon, doublestranded RNA, and protein phosphorylation. Proc. Nat. Acad. Sci. USA **73:** 3107–3111.
28. ZILBERSTEIN, A., P. FEDERMAN, L. SHULMAN & M. REVEL. 1976. Specific phosphorylation *in vitro* of a protein associated with ribosomes of interferon-treated mouse L cells. FEBS Lett. **68:** 119–124.
29. ROBERTS, W. K., A. HOVANESSIAN, R. E. BROWN, M. J. CLEMENS & I. M. KERR. 1976. Interferon-mediated protein kinase and low-molecular weight inhibitor of protein synthesis. Nature **264:** 477–480.
30. GUPTA, S. L. 1979. Specific protein phosphorylation in interferon treated uninfected and virus-infected mouse L929 cells: Enhancement by double-stranded RNA. J. Virol. **29:** 301–311.
31. SEN, G. C., H. TAIRA & P. LENGYEL. 1978. Interferon, double-stranded RNA and protein phosphorylation: Characteristics of a double-stranded RNA activated protein kinase system partially purified from interferon-treated Ehrlich ascites tumor cells. J. Biol. Chem. **253:** 5915–5921.
32. SAMUEL, C. E. 1979. Mechanism of interferon action: Phosphorylation of protein synthesis initiation factor eIF-2 in interferon-treated human cells by a ribosome-associated kinase possessing site specificity similar to hemin-regulated rabbit reticulocyte kinase. Proc. Nat. Acad. Sci. USA **76:** 600–604.
33. KIMCHI, A., A. ZILBERSTEIN, A. SCHMIDT, L. SHULMAN & M. REVEL. 1979. The interferon-induced protein kinase PK-i from mouse L cells. J. Biol. Chem. **254:** 9846–9853.
34. FARRELL, P. J., K. BALKOW, T. HUNT & R. JACKSON. 1977. Phosphorylation of initiation factor eIF-2 and the control of reticulocyte protein synthesis. Cell **11:** 187–200.
35. SCHMIDT, A., Y. CHERNAJOVSKY, L. SHULMAN, A. FEDERMAN, H. BERISSI & M. REVEL. 1979. An interferon-induced phosphodiesterase degrading (2′–5′) oligoadenylate and the CCA terminus of tRNA. Proc. Nat. Acad. Sci. USA **76:** 4788–4792.
36. BILLETER, M. A., C. WEISSMANN & R. C. WARNER. 1966. Replication of viral nucleic acid. IX. Properties of double-stranded RNA from *Escherichia coli* infected with bacteriophage MS2. J. Mol. Biol. **17:** 145–173.
37. COLBY, C. & P. H. DUESBERG. 1969. Double-stranded RNA in vaccinia virus infected cells. Nature **222:** 940–944.
38. BOONE, R. F., R. P. PARR & B. MOSS. 1979. Intermolecular duplexes formed from polyadenylated vaccinia virus RNA. J. Virol. **30:** 365–374.
39. FARRELL, P., R. BROEZE & P. LENGYEL. 1979. Accumulation of an mRNA and protein in interferon-treated Ehrlich ascites tumour cells. Nature **279:** 523–525.
40. FARRELL, P. J., R. J. BROEZE & P. LENGYEL. 1980. Interferon induced mRNAs and proteins in Ehrlich ascites tumor and HeLa cells. Ann. N.Y. Acad. Sci. This volume.
41. KNIGHT, E., JR. & B. KORANT. 1979. Fibroblast interferon induces synthesis of four proteins in human fibroblast cells. Proc. Nat. Acad. Sci. USA **76:** 1824–1827.
42. GUPTA, S. L., B. Y. RUBIN & S. L. HOLMES. 1979. Interferon action: Induction of specific proteins in mouse and human cells by homologous interferons. Proc. Nat. Acad. Sci. USA **76:** 4817–4821.

PROTEIN KINASE ACTIVITY AND THE NATURAL OCCURRENCE OF 2-5A IN INTERFERON-TREATED EMC VIRUS-INFECTED L-CELLS

R. R. Golgher,*† B. R. G. Williams, C. S. Gilbert,
R. E. Brown and I. M. Kerr

National Institute for Medical Research
Mill Hill
London NW7 1AA, England

Protein synthesis in cell-free systems from interferon-treated cells shows an enhanced sensitivity to inhibition by double-stranded RNA (dsRNA). This cell-free system effect shows exactly the same interferon (IF) dose-response curve as does the antiviral effect in the intact cell, indicating that the two might indeed be closely related.[1] On the basis of these observations and the known effects of dsRNA in the intact cell and cell-free system, we suggested that the production of viral dsRNA in response to infection (even with a DNA virus) could bring about a general inhibition of protein synthesis such as is observed, for example, in IF-treated, vaccinia virus-infected mouse L-cells. The cell dies but little virus is produced: an effective way of limiting a natural infection. Alternatively, the triggering by dsRNA of a more transient or selective inhibition could result in the degradation of viral nucleic acid but permit the ultimate recovery of the cell.[1-4] The mechanism of action of dsRNA in inhibiting protein synthesis was therefore investigated. Two distinct pathways appear to be involved: (1) phosphorylation of the protein synthesis initiation factor eIF-2 by an interferon and dsRNA mediated kinase and (2) degradation of mRNA by a nuclease(s) activated by sub-nanomolar levels of the unusual oligonucleotide pppA2′p5′A2′p5′A (and related oligomers collectively referred to as 2-5A) synthesized by an interferon and dsRNA-mediated synthetase.[5-18]

When artificially introduced into intact cells, 2-5A has also been shown to activate a nuclease and inhibit protein synthesis and virus growth. Both in the cell-free system and when introduced into the intact cell 2-5A is unstable, and in the absence of a regenerating system the activation of the nuclease and inhibition of protein synthesis are transient.[12-16] Thus, cells have a mechanism for coping with 2-5A, and the nuclease that it activates is capable of cyclic activation and deactivation. This, combined with the very low concentrations of 2-5A required for activity, suggested a possible wider significance of the 2-5A system in the control of cell metabolism. In accord with this the 2-5A synthetase can be detected in different amounts in a variety of cells and tissues and the levels of the enzyme can also vary with growth and hormone status.[17] In addition, as was first shown in collaboration with E.M. Martin, the dephosphorylated core of the molecule, A2′p5′A2′p5′A, is capable of inhibiting DNA synthesis and cell growth in the Daudi line of human lymphoblastoid cells. A similar effect of 2-5A *per se*

**Current address:* Departamento de Microbiologia, Instituto de Ciencias Biologicas, Universidade Federal de Minas Gerais, Belo Horizonte, Brasil.

†R.R.G. was supported by a fellowship from the Conselho Nacional de Desenvolvimento Cientifico e Tecnologico, Brasil.

0077-8923/80/0350-0448 $01.75/0 © 1980, NYAS

has been observed by Hovanessian and Wood (personal communication) on its introduction into mouse L-cells using the calcium phosphate co-precipitation technique.[15] The results are consistent with a role for 2-5A both in the antiviral and cell growth inhibitory activities of IF and raise the possibility of a wider involvement of the 2-5A system in the general context of hormone action and the control of cell growth and development. This possible wider role has been further emphasized by the recent demonstration by Ball that an enzyme which is almost certainly the 2-5A synthetase is capable (in cell extracts) of adding AMP in 2′-5′ linkage to a variety of important metabolites such as NAD, ADP ribose and AppppA.[18] On the other hand, this raises inevitable questions concerning the normal function of this enzyme particularly as, to date, there has been no direct evidence for the natural occurrence of 2-5A. (It has only been detected after synthesis in cell extracts or with the partially purified synthetase). Similarly, although it is clear that under appropriate conditions[19] phosphorylation of eIF-2 by the IF-mediated kinase plays a part in the inhibition of protein synthesis by dsRNA in cell-free systems, there is as yet no direct evidence for its involvement in the intact cell. The experiments described here were undertaken, therefore, to try to obtain more direct evidence for a role for the kinase and for the natural occurrence of 2-5A. The most likely system in which to look seemed *a priori* to be the IF-treated virus-infected cell. Accordingly, these initial experiments were carried out in IF-treated, encephalomyocarditis (EMC) virus-infected mouse L-cells. Although it has not yet been possible to obtain direct evidence for kinase activity in the intact cell, extracts from IF-treated virus-infected cells no longer require the addition of dsRNA for the phosphorylation of the 67K protein and added eIF-2: results consistent with the presence of preactivated kinase in these extracts and hence in the intact cell. In the case of 2-5A more direct evidence for the natural occurrence of these 2′-5′ linked oligomers in the IF-treated virus-infected cell is presented.

Results

Protein Kinase Activity in Intact Cells and Presence of a "Preactivated" Kinase in Extracts from Interferon-treated Virus-infected Cells

Interferon-treated and control cells plus and minus infection with EMC virus were pulse-labeled with $^{32}P_i$ for 1.5 hr–3 hr after infection. The cells were lysed with NP40, centrifuged at 2,000 × g and the resultant supernatant fractions analysed by electrophoresis on SDS polyacrylamide gels (FIGURE 1A). Although an infection-specific protein kinase activity resulted in the phosphorylation of two relatively low molecular weight polypeptides (channels 2 and 4, FIGURE 1A) no interferon- and infection-specific enhancement of phosphorylation was apparent (compare channels 2, 3, 4, FIGURE 1A). On the other hand, when extracts prepared from IF-treated infected cells 4.5 hr post infection were incubated *in vitro* with [γ-^{32}P]ATP an enhanced phosphorylation of an endogenous 67K protein and of the 38K subunit of added eIF-2 was observed. In contrast to the situation after IF treatment alone (channels 9–12, FIGURE 1B) and consistent with the "preactivation" of a kinase by small amounts of endogenous viral dsRNA produced in response to infection, the phosphorylation of these two polypeptides in IF-treated, infected cell extracts was no longer dependent on the addition of dsRNA. This is particularly obvious in the case of the 38K subunit of added eIF-2 (channels 13–16, FIGURE 1B).

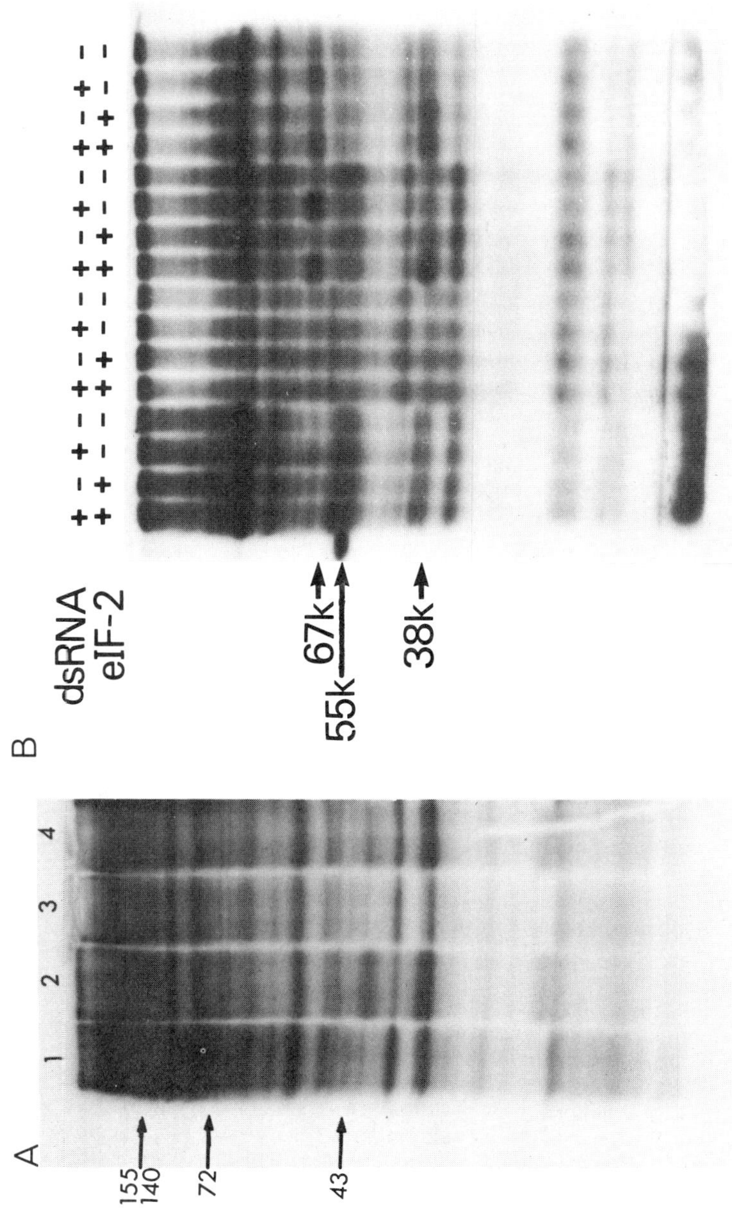
A
155
140
72
43
1
2
3
4
B
dsRNA
eIF-2
67k
55k
38k

FIGURE 1. *In vivo* (A) and *in vitro* (B) protein kinase activity in control or interferon-treated uninfected and EMC-infected mouse L-cells. Confluent monolayers of mouse L-cells (100 mm diameter plates in A) or spinner cultures (B) were treated for 17 hr at 37°C with 400 reference (20 effective) units per ml of partially purified mouse (IF) (5×10^7 reference units per mg of protein), infected with 20 p.f.u. per cell of EMC virus and incubated for 4.5 hr at 37°C. Control cells with or without IF treatment or EMC infection were incubated in parallel.

In (A) the cells were pulsed for 1.5 hr before harvesting by incubating in phosphate-free medium (lml) containing 2% dialyzed calf serum and 250 μCi carrier-free ^{32}P. The cells were washed, scraped into phosphate-buffered saline and centrifuged, and the packed cells were lysed into an equal volume of 0.5% NP40 in dialysis buffer (10 mM HEPES, pH 7.5, 90mM KCl, 1.5mM magnesium acetate). Aliquots of a $2000 \times g$ supernatant were analyzed by SDS polyacrylamide gel electrophoresis (12.5%) and autoradiography. Tracks 1–4 contain extracts from control, infected, IF-treated and IF-treated infected cells respectively. The position of reovirus polypeptide molecular weight markers (155,000, 140,000, 72,000, and 43,000, respectively) run in parallel are indicated.

In (B) the cells were washed and harvested at 4.5 hr and a $2000 \times g$ supernatant (prepared by homogenization as in cell-free system preparation[12]) was centrifuged at $100{,}000 \times g$ and the pellets were resuspended in dialysis buffer 20% glycerol. Protein kinase activity was monitored by incubating the resuspended material (3 μl) with 1 μCi [γ-^{32}P]ATP (specific activity 3000 Ci/mmol) 0.1 mM ATP, 3mM magnesium acetate in the presence or absence of 10^{-6} g/ml poly rI.rC and 1 μg of highly purified eIF-2 (a gift from Dr. W. Merrick). After 15 min at 30°C the samples were analysed by SDS-polyacrylamide gel electrophoresis and autoradiography. The 55K autophosphorylated subunit of eIF-2[5] and positions of the 67K and 38K proteins are indicated on the left.

Tracks 1–4 (from the left) contain extracts from control cells; tracks 5–8, infected cell extracts; tracks 9–12, IF-treated cell extracts; and tracks 13–16, IF-treated infected cell extracts.

Presence of 2-5A in Interferon-treated EMC Virus-infected L-Cells

Interferon-treated and control cells 4 hr after infection with EMC were lysed with the detergent NP40 and the soluble fractions either precipitated with trichloroacetic acid (TCA) or heated to 95°C for 5 min, centrifuged to remove denatured protein and purified on DEAE Sephadex to remove the majority of contaminating mono and oligonucleotides. Fractions corresponding to the known position of elution of 2-5A were pooled, lyophilized, redissolved and assayed for

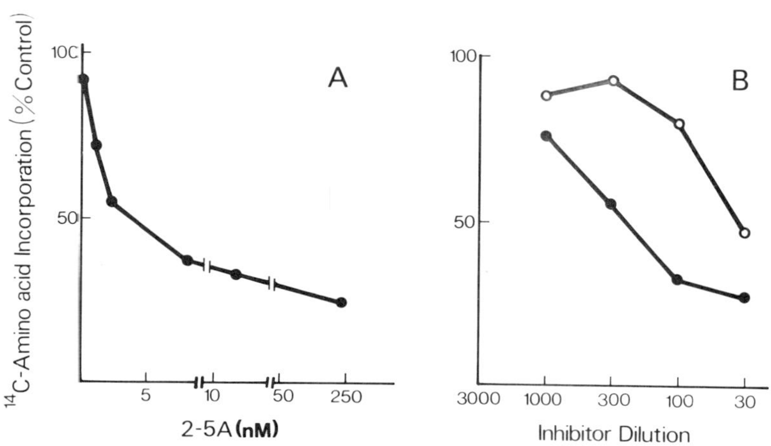

FIGURE 2. Inhibition of cell-free protein synthesis by 2-5A recovered from interferon-treated, EMC-infected cells. Spinner cultures of mouse L-cells were treated with interferon (IF) plus or minus infection with EMC as in FIGURE 1. The cells were harvested at 4.5 hr post infection and washed and the packed cells were lysed into an equal volume of 0.5% NP40 dialysis buffer. The 100,000 × g supernatant fractions were heated to 95°C for 5 min and centrifuged to remove denatured protein and the supernatants were fractionated on DEAE Sephadex.[20] Fractions corresponding to 2-5A were eluted with 1M NH_4HCO_3, lyophilized extensively to remove bicarbonate, and redissolved in 20 μl of H_2O prior to dilution (*abscissa*, B) and assayed in the EMC-RNA-programmed Erhlich ascites tumor cell-free system prepared and incubated for 120 min at 30°C as described for similar systems for mouse L-cells.[12] The *ordinate* gives the incorporation of a mixture of ^{14}C-amino acids into acid-insoluble polypeptides as a percentage of a control incubation (19191 cpm per 10 μl sample). (A) Assay of a reticulocyte 2-5A standard preparation (concentrations are in AMP equivalents). (B) Assay of material prepared from IF-treated (○) and IF-treated EMC infected (●) cells. The inhibition observed at a 1:30 dilution with the IF-treated material in B reflects a nonspecific inhibition seen with all cell extracts of this type at relatively low dilutions.

2-5A either by inhibition of protein synthesis in an EMC RNA programmed cell-free system from Ehrlich ascites tumor (EAT) cells or by activation of a nuclease in rabbit reticulocyte lysates. Whereas material from control, control-infected, or IF-treated cells was without significant effect, that from IF-treated, EMC virus-infected cells inhibited protein synthesis over a range of dilutions in the cell-free system (FIGURE 2). In accord with this, only the material from IF-treated EMC virus-infected cells activated a nuclease in reticulocyte lysates (see FIGURE 3). The material responsible for the activity in both the above assays was sensitive to digestion with bacterial alkaline phosphatase and snake venom phosphodiesterase but resistant to digestion with T2 and micrococcal nuclease as would be expected for 2-5A (data not shown). Further evidence for the identity of this material as 2-5A came from its behavior on high pressure liquid chromatography (HPLC) in comparison with appropriate standards.

Characterization of 2-5A by HPLC

2-5A Synthesized with the synthetase from IF-treated mouse L-cells or rabbit reticulocytes consists of a mixture of oligonucleotides of the general formula ppp $(A2'p)_nA$ with the trimer as the predominant species.[7, 20] The individual components, trimer, tetramer and pentamer ($n = 2$-4, respectively) were isolated by chromatography on DEAE cellulose[20] and subjected to HPLC. In FIGURE 3 the pattern obtained with a recombined mixture of these standard preparations is presented. Peaks 7 to 9 correspond to the trimer, tetramer and pentamer triphosphates respectively. All preparations also contain smaller and variable amounts of the corresponding di- and monophosphates (peaks 4–6 and 1–3, respectively).[20] These are thought to represent breakdown products of the predominant triphosphates. (Throughout the rest of this paper we will use the terms trimer, tetramer, and pentamer to denote preparations of this type consisting largely of the triphosphates, but also containing smaller amounts of the di-and monophosphates. We will use the more complete nomenclature to identify the individual species). We have previously shown that the trimer diphosphate (but not the monophosphate) has essentially the same specific biological activity as the corresponding triphosphate.[20] The same appears to be true for the corresponding tetramer and pentamer species. It is not known whether the diphosphates are active *per se* or are rephosphorylated in the assay system.

An analysis of the putative 2-5A from IF-treated, EMC virus-infected cells (to which ATP and p_4A were added as optical density markers) is shown in FIGURE 3. Since too little 2-5A was present for it to be identified by optical density, appropriate fractions were analyzed for biological activity using nuclease activation in the reticulocyte lysate (FIGURE 3). A broad peak of nuclease activity was obtained in fractions 16 to 21 (FIGURE 3B, channels Q–V, FIGURE 3C) corresponding to the tetramer and pentamer triphosphates (FIGURE 3A). The extent of resolution of these two components is given by the densitometer scan (FIGURE 3D) of the nucleolytic breakdown products of the ^{32}P-RNA in the region between the arrows in FIGURE 3C. For comparison, the results obtained in the nuclease assay with increasing concentrations of a standard preparation of 2-5A are included (channels B–F, FIGURE 3C).

The apparent absence of trimer in the above preparation was initially curious, but further analysis showed that the trimer tri- and diphosphates, in contrast to the tetramer and pentamer, are relatively poor activators of the nuclease and inhibitors of protein synthesis in rabbit reticulocyte lysates although fully active in this respect in other systems.[7, 20] In support of this, in further more detailed studies at higher resolution (manuscript in preparation) biological activities corresponding to the trimer, tetramer, and pentamer di- and triphosphates were recovered from extracts from the IF-treated virus-infected cells. In one such experiment, for example, peak HPLC fractions corresponding to the trimer and tetramer triphosphates were pooled, dialyzed, concentrated and shown to have inhibitory activity in an EMC RNA programmed EAT cell-free system (FIGURE 4).

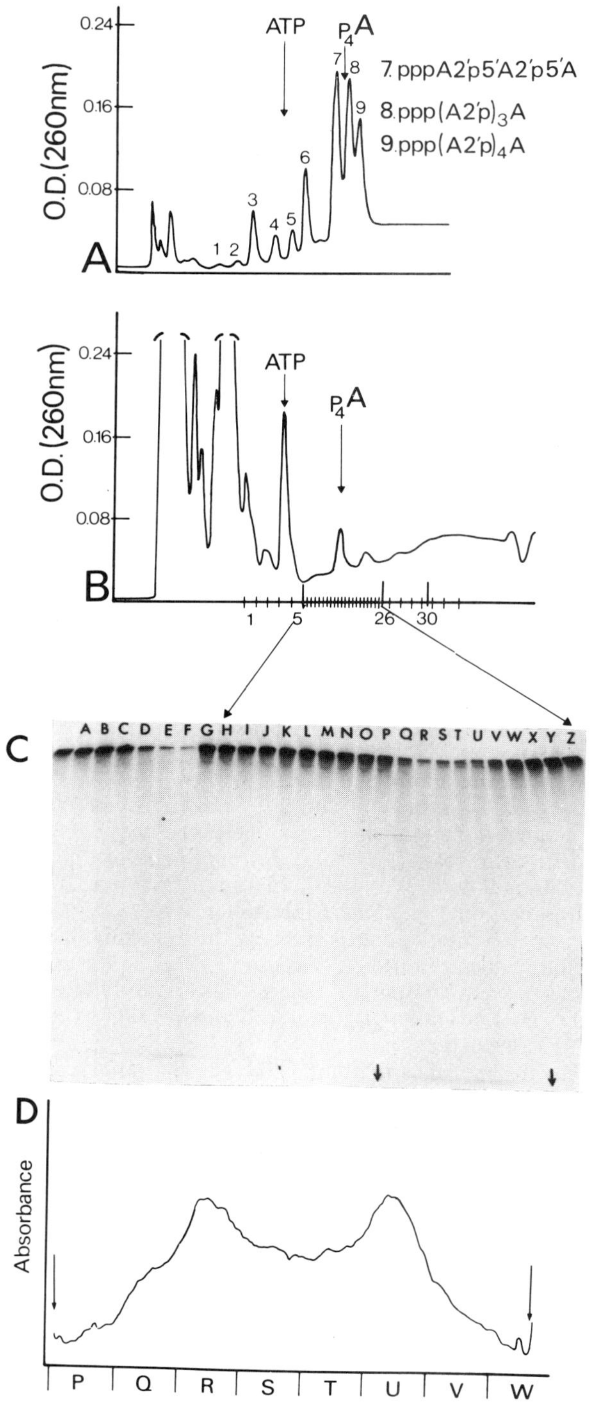
O.D.(260nm)
0.24
0.16
0.08
ATP
P_4A
7. pppA2'p5'A2'p5'A
8. ppp(A2'p)$_3$A
9. ppp(A2'p)$_4$A
A
B
1
5
26
30
C
A B C D E F G H I J K L M N O P Q R S T U V W X Y Z
D
Absorbance
P Q R S T U V W

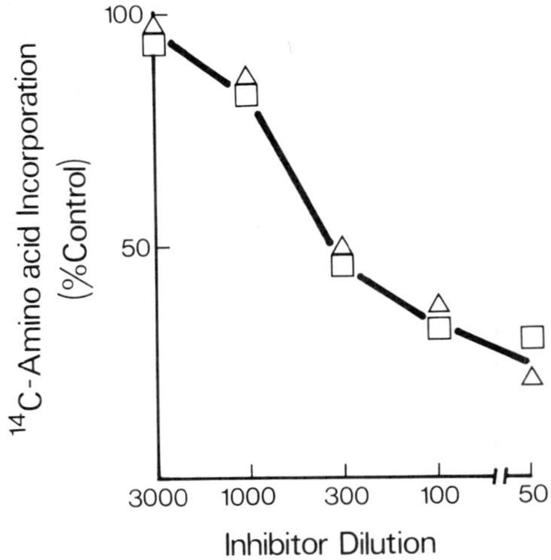

FIGURE 4. Inhibition of cell-free protein synthesis by the trimer and tetramer triphosphate components of 2-5A recovered from interferon-treated EMC virus-infected cells by HPLC. Material from IF-treated, EMC virus-infected cells prepared as described in FIGURE 3 was subjected to analysis by HPLC. Fractions corresponding to the known elution positions of the trimer (△) and tetramer (□) triphosphates were each pooled (750 μl), dialyzed against four changes of 100 volumes of water at 4°C, lyophilized, redissolved in water (20 μl) and assayed at the final dilutions indicated (*abscissa*) in an EMC RNA programmed EAT cell-free system. Standard trimer and tetramer triphosphate preparations (750 μl of 1 μM in HPLC elution buffer) processed in parallel were each recovered in 80% yield. Nonphosphorylated A2′p5′A2′-5′A was added as a "carrier" prior to dialysis: parallel controls confirmed that neither it nor "off peak" fractions from the HPLC analysis processed in parallel had significant inhibitory activity in the cell-free system. Incorporation of ^{14}C-amino acids into acid-insoluble polypeptides is given as a percentage of the control (no inhibitor) value which was 17,100 cpm per 10 μl sample in the system used here. A standard 2-5A preparation gave a 50% inhibition of incorporation at a final concentration of 2.5 nM in the same assay.

FIGURE 3. HPLC analysis of 2-5A from interferon-treated, EMC virus-infected cells. (A) A mixture of reticulocyte 2-5A standards containing the trimer, tetramer, and pentamer triphosphates (peaks 7, 8, and 9, respectively) purified as described.[20] Each contained lesser amounts of the corresponding di- (peaks 4–6) and mono- (peaks 1–3) phosphates. In a parallel run, ATP and p_4A were included with the above components and the positions at which they eluted are indicated on the figure. (B) 2-5A (3μ1) from IF-treated, EMC virus-infected cells prepared as in FIGURE 2 plus 5 μl each of 10 μM ATP and p_4A. (C) Samples (2 μl of threefold dilution) of the column fractions (1, 4, 6, 10–23, 25 and 27, *abscissa*, B) were analyzed (channels G to Z, part C) for their ability to activate a nuclease and degrade ^{32}P-RNA in the reticulocyte lysate system (12.5 μ1).[19] Channels A to F: analysis of the ^{32}P-RNA incubated in the same system in the absence, A, and presence, B to F, of 0.24, 0.8, 2.4, 8 and 24 nanomolar standard 2-5A. An autoradiograph of an SDS polyacrylamide gel analysis of the ^{32}P-RNA is shown. (D) Densitometer scan of the original autoradiograph corresponding to the region between the arrows in Part (C). In the nuclease assay approximately 100 ng (equivalent to 5,000 cpm at a specific activity of 5×10^4 cpm per μg) of ^{32}P-labeled RNA was added per 12.5 μl assay. The concentrations of the standard preparations of 2-5A are given in AMP equivalents. The HPLC analysis was on a LiChrosorb 10 NH_2 column with a linear gradient of 40 to 200 mM ammonium phosphate, pH 7.2, 700 (1–5, 26–32) and 250 (6–25) μl fractions were collected. (In our experience a number of amine columns from different manufacturers all gave excellent separations of the type shown in (A). It appears, however, that these columns have a relatively short life under the conditions used allowing, on occasion, very few runs to be made).

Discussion

Role of the Protein Kinase

To date it has not been possible to obtain direct evidence for enhanced activity of the 67K polypeptide and eIF-2 38K subunit kinase(s) in response to infection in intact IF-treated cells. Nevertheless, the results in cell extracts are consistent with the presence of a "preactivated" kinase in such cells (FIGURE 1B). Also, the fact that this "preactivated" kinase activity is found associated with a sedimentable fraction which might be expected to contain the virus dsRNA replication complex (FIGURE 1) is also consistent with this interpretation. In these respects our results are similar to those of Gupta[21] and Aujean *et al.*,[22] but the "preactivated" kinase activity detected here was not dependent on the presence of NP40 as in the latter study. Results concerning the kinase, however, are complicated by the fact that the dsRNA dependence observed in extracts reflects, in part at least, the presence of a dsRNA inhibitable protein phosphatase (M. Revel and R. M. Friedman, personal communication). In accord with this, the partially purified kinase, although it binds to dsRNA no longer appears to require it for activity.[23] Clearly, a more detailed knowledge of the characteristics of both the kinase and any related phosphatase, their dependence on dsRNA and distribution in the IF-treated virus-infected cell is required. Finally, it is worth noting that it is the phosphorylation of the 38K subunit that is essential for inhibition of protein synthesis, yet this can be clearly detected only when exogenous eIF-2 is added to extracts (FIGURE 1B). The analysis of the extent of phosphorylation of eIF-2 and the establishment of its role in the intact IF-treated virus-infected cell may therefore require the use of larger amounts of material coupled with 2-dimensional gel analysis.

The Significance of the Detection of 2-5A in the Intact Cell

From the data presented in FIGURES 3 and 4 and related experiments, it would appear that the triphosphorylated trimer, tetramer, and pentamer components at least of 2-5A are present in IF-treated mouse L-cells 4 hr post infection with 20 p.f.u. per cell of EMC virus. It is possible that smaller amounts of the diphosphates are also present in the intact cell, but these may reflect partial breakdown products of the corresponding triphosphates. If higher oligomers are present then they are not detectable with the procedures used here. The heterogeneity in the length of the 2-5A synthesized in cell extracts has still to be explained. This, perhaps more than anything else, emphasized the possibility that 2-5A in the form originally isolated might be no more than an intriguing artefact of cell-free systems. The discovery of similar heterogeneity here in the intact cell argues against this, and although providing no explanation for the phenomenon, suggests that it may indeed have some significance.

We have previously shown that 2-5A artificially introduced into cells is capable of activating a nuclease(s) and inhibiting protein synthesis and virus growth.[14–16] Here we have demonstrated the natural occurrence of 2-5A in amounts sufficient for it to be responsible for a similar sequence of events in IF-treated, EMC virus-infected L-cells. Assuming 50% recovery of the 2-5A throughout the isolation procedure (which is reasonable from appropriate control experiments), the yields obtained from experiments completed so far have been consistent with concentrations of 20 to 200 $\times$ 10^{-9} M 2-5A in the IF-treated, EMC virus-infected cells from which the extracts were made. In addition, evidence has been obtained for an enhanced rate of breakdown of preformed mRNA in such cells. There is a 70% decrease in the amount of polyadenylated mRNA recoverable 4 hr after EMC infection of IF-treated cells. In accord with this, there is an overall inhibition of protein synthesis, a significant decrease in the number of polysomes and a corresponding marked increase in the 80S monosome peak (arrowed, FIGURE 5D) in such cells (FIGURE 5). All these results are at least consistent with the activation of a nuclease by 2-5A in IF-treated EMC virus-infected L-cells. The relative importance of this mechanism, however, compared with any effect of the IF- and dsRNA-mediated kinase or alternative mecha-

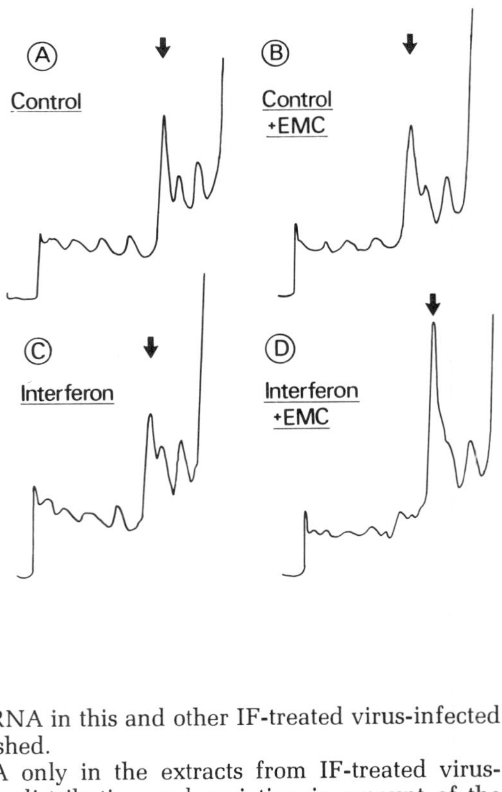

FIGURE 5. Sucrose gradient analysis of polysomes prepared from interferon-treated EMC virus-infected and control cells. Monolayers of mouse L-cells were treated with interferon (IF) and infected with EMC virus as described in FIGURE 1A. Control cells with or without IF treatment or EMC infection were incubated in parallel. At 3.5 hr post infection cycloheximide was added to 400 μg/ml and incubation continued for a further 30 min. The cells were lysed by the addition of 0.5% NP40 dialysis buffer (100 μl per dish) and lysates added directly to 5 ml 15–40% sucrose gradients (in 100 mM KCl, 10 mM Tris-HCl, pH 7.4 1 mM EDTA) and centrifuged for 50 min at 45,000 rpm in the Beckman SW 50.1 rotor. Absorbance at 260 nm was monitored by passing the gradients through a Unicam SP1800 spectrophometer using a flow cell with a 0.1 cm light path.

nism(s) not mediated through dsRNA in this and other IF-treated virus-infected cell systems remains to be established.

Here we have detected 2-5A only in the extracts from IF-treated virus-infected cells, whereas the wide distribution and variation in amount of the synthetase has raised the possibility that it may have a wider significance in the regulation of cell growth or development.[17] It should be emphasized, however, that were 2-5A to have been present in physiological concentrations of less than 10×10^{-9} M we would not have detected it with the procedures used. Clearly, a more sensitive and convenient assay for 2-5A and a much more detailed analysis of this and alternative systems will be required before the full significance of either 2-5A or its synthetase can be assessed. Meanwhile, however, it is unlikely from the results presented here that 2-5A is a mere artefact of the cell-free system and reasonable to assume that it plays some part in the inhibition of virus growth in the IF-treated EMC virus-infected cell.

References

1. Kerr, I. M., R. E. Brown & L. A. Ball. 1974. Nature **250:** 57–59.
2. Joklik, W. K. & T. C. Merigan. 1966. Proc. Nat. Acad. Sci. USA **56:** 558–565.
3. Metz, D. H. & M. Esteban. 1972. Nature **238:** 385–388.
4. Friedman, R. M., D. H. Metz, M. Esteban, D. R. Tovell & I. M. Kerr. 1972. J. Virol. **10:** 1184–1198.
5. Farrell, P. J., K. Balkow, T. Hunt & R. J. Jackson. 1977. Cell **11:** 187–200.
6. Roberts, W. K., A. G. Hovanessian, R. E. Brown, M. J. Clemens & I. M. Kerr. 1976. Nature **264:** 477–480.
7. Kerr, I. M. & R. E. Brown. 1978. Proc. Nat. Acad. Sci. USA **75:** 256–260.
8. Farrell, P. J., G. C. Sen, M. F. Dubois, L. Ratner, E. Slattery & P. Lengyel. 1978. Proc. Nat. Acad. Sci. USA **75:** 5893–5897.
9. Zilberstein, A., A. Kimchi, A. Schmidt & M. Revel. 1978. Proc. Nat. Acad. Sci. USA **75:** 4734–4738.
10. Ball, L. A. & C. N. White. 1978. Proc. Nat. Acad. Sci. USA **75:** 1167–1171.
11. Clemens, M. J. & B. R. G. Williams. 1978. Cell **13:** 565–572.
12. Williams, B. R. G., I. M. Kerr, C. S. Gilbert, C. N. White & L. A. Ball. 1978. Eur. J. Biochem. **92:** 455–462.
13. Minks, M. A., S. Benvin, P. A. Maroney & C. Baglioni. 1979. Nucl. Acid Res. **6:** 767–780.
14. Williams, B. R. G. & I. M. Kerr. 1978. Nature **276:** 88–90.
15. Hovanessian, A. G., J. Wood, E. Meurs & L. Montagnier. 1979. Proc. Nat. Acad. Sci. USA **76:** 3261–3265.
16. Williams, B. R. G., R. R. Golgher & I. M. Kerr. 1979. FEBS Letts. **105:** 47–52.
17. Stark, G. R., W. J. Dower, R. J. Schimke, R. E. Brown & I. M. Kerr. 1979. Nature **276:** 471–473.
18. Ball, L. A. 1979. *In* Regulation of macromolecular synthesis by low molecular weight mediators. G. Koch & D. Richter, Eds. Academic Press. 303–317.
19. Williams, B. R. G., C. S. Gilbert & I. M. Kerr. 1979. Nucl. Acid Res. **6:** 1335–1350.
20. Martin, E. M., N. J. M. Birdsall, R. E. Brown & I. M. Kerr. 1979. Eur. J. Biochem. **95:** 295–307.
21. Gupta, S. L. 1979. J Virol. **29:** 301–311.
22. Aujean, O., J. Sanceau, E. Falcoff & R. Falcoff. 1979. Virology **92:** 583–586.
23. Hovanessian, A. G. & I. M. Kerr. 1979. Eur. J. Biochem. **93:** 515–526.

ROLE OF INTERFERON-INDUCED ENZYMES IN THE ANTIVIRAL AND ANTIMITOGENIC EFFECTS OF INTERFERON

M. Revel, A. Kimchi, L. Shulman, A. Fradin, R. Shuster,†
E. Yakobson,‡ Y. Chernajovsky, A. Schmidt, A. Shure,
and R. Bendori

Department of Virology
Weizmann Institute of Science
Rehovot, Israel

INTERFERON-INDUCED ENZYMES AND THE ANTIVIRAL STATE

Exposure of human or animal cells to their respective interferons (IFs) produces, within a few hours, an increase in several enzymes, whose function appears to be mainly related to regulation of protein biosynthesis. FIGURE 1 summarizes what is known of the mechanism of action of three such enzymes: protein kinase PK-i, (2′-5′) oligo A synthetase E, and phosphodiesterase 2′-PDi. (For a complete review and bibliography see ref. 1). Induction of these enzymes was seen in our laboratory in human fibroblasts and Namalva cells, in monkey BSC-1 cells, in bovine MDBK cells and in mouse L cells and splenic lymphocytes. Using a microassay that allows the determination of the enzyme levels with about 25,000 cells (one well of a 96-hole microplate), the kinetics of induction were determined.[2] A typical lag period of 2-4 hr is observed after IF addition and before the enzyme levels begin to rise. Maximum increase is reached after 18-24 hr. With actinomycin D, it was possible to show that in mouse L cells, the transcription step necessary for induction of the protein kinase and of the (2′-5′) oligo A synthetase takes place during the first 2 hr; actinomycin D inhibits if added during the first 2 hr, but if added later, a phenomenon of superinduction is observed.[2] TABLE 1 shows that, in contrast, cycloheximide inhibits induction even if added late after IF, indicating that translation of the mRNA transcripts continues throughout the induction period. It can also be seen from TABLE 1 that in human fibroblast FS11, the transcription step for the (2′-5′) oligo A synthetase occurs more slowly than in L cells. With anti-IF antibodies, it can be shown (FIGURE 2) that the continued presence of IF on the cell surface is required for induction. Antibodies do not penetrate the cells, and their ability to inhibit even as late as 3 hr after IF addition, indicates that IF is still outside the cell at this point. From the data in FIGURE 2, the induction could be described as a stochastic process: the longer the time allowed for IF action, the higher the level of induction. The discrepancy between the effect of anti-IF shown in FIGURE 2 and

*The research for this paper was supported by grants from the Gesellschaft für Strahlung and Umweltforschung (Munich, FRG) and the National Council for Research and Development (Israel).

†Recipient of a Fogarty Senior International Fellowship. *Present address:* Department of Biochemistry, Emory University, Atlanta, Georgia.

‡*Present address:* Department of Viral Oncology, ICRF, Lincoln's Inn Fields, London, England.

0077-8923/80/0350-0459 $01.75/0 © 1980, NYAS

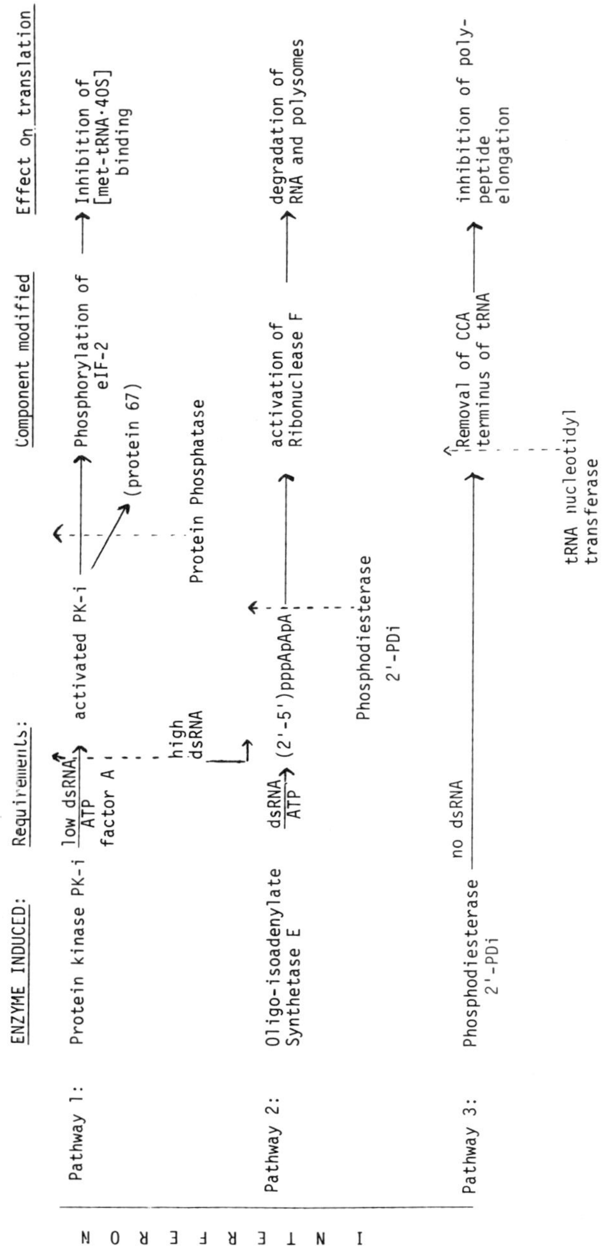

FIGURE 1. Interferon-induced translation inhibitory pathways.

TABLE 1

INDUCTION OF OLIGO-ISOADENYLATE SYNTHETASE*

	Mouse L929 Cells		Human FS11 Cells
Inhibitor Added at Time =	Cycloheximide %	Actinomycin D %	Actinomycin D %
−2 hr	—	0	—
0 hr	—	20	0
1 hr	2	29	—
1.5 hr	—	—	17
2 hr	5	100	—
3 hr	2	145	58
4.5 hr	26	—	—
6 hr	—	133	132
No inhibitor (8hr)	100	100	100

*Monolayer cultures of mouse or human cells were treated at time = 0, with mouse L cell IF (200 U/ml) or with human fibroblast IF (50 U/ml). Cycloheximide (25 μg/ml) and actinomycin D (2 μg/ml) were added at the indicated time before or after interferon. The level of (2′–5′) oligo-isoadenylate synthetase was measured in NP-40 extracts prepared 8 hr after IF, as detailed previously.[2] The 100% value correspond to about 15,000 cpm of [^{32}P]-(2′–5′)ApA produced; a background of 1500 cpm for nontreated cells was subtracted.

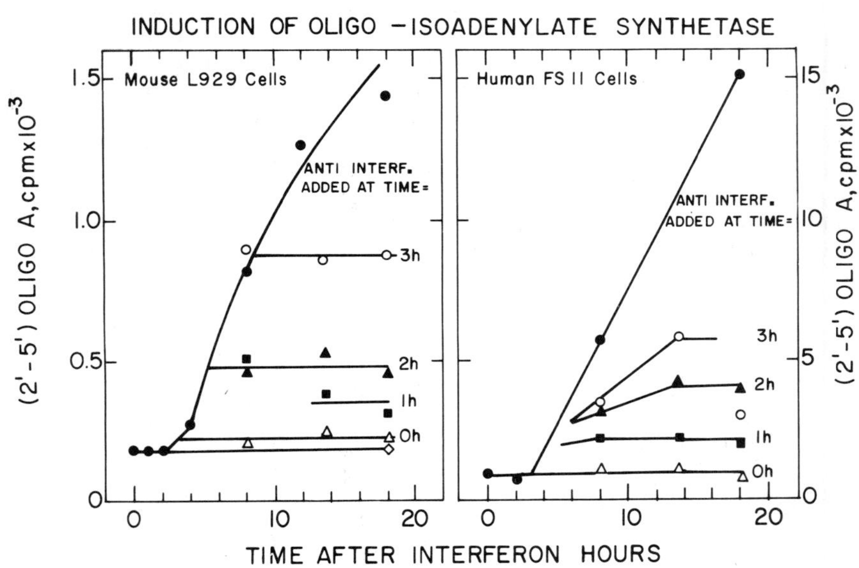

FIGURE 2. Effect of anti-interferon antibodies added after interferon (IF) on oligo-isoadenylate synthetase E induction. Monolayer cultures of L929 or FS11 cells (about 2.5 × 10^4 cells per well of a 96-well microplate) received 50 U/ml mouse L cell IF or 15 U/ml human fibroblast IF, respectively. The level of enzyme E was measured at the indicated time as described.[2] Antibodies to mouse L cell IF (gift from G. Galasso, NIH) or antibodies to human fibroblast IF obtained in rabbits,[24] were added (in amounts sufficient to block the antiviral effects of the concentrations of IF used) at the indicated times after IF addition. The lower activity of the L cells only reflects use of less radioactive ATP in the assay.

1. Rapid binding of interferon — 2. Interaction with species specific receptor — Interferon still on the cell surface — 3. Nuclear response (transcription) — 4. Interferon-induced enzymes start to accumulate (translation)

rapid membrane changes — Internalization of interferon and receptor (?) — Delayed biochemical response

TIME: 0 hr.......................................1 hr... .... 2 hr............. 3 hr .... 12 hr

binding to ganglicsides (even in the cold) — binding to surface component coded by chr 21 — Inhibition by antibodies to interferon or to receptor — Antiviral state and enzyme induction becomes Act D resistant — Superinduction of antiviral state and enzyme by Act D

FIGURE 3. Schematic view of the early events in interferon action. Scheme based on experimental evidence listed below the time scale.

that of actinomycin D shown in TABLE 1, is due to the superinduction phenomenon by actinomycin D. The slower induction in human FS11 cells seen with actinomycin D (TABLE 1) is also seen with anti-IF (FIGURE 2). These data can be summarized as in FIGURE 3, which describes some of the early events in the action of interferon.

By two-dimension gel electrophoresis of proteins labeled with [^{35}S] methionine in the treated cells, it has been possible to demonstrate the induction of about 5-6 proteins by interferon[3,4] (see FIGURE 8, below). It is not yet known which of these proteins corresponds to the identified enzymes.

The induction of the three enzymes in response to different doses of mouse IF on L cells correlates well with the inhibition of vesicular stomatitis virus (VSV) replication in the cells (TABLE 2). Correlation between the antiviral state and the induction of the (2′-5′) oligo A synthetase were reported in chick cells by Ball[4] and HeLa cells by Baglioni *et al.*[5] Monkey BSC-1 cells infected by SV40 allows a more precise kinetic study of the correlation between IF-dependent enzyme induction and the inhibition of viral protein synthesis. In this system,[6] monkey IF is added to cell cultures *already infected* by SV40 for 24 hr. Subsequently, an inhibition of SV40 late viral protein synthesis appears, together with an inhibition of viral DNA replication and virus yield. The kinetics of protein synthesis inhibition are shown in FIGURE 4. The rate of synthesis of the viral T-antigen is

TABLE 2

INTERFERON-INDUCED ENZYMES AND ANTIVIRAL STATE IN L CELLS*

	Experiment I		Experiment II		
Interferon U/ml	VSV-RNA	Protein Kinase PKi	VSV-RNA	Oligo-isoadenylate synthetase E	Phosphodiesterase 2′ PDi
0	100	15	100	4	25
2	24	35	12	5	72
10	6	80	5	20	86
50	0	100	2	42	100
250			0	66	
1,250			0	100	100

*Results are in percent of maximum activity. Cells were treated for 8 hr with interferon. Enzyme assays are as described by Kimchi *et al.*[2] Measure of vesicular stomatitis virus (VSV) RNA synthesis as in Weissenbach *et al.*[24]

inhibited first, while inhibition of capsid proteins develops only after a 10-hr lag period. Most of the host proteins continue to be synthesized,[6] with the exception of host histone synthesis, which is inhibited similarly to the T-antigen (FIGURE 4). Both protein kinase PK-i and (2′-5′) oligo A synthetase are induced in this system; the kinetics of induction of the latter enzyme are shown in FIGURE 4. The enzymes accumulate before viral protein synthesis inhibition. Studies with extracts prepared from IF-treated SV40-infected cells confirm the presence of a

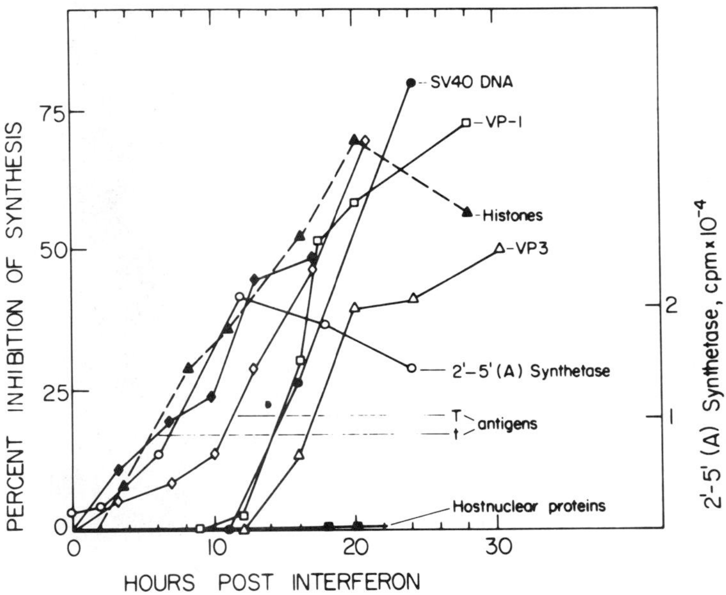

FIGURE 4. Kinetics of inhibition of viral function by monkey interferon given late (24 hr) after SV40 infection of BSC-1 cells. The rate of synthesis of the various proteins was determined by[^{35}S]methionine pulse-labeling and gel electrophoresis analysis as described.[6] Viral DNA synthesis was measured by [^{3}H]thymidine-labeling of Hirt-extractable DNA. Inhibitions were calculated at various times after interferon addition in comparison to appropriate controls. The level of (2′-5′) oligo A synthetase E was measured as described.[2]

dominant inhibitor of translation that can also inhibit protein synthesis when added to control cell extracts.[7]

MECHANISM OF PROTEIN SYNTHESIS INHIBITION IN SV40-INFECTED BSC-1 CELLS BY INTERFERON: SPECIFIC CLEAVAGE OF 28S rRNA

A detailed study of the effects of IF on the expression of SV40 genes in the infected cells showed[6] that the inhibition is most probably at the translational level. SV40 mRNAs still continue to be synthesized at the time when SV40 protein synthesis is maximally inhibited.[6] Normal amounts of SV40 VP-1 mRNA can be extracted from these cells, and it was shown, by translation in reticulocyte

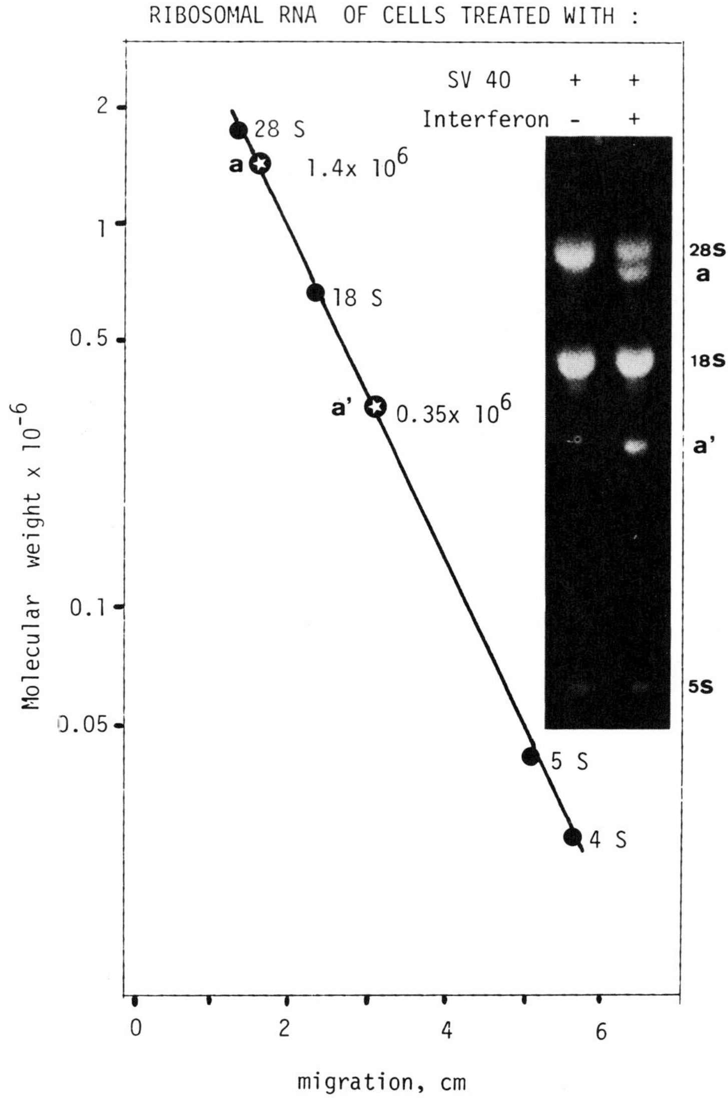

FIGURE 5. Cleavage of 28S ribosomal RNA in interferon-treated SV40-infected BSC-1 cells. Cultures infected for 24 hr were treated with 100 U/ml monkey IF and 24 hours later, RNA was phenol-extracted from NP40 cytoplasmic extracts, heated 30 min to 50°C with 13% glyoxal-44% DMSO and electrophoresed on a 1.5% agarose gel. A UV photograph of the gel stained with ethidium bromide is shown with RNA from untreated *(left)* and IF-treated *(right)* SV40-infected cells. The size of fragments a and a' was calculated from the known ribosomal RNA bands.

lysates, to be fully active.[8] This mRNA is, however, not in polyribosomes.[6] An increased methylation of internal adenine residues in SV40 RNA was, until now, the only noticeable change in mRNA structure.[8] Degradation of the SV40 16S and 19S mRNA was not observed.

One of the methods that we used to study SV40 mRNA in these cells was agarose gel electrophoresis of total cytoplasmic RNA after heating in glyoxal-dimethylsulfoxide, followed by blotting onto diazobenzyloxymethyl (DBM) paper[9] and hybridization of the DBM-paper with nick-translated [^{32}P] SV40 DNA.

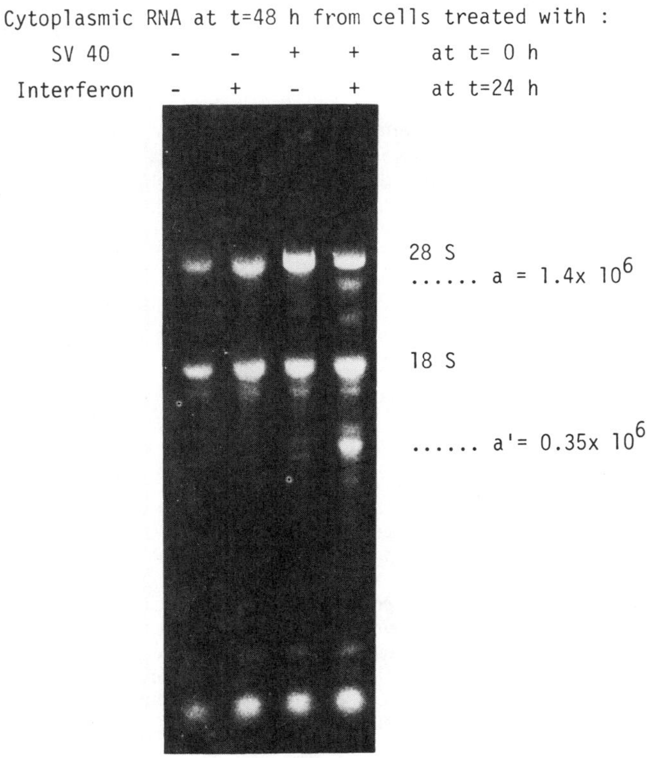

FIGURE 6. Cleavage of ribosomal RNA in interferon-treated SV40-infected BSC-1 cells: Experiments are similar to that in FIGURE 5 comparing RNA from (left to right) uninfected untreated cells, uninfected IF-treated cells, infected untreated cells, infected IF-treated cells.

Even under these conditions, it was possible to show that 24 hr after IF treatment, the cytoplasm still contains the normal amount of 16S SV40 RNA. Surprisingly, however, examination of the agarose gel after ethidium bromide staining showed that the ribosomal RNA pattern from interferon-treated SV40-infected cells was altered.[10] The major alteration, consistently observed after IF treatment of the cells, are two new bands of 1.4 and 0.35 x 10^6 daltons and a reduction in 28S RNA (1.75 x 10^6 daltons) (FIGURE 5). The new bands are best explained as being derived from the 28S RNA by a single cleavage located 20% away from one end. The cleavage is more apparent in RNA prepared from isolated ribosomes or from cytoplasmic extracts prepared after lysis of the cells with Nonidet (NP) P40. It is only barely visible in total cell RNA extracted with dodecylsulfate. There may be several reasons for this: either the NP40 detergent treatment is needed to detect the cleavage, or rather, nuclear RNA is uncleaved and its presence masks the partial cytoplasmic RNA cleavage. The cleavage appears related to the state of activity of the ribosomes, since after fractionation cytoplasmic ribosomes on a sucrose gradient, the cleavage was much more apparent in the 80S monosome peak than in the polysomal region (unpublished). Often additional rRNA fragments may be observed (e.g. FIGURE 6, at 1.0 × 10^6 daltons), but these can

TABLE 3

ACTIVATION OF (2′–5′) OLIGO-ISOADENYLATE SYNTHETASE BY RNA FROM SV40-INFECTED AND UNINFECTED CELLS*

Cells	Treatment	RNA	Amount	(2′–5′)Oligo A Synthesis [^{32}P]-(2′–5′)ApA cpm
I. BSC-1	None	Total cell RNA	1 μg	9,000
	Interferon			7,800
	SV40			13,600
	SV40 + interferon			18,100
BSC-1	SV40 + interferon	Cytop. RNA	1 μg	1,500
—	—	poly(rI):(rC)	0.01 μg	36,100
		None	—	150
II. BSC-1	SV40	polyA$^+$ cytop.RNA	0.8 μg	8,800
Reticulocytes		polyA$^+$ RNA	0.6 μg	145
—	—	poly(rI):(rC)	0.01 μg	9,600

*Where indicated, monolayer cultures of BSC-1 cells infected with SV40 for 24 hr were treated by 100 U/ml monkey IF (Yakobson *et al.*[6,25]) and 24 hr later, total RNA was extracted by phenol and 0.5% SDS, and precipitated with 2 M LiCl. From cytoplasmic extracts prepared with 0.5% NP40, cytoplasmic total RNA was obtained by phenol, 0.5% SDS- 5 mM EDTA. PolyA$^+$ RNA was purified on oligo(dT)-cellulose. RNAs were added to a 25 μl reaction containing purified (2′–5′) oligo-isoadenylate synthetase E (3 μg) and [^{32}P]-α-ATP (1 mM; 150 mCi/mmol), incubated 20 hr, at 30°C and the amount of (2′–5′)ApA cores formed measured after alkaline phosphate as in Kimchi *et al.*[2]

appear also in extracts from control cells. It is unlikely that the specific cleavage of ribosomal RNA extracted from IF-treated cells, shown in FIGURE 5, is produced *in vitro*, since incubation of these extracts under conditions of protein synthesis did not enhance the specific cleavage but produced different patterns of ribosomal RNA degradation in both control and IF-treated extracts. It appears therefore that a rather specific nuclease activity which cleaves 28S RNA at a single site is enhanced in the cytoplasm of IF-treated cells. The specific rRNA cleavage appeared only if cells had been both infected with SV40 and treated with IF (FIGURE 6), under conditions where the inhibition of viral protein synthesis is observed. The nuclease that produces this cleavage has not yet been identified with certainty. One interesting possibility is that RNase F, which is activitated by (2′-5′) oligo A,[11–13] is responsible for this cleavage. Interferon induces the (2′-5′) oligo A synthetase in these cells (FIGURE 4). In addition, poly A$^+$ mRNA from BSC-1 cells fulfills the double-stranded RNA requirement of (2′-5′) oligo A synthetase (and protein kinase) with about 1% the efficiency of poly(rI):(rC) (TABLE 3). Some increase in this dsRNA-like activity was seen in total RNA from SV40 infected cells (TABLE 3). There was, however, no such increase in the cytoplasmic RNA. It is, nevertheless, likely that (2′-5′) oligo A is produced in these IF-treated SV40-infected BSC-1 cells. Hovanessian *et al.*[14] recently observed a similar pattern of ribosomal RNA cleavage in cells treated by (2′-5′) oligo A in the presence of calcium phosphate. This would be in line with a role of the (2′-5′) oligo A-dependent RNase F in the cleavage of ribosomal RNA; another nuclease, such as the RNase M of Herzberg *et al.*,[15] which also splits rRNA, was not found to be increased after IF (Herzberg, personal communication). Interferon's action may thus resemble in some way, that of colicin E_3.[16] The degradation of the 28S rRNA may explain the inhibition of translation observed *in vivo* and *in vitro*. The cleavage may affect only a part of the cell's ribosomes, if the idea of a localized activation of the (2′-5′) oligo A-dependent RNase proposed by Baglioni,[17] as a result of a localization of dsRNA sequences, is valid. In the intact cell, only certain ribosomes would be affected, explaining why a large fraction of the host protein synthesis continues. In the cell extracts, the effect might become more pronounced than it is in the intact cells. Clearly, the mechanism of rRNA cleavage remains to be further elucidated, but the importance of these experiments is that they focus our attention, for the first time, on rRNA rather than on mRNA as the target of IF action, at least for the antiviral effect of interferon on SV40.

ROLE OF (2′-5′) OLIGO A SYNTHESIS AND DEGRADATION IN THE REGULATION OF CELL MITOGENESIS

Interferon synthesis slows down the rate of cell division and the onset of DNA synthesis in a variety of cells (for review see ref. 18). It is not known whether these effects are mediated by an action on protein synthesis similar to that observed in the antiviral effect. Histone biosynthesis is inhibited very early after IF treatment in SV40-infected cells (FIGURE 4), and also in uninfected cells (TABLE 4). We have, however, found that the histone mRNA activity (assayed by translation of poly A$^-$ RNA in reticulocyte lysates) is also reduced by IF (unpublished). But another indication that common pathways operate for the antiviral and antimitogenic effects comes from the observation[19] that (2′-5′) oligo A cores (e.g., micromolar concentrations of (2′-5′)ApApA but not (3′-5′)ApApA) are able to inhibit the onset of DNA synthesis in Concanavalin A (Con A)-stimulated mouse spleen lymphocytes, in the same way as interferon. TABLE 5 shows that inhibition of DNA synthesis by (2′-5′)ApApApA added to the intact lymphocyte cultures is largest when the oligonucleotides, are added together with Con A or 24 hours later, while addition at 48 hr produces only slight inhibition. In all cases, DNA synthesis was measured at 72 hr after Con A. Stimulation of DNA synthesis by Con A in these lymphocyte cultures starts at 48 hr and is maximal at 72 hr. The oligonucleotides have therefore to be added before the cell enters the S phase. This is also true for IF itself (TABLE 5 and ref. 20). Addition of the (2′-5′) oligo A produces after 48 hr a partial inhibition of protein synthesis in these Con A-stimulated lymphocytes; polyacrylamide gel

TABLE 4

INHIBITION OF HISTONE SYNTHESIS BY INTERFERON IN UNINFECTED MONKEY KIDNEY CELLS*

Hours After Interferon	Inhibition of [^{35}S]Methionine Label Histones (%)	Actin (%)
7 hr	30	10
12 hr	35	3
18 hr	50	10

*Duplicate cultures of BSC-1 cells were treated with 200 U/ml monkey interferon,[25] about one day before confluency. Cells were labeled for 2 hr with [^{35}S]methionine (40 μCi/ml) and nuclear proteins were subjected to electrophoresis on 12% polyacrylamide gel in SDS. After autoradiography the intensity of the histone and actin bands were measured by scanning at 600 mμ. The percent decrease in band intensity after IF is given.

electrophoresis showed that among others, histone synthesis is particularly affected, while many other proteins are unaffected (unpublished results). Inhibition of DNA synthesis by (2′-5′)ApApA was also reported by Martin[21] in cultures of lymphoblastoid Daudi cells.

A further line of evidence indicating that the (2′-5′) oligo A plays a role in the regulation of cell mitogenesis is derived from the observation that Con A-stimulated lymphocytes have a much higher level of the 2′-phosphodiesterase (2′-PDi) which degrades (2′-5′)pppApApA into ATP and AMP[22] than do lymphocytes maintained without mitogen (TABLE 6). The high level of 2′-phosphodiesterase produces an inhibition of the synthesis of (2′-5′) oligo A in extracts of Con A-stimulated lymphocytes.[19] A similar higher level of 2′-PDi was seen in fast growing BSC-1 cells as compared to confluent cultures of these monkey kidney

TABLE 5

INHIBITION OF DNA SYNTHESIS IN CON A-STIMULATED MOUSE SPLEEN LYMPHOCYTES BY INTERFERON AND BY (2′-5′) OLIGO-ISOADENYLATE*

	Addition to Con A-stimulated Cultures	Time of Addition	DNA Synthesis at 72 hr after (^{3}H)Thymidine Incorporation (cpm)	Inhibition (%)
Experiment 1	None	—	111,020	0
	Interferon	0 hr	13,175	88
	Interferon	24 hr	66,050	41
	Interferon	48 hr	102,060	8
Experiment 2	None	—	66,150	0
	(2′-5′)ApApApA	0 hr	17,665	74
	(2′-5′)ApApApA	24 hr	18,800	72
	(2′-5′)ApApApA	48 hr	56,765	15

*Mouse spleen lymphocytes (8×10^6 cells/ml) were treated with 2.5 μg/ml Con A. Interferon (200 U/ml) or (2′-5′)ApApApA (5 μM) was added 10 min later (0 time) or at various times after Con A. DNA synthesis was measured at 72 hours by a 3-hr pulse of 6 μCi/ml [^{3}H]thymidine (5 Ci/mmol). Cells were then harvested on glass fiber filters (Whatman GFC), washed twice with 5 ml cold PBS, twice with 5 ml 5% TCA then with 95% ethanol, dried, and counted. [^{3}H]thymidine incorporated into the unstimulated lymphocytes (28,750 cpm) was subtracted from that incorporated into the mitogen-treated cells.

TABLE 6

CON A-INDUCED 2′-PHOSPHODIESTERASE IN MOUSE LYMPHOCYTES*

Fraction	Degradation of (2′–5′) Oligo A (dimer + trimer) No Mitogen (cpm)	Con A (cpm)
Crude extract 14 μg	1500	8350
DEAE, 150 mM KCl 2.5 μg	0	10750
5 μg	5050	15550

*Mouse spleen lymphocytes were cultured for 72 hr in RPMi 1640 with or without 2.5 μg/ml Con A. The cells were lysed in a buffer containing 0.5% NP40 and the cytoplasmic crude extract was fractionated on DEAE-cellulose to isolate the fraction containing the 2′-phosphodiesterase as in Schmidt *et al.*[22] Degradation of a mixture of [^{32}P]-(2′-5′)pppApApA and pppApApApA (total cpm = 30,400 cpm) was measured by the amount of AMP released in 1 hr at 30°C as described before,[22] with the indicated amount of protein fractions.

cells (Kimchi, Shure & Revel, in preparation). The basal level of (2′-5′) oligo A synthetase is also quite variable under various cell culture conditions.[23]

These results suggest that a growth stimulus is accompanied by an increase in an enzyme which degrades (2′-5′) oligo A and may prevent its action as an inhibitor of entry in the S phase. Interferon treatment increases the level of (2′-5′) oligo A synthetase E by at least fourfold over its basal level in Con A-treated lymphocytes.[19] This high level of (2′-5′) oligo A synthetase, activated by the endogenous dsRNA-like RNA of the cell, would overcome the effect of the 2′-phosphodiesterase and produce enough accumulation of (2′-5′) oligo A to block

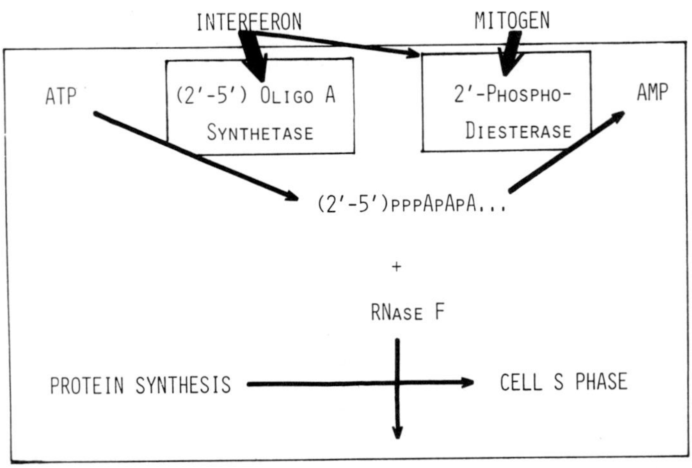

FIGURE 7. Schematic view of the regulation of mitogenesis by (2′-5′) oligo A synthetase E and 2′-phosphodiesterase 2′-PDi. The rectangle symbolizes the cell. Arrows indicate that interferon induces E and to a lesser extent 2′-PDi[2]. A mitogen stimulus as Concanavalin A for lymphocytes leads to an increase in 2′-PDi activity (see TABLE 6).

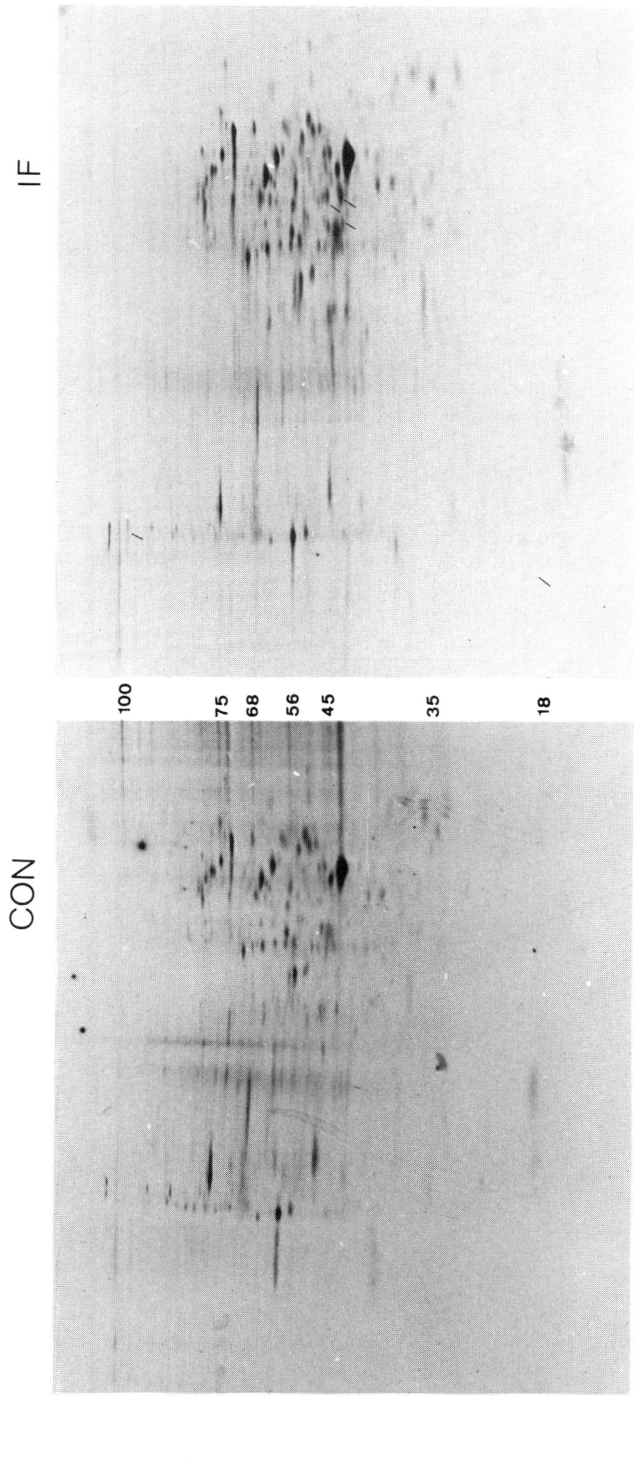

FIGURE 8. Proteins synthesized by mouse spleen lymphocytes treated with interferon. Two dimensional gel electrophoresis of the proteins labeled by [^{35}S]methionine between 22 and 24 hr after exposure of mouse spleen lymphocytes to 1,000 U/ml mouse interferon (IF). From left to right isoelectrofocusing from anode to cathode; vertically SDS-poly acrylamide gel electrophoresis according to O'Farrell.[26] The CON panel shows the analysis of untreated cells. Oblique bars indicate IF-stimulated proteins.

entry in the S phase. The stimulation of 2′-PDi observed in IF-treated L cells (ref. 2 and TABLE 2) may actually be needed to prevent the damage that (2′-5′) oligo A accumulation and RNase F activation could cause to these cells. It may be speculated that cells whose rate of division is less affected by IF treatment utilize this induction of 2′-PDi to balance the increase in (2′-5′) oligo A synthetase. The ratio of (2′-5′) oligo A synthetase over 2′-phosphodiesterase may then be a really significant parameter regulating cell division (FIGURE 7). Actually, the possibility is not excluded that exogenously added (2′-5′)ApApA cores act by competitive inhibition of the 2′-phosphodiesterase, rather than being phosphorylated into the (2′-5′)pppApApA activator of RNase F. The possibility that the (2′-5′) oligo A has other effects in the cell than just activating RNase F has also not been excluded. Nevertheless, it now seems tempting to implicate the intracellular level of (2′-5′) oligo A in both antiviral and antimitogenic effect of interferon. Since, however, IF induces at least 4–5 proteins in these lymphocytes (FIGURE 8), including the dsRNA-dependent protein kinase PK-i (Kimchi and Revel, unpublished), it would not be suprising that more complicated mechanisms are at work to produce the astonishing cell regulatory functions of interferons.

ACKNOWLEDGMENTS

Gifts of (2′-5′) oligo A from Drs. Y. Lapidot and S. Rapoport are gratefully acknowledged.

REFERENCES

1. REVEL, M. 1979. *In* Interferon 1979. I. Gresser, Ed.: 101–163. Academic Press, New York.
2. KIMCHI, A., L. SHULMAN, A. SCHMIDT, Y. CHERNAJOVSKY, A. FRADIN & M. REVEL. 1979. Proc. Nat. Acad. Sci. USA **76:** 3208–3212.
3. KNIGHT, T. E. & B. D. KORANT. 1979. Proc Nat. Acad Sci. USA **76:** 1824–1827.
3a. DELEY, M., A. BILLIAU & P. DE SOMER. 1979. Biochem. Biophys. Res. Commun. **89:** 701–705.
4. BALL, A. 1979. Virology **94:** 282–296.
5. BAGLIONI, C., P. A. MARONEY & D. K. WEST. 1979. Biochemistry **18:** 1765–1768.
6. YAKOBSON, E., C. PRIVES, J. R. HARTMAN, E. WINOCOUR & M. REVEL. 1977. Cell **12:** 73–81.
7. REVEL, M., E. GILBOA, A. KIMICHI, A. SCHMIDT, L. SHULMAN, E. YAKOBSON & A. ZILBERSTEIN. 1977. Proc. FEBS Meet. 11th **43:** 47–58.
8. KAHANA, C., M. REVEL & Y. GRONER. 1979. Ann. Meeting Israel Biochem. Soc. Abstract, p. 40.
9. ALWINE, J. C., D. J. KEMP & G. R. STARK. 1977. Proc. Nat. Acad. Sci. USA **74:** 5350–5355.
10. REVEL, M., A. KIMCHI, A. SCHMIDT, L. SHULMAN, Y. CHERNAJOVSKY, S. RAPOPORT & Y. LAPIDOT. 1979. *In* Regulation of Macromolecular Weight Mediators. G. Kock & D. Richter, Eds.: 341–359. Academic Press. New York.
11. SCHMIDT, A., A. ZILBERSTEIN, L. SHULMAN, P. FEDERMAN, H. BERISSI & M. REVEL. 1978. FEBS Letters **95:** 257–264.
12. CLEMENS, M. J. & B. R. G. WILLIAMS. 1978. Cell **13:** 565–572.
13. BAGLIONI, C., M. A. MINKS & P. A. MARONEY. 1978. Nature **273:** 684–487.
14. HOVANESSIAN, A. G., J. WOOD, E. MEURS & L. MONTAGNIER. 1979. Proc. Nat. Acad. Sci. USA **76:** 3261–3265.
15. WRESCHNER, D., D. MELLOUL & M. HERZBERG. 1978. Eur. J. Biochem **85:** 233–240.

16. BOWMAN, C. M. 1972. FEBS Letters **22:** 73–75.
17. NILSEN, T. W. & C. BAGLIONI. 1979. Proc. Nat. Acad. Sci. USA **76:** 2600–2604.
18. GRESSER, I. & M. G. TOVEY. 1978. Biochim. Biophys. Acta **516:** 231–247.
19. KIMCHI, A., H. SHURE & M. REVEL. 1979. Nature **282:** 849–851.
20. WEINSTEIN, Y., B. R. BRODEUR, K. L. MELMON & T. C. MERIGAN. 1977. Immunol. **33:** 313–319.
21. MARTIN, E. M. 1979. Personal communication.
22. SCHMIDT, A., Y. CHERNAJOVSKY, L. SHULMAN, P. FEDERMAN, H. BERISSI & M. REVEL. 1979. Proc. Nat. Acad. Sci. USA **76:** 4788–4792.
23. STARK, G. R., W. J. DOWER, R. T. SHINKER, R. E. BROWN & I. M. KERR. 1979. Nature **278:** 471–473.
24. WEISSENBACH, J., M. ZEEVI, T. LANDAU & M. REVEL. 1979. Eur. J. Biochem. **98:** 1–8.
25. YAKOBSON, E., M. REVEL & D. GURARI-ROTMAN. 1979. Arch. Virol. **59:** 251–255.

MECHANISMS OF INTERFERON-MEDIATED INHIBITION OF PROTEIN SYNTHESIS*

Charles E. Samuel, Susan M. Kingsman, Rivka W. Melamed, Deborah A. Farris, Mark D. Smith, Neil G. Miyamoto, Stephen R. Lasky, and Grace S. Knutson

Section of Biochemistry and Molecular Biology
Department of Biological Sciences
University of California
Santa Barbara, California 93106

INTRODUCTION

Interferons inhibit the production of infectious progeny virions of a wide range of unrelated DNA and RNA viruses.[1,2] In most animal virus-host cell systems the level of virus genome expression inhibited as a result of interferon (IF) treatment is the accumulation or translation, or both, of viral messenger RNAs.[3] Interferon does not block the initial steps of a viral infection—parental virion adsorption to cells, penetration into cells, and uncoating within cells[1]—but the final steps—assembly and release of infectious progeny—may be altered in the case of some enveloped viruses, such as the murine leukemia viruses.[4]

IN VITRO STUDIES

Cell-free extracts prepared from IF-treated cells catalyze the translation *in vitro* of a variety of exogenously added viral mRNAs much less efficiently than extracts prepared from untreated cells.[5-8] The inhibitor(s) of protein synthesis observed in extracts of IF-treated murine cells is associated with the ribosomal system, and can be separated from ribosomes by washing with buffers containing concentrated salt.[8,9] The IF-mediated ribosome-associated inhibitors of translation are not species-specific, even though certain IFs are relatively species-specific.[10] As the duration of IF treatment of murine cells is increased, the phosphorylation of certain proteins present in the ribosomal salt-wash fraction as well as the degradation of reovirus mRNA is increased in extracts prepared from IF-treated cells; the increases in protein phosphorylation and mRNA degradation correlate with the appearance of the ribosome-associated inhibitor(s) of translation.[9] Recent studies indicate that the inhibition of protein synthesis observed in cell-free extracts prepared from IF-treated cells is due to the induction by IF of at least two enzymic activities.[11] Both of the recently identified IF-induced enzymes, a protein kinase and 2′,5′-oligoadenylate synthetase, utilize ATP as a substrate and are apparently dependent upon the presence of RNA with double-stranded character for activation.

The IF-mediated protein kinase activity[9,12-14] is ribosome-associated and

*This work was supported in part by research grants from the National Institute of Allergy and Infectious Disease and the American Cancer Society, and by a Research Career Development Award from the United States Public Health Service.

0077-8923/80/0350-0473 $01.75/0 © 1980, NYAS

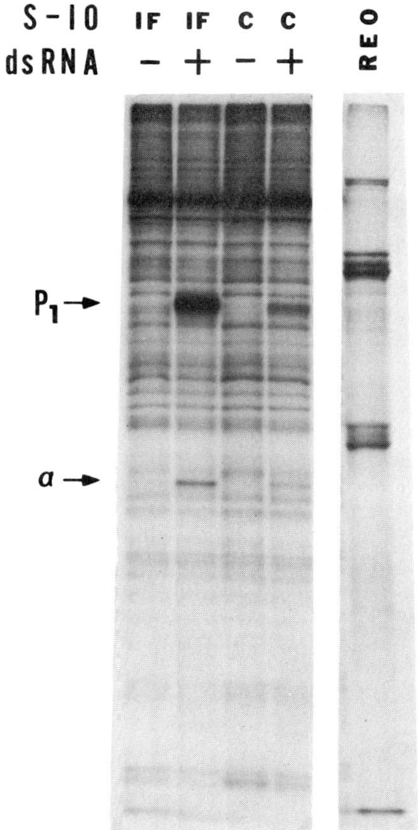

FIGURE 1. Autoradiogram showing the effect of interferon (IF) treatment and dsRNA on [γ-32p] ATP-mediated phosphorylation of ribosome-associated protein P_1 and endogenous initiation factor eIF-2α. Phosphorylation was catalyzed by S-10 cell-free extracts prepared from untreated (C) or IF-treated (IF) mouse fibroblast L cells in the presence (+) or absence (−) of reovirus genome dsRNA (1 μg/ml).

catalyzes the phosphorylation of a 67 to 69,000-dalton ribosome-associated protein (designated P_1) as well as the phosphorylation of the 38,000 dalton α-subunit of protein synthesis initiation factor eIF-2[15-17] (FIGURE 1). As shown in FIGURE 2 the *in vitro* activation of the IF-mediated kinase by reovirus genome dsRNA as measured by the phosphorylation of protein P_1 and eIF-2α can also be obtained with reovirus ssRNA. However, the phosphorylation of at least two other proteins, designated P_{ds}, is also observed in the presence of reovirus dsRNA but not reovirus ssRNA. The differential effects of reovirus dsRNA and ssRNA on protein phorphorylation suggest that either different kinase or phosphatase activities or both may be affected by the viral RNAs. Conceivably, dsRNA regions of mRNA resulting from the secondary structure of the ssRNA or, alternatively, dsRNA *per se* produced during virus genome replication and transcription, may fulfill the apparent requirement for dsRNA in the activation of the kinase *in vivo*. The effect of the duration of IF treatment on the ability of ribosomal salt-wash fractions to catalyze the phosphorylation of proteins P_1 and eIF-2α[18] correlates with the appearance of an interferon-mediated ribosome-associated inhibitor of translation.[9] Translational control under a seemingly quite different physiological condition, hemin deficiency in rabbit reticulocytes, also involves the phorphorylation of eIF-2α which significantly reduces the ability of the factor to function efficiently at the level of initiation of protein synthesis.[19] Interestingly, the IF-induced ribosome-associated protein kinase from human cells catalyzes the phosphorylation of eIF-2α in a site-specific manner that is apparently identical with the hemin-regulated rabbit reticulocyte kinase.[16] The IF-induced protein kinase has been extensively purified; fractions that contain phosphoprotein P_1 possess kinase activity and inhibit reovirus mRNA translation *in vitro*.[20]

The 2′,5′-oligoadenylate synthetase catalyzes the synthesis of a very unusual oligonucleotide that contains 2′,5′-phosphodiester bonds, pppA(2′p5′A)$_n$.[21] 2′,5′-oligo A derivatives appear to function as a positive effector in the activation of an inactive latent endoribonuclease present in untreated cells as well as IF-treated cells.[22-25] The activated endoRNase efficiently catalyzes the degradation of viral mRNA as shown in FIGURE 3. The low-molecular-weight 2′,5′-oligo A effectors are not species-specific in their ability to activate the endoribonuclease, and they are inactivated relatively rapidly ($t_{1/2}$ < 10 min) by cell-free extracts.[26] The IF-induced synthetase involved in the synthesis of 2′,5′-oligo A may have a wider regulatory role than in IF action as different cells and tissues have widely differing levels of the enzyme.[27]

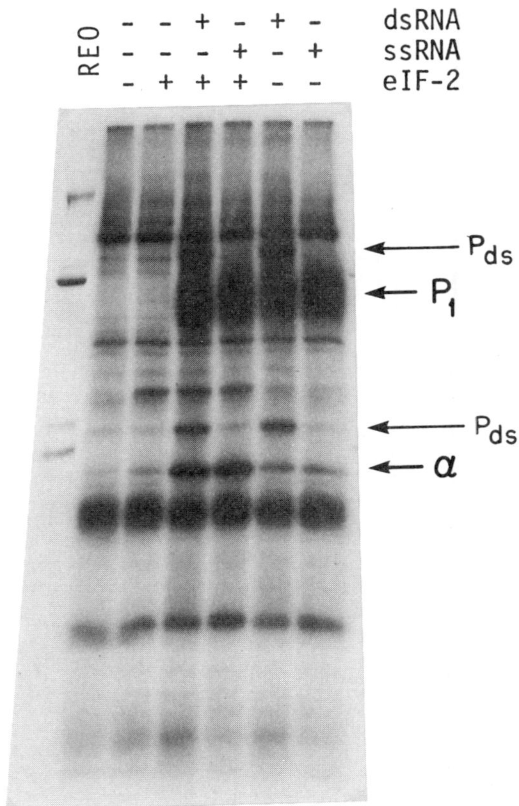

FIGURE 2. Effects of reovirus dsRNA and ssRNA on the phosphorylation of ribosome-associated protein P_1 and the α subunit of initiation factor eIF-2 catalyzed by 0.8M ribosomal salt-wash fraction prepared from interferon-treated human cells. The incubation mixture contained where indicated (+): eIF-2 (0.5 μg protein), reovirus genome dsRNA (1 μg/ml), and reovirus ssRNA (60 μg/ml). (From Samuel.[16])

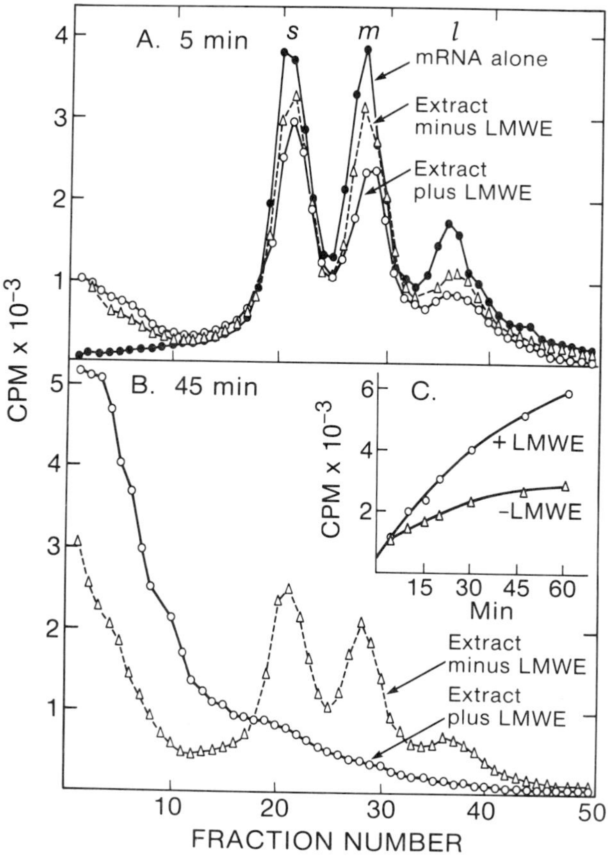

FIGURE 3. Effect of 2′, 5′-oligoadenylate (LMWE) on the degradation of reovirus [^{3}H]mRNA catalyzed by S-10 cell-free extracts prepared from untreated mouse L_{929} cells. Reaction mixtures containing reovirus [^{3}H]mRNA were incubated for either (A) 5 min or (B) 45 min in the presence (O) or absence (△) of 5 × 10^{-8}M LMWE before analysis by centrifugation using 15–30% linear sucrose gradients. The insert (C) shows the formation of acid soluble oligonucleotides from the same reaction mixtures. (From Eppstein *et al.*[26] Reproduced by permission.)

TABLE 1

EFFECT OF INTERFERON ON SV40 AND REOVIRUS MULTIPLICATION IN CV-1 MONKEY KIDNEY CELLS

Interferon Dose units/ml	Virus Yield: Reovirus pfu/ml	Reovirus %	SV40 pfu/ml	SV40 %
0	2.6×10^8	100	8.1×10^7	100
30	2.8×10^7	11	4.1×10^7	51
100	5.1×10^6	2	1.0×10^7	12
300	4.4×10^6	2	1.7×10^6	2

Although the IF-induced protein kinase and 2′,5′-oligo A synthetase appear to inhibit the synthesis of viral proteins by two independent mechanisms, the kinase directly by phosphorylation of eIF-2, which inhibits the initiation of mRNA translation, and the synthetase indirectly by production of an effector that activates a nuclease which degrades the messenger RNA, the two enzymes may conceivably work in concert as well as independently to inhibit protein synthesis. Messenger RNAs that are not efficiently utilized in the formation of polyribosomes because of an initiation block may otherwise be more susceptible to endonuclease degradation.

In Vivo Studies

The above *in vitro* results suggest that at least two mechanisms may operate to inhibit viral gene expression in IF-treated cells: one at the level of RNA accumulation, and the other at the level of protein accumulation. In view of the apparent contradictions concerning the mechanism of IF action in virus-infected cells in culture,[1,2] the effect of homologous IF treatment on the synthesis and degradation, and translation, of the virus-specific mRNAs of two quite different viruses, reovirus and simian virus 40, was examined in monkey kidney CV-1 cells, a host cell permissive to both viruses. In addition, results obtained for reovirus in CV-1 cells were compared to those obtained in mouse L_{929} cells.

TABLE 2

EFFECT OF INTERFERON ON THE ACCUMULATION OF EARLY SV40 RNA*

Experiment	Interferon Dose units/ml	Cellular Fraction	SV40-Specific RNA (%)	Reduction (%)
A	0	nucleus	0.0074	
	0	cytoplasm	0.0052	
	50	nucleus	0.0011	85
	50	cytoplasm	0.0013	75
B	0	nucleus	0.0077	
	0	cytoplasm	0.0046	
	50	nucleus	0.0032	58
	50	cytoplasm	0.0017	63

*Interferon treatment was at 37°C for 24 hr before infection with 5 pfu/cell tsA30 at 41°C in the presence of cytosine arabinoside. (Adapted from Kingsman and Samuel[30].)

Interferon Dose and Virus Yield

The effect of IF dose on reovirus and SV40 multiplication in monkey kidney CV-1 cells is shown in TABLE 1. An interferon dose of 300 units/ml inhibited the yield of both viruses by about 98%. However, at lower doses of interferon, the reduction in reovirus yield was somewhat greater than the reduction in SV40 yield.

The Effect of Interferon on the Accumulation of Early SV40 RNA

The effect of IF on the accumulation of early SV40 mRNA was studied in CV-1 cells infected with SV40 temperature sensitive mutant tsA30 at 41°C in the presence of cytosine arabinoside. As shown in TABLE 2, treatment with 50 units/ml IF resulted in a 58–85% reduction in SV40-specific RNA in two independent experiments when nuclear and cytoplasmic RNA fractions were analyzed separately. A comparable reduction, 76%, was obtained with 50 units/ml when total cell RNA was analyzed. A marked reduction in the accumulation of SV40 early RNA during lytic infection in IF-treated cells was reported some time ago by Oxman and Levin[28] and more recently by Yakobson *et al.*[29] Under our experimental conditions greater than 90% of the SV40-specific RNA hybridized to the fragment of SV40 DNA corresponding to map position 0.14–0.67 of the genome.[30] The 0.14–0.67 fragment was obtained by digestion of SV40 DNA with restriction endonucleases *Eco*RI (0.0), *Bam*HI (0.14) and *Bgl*I (0.67), and spans the early region which has been mapped between 0.67 and 0.14.[31]

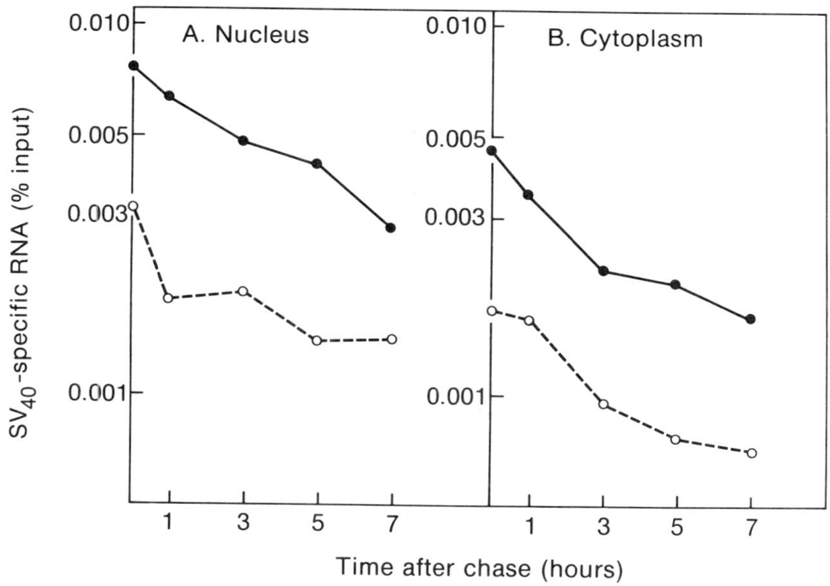

FIGURE 4. The decay of SV40 early RNA in the nucleus and cytoplasm of untreated and interferon-treated cells. CV-1 cells were pretreated with 50 units/ml of IF for 24-hr before infection with 5 pfu/cell of *tsA30* at 41°. Cells were pulse-labeled at 24 hr post-infection with [5,6-^{3}H] uridine for 15 hr and then chased for various times. (A) nuclear and (B) cytoplasmic RNA was isolated and analyzed by hybridization to SV40 DNA. (●———●), SV40 early RNA, no IF treatment. (O---O), SV40 early RNA, IF-treated. (From Kingsman and Samuel.[30] Reproduced by permission.)

To resolve whether the IF-mediated reduction in early SV40 RNA accumulation was due to an effect on RNA synthesis or on RNA degradation, the rate of decay of early SV40-specific RNA was measured under pulse-chase conditions.

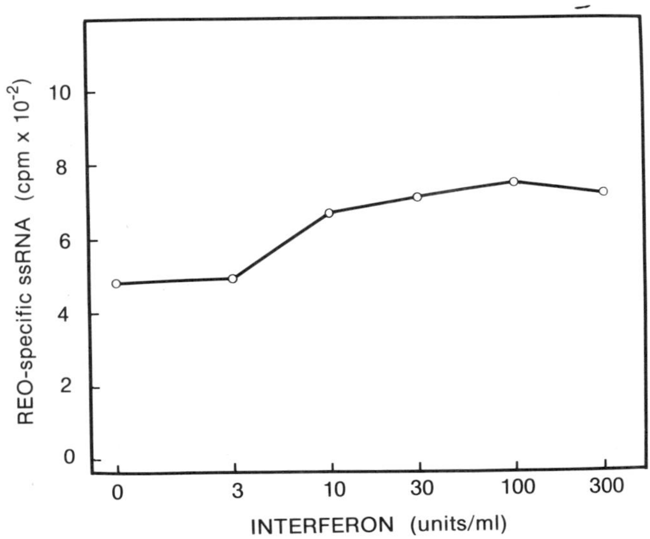

FIGURE 5. Effect of interferon dose on the synthesis of reovirus early RNA in monkey kidney cells. CV-1 cells were pretreated with homologous monkey IF for 24 hr before infection; cells were pulse-labeled with [5,6-^{3}H] uridine from 3 to 6 hours post-infection. Cytoplasmic RNA was isolated and analyzed by hybridization to reovirus dsRNA.

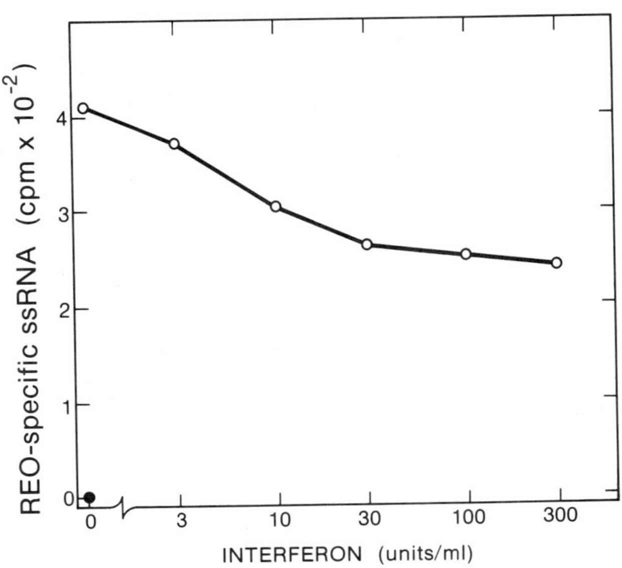

FIGURE 6. Effect of interferon dose on the synthesis of reovirus early RNA in mouse fibroblast cells. L_{929} cells were pretreated with homologous mouse IF for 24 hr at 37°C before infection with 10 pfu/cell of *ts447* at 39°C; cells were labeled and RNA analyzed as described for FIGURE 5.

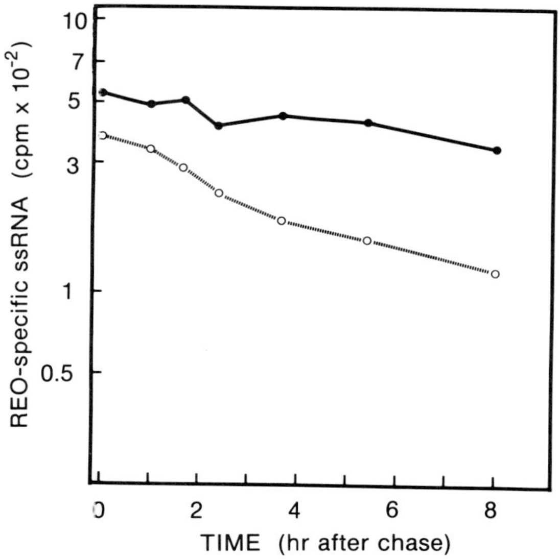

FIGURE 7. The decay of reovirus early RNA in the cytoplasm of untreated and interferon-treated mouse fibroblast cells. L_{929} cells were pretreated with 300 units/ml of IF for 24 hr before infection, pulse-labeled from 3 to 6 hours post-infection, and then chased for various times before analysis for virus-specific RNA.

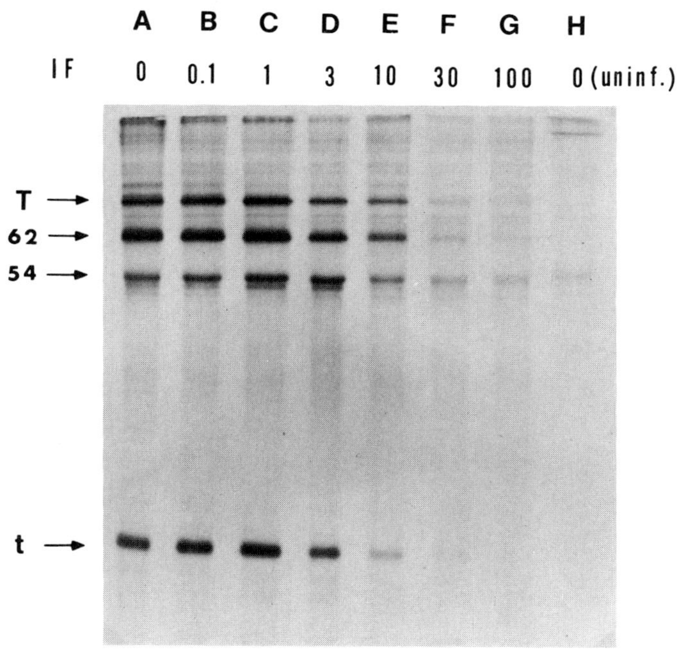

FIGURE 8. Effect of interferon dose on the synthesis of early SV40 proteins in *tsA30*-infected CV-1 cells. Treatment with (A,H) 0; (B) 0.1; (C) 1; (D) 3; (E) 10; (F) 30; and (G) 100 units/ml IF was at 37°C for 24 hr before infection (A-G) at 41°C in the presence of cytosine arabinoside. Cultures were labeled with [^{35}S] methionine for 1 hr from 34 to 35 hr post-infection. Proteins were precipitated with anti-T serum and analyzed by SDS-polyacrylamide gel electrophoresis and fluorography.

As shown in FIGURE 4, there was no significant difference between IF-treated and untreated CV-1 cells in the decay characteristics of either nuclear or cytoplasmic SV40-specific RNA. The decay curves were essentially parallel throughout the 7-hour chase with a half-life of about 4 hr. These results suggest that the IF-mediated reduction in early SV40 RNA accumulation may be due to an effect on RNA synthesis rather than RNA degradation.

The Effect of Interferon on the Accumulation of Early Reovirus mRNA

The effect of interferon on the accumulation of early reovirus mRNA was studied in CV-1 and L_{929} cells infected with reovirus temperature-sensitive mutant *ts447* at 39°C. Under such experimental conditions essentially all viral mRNA is transcribed by parental subviral particles which, by definition, is early RNA.[32,33] As shown in FIGURE 5, the accumulation of reovirus-specific early RNA in virus-infected CV-1 cells was not reduced by IF treatment but rather appeared to be slightly increased as measured by hybridization of extracted ^{3}H-labeled

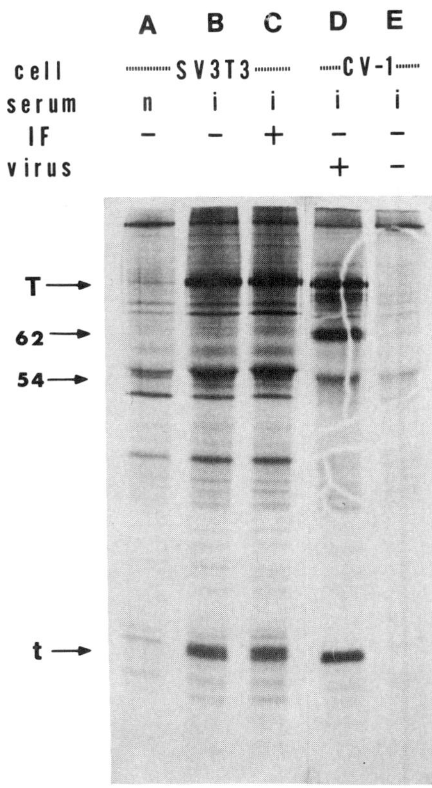

FIGURE 9. Effect of interferon on proteins immunoprecipitated from SV40-transformed 3T3 cells. SV3T3 transformed mouse cells were treated for 24 hr with 300 units/ml IF and then labeled for 22 hr with [^{35}S] methionine. Proteins were precipitated with either normal (n) or SV40 anti-T immune (i) serum. (A) Untreated SV3T3, normal serum; (B) untreated SV3T3, anti-T serum; (C) IF-treated SV3T3, anti-T serum; (D) untreated, *tsA30*-infected CV-1; (E) untreated, uninfected CV-1. (From Kingsman *et al.*[38])

RNA to an excess of unlabeled genome dsRNA.[34] The reason for the apparent increase in reovirus-specific transcripts in IF-treated CV-1 cultures is not known; an apparent increase in vaccinia virus early RNA has also been observed in IF-treated virus-infected cells.[35] By contrast to the results observed in reovirus-infected CV-1 cells, treatment of mouse L_{929} cells with homologous IF resulted in a dose-dependent reduction in accumulation of early reovirus-specific mRNA (FIGURE 6). An IF-dependent reduction in early reovirus RNA was also observed by Wiebe and Joklik.[36]

The kinetics of decay of labeled reovirus-specific mRNA was measured in untreated and IF-treated virus-infected L_{929} cells. As shown in FIGURE 7, reovirus ssRNA decayed more rapidly in IF-treated as compared to untreated cells. The apparent average half-life was about 4.5 hr in IF-treated and 12.5 hr in untreated L_{929} cells. These results suggest that the IF-mediated reduction in early reovirus-specific RNA accumulation in L_{929} cells may be due to an effect on RNA degradation rather than RNA synthesis. The enhanced turnover of reovirus mRNA in IF-treated L_{929} cells may possibly be mediated by the 2′,5′-oligo A-activated endoribonuclease.[23,26]

TABLE 3

EFFECT OF INTERFERON ON VSV MULTIPLICATION IN SV3T3 CELLS

Interferon Dose (units/ml)	Virus Yield (pfu/ml)
0	2.4×10^8
30	1.6×10^5
300	1.0×10^4

The Effect of Interferon on the Accumulation of Early SV40 Tumor Antigens and Reovirus Polypeptides

In addition to previously described large T (94K) and small t (19K) antigens, a 62K polypeptide was immunoprecipitated by SV40 anti-T serum from extracts of CV-1 monkey kidney cells infected with *ts*A30 at 41°C. The 94K, 62K and 19K polypeptides were not precipitated with normal serum from extracts of infected cells, and they were not present in extracts of uninfected cells. However, a 54K species was immunoprecipitated with both normal and anti-T serum from uninfected and infected cells. As shown in FIGURE 8, there was a dose-dependent reduction in the accumulation at early times after infection of newly synthesized large T and small t antigens as well as the 62K polypeptide in CV-1 cells pretreated with interferon. This has also recently been shown by Mozes and Defendi[37] for large T under similar conditions, and by Yakobson *et al.*[29] for both T and t under quite different conditions of IF treatment late in the infection cycle. The 94K, 62K and 19K antigens possessed comparable sensitivity to IF in lytically infected cells; a dose of about 3 units/ml reduced the amount of radioactivity in each of the tumor antigens by about 50 percent. Less than a twofold change in the amount of the 54K cellular protein was observed with an IF dose of 100 units/ml. In SV40-transformed mouse 3T3 cells the synthesis of large T and small t antigens was readily detected but was not affected by treatment with 300 units/ml IF for 24 hr (FIGURE 9). However, the SV3T3 cells were sensitive to the

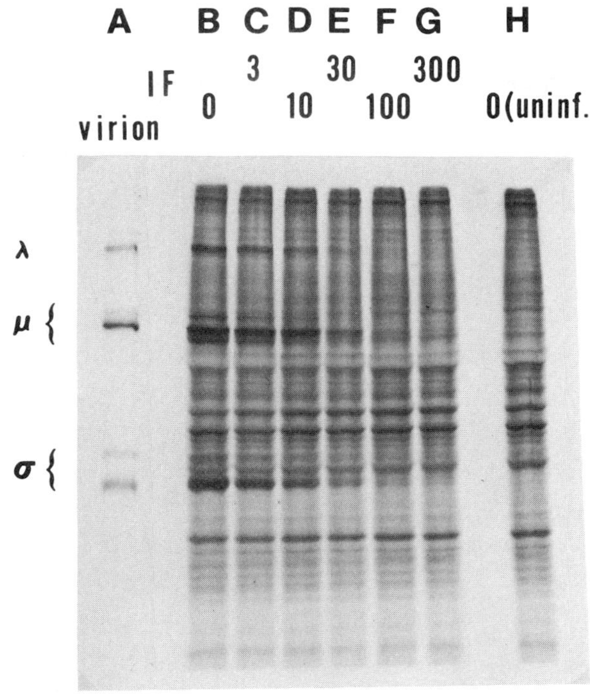

FIGURE 10. Effect of interferon dose on the synthesis of reovirus proteins in wt-infected CV-1 cells. Treatment with (B,H) 0; (C) 3; (D) 10; (E) 30; (F) 100; and (G) 300 units/ml interferon was at 37°C before infection (B-G). Cultures were labeled with [^{14}C] valine for 1 hr from 14 to 15 hr post-infection. Proteins were analyzed by SDS-polyacrylamide gel electrophoresis and autoradiography.

antiviral action of interferon as evidenced by the IF-mediated reduction in vesicular stomatitis virus yield in superinfected cells (TABLE 3).

Although the accumulation of early reovirus mRNA was not reduced by IF in CV-1 cells, the accumulation of reovirus λ, μ and σ polypeptides was reduced in a dose-dependent manner (FIGURE 10). By contrast, overall cellular protein synthesis was unaffected in IF-treated virus-infected cells.

TABLE 4

EFFECT OF INTERFERON ON EARLY SV40- AND REOVIRUS-SPECIFIC RNA AND PROTEIN ACCUMULATION IN CV-1 AND L929 CELLS

		Interferon-mediated Reduction	
Virus	Host Cell	RNA	Protein
SV-40	CV-1	yes (synthesis?)	yes
Reovirus	CV-1	no	yes
	L929	yes (degradation?)	yes

Conclusion

Interferon inhibits the production of infectious progeny virions of SV40 and reovirus. However, as summarized in Table 4, the results of this study suggest that the level of virus genome expression affected by IF may be dependent upon both the nature of the virus and the host cell. The reduction in accumulation of viral polypeptides in IF-treated virus-infected cells may be the result of an IF-mediated effect on the accumulation or translation or both of viral messenger RNAs.

References

1. Finter, N. B., Ed. 1973. Interferons and interferon inducers. *In* Frontiers of Biology, Vol. 2, American Elsevier, New York.
2. Stewart, II, W. E. 1979. The interferon system. Springer-Verlag. Vienna-New York.
3. Samuel, C. E. 1980. Microbiology 1980. Am. Soc. Microbiol. :211-213.
4. Friedman, R. M. 1980. Microbiology 1980. Am. Soc. Microbiol.: 214–216.
5. Falcoff, E., R. Falcoff, B. Lebleu & M. Revel. 1973. J. Virol. **12:** 421–430.
6. Friedman, R. M., D. H. Metz, R. M. Esteban, D. R. Tovell, L. A. Ball & I. M. Kerr. 1972. J. Virol. **10:** 1184–1198.
7. Gupta, S. L., W. D. Graziadei, H. Weideli, M. L. Sopori & P. Lengyel. 1974. Virology **57:** 49–63.
8. Samuel, C. E. & W. K. Joklik. 1974. Virology **58:** 476–491.
9. Samuel, C. E., D. A. Farris & D. A. Eppstein. 1977. Virology **83:** 56–71.
10. Samuel, C. E. & D. A. Farris. 1977. Virology **77:** 556–565.
11. Baglioni, C. 1979. Cell **17:** 255–264.
12. Lebleu, B., G. C. Sen, S. Shaila, B. Cabrer & P. Lengyel. 1976. Proc. Nat. Acad. Sci. USA **73:** 3107–3111.
13. Roberts, W. K., A. Hovanessian, R. E. Brown, M. J. Clemens & I. M. Kerr. 1976. Nature **264:** 477–480.
14. Zilberstein, A., P. Federman, L. Schulman & M. Revel. 1976. FEBS. Lett. **68:** 119–124.
15. Farrell, P. J., G. C. Sen, M. F. Dubois, L. Ratner, E. Slattery & P. Lengyel. 1978. Proc. Nat. Acad. Sci. USA **75:** 5893–5897.
16. Samuel, C. E. 1979. Proc. Nat. Acad. Sci. USA **76:** 600–604.
17. Zilberstein, A., A. Kimchi, A. Schmidt & M. Revel. 1978. Proc. Nat. Acad. Sci. USA **75:** 4734–4738.
18. Samuel, C. E. 1979. Virology **93:** 281–285.
19. Safer, B. & W. F. Anderson. 1978. CRC Crit. Rev. Biochem. **5:** 261–290.
20. Lasky, S. R., M. J. Berry, G. S. Knutson & C. E. Samuel. Unpublished observation.
21. Kerr, I. M. & R. E. Brown. 1978. Proc. Nat. Acad. Sci. USA **75:** 256–260.
22. Eppstein, D. A. & C. E. Samuel. 1977. Biochem. Biophys. Res. Commun. **79:** 145–153.
23. Eppstein, D. A. & C. E. Samuel. 1978. Virology **89:** 240–251.
24. Ratner, L., R. C. Wiegand, P. J. Farrell, G. C. Sen, B. Cabrer & P. Lengyel. 1978. Biochem. Biophys. Res. Commun. **81:** 947–953.
25. Schmidt, A., A Zilberstein, L. Shulman, P. Federman, H. Berissi & M. Revel. 1978. FEBS Lett. **95:** 257–264.
26. Eppstein, D. A., T. C. Peterson & C. E. Samuel. 1979. Virology **98:** 9–19.
27. Stark, G. R., W. J. Dower, R. T. Schimke, R. E. Brown & I. M. Kerr. 1979. Nature **278:** 471–473.
28. Oxman, M. N. & M. J. Levin. 1971. Proc. Nat. Acad. Sci. USA **68:** 299–302.
29. Yakobson, E., C. Prives, J. R. Hartman, E. Winocour & M. Revel. 1977. Cell **12:** 73–81.
30. Kingsman, S. M. & C. E. Samuel. 1980. Virology **101:** 458–465.
31. Berk, A. J. & P. A. Sharp. 1978. Proc. Nat. Acad. Sci. USA **75:** 1274–1278.

32. MATSUHISA, T. & W. K. JOKLIK. 1974. Virology **60:** 380–389.
33. JOKLIK, W. K. 1974. Comprehensive Virology **2:** 231–334.
34. ITO, Y. & W. K. JOKLIK. 1972. Virology **50:** 202–208.
35. JOKLIK, W. K. & T. C. MERIGAN. 1966. Proc. Nat. Acad. Sci. USA **56:** 558–565.
36. WIEBE, M. E. & W. K. JOKLIK. 1975. Virology **66:** 229–240.
37. MOZES, L. W. & V. DEFENDI. 1979. Virology **93:** 558–568.
38. KINGSMAN, S. M., M. D. SMITH & C. E. SAMUEL. 1980. Proc. Nat. Acad. Sci. USA **77:** 2419–2423.

INDUCTION, PURIFICATION, AND PROPERTIES OF 2′5′ OLIGOADENYLATE SYNTHETASE

L. Andrew Ball

Biophysics Laboratory
University of Wisconsin–Madison
Madison, Wisconsin 53706

INTRODUCTION

Treatment of cells with homologous interferon (IF) causes several profound changes in their properties, the best characterized of which is the development of resistance to viral infection.[1] While it is clear from studies using inhibitors and enucleated cells that IF exerts many of its effects by causing the derepression of cellular genes, none of its biological actions is yet understood at the molecular level. Even the products of the IF-inducible genes have yet to be identified unambiguously.

Recent progress in this area has come from studies of the biochemical properties of extracts of IF-treated cells.[2,3] The ability of such extracts to carry out cell-free protein synthesis is severely inhibited by double-stranded RNA (dsRNA), under conditions where extracts of non-IF-treated cells are insensitive to inhibition.[4] This effect of dsRNA can be ascribed to the presence, in the extracts of IF-treated cells, of two dsRNA-activated enzymes which are relatively lacking from extracts of untreated cells. The first of these enzymes is a protein kinase that is able to phosphorylate the small subunit of protein synthesis initiation factor 2 (eIF2α). Since polypeptide chain initiation is one of the steps at which dsRNA inhibits protein synthesis under these conditions, it seems likely that the phosphorylation of eIF2 is responsible; but this has yet to be proved. The second enzyme is 2′5′ oligoadenylate synthetase (2-5A synthetase), an enzyme which, upon activation by dsRNA, uses ATP to make a series of 2′-5′-linked oligonucleotides with the general structure pppA$^{2'}$ (p$^{5'}$ A)$_n$, where n lies between one and about seven.[5] The trimer and higher oligomers are very potent inhibitors of protein synthesis, both in cell-free systems[5,6] and when introduced into intact cells.[7,8] In both situations, they activate a latent pre-exisiting endoribonuclease that degrades messenger RNA.[8–11] Basal levels of 2-5A synthetase have been found in a wide variety of eukaryotic cells, and these levels vary in response not only to IF treatment, but also to hormones and the growth state of the cells.[12] Thus 2-5A synthetase emerges as an intriguing enzyme in that the level of its activity is subject to multiple controls, and its products modulate mRNA degradation.

Clearly, the dsRNA-activated kinase and 2-5A synthetase are good candidates for products of IF-inducible genes, since their enhancement in IF-treated cells requires *de novo* synthesis of RNA and protein.[13–15] However, proof of induction requires assay of their corresponding mRNAs, and this has not yet been accomplished. Moreover, the roles of these enzymes in the many actions of IF on cells are not yet clear. For these reasons, we have undertaken the purification and characterization of 2-5A synthetase from IF-treated chick cells in order to define its polypeptide composition and enzymatic properties. Some of these results were presented at a meeting entitled "Regulation of Macromolecular Synthesis by Low Molecular Weight Mediators" held in Hamburg, Germany, in May 1979.[19]

Results and Discussion

Assay of 2-5A Synthetase

The original assay for 2-5A synthetase[5,6] was based on the ability of the reaction products to inhibit cell-free protein synthesis. Although extremely sensitive, this assay was laborious and expensive. A simpler radiochemical assay was developed subsequently,[13] and has now been further simplified.[19] As shown in FIGURE 1, the assay measures the incorporation of ^{3}H label from [^{3}H]ATP into material that is able to bind to DEAE-cellulose paper after digestion with bacterial alkaline phosphatase (EC 3.1.3.1). The incorporation that occurs in the absence of dsRNA (which is very low) is used as a control and subtracted from the experimental values. Under the conditions described in the legend to FIGURE 1, this assay is capable of detecting 2-5A synthetase levels down to about 5000 units per 10^{5} cells (where one enzyme unit is defined as the incorporation of 10^{-14} mol of AMP per hour at 30°C). This is about 1000 times the basal enzyme level in untreated chick embryo cells, and corresponds to the level found in cells treated for 12 hr with about 10 units of IF per ml.[13] Clearly, therefore, this assay is not sufficiently sensitive for general use, but was well suited to monitoring the purification of 2-5A synthetase.

Purification of 2-5A Synthetase

Treatment of primary cultures of chick embryo cells with 100–300 units of IF per ml caused a 5000–10,000-fold increase in their level of 2-5A synthetase activity.[13] Moreover, a new 56,000 dalton polypeptide was detected in the post-ribosomal supernatant of IF-treated cells. This polypeptide was synthesized in response to IF treatment and resembled 2-5A synthetase in its molecular weight under non-denaturing conditions (50,000-60,000 MW) and in its affinity for dsRNA.[13] Purification of 2-5A synthetase was undertaken in order to study the relationship between the enzyme and the 56K polypeptide.

Post-ribosomal supernatants of IF-treated cells that had been labeled by incorporation of [^{35}S]methionine were subjected to fractional methanol precipitation at −5°C, reprecipitation at pH 5.0 in the presence of poly(I)·poly(C), and chromatography on columns of DEAE-cellulose. Together, these steps provided a 150–200-fold purification of 2-5A synthetase. Extracts of non-IF-treated cells were fractionated in parallel. The fractions corresponding to the peak of 2-5A synthetase activity that eluted from the DEAE-cellulose column were subjected to polyacrylamide gel electrophoresis in the presence of sodium dodecyl sulfate (SDS). FIGURE 2 shows that the major labeled polypeptide present in the partially purified 2-5A synthetase preparation was the 56K species, and that this polypeptide was undetectable in extracts of non-IF-treated cells. The simplest interpretation of these results is that the 56K polypeptide is 2-5A synthetase, and that its synthesis in response to IF treatment of cells is the result of derepression of the corresponding structural gene. However, proof of these interpretations will

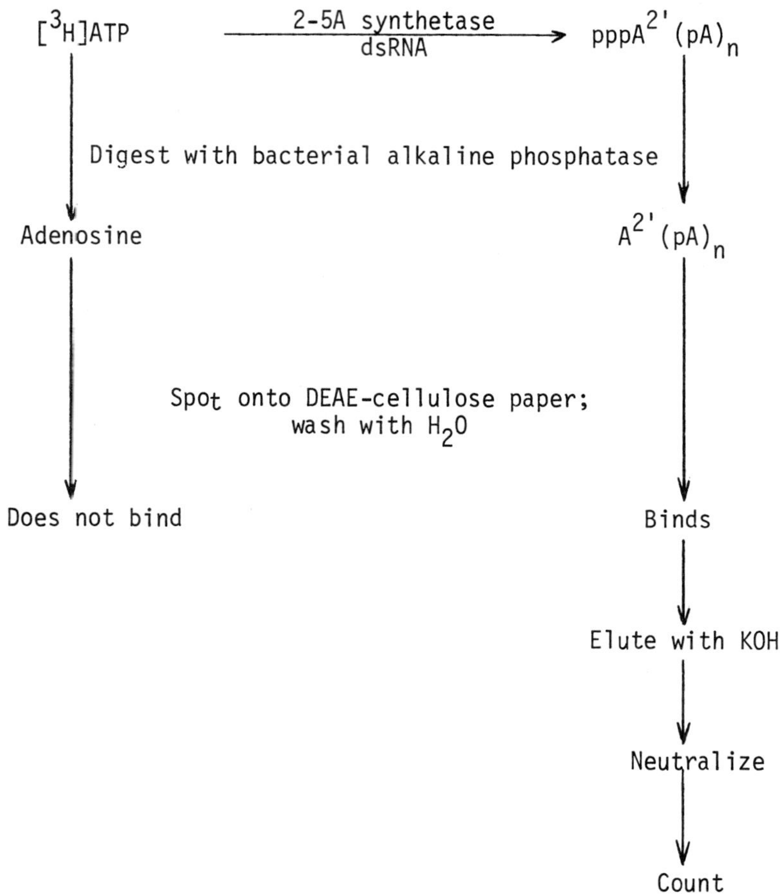

FIGURE 1. A simple radiochemical assay for 2–5A synthetase. Reaction mixtures (10 μl) contained 50 mM magnesium acetate, 1.5 mM [^{3}H]ATP (16.7 Ci/M; Amersham), 10 μg/ml poly(I) · poly(C) (P-L Biochemicals) and 5 μl of a 100,000 × g supernatant extract of interferon-treated chick embryo cells. Incubation was at 30° for 2 hr and the reaction was terminated by heating at 95° for 5 min. Precipitated protein was removed by brief centrifugation, and 7.5 μl aliquots of the supernatants were digested with 6 units per ml of bacterial alkaline phosphatase (EC 3.1.3.1; Sigma, type III) at 37°C for 2 hr. Aliquots (6 μl) of the digests were spotted onto 1 cm^2 squares of DEAE-cellulose paper (Whatman DE81), dried, and washed with several changes of distilled water to remove [^{3}H]adenosine, the phosphatase digestion product of unincorporated [^{3}H]ATP. The incorporated label was eluted from the filters with 0.3 M KOH, and measured by liquid scintillation counting in Aqueous Counting Scintillant (Amersham). Reaction mixtures lacking poly(I) · poly(C) were used as controls and their incorporation was subtracted from the experimental values.

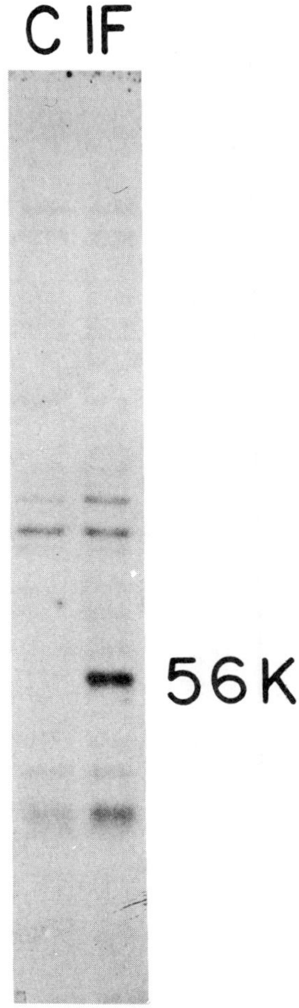

FIGURE 2. SDS polyacrylamide gel electrophoresis of partially purified 2-5A synthetase. The enzyme was purified from the post-ribosomal supernatants of chick embryo cells that had been treated for 8 hours with 250 units of interferon (IF) per ml, and labeled with [^{35}S]methionine from 3 to 8 hours after IF treatment.[13,19] The initial steps in the purification have been described before.[19] Following precipitation at pH 5.0 in the presence of 10 μg/ml of poly(I) · poly(C), the enzyme was subjected to DEAE-cellulose chromatography in a buffer containing 50 mM KCl. The enzyme activity eluted in the void volume of the column, and an aliquot of the peak fraction was subjected to SDS polyacrylamide gel electrophoresis as described before[13] (IF). The corresponding fraction from the purification of a mock enzyme preparation from non-IF-treated cells was electrophoresed in parallel for comparison (C). An autoradiograph of the dried gel is shown.

depend on further purification of the enzyme and on the development of assays for its mRNA.

Degradation of 2-5A

The assay for the synthesis of 2-5A, by binding the phosphatase-resistant products to DEAE-cellulose paper, can also be used to follow 2-5A degradation. Since the 5′-terminal phosphates are removed and do not contribute to the binding, this assay measures cleavage of the 2′-5′ bonds. However, being a radiochemical assay, it is suitable only for 2-5A concentrations that are far above those required for nuclease activation *in vitro*, and the results must be interpreted with this in mind.

2-5A was degraded at the same rate in extracts of IF-treated and non-IF-treated chick cells, with a half-life of about 4 min (FIGURE 3a). These results

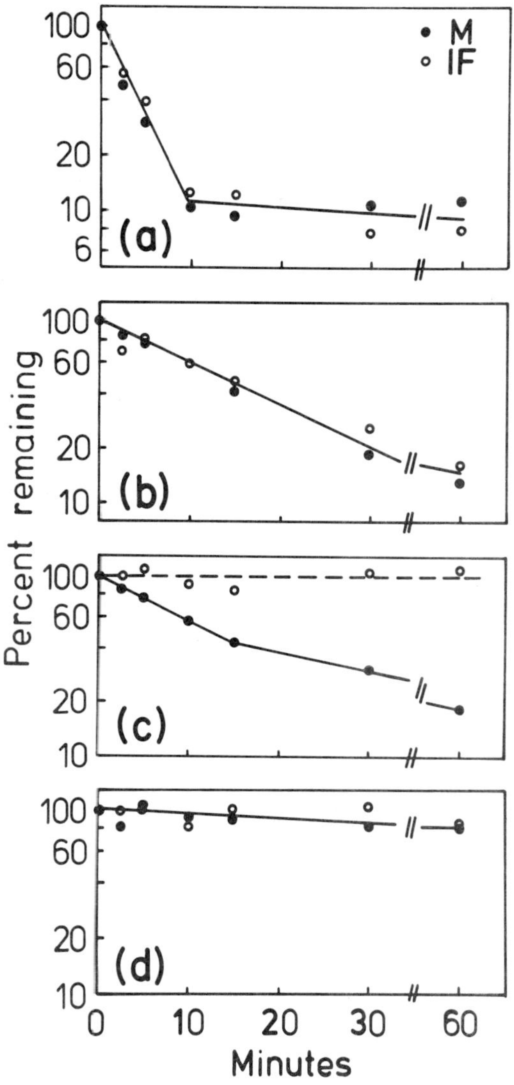

FIGURE 3. Kinetics of degradation of 2-5A under various conditions. A mixture of 2-5A oligomers in which the trimer was the major species was incubated with a post-ribosomal supernatant extract of IF-treated (open circles) or non-IF-treated (closed circles) chick embryo cells under the following conditions: HEPES, 6 mM, pH 7.6; magnesium acetate, 50 mM; NH_4Cl, 30 mM; dithiothreitol, 0.3 mM; postribosomal supernatant, 30% (v/v); [^{3}H]2-5A, 3.3 μM (AMP equivalents), 1370 cpm per μl; ATP and AMP (where indicated), 3 mM; poly(I) · poly(C) (where indicated), 10 μg/ml. Samples (10 μl) were taken at the times shown and assayed for their content of 2-5A as described in the legend to TABLE 1. (a) no addition; (b) + ATP; (c) + ATP + poly(I) · poly(C); (d) + 5′ AMP.

differ from those found in the mouse system, where extracts of IF-treated cells degraded 2-5A significantly faster than extracts of untreated cells.[15] Schmidt *et al.*[16] have found that the enzyme responsible for 2-5A breakdown is a phosphodiesterase which can also degrade the 3′-CpCpA terminus of tRNA. These authors have suggested that the previously described tRNA-reversible inhibition of protein synthesis in extracts of IF-treated mouse cells[17] can be attributed to the action of this phosphodiesterase on tRNA. In chick cell extracts, no tRNA-reversible inhibition was observed,[18] and this result now becomes explicable in light of the apparent failure of IF to enhance the phosphodiesterase activity in these cells. The massive increase in 2-5A synthetase activity in the chick system and the absence of an effect on the phosphodiesterase suggest that different cells may respond differently to interferon treatment, expressing various members of a family of IF-inducible genes to different extents.

The rate of degradation of 2-5A was profoundly affected by the conditions, and in particular by the other nucleotides present. Thus, ATP (3 mM) reduced the rate of 2-5A degradation by about threefold (FIGURE 3b) while 5′-AMP (the end-product of 2-5A breakdown[20]) inhibited degradation almost completely (FIGURE 3d). A variety of other nucleotides were also found to influence the rate of degradation (TABLE 1). Under all these conditions, extracts of IF-treated and non-IF-treated cells behaved identically. The only situation in which they differed was in the presence of ATP and poly(I)-poly(C). Here, 2-5A was almost completely stable in extracts of IF-treated cells, whereas it was rapidly degraded in extracts of non-IF-treated cells (FIGURE 3c).

TABLE 1

EFFECT OF NUCLEOTIDES ON THE DEGRADATION OF 2-5A*

Nucleotide	% 2-5A Remaining After 1 Hour at 30°
None	4.8
Adenosine	4.8
2′ AMP	17.0
3′ AMP	8.0
5′ AMP	98.5
2′ OMe5′ AMP	5.7
2′3′ cyclic AMP	6.1
3′5′ cyclic AMP	6.0
5′ GMP	55.0
5′ IMP	54.6
5′ CMP	40.3
5′ UMP	57.2
2′5′ ADP	73.2
3′5′ ADP	78.7
A2′p5′A	49.4
A3′p5′A	87.3
5′ ADP	49.0
5′ ATP	12.4
Poly(A)	5.5
Poly(C)	7.0
Poly(U)	76.1

*A mixture of 2-5A oligomers, in which the trimer was the major species, was incubated with a post-ribosomal supernatant extract of IF-treated (125 units/ml; 17 hours) chick embryo cells under the following conditions: HEPES, 6 mM, pH 7.6; magnesium acetate, 50 mM; NH_4Cl, 30 mM; dithiothreitol, 0.3 mM; post-ribosomal supernatant, 30% (v/v); [^{3}H]2-5A, 4.2 μM (AMP equivalents), 1200 cpm per μl; adenosine, mono- and dinucleotides, 3 mM; poly(A), poly(C), poly(U), 1.4 mg/ml. After incubation for 1 hr at 30°C, the reactions were terminated by heating at 95° for 5 min, and the precipitated protein was removed by centrifugation. Aliquots of the supernatants were digested with bacterial alkaline phosphatase (6 units/ml; 37°C; 2 hours) and then assayed for their ability to bind to DEAE-cellulose paper as described in the legend to FIGURE 1.

Mechanism and Direction of Polymerization

The preceding result suggested that the activated synthetase was able to interact with its preformed product. Indeed, an experiment designed to follow the fate of purified $pppA^{2'}p^{5'}A^{2'}p^{5'}A$ showed that on exposure to the activated synthetase, the trimer was further elongated to form tetramer (FIGURE 4b). On the other hand, when 2-5A degradation was inhibited by 5′AMP no such chain growth was observed (FIGURE 4c). The activated synthetase was therefore able to catalyze elongation by a non-processive mechanism. The distribution of ^{3}H-labeled residues in 2-5A tetramer that had been formed by the addition of an unlabeled residue to a uniformly labeled trimer showed that the newly incorporated residue was at the 2′ terminus.[19] This indicated that polymerization occurred in a 5′ to 2′ direction.

Use of Primers by 2-5A Synthetase

The non-processive mechanism of elongation that was catalyzed by 2-5A synthetase raised the possibility that the activated enzyme could add AMP residues to molecules other than the shorter oligomers of 2-5A itself. A synthetase reaction carried out in the presence of $A^{3'}p^{5'}A$ resulted in the synthesis of two oligomeric series of nucleotides–normal 2-5A and, in addition, a series with the general structure $A^{3'}p^{5'}A^{2'}(p^{5'}A)_n$ (see ref. 19). Other dinucleoside monophosphates, linked either 3′-5′ or 2′-5′, could also act as primers for the addition of AMP residues in 2′-5′ linkage, but the presence of a 2′ (or 3′)-terminal AMP residue with unsubstituted 2′ and 3′ hydroxyl groups appeared to be essential for this primer activity.[19] ADP-ribose and nicotinamide adenine dinucleotide (NAD^+) also served as primers for the activated synthetase.[19]

The ability of the enzyme to use primers *in vitro* raises the possibility that it can catalyze similar reactions in intact IF-treated cells. No data are yet available on this point, but the possibility is intriguing because 2′-adenylated NAD^+, for example, is unable to function as a redox coenzyme.[19] Alterations in the level of functional NAD^+ could have profound affects on various aspects of cellular metabolism, and this might be one way in which several actions of IF could be elicited by a single cause. At present, these ideas are wholly speculative, but experiments are planned to test their validity.

α,β and β,γ-Methylene 2-5A

2-5A depends on the presence of at least some of its 5′-terminal phosphate groups for its ability to activate the latent ribonuclease and to inhibit protein synthesis, since phosphatase-digested 2-5A is inactive.[5] However, it is not known whether cleavage of any of the bonds linking the terminal phosphates is involved in its mechanism of action. This question was approached by synthesizing two analogues of 2-5A with methylene bridges between the α and β phosphates, and the β and γ phosphates, respectively. To make the latter analogue, for example, 2-5A synthetase reactions were carried out in the presence of β,γ-methylene ATP. In addition to 2-5A, the products included an oligomeric series of molecules that appeared to result from the incorporation of the methylene-bridged ATP analogue at the 5′ end of the oligonucleotides. These molecules incorporated

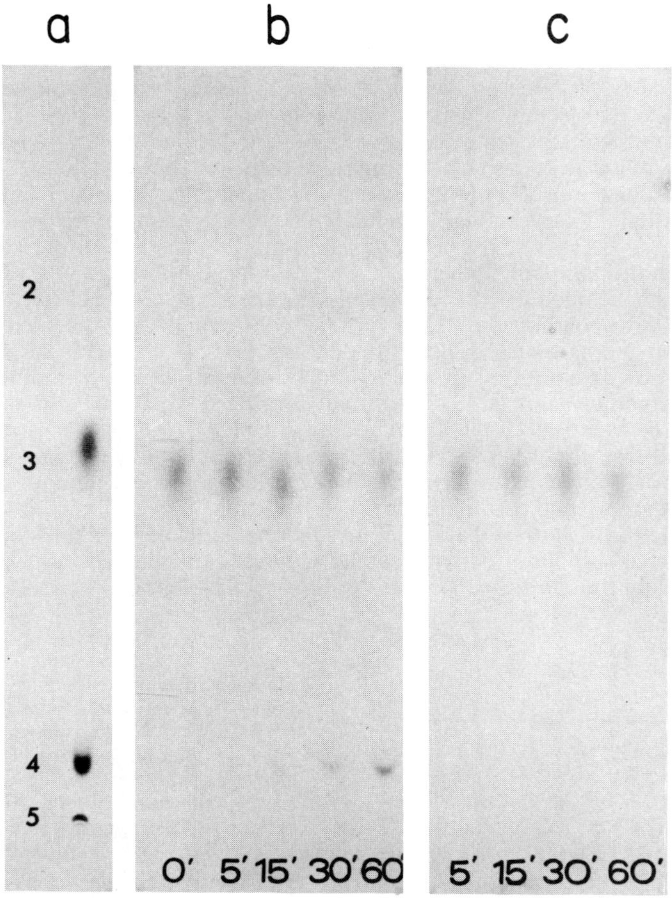

FIGURE 4. Reaction products of pppA$^{2'}$ (p$^{5'}$A)$_n$ during the inhibition of degradation mediated by activated 2-5A synthetase (b), and 5′AMP (c). Purified [^{3}H]pppA$^{2'}$ (p$^{5'}$A)$_2$ (24 μM, 1500 cpm/μl) was incubated with a post-ribosomal supernatant extract of interferon-treated (250 units/ml, 18 hours) chick embryo cells. The conditions were as described in the legend to FIGURE 3 except that in (b), ATP was present at 6 mM and poly(I) · poly(C) at 10 μg/ml, and in (c), 5′AMP was present at 3 mM. Samples were taken at the times shown, digested with bacterial alkaline phosphatase, and 1 μl aliquots of the digests were subjected to thin-layer chromatography on sheets of polyethyleneimine (PEI)-cellulose, in 1.0 M acetic acid.[5] A mixture of phosphatase-resistant 2-5A cores was included to provide markers (a). Fluorographs of the TLC plates are shown.

^{3}H-label from both [^{3}H]β,γ-methylene ATP and [^{3}H]ATP, were resistant to digestion with alkaline phosphatase, and had net negative charges consistent with the proposed structure p(CH$_2$)ppA$^{2'}$(p$^{5'}$A)$_n$ (data not shown). The α,β-methylene-bridged analogue of ATP was used to make a similar oligomeric series of molecules, but in this case, digestion with alkaline phosphatase removed the

γ-phosphate group to give a series of molecules with the proposed structure $p(CH_2)pA^{2'}(p^{5'}A)_n$.

The resistance to phosphatase digestion of these methylene-bridged analogues of 2-5A provided an easy way to test their ability to activate the latent ribonuclease and to inhibit protein synthesis. The products derived from analogue-primed synthetase reactions were digested exhaustively with alkaline phosphatase and then assayed for nuclease activation activity. FIGURE 5 shows that the analogue-derived products were able to enhance the rate of degradation of viral mRNA, whereas those from a synthetase reaction primed with NAD^+ were not.

For a more thorough analysis of their activities, the analogue-derived products were fractionated by DEAE-cellulose column chromatography in 7 M urea.[5,6] The peak corresponding to $p(CH_2)pA^{2'}(p^{5'}A)_2$ was contaminated with $A^{2'}(p^{5'}A)_4$ and that corresponding to $p(CH_2)ppA^{2'}(p^{5'}A)_2$ was contaminated with $A^{2'}(p^{5'}A)_5$, but since the contaminants were inactive, any residual ability to inhibit protein synthesis could be ascribed to the methylene-bridged analogues. The results are shown in FIGURE 6. Both $p(CH_2)pA^{2'}(p^{5'}A)_2$ and $p(CH_2)ppA^{2'}(p^{5'}A)_2$ were able to inhibit cell-free protein synthesis at concentrations in the nanomolar range. However, both appeared to have a somewhat lower specific inhibitory activity than $pppA^{2'}(p^{5'}A)_2$, and to inhibit less fully.

Martin *et al.*[21] showed that the diphosphorylated trimer, $ppA^{2'}(p^{5'}A)_2$ had the same specific inhibitory activity as the triphosphorylated species, but these workers were unable to exclude the possibility that the activity depended on

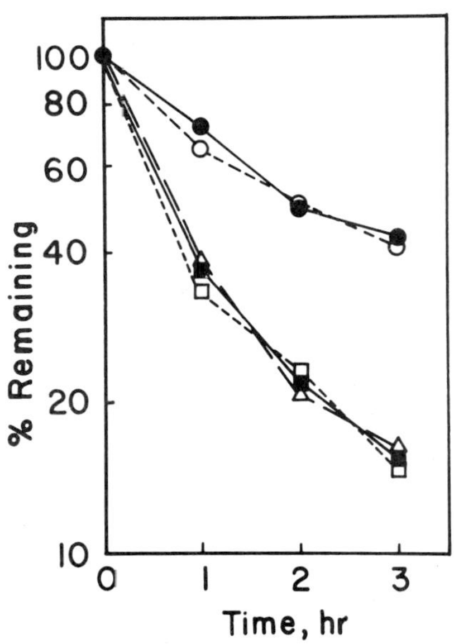

FIGURE 5. Enhancement of ribonuclease activity by 2-5A and its analoques. The rate of degradation of [^{3}H] VSV mRNA to yield oligonucleotide fragments soluble in 5% trichloroacetic acid was monitored as described before.[23] Reaction mixtures contained 25% (v/v) of a 10,000 × g supernatant extract of non-IF-treated chick embryo cells, and 2 μg/ml of [^{3}H] VSV mRNA, 1100 cpm/μl. 2-5A and its analogues were added as follows: (—●—), no addition; (—■—), unfractionated 2-5A at 2×10^{-8} M; (--○--), unfractionated NAD^+-primed products, digested with alkaline phosphatase (8.5 units/ml, 37°, 2 hours), at 2×10^{-7} M (AMP equivalents); (--□--), unfractionated α,β-methylene ATP-primed products, digested with alkaline phosphatase as above, at 2×10^{-7} M; (--▵--), β,γ-methylene ATP-primed products, digested with alkaline phosphatase as above, at 2×10^{-7} M. The primed products were synthesized under the conditions described in the legend to FIGURE 1, with the inclusion of the appropriate primer at 2 mM. [^{14}C]ATP was included during the phosphatase digestion reactions in order to check for complete digestion.

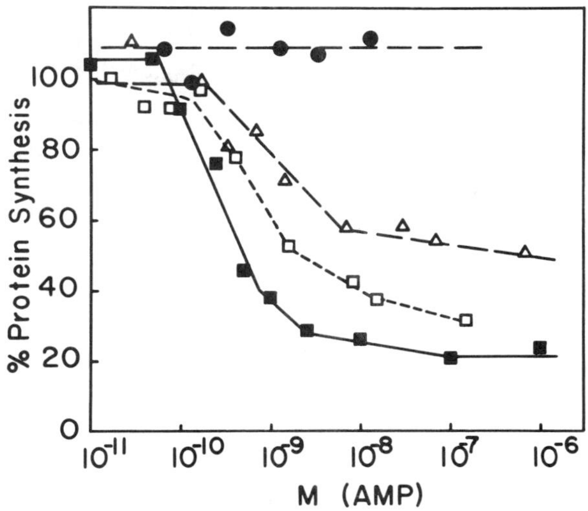

FIGURE 6. Inhibition of cell-free protein synthesis by methylene-bridged analogues of 2-5A. The methylene-bridged analogues of 2-5A were synthesized as described, digested with alkaline phosphatase (8 units/ml, 37°, 2 hours) and fractionated by chromatography on columns of DEAE-cellulose in 7 M urea.[5,6] Because of the inductive effect of the methylene group, adjacent secondary phosphate ionizations are suppressed at pH 8.0, so, for example, $p(CH_2)ppA$ has a net negative charge of −3 under these conditions. The peak fractions corresponding to $p(CH_2)pA^{2'}p^{5'}A^{2'}p^{5'}A$ (net charge, −3.7) andp$(CH_2)ppA^{2'}p^{5'}A^{2'}p^{5'}A$ (net charge, −4.7) were collected from the $\alpha,\beta(CH_2)$ATP and $\beta,\gamma(CH_2)$ATP-primed reaction products, respectively. As discussed in the text, they were contaminated with the pentamer and hexamer cores of 2-5A, respectively, and this was confirmed by further analysis using PEI-cellulose thin-layer chromatography. The column fractions were dialyzed against water, lyophilized, redissolved, and assayed for their ability to inhibit cell-free protein synthesis directed by VSV mRNA in extracts of primary chick embryo cells.[6,13] Inhibition by: (—●—), $A^{2'}(p^{5'}A)_4$; (—■—), $pppA^{2'}(p^{5'}A)_2$; (—□—), $p(CH_2)pA^{2'}(p^{5'}A)_2$; (—Δ—), $pCH_2ppA^{2'}(p^{5'}A)_2$.

prior replacement of the γ-phosphate group. However, the results shown in FIGURES 5 and 6 indicate that cleavage of neither the α-β nor the β-γ phosphate bonds is obligatory for nuclease activation by 2-5A. This would appear to eliminate the possibility[22] that 2-5A functions as a phosphate donor in a kinase reaction, and suggests, rather, that a minimum of two phosphate groups is required at the 5′ terminus of 2-5A for successful interaction with a binding site.

SUMMARY

The results presented above relate to several aspects of the 2-5A system. A simple but insensitive radiochemical assay for 2-5A and its synthetase is described. Progress towards the molecular characterization of the synthetase suggested that it is composed of a single 56,000 dalton polypeptide chain that is synthesized in reponse to IF treatment. Degradation of 2-5A occurs at the same rapid rate in extracts of IF-treated and untreated chick cells. However, this breakdown can be inhibited by its end-product, 5′AMP, or by the activated synthetase which can further elongate 2-5A and thereby protect it from degradation. The direction of elongation is from the 5′ to the 2′ terminus. Molecules other than 2-5A can act as substrates for 2′-adenylation by the activated synthetase. These include some dinucleoside monophosphates, ADP-ribose and NAD^+, and methylene-bridged analogues of ATP. The methylene-bridged analogues of 2-5A that are synthesized in the latter case retain some of the biological activity of authentic 2-5A, indicating that cleavage of the 5′-terminal phosphate group(s) is not involved in the mechanism of nuclease activation by 2-5A.

References

1. Stewart, W. E., II. 1979. The Interferon System. Springer-Verlag, New York.
2. Revel, M. & Y. Groner. 1978. Ann. Rev. Biochem. **47:** 1079–1126.
3. Baglioni, C. 1979. Cell **17:** 255–264.
4. Kerr, I. M., R. E. Brown & L. A. Ball. 1974. Nature (London) **250:** 57–59.
5. Kerr, I. M. & R. E. Brown. 1978. Proc. Nat. Acad. Sci. USA **75:** 256–260.
6. Ball, L. A. & C. N. White. 1978. Proc. Nat. Acad. Sci. USA **75:** 1167–1171.
7. Williams, B. R. G. & I. M. Kerr. 1978. Nature (London) **276:** 88–89.
8. Hovanessian, A. G., J. Wood, E. Meurs & L. Montagnier. 1979. Proc. Nat. Acad. Sci. USA **76:** 3261–3265.
9. Clemens, M. J. & B. R. G. Williams. 1978. Cell **13:** 565–572.
10. Williams, B. R. G., R. R. Golgher & I. M. Kerr. 1979. FEBS Lett. **105:** 47–52.
11. Farrell, P. J., G. C. Sen, M. F. Dubois, L. Ratner, E. Slattery & P. Lengyel. 1978. Proc. Nat. Acad. Sci. USA **75:** 5893–5897.
12. Stark, G. R., W. J. Dower, R. T. Schimke, R. E. Brown & I. M. Kerr. 1979. Nature (London) **278:** 471–473.
13. Ball, L. A. 1979. Virology **94:** 282–296.
14. Baglioni, C., P. A. Maroney & D. K. West. 1979. Biochemistry **18:** 1765–1770.
15. Kimchi, A., L. Shulman, A. Schmidt, Y. Chernajovsky, A. Fradin & M. Revel. 1979. Proc. Nat. Acad. Sci. USA **76:** 3208–3212.
16. Schmidt, A., Y. Chernajovsky, L. Shulman, P. Federman, H. Berissi & M. Revel. 1979. Proc. Nat. Acad. Sci. USA **76:** 4788–4792.
17. Content, J., B. Lebleu, A. Zilberstein, H. Berissi & M. Revel. 1974. FEBS Lett. **41:** 125–130.
18. Ball, L. A. & C. N. White. 1978. Virology **84:** 496–508.
19. Ball, L. A. & C. N. White. 1979. *In* Regulation of Macromolecular Synthesis by Low Molecular Weight Mediators. G. Koch & D. Richter, Eds.: 303–317. Academic Press.
20. Williams, B. R. G., I. M. Kerr, C. S. Gilbert, C. N. White & L. A. Ball. 1978. Eur. J. Biochem. **92:** 455–462.
21. Martin, E. M., N. J. M. Birdsall, R. E. Brown & I. M. Kerr. 1979. Eur. J. Biochem. **95:** 295–307.
22. Eppstein, D. A., T. C. Peterson & C. E. Samuel. 1979. Virology **98:** 9–19.
23. Ball, L. A. & C. N. White. 1979. Virology **93:** 348–356.

INTERFERON-INDUCED ENZYMES: ACTIVATION AND ROLE IN THE ANTIVIRAL STATE*

Corrado Baglioni, Susan Benvin, Patricia A. Maroney, Michael A. Minks, Timothy W. Nilsen, and Deborah K. West

Department of Biological Sciences
State University of New York at Albany
Albany, New York 12222

Two enzymes are induced in mammalian and avian cells by interferon (IF): an oligoadenylate polymerase and a protein kinase.[1] Both enzymes are activated by double-stranded RNA (dsRNA) and utilize ATP as substrate. The oligoadenylate polymerase converts ATP into a series of oligonucleotides characterized by 2′5′phosphodiester bonds and designated 2′5′oligo(A) or 2,5A. The 2,5A in turn activates an endonuclease present in extracts of control and IF-treated cells, which degrades RNA.[1] The protein kinase (PK_{ds}) phosphorylates two polypeptides of M_r 38,000 and about 70,000. The first is the α subunit of initiation factor eIF-2; this phosphorylation is thought to inhibit the initiation of protein synthesis.

We have reported studies on the activation of the endonuclease by 2,5A in HeLa cell extracts[2] and on the kinetics of induction by IF of the 2,5A polymerase and PK_{ds}[3,4]; we have developed sensitive and quantitative assays for these enzymatic activities[4,5] and have proposed a mechanism that accounts for the preferential degradation of viral RNA at the level of the viral replicative complexes of RNA viruses.[6] More recently, we have investigated the structural requirements of dsRNA for the activation of 2,5A polymerase and PK_{ds}[7,8] and the substrate specificity of the 2,5A-activated endonuclease.[9] These studies have allowed us to define some possible roles of these enzymatic activities in the antiviral state. We present here a concise description of this recent work from our laboratory. The limitation of space does not allow us to review this active field of research in a comprehensive way; only references to work directly related to our findings will be given. Other relevant references can be found in a recent review.[1]

Activation of 2′5′Oligo(A) Polymerase and Protein Kinase

The rationale of this line of research is to define the molecular features of polynucleotides that may be responsible for the activation of 2,5A polymerase and PK_{ds} in virus-infected cells. By identifying these features, we can implicate specific viral structures in the activation of the IF-induced enzymes. The activated enzymes may inhibit virus replication via inhibition of protein synthesis or cleavage of viral RNA. Here we briefly describe the assay for these enzymes and summarize data on the activation observed with different polynucleotides.

*Supported by research Grants AI-11887 and AI-16076 from the National Institute of Allergy and Infectious Diseases.

0077-8923/80/0350-0497 $01.75/0 © 1980 NYAS

Synthesis of 2,5A was initially observed in extracts of IF-treated L cells upon incubation with dsRNA and ATP.[10] Subsequently, the enzyme was adsorbed to poly(I) · poly(C)-agarose and conversion of ATP into 2.5A was observed with the bound enzyme.[11] This assay could not easily be adapted to a study of the structural requirements of dsRNA for activation of 2,5A polymerase. Therefore, a systematic study of the conditions that favor synthesis of 2,5A with dsRNA in solution was undertaken.[5] Up to 60% conversion of ATP into 2,5A was obtained in 1- to 2-hr incubations of extract from IF-treated HeLa cells under optimal conditions.[5] These include relatively high concentrations of dsRNA (20 μg/ml), ATP (5 mM), and $Mg(OAc)_2$ (20 mM). At the end of the reaction 2,5A was separated from ATP by DEAE-cellulose column chromatography; ATP was eluted with 90 mM KCl and 2,5A with 0.35 M KCl.[5]

The PK_{ds} was initially assayed in cell extracts.[10,12] However, a phosphatase present in cell sap dephosphorylates polypeptides phosphorylated by PK_{ds}.[13] For this reason, it is convenient to isolate ribosomes from extracts of IF-treated cells and assay the ribosome-bound PK_{ds} either by its inhibition of protein synthesis or by the extent of phosphorylation of the 70,000 M_r polypeptide.[4,14] The latter assay was used throughout our studies of the activation of PK_{ds} by dsRNA.[7,8]

The synthetic polynucleotides tested and the activation of 2,5A polymerase and PK_{ds} observed with these polymers are shown in TABLE 1. Unmethylated polynucleotides were either commercially available or were prepared in our laboratory[7]; dsRNAs methylated in either strand were obtained from Greene *et al.*[15] One triple-stranded RNA tested and hybrid polymers containing a polydeoxyribonucleotide in one strand were completely inactive. The dsRNAs containing randomly mismatched G residues, which cannot form Watson-Crick base pairs with I residues in the complementary strand, were inactive when on average one or more out of 15 base pairs were mismatched.[7] Polymers with fewer mismatches showed increasing activity. The dsRNAs containing long poly(I) strands annealed to complementary short strands of increasing size showed a clear threshold for enzyme activation (FIGURE 1). Full activity was observed with a short strand longer than 60 to 80 nucleotides.[7] The same threshold effect was observed with dsRNAs formed with complementary poly(A) and poly(U) strands of known size; in this case full activity was obtained when dsRNA was formed with both strands longer than 160 nucleotides. Finally, dsRNAs containing one fully 2′-O-methylated strand were inactive, whereas partially methylated dsRNAs showed a characteristic pattern of activation.[8]

These results indicate that the structural requirements for activation of the IF-induced enzymes are: (1) the absence of mismatches within a critical length of dsRNA; (2) a minimum length of dsRNA, uninterrupted by discontinuities in either strand; and (3) the presence of a sufficient number of 2′-*OH* groups in both strands. These structural requirements are identical to those necessary for IF induction by synthetic dsRNA.[16] The reasons for this close correlation between IF-inducing activity and ability to activate 2,5A polymerase and PK_{ds} are presently unexplained. We have suggested, however, that an IF-induced enzyme may be part of a cellular recognition system for dsRNA.[7,8] This could explain the similar structural requirements of dsRNA for IF induction and enzyme activation.

It should be pointed out that the structural requirements of dsRNA for activation of 2,5A polymerase are different from those required for activation of PK_{ds}.[7,8] Full activation of the PK_{ds} is observed with dsRNAs that contain fewer mismatches, have a larger size, and contain fewer 2′-O-methylated residues than the dsRNAs that activate the 2,5A polymerase (see TABLE 1). There are other

TABLE 1

ACTIVATION OF 2′5′OLIGO(A) POLYMERASE AND PROTEIN KINASE BY SYNTHETIC POLYNUCLEOTIDES

Polynucleotides	Composition	Activation of 2′5′Oligo(A) Polymerase	Activation of Protein Kinase
1. Perfectly matched dsRNA	$(I)_n \cdot (C)_n$ or $(A)_n \cdot (U)_n$	Most active	Most active
2. Triple-stranded RNA	$(A)_n \cdot (U)_n \cdot (U)_n$	Inactive	Inactive
3. Heteropolymers RNA/DNA	$(I)_n \cdot (dC)_n$ or $(dI)_n \cdot (C)_n$	Inactive	Inactive
4. Mismatched dsRNA	$(I)_n \cdot (C_x, G)_n$	Activity inversely related to the N. of mismatches (Fully active for C/G > 35)	Activity inversely related to the N. of mismatches (Fully active for C/G > 50)
5. dsRNA with one strand of known size	$(I)_n \cdot (C_x G)_n$	Active for x > 60	Fully active for x > 80
6. dsRNA with both strands of known size	$(A_x)_n \cdot (U_y)_n$	Inactive for x < 33; partially active for x = 54 and y = 120; fully active for x and y > 160	Inactive for x < 33; partially active for x = 54 and y = 120; fully active for x and y > 160
7. dsRNA methylated in either strand	$(I)_n \cdot (Cm_x, C)_n$ & $(Im_x, I)_n \cdot (C)_n$	Inactive if fully methylated in either strand Active if x < 60	Inactive if fully methylated in either strand Active if x < 20%

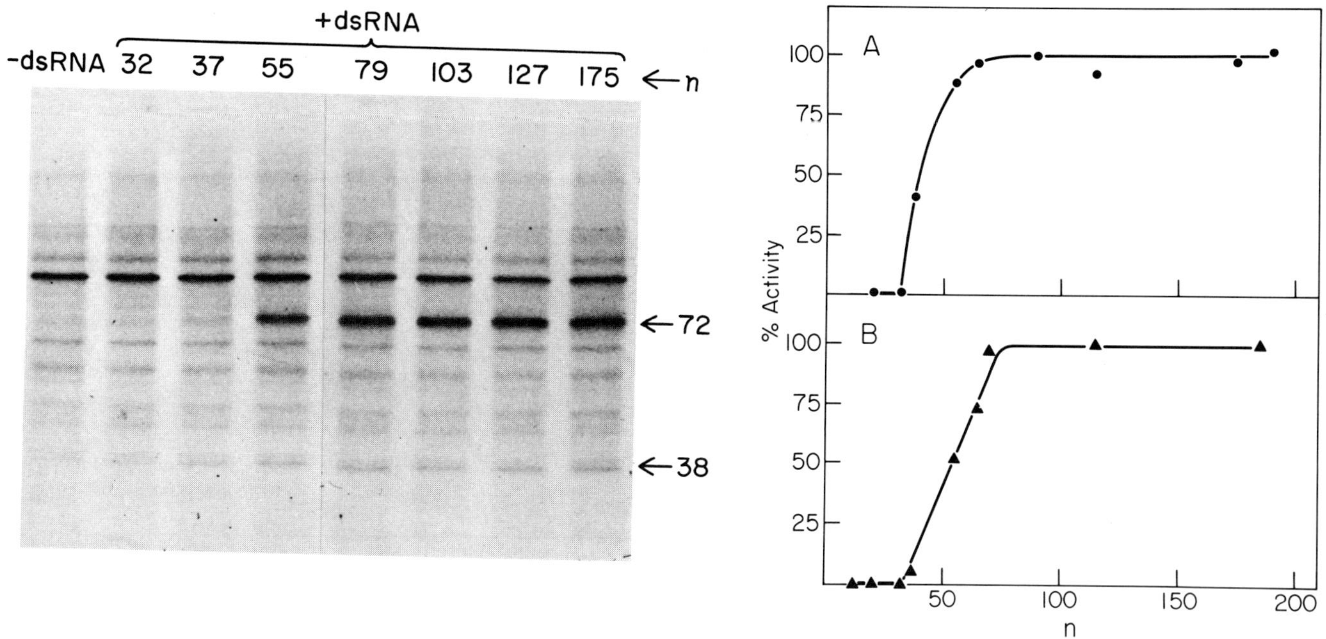

FIGURE 1. Phosphorylation of the 72,000 M_r polypeptide (*left*) and activation (*right*) of the 2′5′oligo(A) polymerase (*A*) and protein kinase (*B*) by poly(I) annealed to sized poly(C). For the PK_{ds} assay ribosomes from interferon-treated HeLa cells were incubated with 0.1 μg/ml of dsRNA for 7 min at 30°C and analyzed by gel electrophoresis and autoradiography as described.[4] The tracks show from left to right: an incubation without added dsRNA; incubations with poly(I) annealed to poly(C) of the length indicated for each track (n). The position of the 72*k* and 38*k* polypeptides is indicated. The 2′5′oligo(A) polymerase was assayed with 10 μg/ml of dsRNA as described.[5] With poly(I)·poly(C), 33 nmol of ATP were converted to 2′5′oligo(A) in 60 min from an imput of 125 nmol per reaction; this value was taken as 100% in *A* and the activation with different dsRNAs is shown as a percentage activity. In the PK_{ds} assay, phosphorylation of the 72*k* polypeptide was determined by scanning autoradiographs of gels, like those shown at left. Activation of the PK_{ds} is shown as a percentage of that obtained with poly(I)·poly(C). The length in nucleotides of the poly(C) annealed to poly(I) is indicated in the abscissa. The data shown are taken from Minks *et al.*[7]

major differences between the activation of the 2,5A polymerase and that of the PK_{ds}. The polymerase is fully activated by dsRNA concentrations higher than 10 μg/ml,[5] whereas the kinase is fully activated by 0.1 μg/ml of dsRNA and high concentrations of dsRNA are inhibitory.[17] Furthermore, dsRNAs that do not activate the IF-induced enzymes do not compete with active dsRNAs in the 2,5A polymerase assay, whereas they compete in the PK_{ds} assay.[7,8] Some of the competition data obtained with inactive dsRNA are shown in FIGURE 2. The most active competitors are dsRNAs that are structurally related to active dsRNAs: i.e., a partially methylated dsRNA competes better than a fully methylated dsRNA. There results suggest that the PK_{ds} may bind to inactive dsRNA with a high enough affinity to form stable complexes, whereas the 2,5A polymerase either does not bind to inactive dsRNAs or can easily dissociate to interact with active dsRNAs. Two other lines of evidence suggest that the IF-induced enzymes may bind to dsRNA with different affinities: (1) the 2,5A polymerase is eluted from

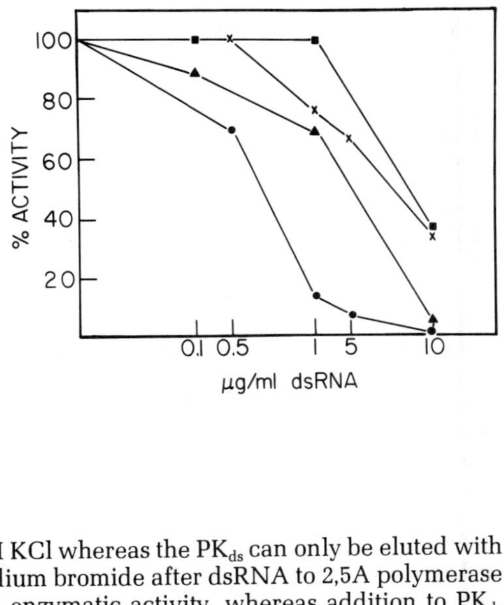

FIGURE 2. Competition for protein kinase activation by inactive dsRNAs. The activation of the PK_{ds} was measured as described in FIGURE 1 with poly(I)·poly(C). The phosphorylation of the 72*k* poypeptide obtained with this dsRNA was taken as 100%. Double-stranded RNAs inactive in promoting phosphorylation of this polypeptide[7,8] were tested as competitors of poly(I)·poly(C) by adding increasing amounts of these polymers to reactions containing 0.1 μg/ml of poly(I)·poly(C). The PK_{ds} activity in the presence of competitors is expressed as a percentage of maximal phosphorylation. The μg of competitor dsRNA added are indicated in the abscissa. ■——■, $(I)_n \cdot (C_7,G)_n$; x——x, $(I)_n \cdot (C_{32}G)_n$; ▲——▲, $(I)_n \cdot (Cm)_n$; ●——●, $(Im_{78}, I_{22})_n \cdot (C)_n$.

poly (I)·poly(C)-agarose with 0.2 M KCl whereas the PK_{ds} can only be eluted with 1 M KCl[18]; and (2) addition of ethidium bromide after dsRNA to 2,5A polymerase assays causes an inhibition of the enzymatic activity, whereas addition to PK_{ds} assays does not result in inhibition.[19] Ethidium bromide intercalates between adjacent base pairs of double-stranded regions of nucleic acids.[20] This intercalation results in an unwinding and a local extension of the duplex structure. These structural changes presumably cause the 2,5A polymerase to dissociate from dsRNA, since further addition of a dsRNA that binds less ethidium restores the enzymatic activity.[19] In the case of PK_{ds}, when the enzyme is allowed to interact with dsRNA before addition of ethidium no inihibition is observed.[19] This suggests that either ethidium cannot intercalate in duplex regions which are complexed with PK_{ds}, or that, once the PK_{ds} interacts with dsRNA, ethidium intercalation does not inhibit enzyme activity.

THE ROLE OF THE INTERFERON-INDUCED ENZYMES IN THE ANTIVIRAL STATE

Our present tenet is that activation of 2,5A polymerase and PK_{ds} is at least in part responsible for inhibition of virus replication in intact cells, even though no evidence is yet available that such an activation takes place in IF-treated cells infected by viruses. Until the role of these enzymes is established by experiments with intact cells, we can only extrapolate from *in vitro* experiments as to what may be going on in intact cells. The 2,5A polymerase and PK_{ds} are activated in cell extracts by relatively long stretches of perfectly matched dsRNA, which are not found among the cytoplasmic RNA species of mammalian cells. RNA duplexes may be formed during the replication of RNA viruses in structures called replicative complexes (RC). These structures contain a viral RNA strand that is transcribed or replicated in a complementary strand by a virally coded enzyme. The presence of dsRNA in native RC has been a matter of controversy for some time.[21,23] Upon deproteinization of RC and isolation of the RNA component designated replicative intermediate or RI, the complementary strands are found base-paired. In intact cells, however, association of viral or cellular proteins with the viral RNA strands may effectively prevent dsRNA formation.[22] Recently, we have shown that complementary strands in RC of encephalomyocarditis virus (EMCV) can be cross-linked in intact cells by aminomethyltrioxsalene.[9] This suggests that the complementary strands of EMCV are at least in part base-paired and possibly form relatively long stretches of dsRNA. In agreement with this finding, the subcellular fraction containing RC obtained from EMCV-infected cells activates the 2,5A polymerase.[24] Once 2,5A is synthesized, an endonuclease is presumably activated in such a way that only viral and not cellular RNA is cleaved, since no generalized breakdown of RNA is observed in virus-infected IF-treated cells.

The mechanism by which the activation of 2,5A polymerase results in preferential cleavage of viral RNA has recently been investigated in extracts of IF-treated HeLa cells.[6] The RI prepared from EMCV-infected cells is almost completely degraded in these extracts to an RNase A resistant double-stranded "core," whereas it is not appreciably degraded in extracts of control cells.[6] Several lines of evidence indicate that the dsRNA in RI is responsible for this preferential degradation. Most of these results have been obtained with model substrates containing dsRNA covalently linked to mRNA, rather than with RI, because degradation of these substrates can be accurately quantitated.[6] The 35S EMCV RNA contains a poly(C) sequence approximately 100 nucleotides long near the 5′-terminus of the molecule.[25] This poly(C) can be annealed to poly(I) to form a structure partially double-stranded near the 5′-terminus. Viral RNA containing this dsRNA structure is preferentially degraded in extracts of IF-treated cells, in a manner similar to the RI degradation.[6] In all the other experiments cytoplasmic mRNA obtained from HeLa cells or vesicular stomatitis virus (VSV) mRNA synthesized *in vitro* was annealed with poly(U), to form a single-stranded polynucleotide linked to a 3′-terminal double-stranded "tail."[6] Molecules containing this dsRNA tail are preferentially degraded in extracts of IF-treated HeLa cells, whereas mRNA not covalently linked to dsRNA is not appreciably cleaved by endonucleases.[6] The preferential cleavage of RNA linked to dsRNA, therefore, occurs independently of the 3′ or 5′-terminal location of the dsRNA.

The endonucleolytic cleavage of mRNA can be measured by determining the fraction that remains attached to the 3′-terminal poly(A) (see following section). With this covenient assay, we obtained evidence that the cleavage is mediated by the 2,5A-activated endonuclease and investigated the structural requirements of the dsRNA tail. Synthesis of 2,5A requires Mg^{2+} and ATP[5]; accordingly, when Mg^{2+} was chelated with EDTA the endonucleolytic degradation of mRNA was abolished, whereas addition of ATP resulted in increased degradation of mRNA.[6] In this latter case, however, all the RNA present in the incubation was degraded and preferential cleavage of the RNA linked to dsRNA was no longer observed. In order to obtain the preferential degradation of this RNA, the dsRNA tail must have a minimal size. The VSV mRNA can be fractionated into molecules containing poly(A) shorter or longer than 60 nucleotides.[6] The mRNA with the short poly(A) annealed to poly(U) is not preferentially degraded, presumably because it cannot activate the 2,5A polymerase.[9] Alternatively, VSV

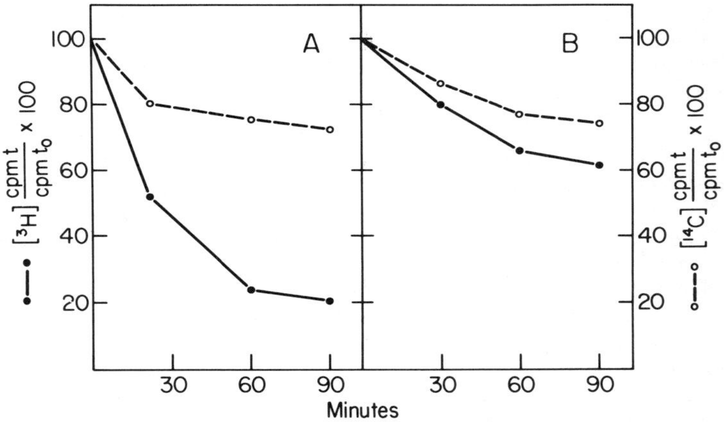

FIGURE 3. Time course of mRNA degradation in extracts of interferon-treated (*A*) and control (*B*) cells. The incubations contained in a 0.1 ml vol: 1,000 cpm of VSV [^{14}C]mRNA not annealed with poly(U) (o--o), 10,000 cpm of VSV [^{3}H]mRNA annealed with poly(U) (●——●), 30 μl of extract from control HeLa cells or from cells treated for 20 hr with 100 units/ml of human fibroblast interferon, 0.12 M KOAc, 4 mM fructose 1,6-*bis*phosphate and 2 mM $Mg(OAc)_2$. The VSV mRNA was synthesized as described[6] in reactions containing 0.32 mM S-adenosylhomocysteine; the presence of long poly(A) sequences was confirmed by gel analysis of RNase A digested [^{3}H]adenosine-labeled RNA.[26] Aliquots of the incubations were taken at the times indicated to measure poly(A)-containing RNA by oligo(dT)-cellulose chromatography.[2,6] The percentage of poly(A)-containing RNA remaining after incubation is shown on the ordinate relative to a control sample not incubated (equal 100%).

mRNA can be transcribed in the presence of the inhibitor of methylation S-adenosylhomocysteine[26]; the viral mRNA synthesized in this way contains only very long poly(A) and is effectively cleaved in extracts of IF-treated cells upon annealing with poly (U) (FIGURE 3). However, this mRNA annealed with enough poly(U) to form a triple-stranded structure is not degraded.

The structural requirements of dsRNA necessary to observe the preferential degradation of covalently linked RNA are essentially identical to those required to activate the 2,5A polymerase. In agreement with this observation, addition of ethidium bromide either to mRNA linked to a dsRNA tail or to the replicative intermediate of EMCV prevents the preferential degradation of these substrates

TABLE 2

SUBSTRATE SPECIFICITY OF THE 2′5′OLIGO(A)-ACTIVATED ENDONUCLEASE*

Substrate Tested	Assay	Effect of 2′5′Oligo(A)
HeLa cell mRNA	Oligo(dT)-cellulose	Cleaved
VSV mRNA	Oligo(dT)-celulose	Cleaved
Vaccinia mRNA	Oligo(dT)-cellulose	Cleaved
dsDNA	Sedimentation analysis	None
ssDNA	↑	None
Poly(A)	↕	None
Poly(U) · $(A33)_n$	↓	None
Poly(C) · $(I_{48})_n$	Sedimentation analysis	None

*The assay for mRNA cleavage by oligo(dT)-cellulose chromatography has been described.[2] Cleavage of the other substrates was assayed under identical incubation conditions but the reaction products were analyzed by velocity sedimentation on sucrose gradients as described.[9] The A_{33} and I_{48} were purchased from Miles and PL-Biochemicals, respectively; the approximate size of I_{48} was estimated from its sedimentation ($S_{20,w}$ = 2.5).

in extracts of IF-treated cells. The structural changes caused by the intercalation of ethidium presumably prevent the activation of 2,5A polymerase.[9]

We have proposed a mechanism that accounts for the preferential degradation of viral RNA in IF-treated cells.[2,6] The activation of the 2,5A polymerase may be localized to viral replicative complexes. In this case the 2,5A would be most concentrated and the endonuclease would be preferentially activated near the site of synthesis of viral RNA; this RNA may be cleaved as it is being synthesized or soon afterward. The concentration of 2,5A initially decreases with the third power of the distance from its site of synthesis and could decrease even further because of its degradation by phosphodiesterase(s) which cleave 2′–5′ bonds.[28] The 2,5A-activated endonuclease reverts to an inactive state in the absence of the oligonucleotides.[1] Therefore, if the 2,5A concentration is limited by diffusion and degradation, a localized activation of the endonuclease may prevent cleavage of cellular RNA. This mechanism for discrimination between viral and cellular RNA has only been shown *in vitro* and it has not yet been possible to obtain evidence for this mechanism *in vivo*. Its validity, therefore, remains to be established in intact cells.

SPECIFICITY OF THE ENDONUCLEASE ACTIVATED BY 2′5′OLIGO(A)

Addition of nM concentrations of 2,5A to cell extracts results in the degradation of cellular and viral mRNA.[2] We have established that the poly(A)-containing mRNA obtained from HeLa cells and various viral mRNAs are cleaved at an apparently similar rate by the activated endonuclease (TABLE 2). This enzyme does not seem to cleave specific nucleotide sequences present only in some mRNAs, but has a rather broad substrate specificity. However, under the conditions of our assay for 2,5A-activated endonuclase with nM concentrations of 2,5A, relatively few cleavages per mRNA molecule are observed (see below). It is not clear whether this results from a limited enzymatic activity, the most likely explanation, and/or from the presence of relatively few nucleotide sequences or conformational features of mRNA which are particularly susceptible to endonucleolytic attack.

The endonuclease assay is based on the isolation of poly(A)-containing RNA by oligo(dT)-cellulose chromatography after incubation with cell extract with or without added 2,5A.[2] Endonucleolytic cleavages are estimated by the decrease in the RNA fraction which binds to oligo(dT)-cellulose. This assay is extremely sensitive, since one random endonucleolytic break per RNA molecule decreases the bound fraction by 50 percent. A measurement of the average number of cleavages per RNA molecule can be obtained by the following calculation.

The 2,5A-activated endonuclease reduces RNA molecules of length L to fragments of average size $\bar{l}$ by introducing $\bar{X}$ cleavages. If $\bar{X} \geqslant 10$, then $\bar{l}/L = 1/(1 + \bar{X})$ for all practical purposes. For smaller values of $\bar{X}$, however, the probability that an RNA molecule is cleaved X times follows a Poisson distribution and the relationship between $\bar{X}$ and $\bar{l}$ can be derived in the following way. Assuming that the RNA fragment which remains linked to poly(A) is equal to $\bar{l}$ (i.e., cleavages occur randomly), a measurement of the RNA fraction which binds to oligo(dT)-cellulose after incubation with 2,5A provides a value for $\bar{l}$ and a measurement of the fraction that binds after incubation without added 2,5A provides a value for L. The distribution of lengths of RNA molecules attached to poly(A) after incubation with 2,5A can be described by the probability P_l of finding fragments of length l. Then $\bar{l} = \Sigma_{l=1}^{L}\, l\, P_l$ by definition. The probability of finding a fragment of size l is the product of the probability that there were no cleavages at the $l - 1$ phosphodiester bonds linking the fragment to poly(A) and that a cut was made at the lth bond. If p is the probability of a cleavage and $1 - p$ the probability of no cleavage, then $P_l = (1 - p)^{l-1}p$. Substitution of P_l in terms of p into the expression for $\bar{l}$ and integration gives:

$$\bar{l}/L = (1 - e^{-X}) / X$$

In practice, $\bar{l}$ and L are estimated by the amount of radioactive poly(A)-containing RNA found respectively in incubations with 2,5A and without added 2,5A. The amount of radioactive RNA is expressed as C (=cpm + 2,5A) and C_0 (=cpm − 2,5A) respectively, and values of $\bar{X}$ for different ratios of C/C_0 have been calculated and are shown in FIGURE 4. A linear increase in the value of $\bar{X}$ is

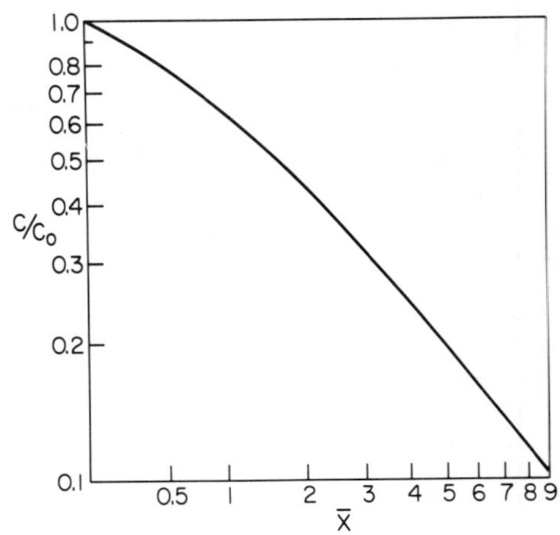

FIGURE 4. Relationship between the ratio of the final concentration of RNA over the initial concentration (C/C_0) and the average number of random endonucleolytic cleavages ($\bar{X}$). See text for explanations.

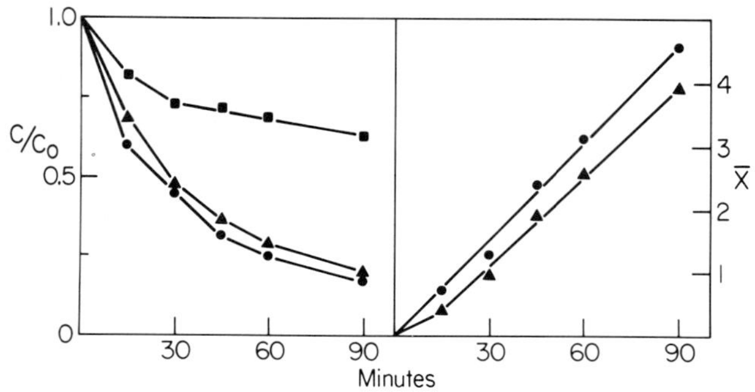

FIGURE 5. Time course of mRNA degradation in extracts of control (●——●) and interferon-treated (▲——▲) cells with added 280 nM 2′5′ oligo(A), or in extract of control cells without added 2′5′oligo(A) (■——■). The preparation of mRNA from VSV-infected cells, the composition of the incubations and the assay for mRNA cleavage by oligo(dT)-cellulose chromatography have been described.[2] In the *left panel* the loss of poly(A)-containing RNA is shown as the ratio of the cpm at time = t over the cpm at time = t_0 (C/C_0). In the *right panel* the average number of cleavages per RNA molecule ($\overline{X}$) have been calculated as described in the text. The loss of poly(A)-containing RNA in the absence of added 2′5′oligo(A) was subtracted from that observed with added 2′5′oligo(A) and the value C/C_0 converted into $\overline{X}$ as described in FIGURE 4.

observed with incubation time; this indicates that cleavages of mRNA occur with a regular frequency in the course of an incubation with added 2,5A (FIGURE 5).

The method used to calculate the average number of cleavages $\overline{X}$ can be applied to mixtures of RNA molecules of different length with identical results. The theoretical value for $\overline{X}$ corresponds to the experimentally determined value of $\overline{X}$ only if: (1) the RNA is uniformly labeled; (2) the 3′-poly(A) is unlabeled and is not cleaved by the 2,5A-activated endonuclease; and (3) the RNA fragments produced by endonucleolytic cleavage are not degraded by exonucleases. The first two conditions are obtained since the RNA analyzed is uniformly labeled with [^{3}H]uridine and poly(A) is not cleaved by the endonuclease (see below). The degradation of RNA by exonucleases, however, presents a more serious problem and has been investigated in some detail.

Some RNA degradation is observed in incubations without added 2,5A and the products are mono- or oligonucleotides soluble in trichloroacetic acid.[2] Only 20 to 30% of poly(A)-containing RNA is degraded in this way and predominantly in the first 30 min of incubation (FIGURE 5). Other RNAs are more susceptible to this type of degradation; for example, ribosomal RNA is extensively and rapidly degraded when added to HeLa cell extracts.[29] Labeled synthetic poly(A), on the other hand, is degraded less than rRNA. Structural differences among these RNAs may account for the different patterns of degradation. Ribosomal RNA can be attacked by both 3′- and 5′-exonuclease and does not seem to be protected by an interaction with cytoplasmic proteins. Poly(A) is partially resistant to exonucleases either because it binds to specific proteins[30] or because of secondary structure. Poly(A)-containing mRNA is "capped" and therefore resistant to 5′-exonucleases; the presence of poly(A) at the 3′-terminus confers protection against 3′-exonucleases.

When cleavages are introduced in mRNA by the 2,5A-activated endonuclease, new unprotected 3′- and 5′-termini are formed. The cleaved mRNA molecules, however, do not seem to be susceptible to a rapid exonucleolytic degradation since large RNA cleavage fragments can be detected by sedimentation analysis.[2] The degradation of mRNA fragments produced by endonucleolytic cleavage has been investigated.[29] The 12-16S VSV mRNA was cleaved by 18-min treatment with 25 mM Na_2CO_3[31] and 28S VSV mRNA was cleaved by radiochemical decay upon prolonged storage at −70°C. In both cases, a few random breaks are introduced and new ends are generated. The fragments linked to poly(A) can be separated by oligo(dT)-cellulose chromatography from those not containing poly(A). The degradation of these fragments upon addition to cell extracts has been investigated (FIGURE 6). Both fragments containing poly(A) and not containing poly(A) are degraded to acid-soluble material at a relatively slow rate, regardless of the way in which the fragments are produced (data not shown). It should be pointed out that the rate of degradation is characteristic of each cell extract and that vastly different rates have been observed in HeLa cell extracts. It seems possible that exonucleases are released into the cell sap during homogenization and that different homogenization procedures result in marked differences in the exonuclease activity of cell extracts. For example, when detergents are used to lyse the cells, the exonuclease activity of the lysate is too high to allow detection of endonucleolytic activity upon addition of 2,5A.[29] It is important, therefore, to prepare cell extracts by gentle mechanical homogenization and to test these extracts for exonuclease activity with a suitable substrate; only those extracts with low exonuclease activity can be used in the assay described above.

The 2,5A-activated endonuclease degrades many different mRNAs and does not show a clear substrate preference.[2] We have established that the activated endonuclease cleaves only single-stranded RNA, but does not cleave poly(A),

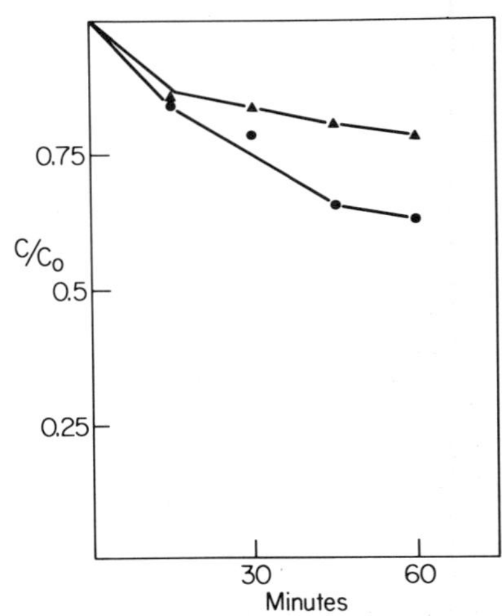

FIGURE 6. Degradation of poly(A)-containing (●——●) and poly(A)-free (▲——▲) fragments of 28S VSV mRNA. The RNA was prepared from HeLa cells infected with VSV and incubated with [^{3}H]uridine as previously described[2]; the poly(A)-containing RNA was isolated and the mRNA for the L protein fractionated by sucrose gradient centrifugation, ethanol precipitated, and stored at −70°C for 9 months. The 28S L mRNA was again fractionated by oligo(dT)-cellulose chromatography into a poly(A)-containing fraction and a poly(A)-free fraction. These fractions were analyzed by velocity sedimentation to verify that the RNAs had a reduced size because of fragmentation. Aliquots of each RNA preparation (30,000 cpm) were incubated with HeLa cell extract under the same conditions used in the assay for endonuclease.[2] Samples taken at the indicated times were precipitated with 5% trichloroacetic acid and counted. The ratio C/C_0 indicates that fraction of RNA which has remained acid-precipitable upon incubation.

poly(C) or poly(U) (TABLE 2). Cleavage of these substrates was assayed by incubating labeled polynucleotides with HeLa cell extract with or without 2,5A and analyzing the reaction products by velocity sedimentation. This assay was satisfactory with ssDNA, dsDNA, and dsRNA, and poly(A). Only the latter polynucleotide is appreciably degraded to acid-soluble nucleotides, presumably by exonucleases, but addition of 2,5A did not increase the rate of degradation.[9] With poly(U) and poly(C), however, degradation in the absence of added 2,5A was rapid and complete. This degradation could be prevented by annealing these polynucleotides with short (less than 50 bases) complementary strands of poly(A) and poly(I) respectively. Partially double-stranded polymers could be formed by adding enough complementary short strands to obtain about 50% resistance to RNase A.[9] These polymers were resistant to exonuclease digestion, since they were not degraded to acid-soluble material upon incubation with cell extract and were also resistant to cleavage by 2,5A-activated endonuclease. However, the same polymers were susceptible to endonucleolytic attack by RNase A. We conclude, therefore, that the 2,5A-activated endonuclease does not cleave the homopolymers tested.

CONCLUSION

The molecular features of dsRNA that are required for the activation of two IF-induced enzymes have been defined by using synthetic mismatched, sized and 2′-*O*-substituted dsRNAs. About 50 base pairs of perfectly matched dsRNA are necessary to activate the 2,5A polymerase and PK_{ds} *in vitro*. A similar structure may therefore activate these enzymes in cells infected by viruses. We have argued that such a structure may only be formed in the process of viral replication. Replicative complexes isolated from infected cells do indeed activate the 2,5A polymerase and the ssRNA components of such structures (RI) are degraded in extracts of IF-treated cells. A series of experiments with RNA covalently linked to dsRNA conclusively show that the dsRNA portion of the RNA activates the 2,5A polymerase and that a local activation of the 2,5A-dependent endonuclease is responsible for the preferential cleavage of the linked ssRNA. We postulate that a similar mechanism may be responsible for the cleavage of nascent viral RNA in IF-treated cells infected by some RNA viruses. The 2,5A-activated endonuclease possesses a broad specificity toward RNA, though it does not cleave the homopolymers tested. It is possible, therefore, that the endonuclease may cleave specific nucleotide sequences, but these sequences must be present in most mRNAs, both cellular and viral. The substrate specificity of the endonuclease cannot account for the preferential degradation of viral RNAs in IF-treated cells. Such degradation, however, needs to be directly documented *in vivo*. Moreover, the 2,5A polymerase/endonuclease system is not the only line of defense against viral infections in IF-treated cells. The role of the PK_{ds}, for example, is still undetermined and there are other possible mechanisms that may interfere with viral replication.

REFERENCES

1. BAGLIONI, C. 1979. Cell **17:** 225–265.
2. BAGLIONI, C., M. A. MINKS & P. A. MARONEY. 1978. Nature **273:** 684–687.
3. BAGLIONI, C., P. A. MARONEY & D. K. WEST. 1979. Biochemistry **18:** 1765–1770.

4. WEST, D. K. & C. BAGLIONI. 1979. Eur. J. Biochem. **101:** 461–468.
5. MINKS, M. A., S. BENVIN, P. A. MARONEY & C. BAGLIONI. 1979. J. Biol. Chem. **254:** 5058–5064.
6. NILSEN, T. W., & C. BAGLIONI. 1979. Proc. Nat. Acad. Sci. USA **76:** 2600–2604.
7. MINKS, M. A., D. K. WEST, S. BENVIN & C. BAGLIONI. 1979. J. Biol. Chem. In press
8. MINKS, M. A., D. WEST, S. BENVIN, J. J. GREENE, P. O. P. TS'O & C. BAGLIONI. 1980. Submitted for publication.
9. NILSEN, T. W. & C. BAGLIONI. In preparation.
10. ROBERTS, W. K., A. HOVANESSIAN, R. E. BROWN, M. J. CLEMENS & I. M. KERR. 1976. Nature **264:** 477–480.
11. KERR, I. M., R. E. BROWN & A. G. HOVANESSIAN. 1977. Nature **268:** 540–542.
12. LEBLEU, B., G. C. SEN, S. SHAILA, B. CABRER & P. LENGYEL. 1976. Proc. Nat. Acad. Sci. USA **73:** 3107–3111.
13. KIMCHI, A., A. ZILBERSTEIN, A. SCHMIDT, L. SHULMAN & M. REVEL. 1979. Submitted for publication.
14. ZILBERSTEIN, A., P. FEDERMAN, L. SHULMAN & M. REVEL. 1976. FEBS Lett. **68:** 119–124.
15. GREENE, J. J., J. L. ALDERFERDER, I. TAZAWA, S. TAZAWA, P. O. P. TS'O, J. A. O'MALLEY & W. A. CARTER. 1978. Biochemistry **17:** 4214–4220.
16. TORRENCE, P. F. & E. DE CLERCO. 1977. Pharmacol. Therap. Part **2:** 1–88.
17. FARREL, J., K. BALCOW, T. HUNT & R. JACKSON. 1977. Cell **11:** 187–200.
18. HOVANESSIAN, A. G. & I. M. KERR. 1978. Eur. J. Biochem. **93:** 515–526.
19. MARONEY, P. A. & C. BAGLIONI. In preparation.
20. WARING, M. J. 1965. J. Mol. Biol. **27:** 87–106.
21. WEISSMAN, C., G. FEIX & H. SLOR. 1968. Cold Spring Harbor Symp. Quant. Biol. **33:** 83–100.
22. OEBERG, B. & L. PHILIPSON. 1971. J. Mol. Biol. **58:** 725–737.
23. LEVINTOW, L. 1974. *In* Comprehensive Virology. H. Fraenkel-Conrat & R. R. WAGNER, Eds. Vol. **3:** 109–169. Plenum Press. New York and London.
24. NILSEN, T. W., P. A. MARONEY & C. BAGLIONI. 1979. *In* Regulation of Macromolecular Synthesis by Low Molecular Weight Mediators. H. Koch & D. Richter, Eds.: 329–339. Academic Press. New York
25. CHUMAKOV, K. M. & V. I. AGOL. 1976. Biochem. Biophys. Res. Commun. **71:** 551–557.
26. ROSE, J. K., H. F. LODISH & M. L. BROCK. 1977. J. Virol. **21:** 683–693.
27. SCHMIDT, A., A. ZILBERSTEIN, L. SHULMAN, P. FEDERMAN, H. BERISSI & M. REVEL. 1978. FEBS Lett. **95:** 257–264.
28. MINKS, M. A., S. BENVIN, P. A. MARONEY & C. BAGLIONI. 1979. Nucleic Acid Res. **6:** 767–780.
29. BAGLIONI, C., P. A. MARONEY & T. W. NILSEN. 1980. Methods in Enzymology. In press.
30. BERGMANN, I. E. & G. BRAWERMAN. 1977. Biochemistry **16:** 259–264.
31. RABBITS, T. H. & C. MILSTEIN. 1975. Eur. J. Biochem. **52:** 125–133.

PROPERTIES OF 2′5′ OLIGOADENYLATE SYNTHETASE*

J. Justesen, D. Ferbus, and M. N. Thang

Institut de Biologie Physico-chimique
Fondation Edmond de Rothschild
75005 Paris, France

Introduction

Since its discovery two years ago, many investigators[1-7] have focused their attention on the 2′5′ oligo-A synthetase. This is the first known enzyme that catalyzes the synthesis of a natural nucleic acid with 2′5′ phosphodiester linkage. It is primarily interesting because the enzyme activity is induced in cells treated by interferons (IFs).[1] Other regulatory functions of this enzyme may be expected because of its wide occurrence in mammalian cells, where its activity appears to be dependent on the growth conditions, hormone responses, or the state of differentiation.[8] While much study has been devoted to this enzyme, its mechanism of action is still unknown.

The nucleic acid polymerizing enzymes can be classified into categories according to their mode of action. One class, such as DNA or RNA polymerase, copies the template for the synthesis of nucleic acids. Another class, including terminal transferase, poly A synthetase, and CTP:ATP transferase, adds nucleotide units to a nucleic primer. Only polynucleotide phosphorylase or deoxynucleoside diphosphate polymerase catalyse the *de novo* formation of polynucleotide without a template or a primer. In the present work, we have investigated the mechanism of elongation of the 2′5′ oligo-A synthetase isolated from rabbit reticulocyte lysate.

Materials and Methods

Assay of Oligo-A Synthetase

An aliquot of enzyme extract was incubated with the following mixture: 20 mM Tris-Cl pH 8.0, 20 mM $Mg(OAc)_2$, 0.1 mg/ml BSA, 4 μg/ml poly I poly C, 1 mM DTT, 1 mM ATP and ca. 1 μCi/ml α-^{32}P-ATP. The volume was normally 20 μl with incubation at 30°C or 37°C as stated. The reaction was stopped by heating to 72°C for 2 min.

Four to ten microliters of the mixture were applied directly to PEI-cellulose thin-layer plates. The PEI-cellulose plates were prepared in our laboratory as described by Randerath and Randerath[9] and could not be replaced by commercially obtainable plates to give a separation of ATP and 2′-5′ oligo-As in our systems.

*This work was supported by grants from CNRS (E.R. 238), INSERM (C.R.L. 80.12.20), DGRST (MREM 80.7.0148), and Commissariat à l'Energie Atomique.

0077-8923/80/0350-0510 $1.75/0 © 1980, NYAS

Composition of Oligomers

Separation of the 2′-5′ Oligo-A

We have developed a new system that permits direct separation of the 5′ phosphorylated oligonucleotides according to chain lengths.[11]

After sample application, the PEI-plate was dried and washed in water for 10 min and in methanol for 5 min with drying in between. The plate was developed in methanol to 1 cm above the application line and transferred directly to a solvent of 2M Tris-Cl pH 8.6.[11] To the top of the 18 × 18 cm plate was attached a 6-cm broad piece of filter paper and the chromatography was continued to the top of the paper wick (4–6 hr). The plate was dried and exposed to an x-ray film overnight (FIGURE 1). The spots containing ATP and oligo-A were localized, cut

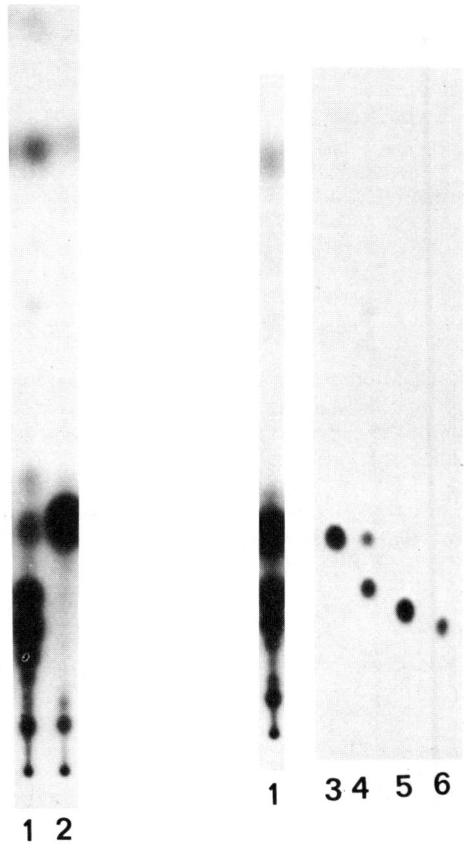

FIGURE 1. Autoradiograms of oligomers, composition analysis.
PEI-cellulose thin-layer sheet after chromatography in 2 M Tris pH 8.6.
1 : total mixture after long incubation of oligo A synthetase with α^{32}P-ATP;
2 : Sample of the commercially obtainable α^{32}P-ATP preparation;
3 : ATP;
4 : ppp5′A2′p5′A (the dimer);
5 : ppp5′A $(2'p5'A)_2$ (the trimer);
6 : ppp5′A $(2'p5'A)_3$ (the tetramer).

The production of oligo-As was as outlined in METHODS. The preparation of the ATP, dimer, trimer and tetramer followed the procedure of Martin et al.[12] using a DEAE Sephadex column. The TLC chromatography is described under METHODS.

by scissors and counted. One unit of enzyme is defined as incorporating 1 nanomole of AMP residues into 2′-5′ oligo-A per min at 37°C.

Separation of the Core Oligonucleotides

The incubation mixture was treated with alkaline phosphatase (AP) to remove the terminal triphosphate group. After 2 hr at 37°C with 25 μg/ml AP, 5-10 μl samples were applied to PEI-cellulose plates as above. The plates were dried, washed 10 min in methanol, and dried. The chromatography procedure, based on a method of Gupta and Randerath[10] using Tris-Cl and urea as solvent systems for the development, is described elsewhere.[11]

Standard Buffer

The standard buffer was 20 mM Tris-Cl pH 8.0, 5 mM $Mg(OAc)_2$, 25 mM KCl, 1 mM DTT, and 10% (v/v) glycerol.

RESULTS

Purification of Oligo-A Synthetase

Crude rabbit reticulocyte lysate was passed through a DEAE-cellulose (DE 52) column in standard buffer. The passed-through fractions were collected and applied to a 3 ml poly I · poly C-agarose column. After washing thoroughly with buffer and buffer plus 0.1 M KCl, the 2′5′ oligo-A-forming activity was eluted by 0.2 M KCl in standard buffer. Ammonium sulfate was added up to 46% to the active fractions. The precipitate was discarded by centrifugation. To the supernatant was added poly I · poly C to 50 μg/ml, and the active portion was

TABLE 1

PURIFICATION OF OLIGO-A SYNTHETASE

		Volume (ml)	Protein Conc. (mg/ml)	Activity (units/ml)	Specific Activity (units/mg protein)	Total Activity	Fold Activity	Yield (%)
Reticulocyte		85	160	—	—	—	1	—
DE-52 pass-through	I	105	32	4.2	0.13	440	4*	100
PolyI–PolyC-agarose chromatography		9.7	0.35	—	—	—	—	—
46% Am. sulfate + 50 μg/ml polyI-polyC	II	0.90	2.7	88	32	79	1010	18

*The fold purification is calculated from the loss of protein assuming that the activity is totally recovered.

The activity was measured as initial velocity at 37°C with 1.5 mM ATP to start with under standard conditions.

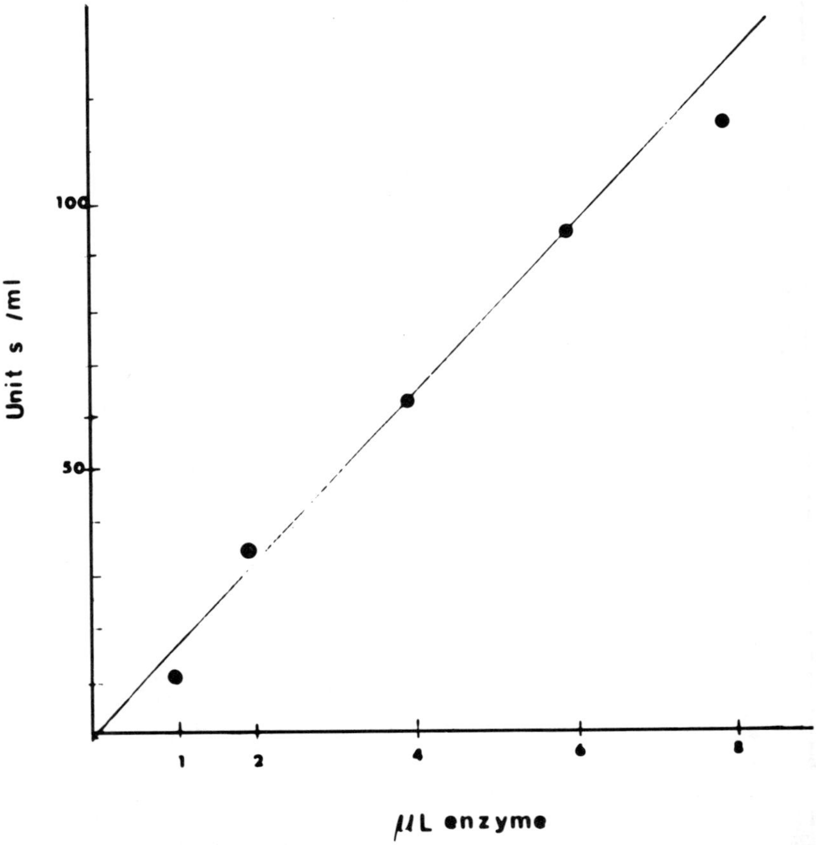

FIGURE 2. Enzyme dependence. The indicated amount of enzyme was incubated at 30°C in a total volume of 40 μl and a concentration of ATP of 1 mM. Of this 6 μl samples were removed and applied directly onto PEI-cellulose sheets at 30, 60, 130 and 210 min. After chromatography and counting the percentage of conversion was calculated. From this, the activity was determined.

precipitated and redissolved in standard buffer and stored at −80°C. The purification is summarized in TABLE 1.

The enzyme obtained at this step contained no detectable interfering enzymatic activities for the reaction studied, such as ATPase, phosphatase or nucleolytic activities degrading the 2'5' oligo-A.

Characterization of Oligo-A Synthetase

The enzyme assay based on separation of ATP from the produced 2'-5' oligomers, showed a linear correlation between amount of enzyme and activity (FIGURE 2). As for many enzymes there is a considerable variation with temperature so that the maximum rate is obtained between 37 and 42°C (FIGURE 3). The

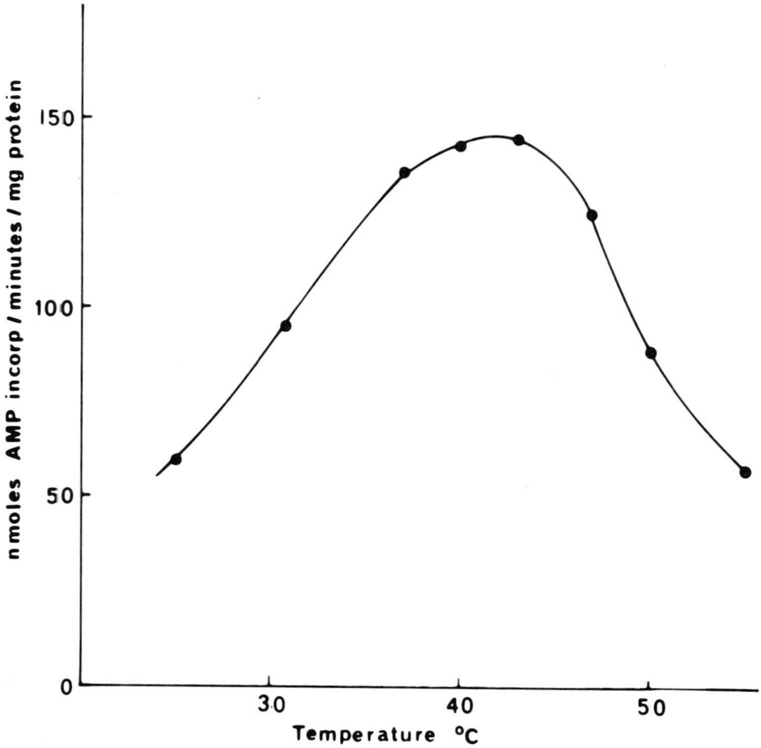

FIGURE 3. Temperature. The standard mixture with purified oligo-A synthetase was incubated for 2 hr at the indicated temperatures in volumes of 18 μl. The reaction was stopped by 5 min at 72°C. 5μl were applied onto a PEI-cellulose sheet that chromatographed in 2 M Tris pH 8.6. After localization by autoradiography, the ATP and oligo-A spots were cut and counted to give the percent conversion. The resulting measure of activity is represented as units per mg protein.

optimum pH value is around 8 (FIGURE 4) with a typical shape of a pH-curve. The Mg^{++} ions are required, and addition up to 20 mM still gives a stimulation (FIGURE 5). The effect of KCl (FIGURE 6) and other inorganic salts (TABLE 2) is very strongly inhibitory, when the KCl concentration is more than 0.1 M; presumably the same is true for the other salts. The phosphates though seem to be even stronger inhibitors, no doubt because of their high ionic strength.

Characterization of 2′-5′ Oligo-As

To test our system, we have verified that the product seen after PEI-cellulose chromatography really is ppp5′A(2′p5′A)$_n$ (n = 1,2,3, . . .). We have separated the oligomers formed by our enzyme preparation by DEAE-sephadex chromatography[12] (FIGURE 1). The products called dimer, trimer, and tetramer were tested for the following characteristics of 2′-5′ compounds in contrast to 3′-5′ compounds:

(1) The dimer and trimer were resistant to the nucleases P1 and U2.[12]

(2) The mobility of the alkaline phosphatase treated dimer was identical to a reference A2′p5′A.

(3) The mobility of the alkaline phosphatase-treated trimer and pentamer was very different from reference 3′-5′ trimer and pentamer.

K_m *Determination*

ATP, the substrate that so far has been considered the only one, has been examined for its K_m value, assuming that the enzyme in a first approximation shows simple Michaelis-Menten kinetics. The straightforward plot shows that even at concentrations as high as 5 mM the plateau has not been reached. A Hanes plot (s/v versus s) on the other hand shows a straight line (FIGURE 7). The advantage of this plot is that the relative error is the same for all points as in a linear plot, whereas the points in a Lineweaver-Burke plot must be weighted with a factor v^4 according to Cleland.[14] From the curve are read the following values of K_m of 2.4 mM ATP and a Vmax value of 86 units/mg protein, which is three times the rate at 1 mM ATP.

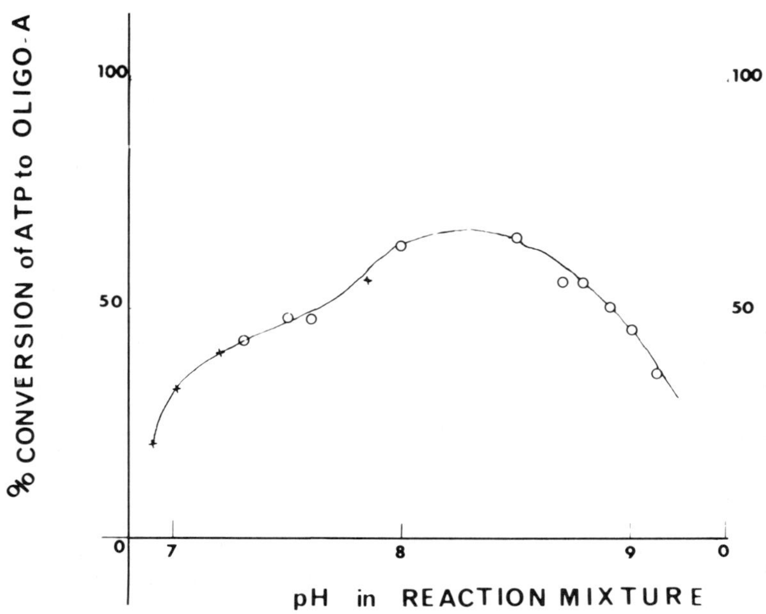

FIGURE 4. pH Curve. Oligo-A synthetase was incubated under standard conditions (1mM ATP) except that 0.05 M Tris at different pH was added to give the indicated pH. After incubation for 16 hr at 30°C, 6μl samples were chromatographed. The spots were cut and counted to give the percent conversion of ATP into oligo-As.

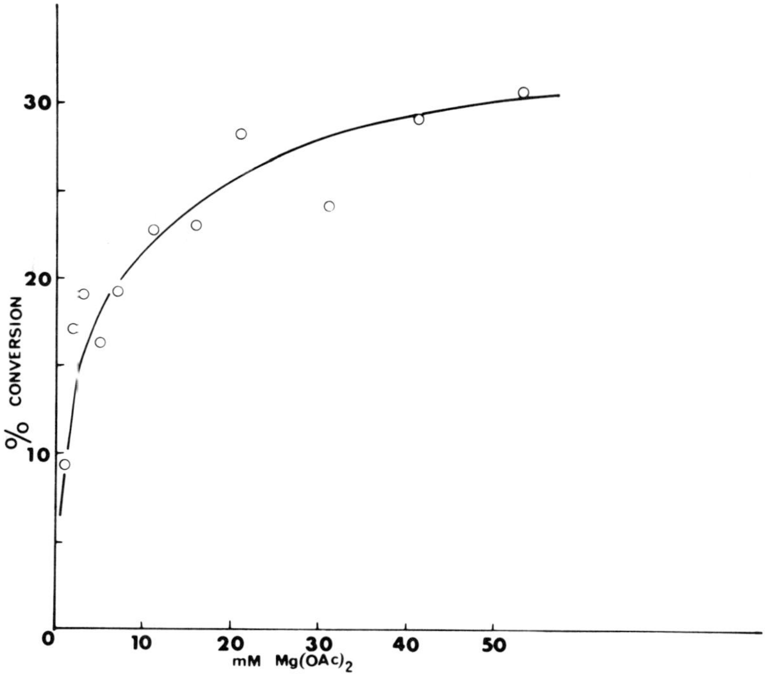

FIGURE 5. Mg^{++} dependence. Oligo-A synthetase was incubated under standard conditions varying the $Mg(OAc)_2$ concentrations. After a 16-hr incubation the samples were chromatographed.

Mechanism of Oligomer Formation

The elongation mechanism was studied[15] by incubating oligo-A synthetase for different periods and analyzing the composition of the oligomers that are formed (FIGURE 8). It is evident that the dimer is the first product and the trimer only occurs when there is a certain amount of dimer. These results, together with other observations described elsewhere,[15] indicate that the products of polymerization are released to the reaction mixture during the elongation and can be reattached to the enzyme on the acceptor side as well as ATP. The elongation of oligomers catalyzed by the 2′5′ A synthetase does not thus follow the processive mechanism that implies the non-dissociation of the intermediates of the polymerization during the elongation process. Rather, the elongation mechanism of this enzyme seems to be of a dissipative nature. There are, however, faint spots that might be long chains formed by a processive mechanism; but this can only explain a very small part of the activity.

Specificity of Substrate

The 2′5′ A synthetase, isolated from different cells, has been shown to be specifically an ATP polymerase. With the purified reticulocyte enzyme, we

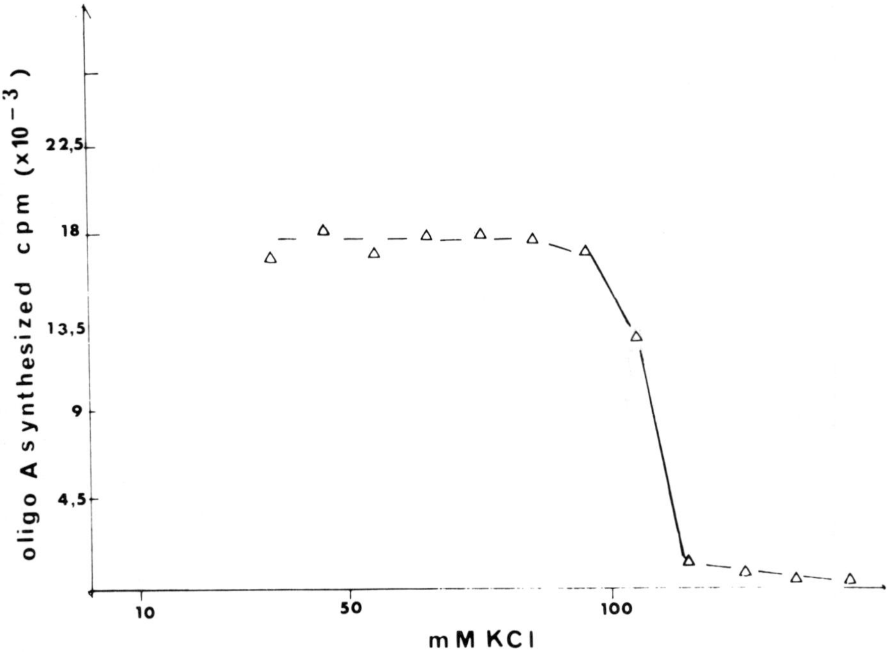

FIGURE 6. KCl dependence. Oligo-A synthetase was incubated under standard conditions with addition of the indicated amount of KCl. After 17 hr of incubation at 30°C, 6 μl samples were chromatographed. The spots were cut and counted.

TABLE 2
SALT EFFECTS
(Activity with Addition of Salts)

	Final Concentration 50 mM	Final Concentration 200 mM
NH_4Cl	+	−
NaCl	+	−
LiCl	+	−
Tris-Cl, pH8	+	−
Sodium phosphate	−	−
Potassium phosphate	−	−
$(NH4)_2SO_4$	(+)	−
KCl	+	−
NH_4HCO_3	+	−

*Oligo-A synthetase was incubated under standard conditions for 3½ hr at 30°C with the addition of the various salts. Symbols + and − mean full activity or no activity, respectively.

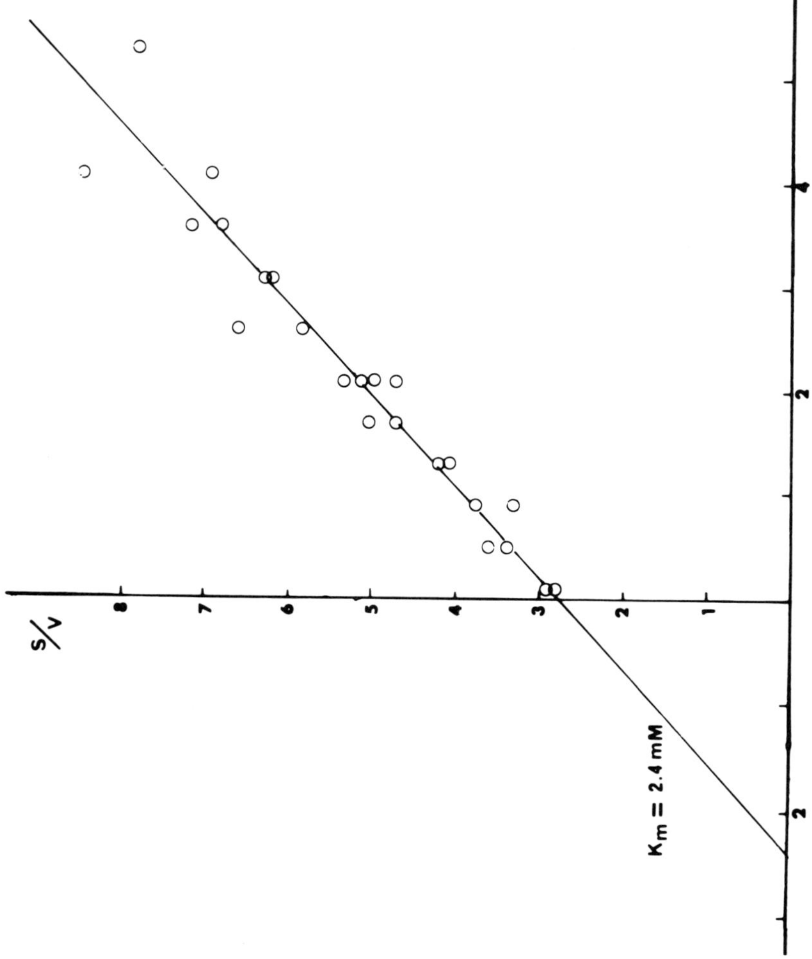

FIGURE 7. K_m for ATP. Oligo-A synthetase was incubated in amounts to give 20 to 40% conversion of ATP into oligo-As in two hours. The standard conditions were used except for the ATP that was added as stated in various amounts. Two-hr incubations at 37°C with doubles of all concentrations were performed. Then 4 μl samples were chromatographed and the percent conversion of ATP into 2′-5′ oligo-As was the basis for calculating the specific activity that is shown. The figure represents the Hanes plot (v/s is plotted versus s).

assayed the substrate specificity in the following way. We used a purified ^{32}P-labeled pppA 2′p5′A2′p5′A as an acceptor and different nucleoside triphosphates as donors for the synthetase.[15] The reaction was carried out under the conditions for 2′5′ A synthesis, and the incubation mixtures were analyzed on PEI-cellulose plates. The autoradiography of such an experiment indicates clearly that there is conversion of the initial trimer to an oligonucleotide with lower mobility by addition of a GMP or UMP moiety onto the (2′5′) pppApApA primer. In the absence of nucleoside triphosphate substrates, there is no change of the mobility of trimer incubated under identical conditions. With the dimer pppA2′p5′A the same pattern is seen with even higher yields of oligonucleotides, to which a GMP or UMP moiety is added. The enzyme also catalyzes the formation of a series of 2′5′ co-oligonucleotides in the presence of a mixture of ATP and another nucleoside triphosphate.

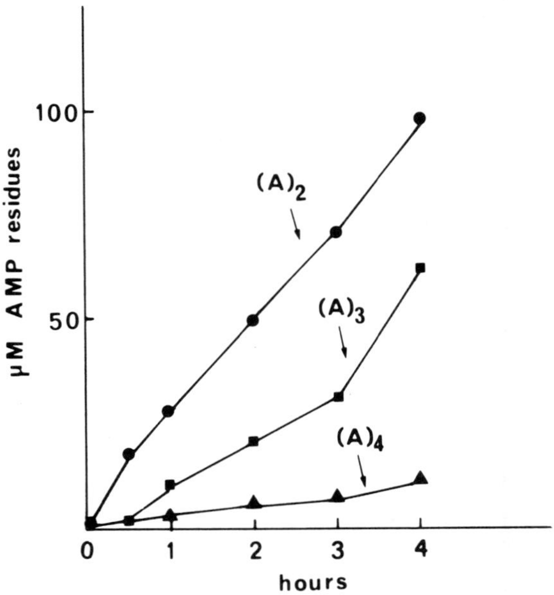

FIGURE 8. Time curve. In a 100 μl volume oligo-A synthetase was incubated at 37°C with 1.5 mM ATP under standard conditions. At times indicated 10 μl samples were taken out and treated with alkaline phosphatase; chromatography was as described in MATERIALS AND METHODS.

DISCUSSION

We have studied the mode of action of the 2′5′ oligo-A synthetase purified from the rabbit reticulocyte lysate. The enzyme is pure enough for such study because the preparation contains no detectable contaminating activities that could affect the substrate ATP or the oligomers produced. In addition, we have developed a rapid, simple and reproducible assay for the enzymatic activity. The assay is based on the separation of ATP from the oligomeric products in the incubation mixture directly spotted on PEI-cellulose thin-layer plates. This procedure allows avoidance of any additional treatment such as alkaline phosphatase digestion, thereby preventing any eventual artefacts. The conditions described here also permit separation of the dimer, trimer, tetramer etc, in a single run.

Using this procedure, we succeeded in following the kinetics of formation of the different oligomers and in determining quantitatively the distribution of chain lengths among the products of reactions as a function of time. The results show that the dimer is the predominant product during the first period of the reaction. The proportion of trimer to dimer present in the reaction medium increases with the time of incubation rather linearly up to 60% of ATP conversion. At the end of the reaction, the trimer becomes the main product. These results cannot fit with a processive mechanism that the compounds found should be predominantly the longest polymeric product. Rather, these observations strongly suggest an elongation mechanism of a dissipative nature.

On the other hand, the 2′5′ oligo-A synthetase has been described as an enzyme using only ATP as substrate. We show in the present work that the substrate specificity is not absolute. When a pppA5p2A (or the trimer) is used as a primer, the enzyme can catalyze in the presence of GTP, or UTP, the incorporation of one unit of GMP or UMP onto the primer. These results lead one to question whether in the cells 2′5′ oligonucleotides containing nucleotides other than AMP could exist. The significance and the biological activities of these co-oligonucleotides are under study.

Summary

2′5′ Oligoadenylate synthetase has been purified from rabbit reticulocyte lysate to a specific activity of 37 units per mg protein (1 unit incorporates 1 nmole of AMP residue into oligoadenylate per min at 37°C) by DEAE-cellulose and rI:rC-agarose chromatography and $(NH_4)_2SO_4$ precipitations. For this a rapid and quantitative assay was developed, based on TLC with PEI-cellulose. In a single step ATP and the 2′5′ oligoadenylates ($pppA(2p5A)_n$ $1 < n < 14$) are separated. The enzyme showed the following properties: a pH optimum around 8, a Mg^{++} requirement with full activation at 20 mM, no effect of KCl between 25 and 100 mM but complete inactivation at 120 mM, 30% stimulation by 10% ethanol, and a half-life at 52°C of around 5 min. The maximum yield of the reaction was 95% conversion of ATP into 2′5′ oligoadenylates.

The mechanism of elongation is not processive. Kinetic studies on the formation of different oligomeric intermediates suggest a mechanism of a dissipative nature. The products are mainly dimers, trimers and tetramers. The longest oligomer seen had about 15 AMP residues.

The enzyme has no absolute substrate specificity for ATP. GTP or UTP can also be incorporated, in the presence of ATP, by the enzyme into a co-oligonucleotide containing A and G or A and U. The enzyme can also add one unit of GMP or UMP onto a primer 2′5′ pppApA or pppApApA.

References

1. Kerr, I. M. & E. B. Brown. 1978. PppA2′p5′A2′p5′A: An inhibitor of protein synthesis synthesized with an enzyme fraction from interferon treated cells. Proc. Nat. Acad. Sci. USA **75:** 256–260.
2. Hovanessian, A. G. & I. M. Kerr. 1978. Synthesis of an oligonucleotide inhibitor of protein synthesis in rabbit reticulocyte lysates analogous to that formed in extracts from interferon treated cells. Eur. J. Biochem. **81:** 149–159.
3. Zilberstein, A., A. Kimchi, A. Schmidt & M. Revel. 1978. Isolation of two interferon-

induced translational inhibitors: A protein kinase and an oligoisoadenylate synthetase. Proc. Nat. Acad. Sci. USA **75:** 4734–4738.
4. BALL, A. L. 1979. Induction of 2′5′-oligoadenylate synthetase activity and a new protein by chick interferon. Virology **94:** 282–296.
5. BAGLIONI, C. 1979. Interferon induced enzymatic activities and their role in the antiviral state. Cell **17:** 255–264.
6. MINKS, M. A., S. BENVIN, P. A. MARONEY & C. BAGLIONI. 1979. Synthesis of 2′5′-oligo(A) in extracts of interferon treated Hela cells. J. Biol. Chem. **254:** 5058–5064.
7. FARRELL, P. J., G. C. SEN, M. F. DUBOIS, L. RATNER, E. SLATTERY & P. LENGYEL. 1978. Interferon action: Two different pathways for the inhibition of protein synthesis by double-stranded RNA. Proc. Nat. Acad. Sci. USA **75:** 5893–5897.
8. STARK, G. R., W. J. DOWER, R. T. SCHIMKE, R. E. BROWN & I. M. KERR. 1979. PppA2′p5′-A2′p5′A synthetase: Convenient assay, species and tissue distribution and variation upon withdrawal of oestrogen from chick oviducts. Nature **278:** 471–473.
9. RANDERATH, E. & K. RANDERATH. 1967. Ion-exchange thin layer chromatography. J. Chromatog. **31:** 485–499.
10. GUPTA, R. C. & K. RANDERATH. 1977. Use of specific endonuclease cleavage in RNA sequencing. Nucl. Acid. Res. **4:** 1957–1978.
11. JUSTESEN, J., D. FERBUS & M. N. THANG. 1980. 2′5′ oligo-A synthetase, an interferon induced enzyme: Direct assay methods for the products, 2′5′ oligo-A and 2′5′ co-oligonucleotides. Nucl. Acid. Res. **8:** 14.
12. MARTIN, E. M., N. J. M. BIRDSALL, R. E. BROWN & I. M. KERR. 1979. Enzymic synthesis, characterization and nuclear-magnetic resonance spectra of pppA2′p5′A2′p5′A and related oligonucleotides: Comparison with chemically synthesised material. Eur. J. Biochem. **95:** 295–307.
13. KERR, I. M., R. E. BROWN & A. G. HOVANESSIAN. 1977. Nature of inhibitor of cell-free protein synthesis formed in response to interferon and double-stranded RNA, Nature **268:** 540–542.
14. CLELAND, W. W. 1967. The statistical analysis of enzyme kinetic data. Adv. Enzymol. **29:** 1–32.
15. JUSTESEN, J., D. FERBUS & N. N. THANG. 1980. Elongation mechanism and substrate specificity of 2′5′ oligoadenylate synthetase. Proc. Nat. Acad. Sci. USA. In press.

RECOVERY BY INTERFERON OF MENGOVIRUS-INDUCED SHUTOFF OF HOST PROTEIN SYNTHESIS*

R. Falcoff, J. Sancéau, O. Aujean, and C. Vaquero.

Institut Curie
75231 Paris, Cédex 05 France

In preincubated cell-free extracts prepared from interferon-treated cells the translation of exogenous viral or cellular mRNAs is inhibited equally.[1,2]

It is also known that the addition to such extracts of dsRNA activates at least two specific enzymes, the consequence being the inhibition of translation. (Reviewed by C. Baglioni.[3])

Since dsRNA seems to play a major role in stimulating interferon-dependent enzymes, it was interesting to study a functional system in which the challenge virus would provide dsRNA molecules. We have chosen as model L cells infected with mengovirus.

It is known that soon after infection by a picornavirus there is an inhibition of cellular RNA and protein synthesis. Later in infection, the synthesis of DNA is also decreased.[4] The inhibition of the synthesis of macromolecules is often referred to as "shutoff."

We decided to study first, the possible action of interferon (IF) on the establishment of the shutoff.

Since the level of shutoff varies with the cell lines and with the multiplicity of infection we established our experimental conditions. (FIGURE 1). Confluent monolayers of L cells were infected with different multiplicities of infection (MOI) of mengovirus; after 4 hr cells were pulse-labeled for 30 min with methionine, lysed with detergents (NP40 and DOC) and the proteins analyzed by slab gel electrophoresis.

The first lane to the left shows the pattern of host proteins; in the second lane, with 5 pfu/cell viral proteins are very easily recognized, although cellular proteins are also present. It should be remembered that the viron RNA acts as messenger and it is translated from one single initiation site. The unique translation product is a "polyprotein" of about 270,000 MW. Primary and secondary cleavages of this protein give rise to precursors, and finally capsid and noncapsid stable proteins. With 20 and 50 pfu/cell the shutoff of host protein synthesis is markedly established.

The counts of this experiment are shown in FIGURE 2, represented by the filled circles. With 5 pfu/cell, although viral proteins are actively synthesized, the total amount of methionine is already lower than in the control noninfected cells. Both, host and viral proteins contributed to the total counts. With 20 pfu cellular proteins are almost absent, the counts correspond principally to viral proteins. With 50 pfu/cell more viral proteins are synthesized, which explains the higher incorporation of the label. When we repeated the experiment with cells pretreated with 200 units IF/ml, we were unable to detect viral proteins.

*This work was supported by grants from the Institut National de la Santé et de la Recherche Médicale (77.4064.1) and Délégation Générale à la Recherche Scientifique et Technique (79.7. 1037).

0077-8923/80/0350-0522 $01.75/0 © 1980, NYAS

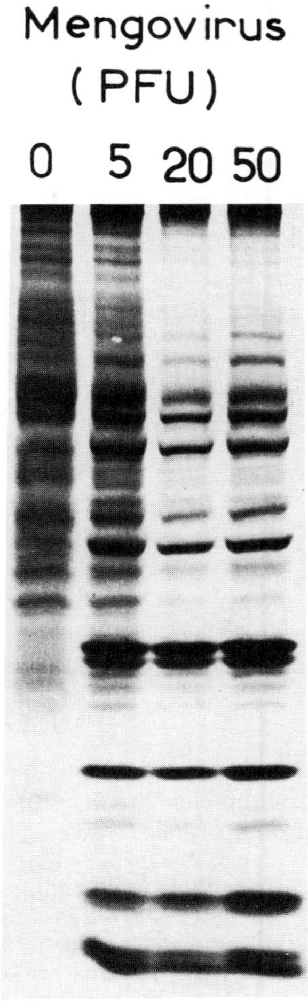

FIGURE 1. Pattern of pulse-labeled cytoplasmic proteins from monolayers of L cells infected with different multiplicities of mengovirus. Cultures were labeled with [^{35}S]methionine for 30 min, 4 hr after infection. Proteins were analyzed by electrophoresis on slab gels of a linear 10–20 % polyacrylamide gradient.

However, as shown by the empty circles, cell protein synthesis was also inhibited and the inhibition appears to be an exponential function of the MOI.

From these results we decided to use 50 pfu/cell for the ensuing experiments.

In 1964, H. Levy[5] published the data showing that IF did not prevent the shutoff. But since the preparations available at that time were of very low titers, we decided to study the effect of higher doses of IF (FIGURE 3).

Cultures were treated over night with 10, 100, 1,000 or 5,000 units IF per ml and infected or not with 50 pfu/cell of mengovirus. The pulse with [^{35}S]methionine was done at 5 hr post-infection; the labeled proteins are shown in this figure. The left side of the figure shows the proteins from noninfected cells, the right side those from infected cells.

Ten units of IF were unable to block completely the multiplication of the

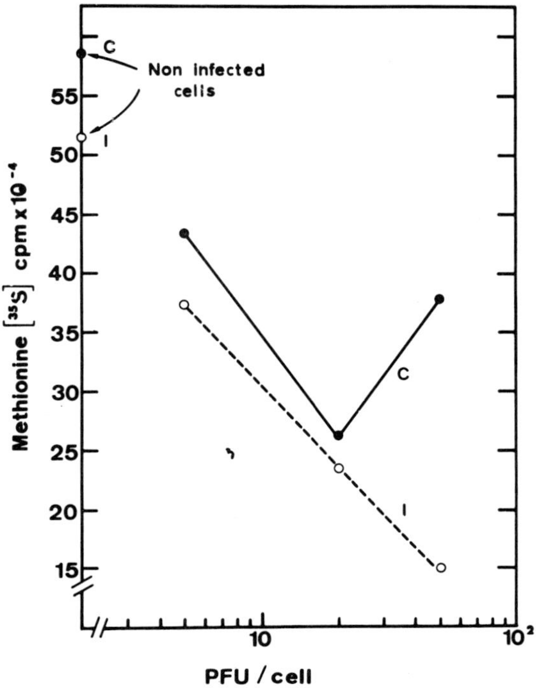

FIGURE 2. Total counts (10-μl aliquots) of pulse-labeled proteins from monolayers of L cells treated (I) or not treated (C) with interferon and infected with different multiplicities of mengovirus. Labeling conditions were the same as for FIGURE 1.

virus. Some faint bands of viral proteins are seen. However, the shutoff of cellular protein synthesis was observed with all the doses of IF, even with as much as 5,000 units/ml.

From this experiment we can conclude that, at 5 hr post-infection, the protein synthetic activity of the IF-treated infected cell is blocked: neither viral nor cellular messengers seem to be translated.

The next question obviously was: what happens after 5 hr of infection? In other words which is the final outcome for the cell?

FIGURE 4 shows the experimental design we adopted to answer this question. Cells were treated 18 hr with 500 units IF/ml infected with 20 pfu/cell, and after 1 hr, replenished with medium containing IF. Proteins were labeled at various times after infection, and gels are shown in the next two figures.

In control infected cells (FIGURE 5) mengovirus proteins are already present 2 hr after infection and their amount increases with the incubation time; at 8 hr, which corresponds to the single-cycle virus multiplication, synthesis stops.

In IF-treated cells (FIGURE 6) inhibition of cell protein synthesis is already observed at 2 hr post-infection, increasing at 4 and is apparently unchanged at 8 hr. Between 8 and 15 hr, the situation is reversed and at 24 hr, cell protein synthesis reaches the level of the IF-treated noninfected cells.

The counts from each point of this experiment are plotted as a percentage of the corresponding counts from IF-treated noninfected cells (FIGURE 7). Results of two other experiments, lasting 48 hr, are also shown in the same figure. Curve inflection occurs after 6–8 hr in all three experiments. Results are different with

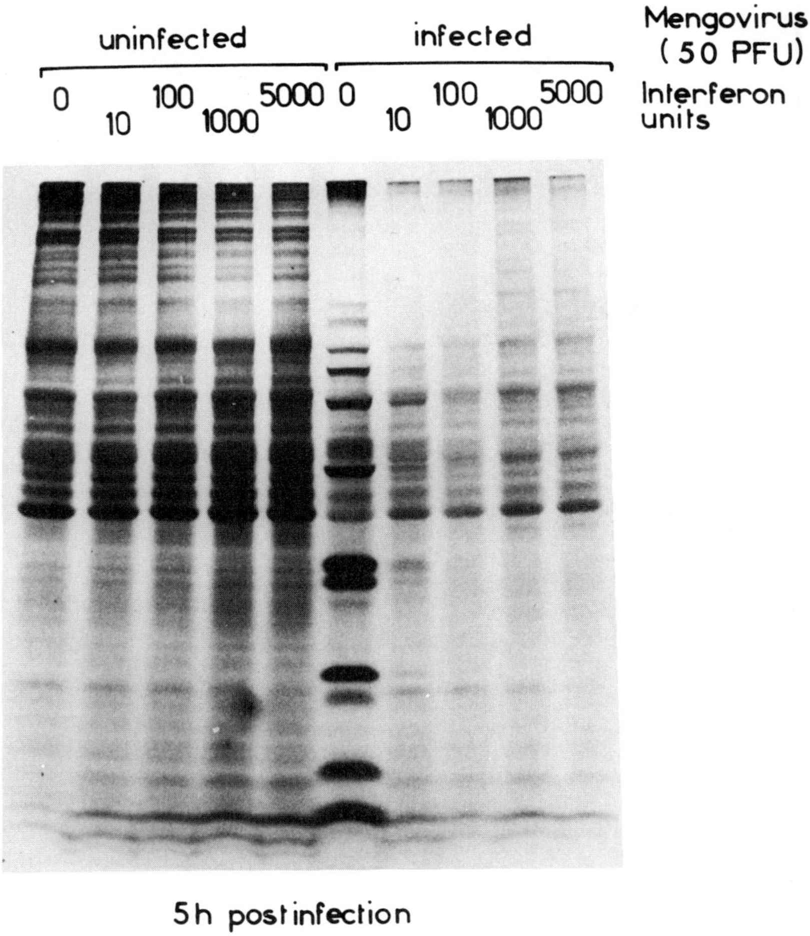

FIGURE 3. Pattern of pulse-labeled proteins from monolayers of L cells pretreated with different doses of interferon for 18 hr and subsequently infected with 50 pfu mengovirus/cell. Cells were labeled at 5 hr after infection.

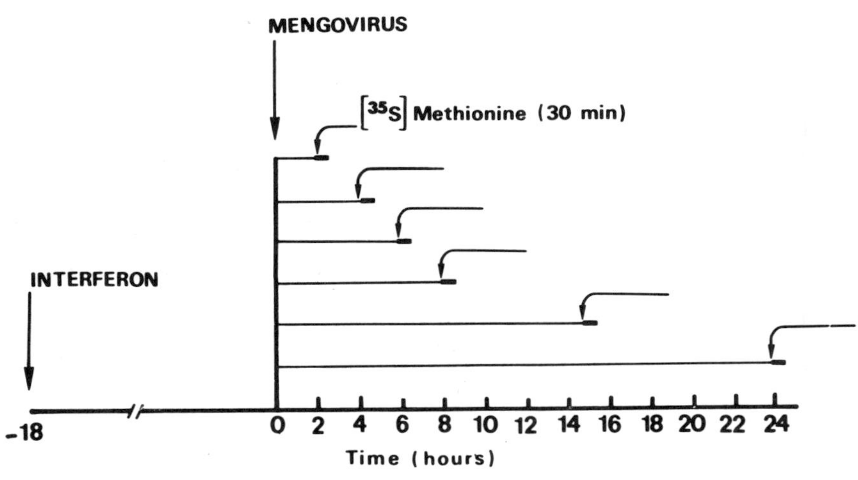

FIGURE 4. Design for the experiment shown in FIGURES 5 and 6.

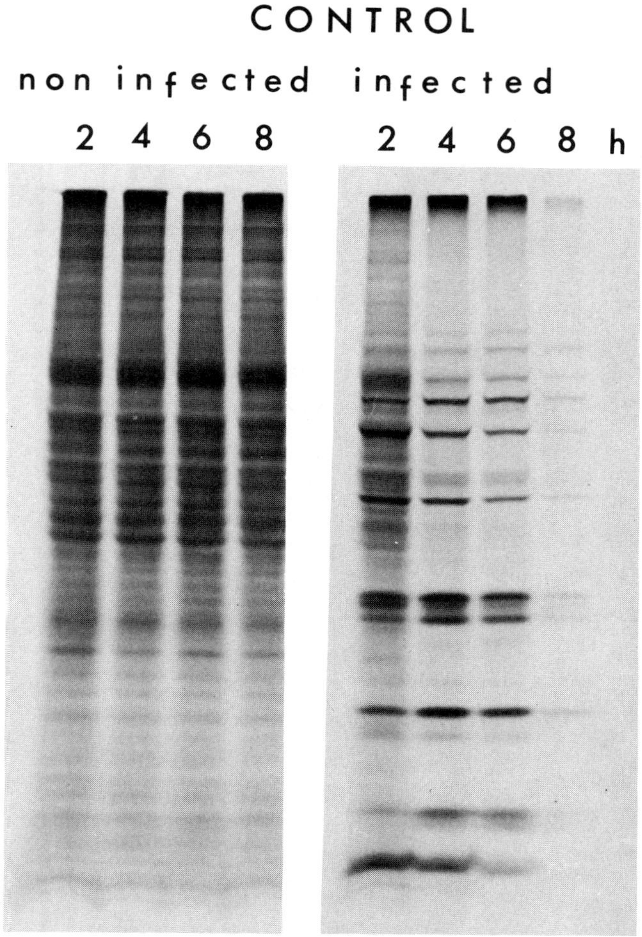

FIGURE 5. 24 hr kinetics of pulse-labeled proteins from L cells infected or not with mengovirus (20 pfu/cell).

low doses of IF even with a lower multiplicity of infection. For instance with 10 units/ml, although there is a 90% inhibition of viral multiplication, the recovery of host protein synthesis is not observed (FIGURE 8).

Microscopic observation of control infected cells showed a cytotoxic effect which increased very rapidly after infection. Cells were lysed after a single-cycle of viral multiplication, at about 8–10 hr of infection. It has been reported[6] that the cytopathic effect of poliovirus on HeLa cells occurs even when virus production is suppressed by guanidine. In IF-treated cells the virus multiplication was also blocked. However, some cytotoxicity appeared at 4–6 hr but it was transient and cultures seemed normal at 24–48 hr. When interferon was washed at the time of

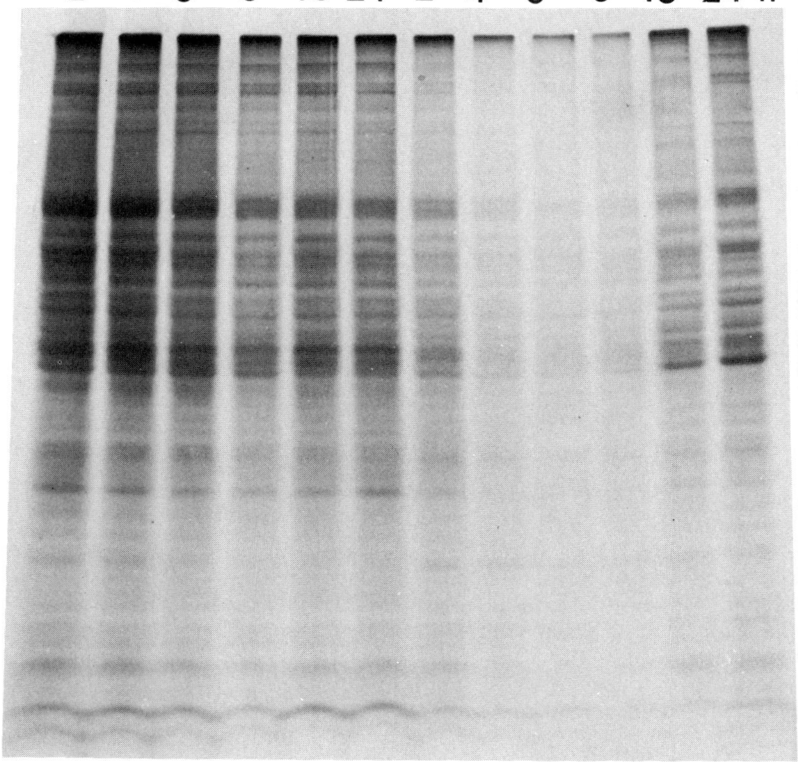

FIGURE 6. 24 hr kinetics of pulse-labeled proteins from interferon-treated (500 units/ml) infected or not with mengovirus (20 pfu/cell).

infection the results were almost similar during the first 24 hr but later on the cytotoxicity increased and virus appeared in the culture medium.

One interesting fact is that some proteins are synthesized with different kinetics.

For instance in FIGURE 9 one protein of 100,000 MW is seen at 36 hr after infection. This protein is not specific for IF since it is also present in control cells. We do not know its significance.

As I have already said, cellular RNA synthesis is also inhibited very shortly after infection. Again, this inhibition is not prevented by IF.

In the experiment shown in FIGURE 10 we measured the incorporation of uridine after pulse of 30 min at different incubation times.

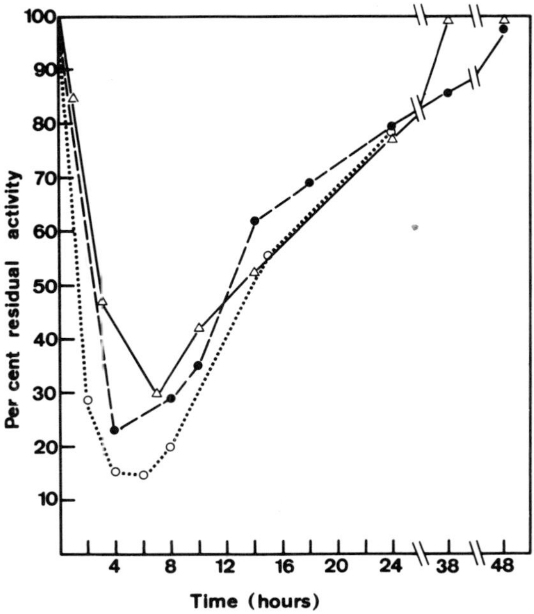

FIGURE 7. Radioactivity at different times from interferon-treated infected cells (shown in FIGURE 6) is plotted as percentage of the corresponding interferon-treated noninfected cells (○ . . . ○) Two other similar experiments prolonged for 48 hr are also shown (●——●; △——△).

The shutoff of RNA synthesis in control infected cells is already detected 1 hr after infection. In IF-treated infected cells the inhibition of RNA synthesis is also present. Later on, in control infected cells incorporation of uridine increases as a consequence of the virus replication, whereas in IF-treated infected cells no changes appear until 8 hr. After this moment, the synthesis of RNA increases reaching the rate of noninfected cells.

Therefore, the recovery of the synthesis of cellular RNA and cellular proteins seems to have similar kinetics.

In consequence one possible explanation of the prolonged shutoff of host protein synthesis in IF-treated infected cells might be the degradation of host mRNA. In control infected cells several authors have shown that the shutoff of host protein synthesis was present although cellular mRNAs were undegraded.[4]

However in IF-treated infected cells the situation could be different since, as we have already shown,[7] there is an increased ribonuclease activity associated with membrane structures. Therefore, the degradation of cellular mRNA could not be excluded. In fact we have some preliminary results, that tell against this hypothesis.

We extracted total RNA at various times after infection and measured the poly A-containing RNA by hybridization with tritiated poly U (FIGURE 11).

Here again, noninfected cell controls and IF-treated cells show parallel curves. In control infected cells, at 4 hr post-infection poly A is principally from virus RNA, increasing with the time of incubation. The poly A of RNA from IF-treated infected cells corresponds to 60% of the control, whereas the synthesis of proteins is reduced to 20 percent.

Of course, the presence of poly A segments is not enough to consider the RNA as undegraded. However all these RNAs are translatable in reticulocyte extracts:

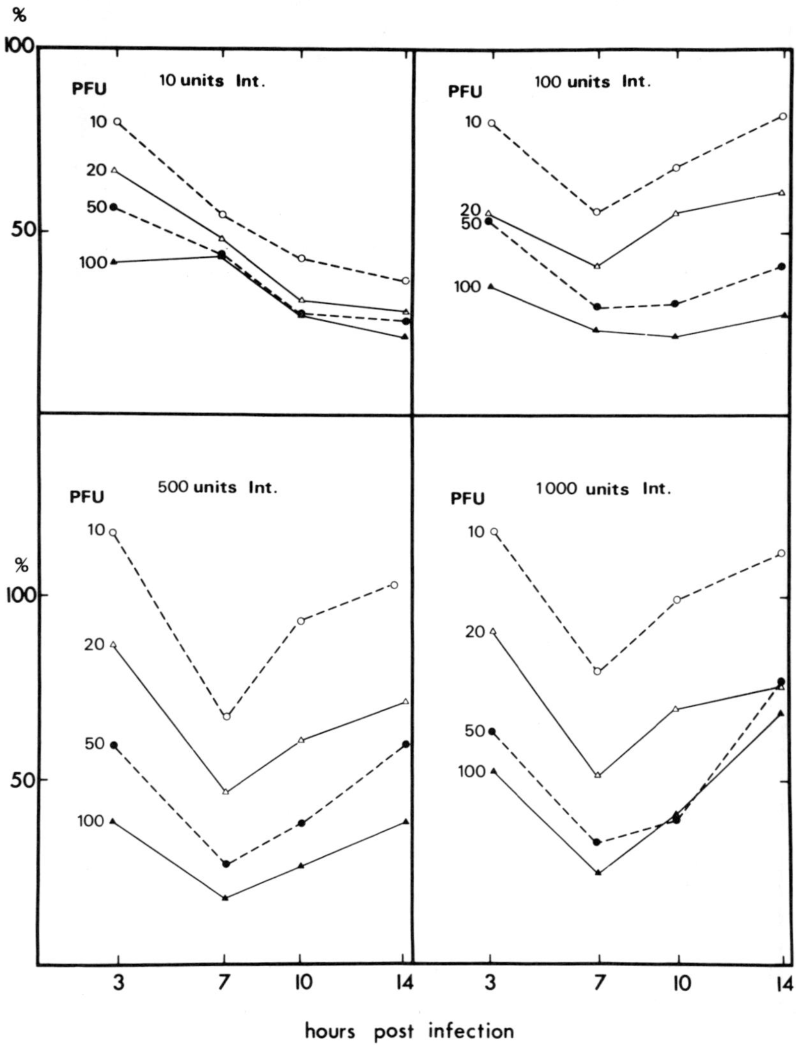

FIGURE 8. Monolayers of L cells were treated overnight with different doses of interferon and infected thereafter with 10, 20, 50, or 100 pfu/cell of mengovirus. Radioactivity of pulse-labeled proteins, at the indicated times, are expressed as percentage of the corresponding interferon-treated noninfected cells.

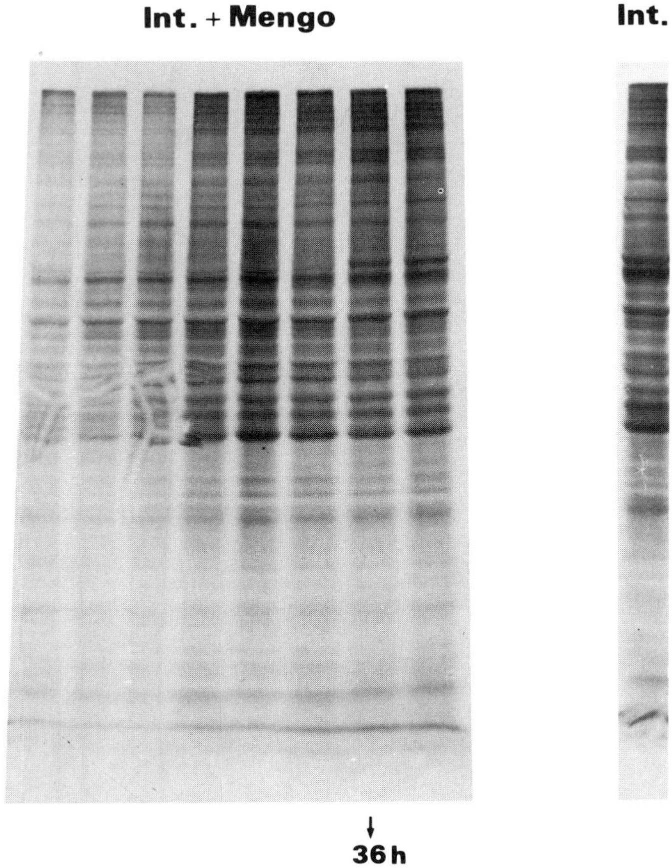

FIGURE 9. Patterns of pulse-labeled proteins from interferon-treated infected cells.

the RNA from control infected cells programmed viral proteins while all the other samples gave host proteins and were apparently of similar activity.

We can summarize these results as follows:

(1) Even very high doses of IF, such as 5,000 units/ml do not prevent the shutoff of host protein and RNA synthesis induced by infection with mengovirus and;

(2) Although a general block of translation was established after infection with a picornavirus, under continuous treatment with IF, cells did not die, they recovered from the infection.

The input virus is apparently responsible for the shutoff, which is rapidly established with 20 pfu/cell or more.

Interferon pretreatment of the cell would not impair a first-run translation of the viral RNA. As a result small amounts of viral replicase would be synthesized and the viral dsRNA replicative and intermediate forms would appear.

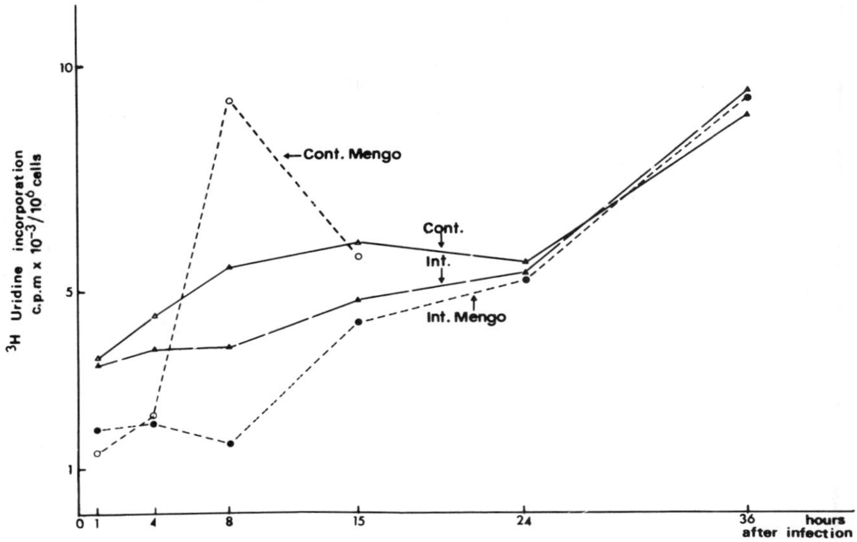

FIGURE 10. Radioactivity of pulse-labeled cytoplasmic RNA. Monolayers of L cells, interferon-treated and controls, infected and noninfected with mengovirus were labeled with 10 μCi/ml of [^{3}H]uridine for 20 min. Cells were washed with isotonic buffer, treated for 2 hr at 4°C with 5% trichloroacetic acid and dissolved with OH Na 0.1 M, 1 hr at 37°C. Aliquots were neutralized with HCl 1 M before measurement of the radioactivity.

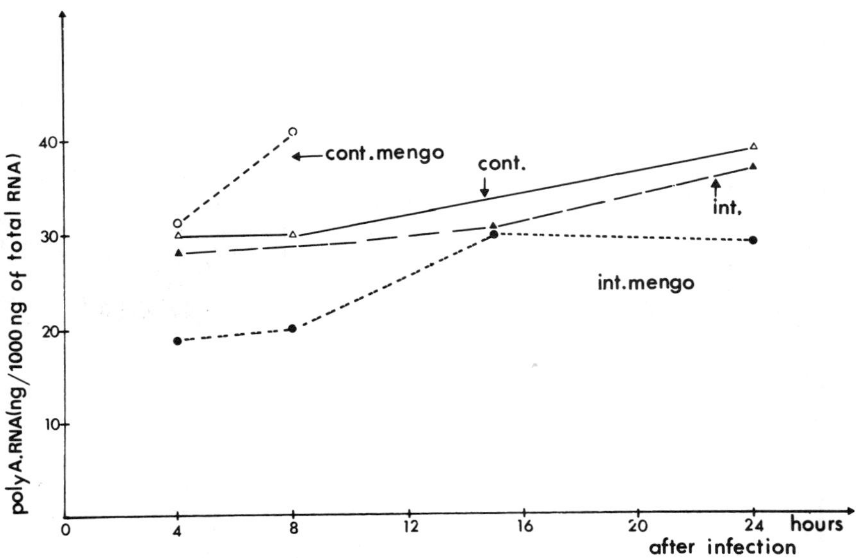

FIGURE 11. Titration of cytoplasmic poly A-containing RNA by hybridization with [^{3}H]poly U. The quantity of poly A-containing RNA was determined assuming an average ratio of 10% poly A in cytoplasmic poly A-containing RNA.[9]

These dsRNA molecules would activate *in vivo* the same enzymes shown in cell extracts, that is a nuclease and a kinase.

We have found that increased ribonuclease activity is located in IF-treated mengovirus-infected cells, in a fraction which is known to contain the viral replication complex: this nuclease will degrade nascent viral RNA molecules.

Cellular messenger RNA does not seem to be degraded to a greater extent than in the control infected cells, but it is not translated until 6–8 hr post-infection, probably by inhibition of initiation.

The shutoff of host RNA synthesis was shown 20 years ago: the mechanism is still unknown. In the IF-treated cells, we do not yet know if the recovery of RNA synthesis precedes the recovery of protein synthesis. The fate of the enzymes nuclease and kinase induced relatively early after infection is under study.

In conclusion, although the mechanism is not completely understood, IF cures the cell of the most striking manifestation of the viral infection.

References

1. Falcoff, E., R. Falcoff, B. Lebleu & M. Revel. 1973. Correlation between the antiviral effect of interferon treatment and the inhibition of "in vitro," mRNA translation in noninfected L cells. J. Virol. **12:** 421–430.
2. Gupta, S. L., M. L. Sopori & P. Lengyel. 1973. Inhibition of protein synthesis directed by added viral and cellular messenger RNAs in extracts of interferon treated Erlich ascites tumor cells. Location and dominance of the inhibitor(s). Biochem. Biophys. Res. Commun. **54:** 777–783.
3. Baglioni, C. 1979. Interferon-induced enzymatic activities and their role in the antiviral state. Cell **17:** 255–264.
4. Lucas-Lenard, J. M. 1979. *In* Molecular Biology of Picornavirus. R. Perez Bercoff, Ed.: 73–100. Plenum Press. New York and London.
5. Levy, H. B. 1964. Studies on the mechanism of interferon action. II. The effect of interferon on some early events in mengovirus infection in L cells. Virology **22:** 575–579.
6. Lenk, R., & S. Penman. 1979. The cytoskeletal framework and poliovirus metabolism. Cell **16:** 289–302.
7. Aujean, O., J. Sancéau, E. Falcoff & R. Falcoff. 1979. Location of enhanced ribonuclease activity and of a phosphoprotein kinase in interferon-treated mengovirus infected cells. Virology **92:** 583–586.
8. Lewis, J. A., E. Falcoff & R. Falcoff. 1978. Dual action of double stranded RNA in inhibiting protein synthesis in extracts of interferon-treated mouse L cells. Eur. J. Biochem. **86:** 497–509.
9. Jacquet, M., D. Caput, E. Falcoff, R. Falcoff & F. Gross. 1977. The use of complementary DNA probe to detect accumulation of mengo RNA in infected cells pretreated with interferon. Biochimie **59:** 189–195.

MECHANISM OF INTERFERON INHIBITION OF VIRUSES THAT BUD FROM THE PLASMA MEMBRANE

Robert M. Friedman, Radha K. Maheshwari, Francis T. Jay, and Christine Czarniecki

Laboratory of Experimental Pathology
National Institute of Arthritis, Metabolism and Digestive Diseases
National Institutes of Health
Bethesda, Maryland 20205

Virus yields in interferon-treated cells newly infected with murine leukemia viruses (MLV) are significantly decreased.[1] Virus yields were also inhibited in interferon-treated rat and mouse cells chronically infected with a murine RNA tumor virus. This was unexpected because interferon (IF) was thought to be effective only in situations where cells were treated before virus infection.[2-4] Replication of endogenous type C RNA tumor viruses was sensitive to IF treatment[5,6]; however, intracisternal A-particle formation was increased in erythroleukemic cells infected with Friend virus.[7,8] The A particles may have been immature C particles in these systems. Mouse mammary tumor virus (MMTV) (B particles) production was also inhibited by IF treatment.[9]

Inhibition of RNA tumor virus production was not correlated with inhibition of any of the intracellular steps in virus replication that were tested.[5,6,11-12] In IF-treated AKR cells in which there was marked inhibition of production of both endogenous MLV particles and infectious MLV, the intracellular concentration of viral p30, the group-specific (gs) antigen, was unaffected or even increased.[6] Transmission electron micrographs indicated that the number of cell-associated virus particles was not altered in IF treated MO-P cells, which were chronic producers of Kirsten murine sarcoma virus[13]; moreover, synthesis of the viral proteins p30, gp 69/71, and p15 was not inhibited in IF-treated mouse 3T3 fibroblast cells infected with MLV. Synthesis and cleavage of the precursors of these proteins were also unaffected.[14] In IF-treated AKR cells, scanning electron micrograph (SEM) studies confirmed and extended the finding that there was not a decrease in the number of cell-associated virus particles, since the number of surface-associated MLV particles was actually increased.[15] This may explain why cell-associated p30 (gs) antigen was increased in these systems after IF treatment. The production of viral RNA-dependent DNA polymerase was also insensitive to IF treatment in AKR cells; therefore, IF-induced inhibition of MLV production probably does not involve inhibition of virus protein synthesis.

Viral RNA synthesis has also been studied. In IF-treated mouse cells infected with Moloney MLV or AKR-MLV, the intracellular concentration of virus-specific RNA was approximately the same as in untreated cells; the rates of viral RNA synthesis were also about equal.[16,17] Substantially, the same findings have been made in chronic MMTV infection after IF treatment (S. Arya, personal communication).

Pitha *et al.*[12] tested the effect of IF on several types of MLV infection in AKR cells. In the case of exogenous infection, virus production was delayed but not suppressed. During inhibition by IF of exogenous or induced infection, the IF block appeared to occur before virus assembly so that, although there was no inhibition of viral p30 (gs) antigen, there was a decrease in released virus;

0077-8923/80/0350-0533 $01.75/0 © 1980, NYAS

however, while the IF-induced inhibition of assembly seemed to result in a relatively small decrease in the number of MLV particles released, there was a marked inhibition in their infectivity. This observation has since been confirmed in both chronic and acute Moloney MLV infection in TB cells[18,19]; therefore, in some systems IF treatment resulted in marked inhibition of virus release, while in others, particle production was almost normal, but the virus released was quite deficient in infectivity (see TABLE 5). The reason for the decreased infectivity of these virus particles is not clear. In a systemic study of the structural components in these defective virions, the only structural abnormality uncovered thus far is that the amount of viral envelope glycoprotein, gp69/71, is much reduced compared to the control. This conclusion was based on the reduced molar ratio of

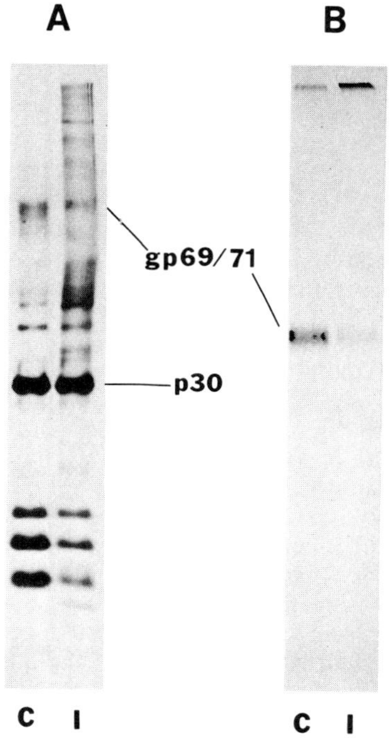

FIGURE 1. **A.** TB cells, either treated with 200 unit/ml mouse interferon (I) or mock treated (C) were labeled with 30 μCi [35S]methionine/ml for 12 hr. The virions produced during that period were pelleted and denatured in SDS/2-mercaptoethanol. Similar amounts of radioactivity (15,000 cpm) were separated by SDS-PAGE on a 12.5% gel to show most of the structural proteins. The samples were visualized by fluorography. **B.** In another experiment, similarly treated cultures were labeled with 50 μCi [3H]glucosamine/ml for 12 hr. Similar amounts of the extracellular virus (40 μg protein) were separated on a 9% SDS-gel. I, interferon-treated; c, mock-treated control.

gp69/71 relative to other structural proteins in [35S]methionine-labeled defective particles (FIGURE 1A) as well as the reduced amount of [3H]glucosamine incorporated into the carbohydrate (gp69/71) of these virions (FIGURE 1B). The deficiency in gp69/71 may account for part, if not all, of the decrease in infectivity of these particles since it has been shown that gp69/71 is responsible for the recognition and binding of the virion to the receptors sites on the cell membrane.[32]

One important question is whether such findings are limited to murine RNA tumor virus systems. We are, therefore, studying vesicular stomatitis virus (VSV) produced by IF-treated L cells. In other studies, which employed IF concentrations often considerably greater than 100 units/ml, there was inhibition of VSV-directed transcription or translation.[21,22] For instance, Ball and White[23] showed that in extracts derived from chick cells treated with 250 units/ml of IF VSV-directed translation was inhibited. In this study mouse cells were treated with 3 to 30 units of IF; under these conditions there was as much as a 200-fold decrease in the production of infectious virus particles, but less than a 10-fold decrease in the level of virus specific extracellular transcriptase activity, viral RNA, or the major viral core protein, N. A significantly larger reduction was found, however, in the amount of glycoprotein (G) and membrane protein (M) associated with VSV from IF-treated cells. A single species of viral RNA (42S) was present in the VSV released into the extracellular fluid, but the inhibition of viral RNA synthesis was about the same as of total viral protein synthesis and transcriptase activity. The VSV particles from IF-treated cells neither interfered with the growth of wild-type VSV, nor induced IF in cell cultures.

Materials and Methods

Virus Stock and Virus Assays.

VSV was the Indiana strain originally obtained from Mr. C. Buckler (National Institute of Allergy and Infectious Diseases, Bethesda, MD). It had been plaque-purified and passaged by us at a multiplicity of 0.01 in VERO cells. The titer was assayed as 50% tissue culture infectious doses ($TCID_{50}$) by cytopathic effect in microtiter plates of BHK or VERO cells; the titer of the pool used was 2×10^9 $TCID_{50}$/ml.

Cells

L-Cells were originally obtained from J. Youngner (University of Pittsburgh); they are very sensitive to the antiviral activity of mouse interferon. VERO cells and baby hamster kidney cells (BHK-21) were obtained from the National Institutes of Health Media Section and were also grown in Eagle's MEM supplemented with 10% fetal calf serum.

Interferon and Interferon Assays

Mouse IF was prepared and partially purified on an antibody affinity column[24] in the laboratory of Dr. K. Paucker (Pennsylvania College of Medicine, Philadelphia, PA). The specific activity of the preparations employed was at least 2×10^7 mouse reference units per milligram of protein. The antiviral activity of this preparation had the physical and chemical properties of mouse interferon. Interferon was assayed by inhibition of VSV-induced cytopathic effect in L-cells.[6]

Preparation and Purification of Virus Samples

L-cells were grown in 150 cm^2 flasks to confluence (2×10^7 cells) and treated with 0-30 units/ml of IF for 14 hr; the cell monolayers were washed 3–4 times to remove the residual interferon. All the monolayers were then infected with VSV at a multiplicity of 5 $TCID_{50}$ per cell. After 16 hr, the supernatant fluids were collected and sedimented at 10,000 × g to remove cell debris. Aliquots of each sample were saved for assay of virus infectivity. All the supernatant fluids were concentrated 100-fold by sedimenting at 48,000 × g for 2 hr or were mixed and stirred with polyethylene glycol (6%) at 4°C. The resultant PEG precipitates were collected by centrifugation at 10,000 × g for 20 min. Virus was further purified in a 20–60% (W/W) equilibrium sucrose gradient in SET buffer (50 mM Tris-HCl pH 7.2, 0.1 M NaCl, and 1 mM EDTA) by centrifugation at 72,000 × g for 18 hr at 4°C in an SW27 rotor. The virus, which banded at 1.16–1.18 g/ml, was sedimented in a Beckman SW27 rotor for 3 hr at 110,000 × g. The pellet containing the purified virus was resuspended in 0.1 M NaCl and 10 mM sodium acetate buffer (pH 7.2) and used for analysis of protein and RNA or transcriptase.

Transcriptase Assay

Samples were assayed for transcriptase activity by the method of Colonno and Banerjee.[25]

Analysis of Virion Proteins

L-cells were treated with IF as described above. After virus adsorption and incubation for 5 hr, the monolayers were washed 2–3 times with leucine-free medium and then [^{3}H] leucine (15 to 20 μCi/ml, specific activity 121.1 Ci/mmol, New England Nuclear, Boston) was added in leucine-free medium, containing 2% dialyzed fetal calf serum; the cells were incubated overnight. The supernatant fluids were then collected and virus was purified by banding on a sucrose gradient as described above. Analysis of viral proteins in these samples was carried out by polyacrylamide gel electrophoresis,[26] in gels composed of 7.5% acrylamide, 0.5 M urea, and 0.1% SDS in 0.1 M phosphate buffer, pH 7.2. The gels were sliced into segments of 1.25 mm and each slice was placed in a scintillation vial with 30% H_2O_2 (100 μl); the vials were kept at 90°C for 3 hr and the radioactivity incorporated into the gel slices was estimated in a liquid scintillation spectrometer.

Extraction and Analysis of Viral RNA

For virion RNA analysis the radioactive virus was prepared as follows: Ly cells were treated with 0–30 units/ml of IF overnight, washed, and then infected with VSV at a multiplicity of 5 $TCID_{50}$ per cell. After 4–5 hr of incubation, the medium was decanted and fresh medium containing actinomycin D (2 μg/ml) (Merck, Sharp & Dohme Res. Lab., Rahway, NJ) was added; [^{3}H]uridine (10 to 15 μCi/ml, specific activity 41.3 Ci/mmol) was added after 1 hr, and the cultures were incubated overnight. VSV was purified from the supernatant fluid by banding on a sucrose gradient as previously described. The RNA was extracted with 0.3% SDS and buffered phenol. The phenol extraction was repeated twice at room temperature and the residual buffer layer was adjusted to 0.4 M NaCl and mixed with 2 vol of 99% ethanol. After 16 hr at −20°C, the resulting precipitate was sedimented at 10,000 × g for 20 min and resuspended in 0.2 ml of SET buffer solution.

Viral RNA was analyzed by electrophoresis on polyacrylamide gels.[27] After electrophoresis the gels were added to test tubes containing 5% TCA for 1 hr, washed twice, sliced, and incubated for 3 hr at 90°C in 100 μl of 30% hydrogen peroxide. Radioactivity was estimated in a liquid scintillation spectrometer.

RNA was also analyzed on 6–30% sucrose density gradients; 200 μl aliquots were layered over a 4.4 ml gradient and sedimented at 248,000 × g at 4°C for 2.5 hr in a Beckman SW65 rotor. Fractions of 0.15 ml were collected and radioactivity was measured in a liquid scintillation spectrometer.

TABLE 1

INHIBITION OF TRANSCRIPTASE ACTIVITY* IN VIRUS† FROM INTERFERON-TREATED CELLS

Interferon Concentration (units/ml)	[^{3}H]GMP Incorporated (cpm)	Inhibition (log)	Virus Titer‡ (TCID 50/ml)	Inhibition (log)
0	8,980 (3.95)	—	6.6×10^8	—
3	5,120 (3.71)	0.24	3.9×10^8	0.27
10	3,630 (3.56)	0.39	3.3×10^7	1.3
30	1,830 (3.26)	0.69	6.4×10^6	2.2

*Reaction mixtures (1 ml) contained the following: 50 mM Tris-HCl (pH 8.0); 0.1M NaCl; 5 mM $MgCl_2$; 4 mM dithiothreitol; 0.05% Triton X-100 plus 1 mM CTP; 0.1 mM GTP; 0.1 mM GTP; 0.1 mM UTP and 100 μCi of 3-H GTP (specific activity 38.0 Ci/mmol). Results are given in cpm of [^{3}H]GMP incorporated; figure in parenthesis represents this in log.

†Supernatant fluid containing virus was concentrated 100-fold by sedimentation at 48,000 × g for 2 hr.

‡Ly cells were treated with 0–30 units/ml of IF for 16 hr followed by washing of the monolayers 3–4 times to remove residual IF. Monolayers were challenged with VSV at a $TCID_{50}$ of 50 particles per cell and incubated for 18–24 hr. The virus assays in these fluids were carried out by, a CPE assay.

RESULTS

Transcriptase Activity in Virus Samples Obtained from Cells Treated with Varying Concentration of Interferon

Culture fluids were concentrated 100-fold and assayed for transcriptase activity as described in METHODS. The results of these experiments (TABLE 1, FIGURE 2) show that with 30 units of IF there was less than a 10-fold decrease in transcriptase activity compared to the control samples not treated with IF; however, inhibition of viral infectivity was 150-fold in samples from cells treated with 30 units of IF (TABLE 1 and FIGURE 2).

In another experiment virus samples were prepared and concentrated 100-fold, serially diluted 2-fold, and tested for transcriptase activity as above. Results indicated that all dilutions tested the transcriptase activity was directly dependent on the virus concentration in the samples (data not presented).

Reaction mixtures were incubated with virus samples for varying periods of

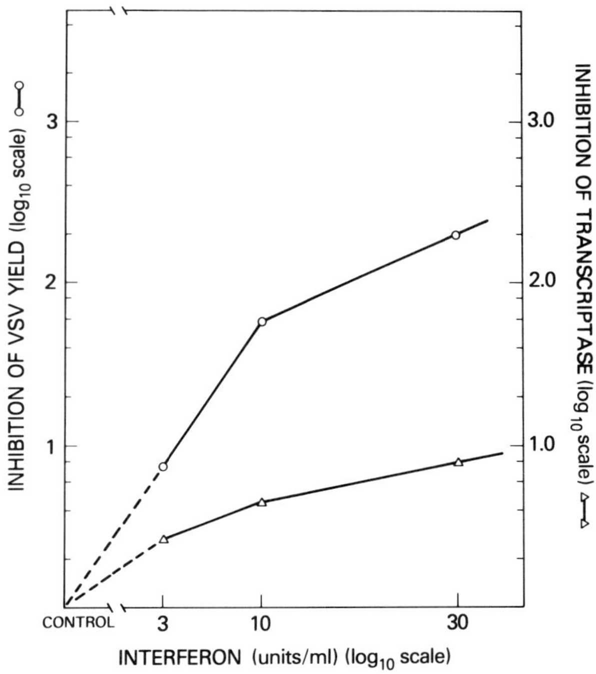

FIGURE 2. VSV transcriptase or infectivity in extracellular fluids from IF-treated and control cells. After IF treatment, cells were infected with 5 $TCID_{50}$ VSV in the presence of actinomycin D (2 μg/ml) for 18 hr. Virus was purified and concentrated as described in METHODS. Transcriptase Δ——Δ and infectivity O——O were assayed as described in METHODS.

time (0, 45, 75, 90, 120, and 150 min) and the transcriptase activity measured. Peak transcriptase activity was present in samples incubated for 90 min (data not presented). Therefore, under the conditions employed there was a direct relationship between the number of virus particles and the transcriptase activity. The time of incubation was optimal for demonstrating enzyme activity.

Effect of Interferon on Viral Protein Production

Analysis of viral proteins was carried out as described in MATERIALS AND METHODS. With 10–30 units of IF there was only a 2–4 fold decrease in the major virion protein (N) compared to untreated control samples (TABLE 2). The ratio of optical density at 260:280 nm in purified VSV indicated a 4-fold decrease in total viral protein concentrations after treatment with 30 units of interferon. This experiment was repeated, and a maximum of a 5-fold decrease was seen in the N protein of VSV obtained from cells treated with 30 units of interferon. Therefore, in VSV from interferon-treated cells the inhibition of these proteins was similar to the reduction in viral transcriptase activity.

During the course of these studies, however, we noted that the content of the glycoprotein (G) and the matrix protein (M) components of VSV derived from IF-treated cells was reduced more than was that of the N protein (TABLE 2). In another experiment equal amounts of radioactive VSV protein of virus derived from IF-treated or untreated cells were analyzed on gels. In the experiments summarized in FIGURE 3 there was a selective decrease in the G and M protein content of the VSV from IF-treated cells as compared to the N protein content.

Effect of Interferon on Viral RNA Synthesis

In samples analyzed for viral RNA according to the method of Peacock and Dingman,[27] only a single species (42S) of viral RNA could be detected in virus from untreated or from IF-treated cells. There was a 2.5 to 6-fold reduction in viral RNA with 3 to 30 units of IF (TABLE 3).

In another experiment viral RNA from virions was analyzed on 6-30% sucrose gradients in SET buffer. Again, only a single 42S peak of RNA was observed. The concentration of RNA was determined by the optical density at 260 nm and the specific activity calculated; there was less than a 2-fold difference in the concentration of RNA in samples treated with 0 to 30 units of IF (TABLE 4). The specific activity of all of the virus samples was similar. Intracellular RNA synthesis was also studied in the presence of actimomycin D (2 μg/ml) in cells treated with 30 units/ml of interferon. No significant reduction in RNA synthesis was observed.

DISCUSSION

Our results indicated that in virus derived from IF-treated Ly cells there was a marked reduction in VSV infectivity compared to transcriptase activity, virion N protein concentration, or virion RNA content. This selective effect was specific for IF and was not seen with a nonspecific inhibitor of protein synthesis. With a

TABLE 2

ANALYSIS OF VIRAL PROTEINS* (N, M OR G) IN SAMPLES OF VIRUS OBTAINED FROM CELLS TREATED WITH INTERFERON

Interferon Concentration (units/ml)	Protein N		Protein M		Protein G		Infectivity	
	[^{3}H] Leucine (cpm)	Inhibition (log)	[^{3}H] Leucine (cpm)	Inhibition (log)	[^{3}H] Leucine (cpm)	Inhibition (log)	Virus Titer ($TCID_{50}$/ml)	Inhibition (log)
0	4,200 (3.62)	—	3,500 (3.54)	—	2,500 (3.39)	—	5.0×10^8	—
30	1,500 (3.18)	0.44	650 (2.81)	0.73	100 (2.00)	1.4	2.5×10^6	2.3

*Viral proteins were labeled by incubating cells with 15 μCi/ml of [^{3}H]leucine (specific activity 121.1 Ci/mmol); the proteins were analyzed by polyacrylamide gel electrophoresis. Values given represent counts in the N, M, or G protein peaks; figures in parenthesis represent this in $\log_{10}$.

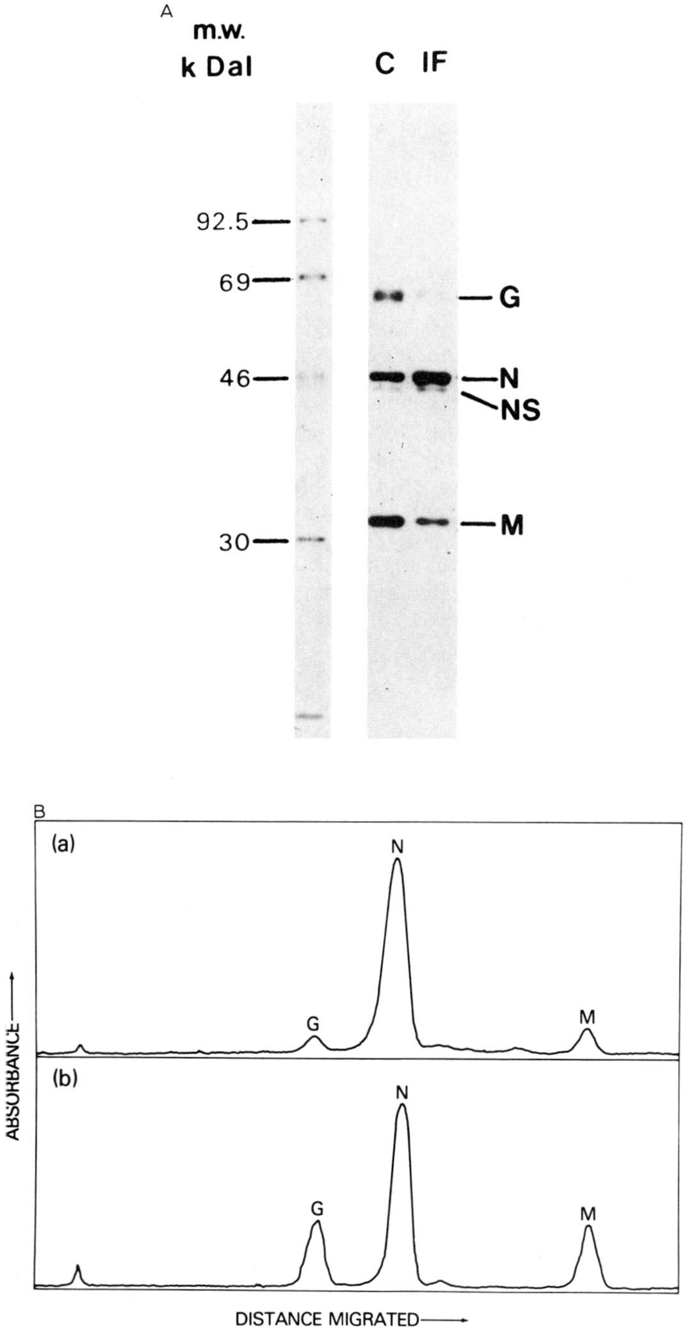
A
m.w.
k Dal
C IF
92.5
69
46
30
G
N
NS
M
B
(a)
N
G
M
(b)
N
G
M
ABSORBANCE
DISTANCE MIGRATED

TABLE 3

ANALYSIS OF VIRAL RNA* BY POLYACRYLAMIDE GEL ELECTROPHORESIS IN SAMPLES OBTAINED FROM INTERFERON-TREATED CELLS

Interferon Concentration (units/ml)	Viral RNA: [^{3}H]Uridine Incorporation (cpm)	Viral RNA: Inhibition (log)	Infectivity: Titer ($TCID_{50}$/ml)	Infectivity: Inhibition (log)
0	4,250 (3.63)	—	3.0×10^9	—
3	1,710 (3.23)	0.40	7.0×10^8	0.6
10	1,430 (3.16)	0.47	1.0×10^8	1.5
30	770 (2.88)	0.75	1.0×10^7	2.5

*Viral RNA was labeled with [^{3}H]uridine (10–15 μCi/ml) in the presence of actinomycin D (2 μg/ml) for 18 hr. Virus was concentrated by stirring the supernatant fluid with polyethylene glycol 6000 at a final concentration of 6%, for 30 min at 4°C. The viral RNA was extracted by SDS-phenol treatment and polyacrylamide gel electrophoresis was carried out as described in METHODS. Values given represent total number of counts in the peak of RNA; the figure in parenthesis represents this in log.

concentration of cycloheximide that inhibited protein synthesis by 95% in L cells, there was a 10-fold reduction in virus yield; there was also a 10-fold reduction in transcriptase activity. These results taken together indicate that in the presence of IF not only is the production of infectious virus particles inhibited, but also the production of noninfectious virus particles is disproportionately enhanced. These results resemble those reported in TB cells infected with MLV,[18,19] as well as in AKR cells chronically infected with MLV[16] and suggest that this mechanism of action of IF may not be restricted to RNA tumor virus infection. It may prove to be an important IF effect on the replication of many viruses. TABLE 5 summarizes the action of IFs on membrane-associated viruses.

A possible mechanism of action that could account for the above observation is that IF treatment may alter a virion structural component(s) such as the viral glycoprotein; this in turn may decrease the production of infectious virus and increase the production of variant particles with low infectivity. The results show

FIGURE 3. Fluorograms and scans of purified VSV proteins with equal amounts of radioactivity (15,000 cpm) applied to each gel:

A. The gels were electrophoresed and then stained with Coomassie brilliant blue r. After destaining the gels were impregnated with 2,5-diphenyloxazole (New England Nuclear, Boston, MA), dried, and exposed to Kodak X-OMAT x-ray film. Phosphorylase B (92,500), bovine serum albumin (69,000), ovalbumin (46,000), carbonic anhydrase (30,000), and cytochrome *c* (12,300) were used as reference protein molecular markers. Lanes: C, proteins of VSV released from cells not treated with interferon; IF, proteins of VSV released from cells treated with interferon (30 reference units/ml).

B. Fluorograms were scanned with a Quick Scan Jr. densitometer (Helena Laboratories). Integrated values are as follows: (a) proteins of VSV released from cells not treated with IF, G (4.0), N (21.0) and M (3.8); (b) proteins of VSV released from cells treated with IF (30 reference units/ml), G (0.1), N (26.7) and M (0.4).

TABLE 4

SUCROSE DENSITY GRADIENT ANALYSIS OF VIRAL RNA* IN VIRUS SAMPLES OBTAINED FROM CELLS TREATED WITH INTERFERON

Interferon Concentration (units/ml)	[^{3}H]Uridine Incorporation (cpm)	Absorption at 260 nm	Concentration of RNA ug/ml	Cpm per μg of RNA (specific activity)
0	22,100	0.210	8.4	2,600
3	18,000	0.182	7.0	2,570
10	16,000	0.170	6.8	2,550
30	13,000	0.140	5.2	2,500

*Viral RNA was labeled with [^{3}H]uridine (specific activity 41.3 Ci/mmol) in the presence of 2 μg/ml of actinomycin D. The virus was concentrated and RNA extracted by phenol as described in METHODS. RNA analysis was carried out on 6–30% sucrose density gradients in SET buffer; 200 μl aliquots were layered over a 4.4 ml gradient and sedimented at 248,000 × g for 2.5 hr in a Beckman SW65 rotor. Fractions of 0.15 ml were collected and radioactivity was measured in a scintillation spectrometer.

that the content of G and M proteins is low in VSV produced by IF-treated L cells. Since previous studies clearly show that VSV particles with reduced amounts of the G protein are low in infectivity,[28] it is likely that at least some of the reduced infectivity of the VSV particles produced by IF-treated L cells is due to the reduced amount of G protein incorporated into such particles. It is possible that IF-induced changes in the cell plasma membrane[29] may be the basis for the alteration in infectivity of both VSV and murine leukemia virus produced after IF treatment, since these viruses bud from the cell surface.

The noninfectious particles produced in IF-treated cells appear to contain only 42S viral RNA; they do not interfere with the growth of wild-type VSV, nor do they produce IF in culture. The profiles of VSV produced by IF-treated and nontreated cells in equilibrium sucrose density gradients are identical. They are, therefore, unlikely to be defective interfering forms of VSV.

TABLE 5

ACTIONS OF INTERFERON ON MEMBRANE-ASSOCIATED VIRUSES

Class of Inhibition	Level of Inhibition	Examples of This Type of Inhibition (ref)
I	Increase in intracisternal A type particles (which may be precursors of C particles)	Friend virus-infected cells[7,8]
II	Virus particles stick to plasma membrane of cell	AKR-MLV in AKR cells[18]; MMTV[9]
III	Particles produced with low infectivity	Moloney MLV in TB cells[18,19]; AKR-MLV in AKR cells[16]; VSV in Ly cells

Abbreviations: MLV—murine leukemia virus; VSV—vesicular stomatitis virus; MMTV—mouse mammary tumor virus.

REFERENCES

1. BADER, J. P. 1962. Production of interferon by chick embryo cells exposed to Rous sarcoma virus. Virology **16:** 436–443.
2. HORVATH, A. E. & R. M. FRIEDMAN. 1971. Nucleic acid and proteins isolated from a strain of murine sarcoma virus (MSV-O). Proc. Soc. Exp. Biol. Med. **137:** 1075–1081.
3. SARMA, P. S., G. SHIU, S. BARON & R. J. HUEBNER. 1969. Inhibitory effect of interferon in murine sarcoma and leukemia virus infection *in vitro*. Nature (London) **223:** 845–846.
4. VAN GRIENSVEN, L. J. D. L., M. F. BAUDELAIRE, J. PERIES, R. EMANOIL-RAVICOVITCH & M. BOIRON. 1971. Studies on the biosynthesis of murine leukemia virus RNA. I. Some properties of Rauscher leukemia virus isolated from interferon treated JLSV5 cells. *In* Lepetit Colloquia on Biology and Medicine, Biology of Oncogenic Viruses. Vol. 2: 145-153. North-Holland. Amsterdam.
5. BILLIAU, A., H. SOBIS & P. DESOMER. 1973. Influence of interferon on virus particle formation in different oncornavirus carrier cell lines. Int. J. Cancer **12:** 646–653.
6. FRIEDMAN, R. M. & J. M. RAMSEUR. 1974. Inhibition of murine leukemia virus production in chronically infected AKR cells: A novel effect of interferon. Proc. Nat. Acad. Sci. USA **71:** 3542–3544.
7. KRIEG, C. J., W. OSTERTAG, V. CLAUSS, I. B. PRAGNALL, P. SWETLY, G. ROESLER & B. J. WEIMANN. 1978. Increase in intracisternal A-type particles in Friend cells during inhibition of Friend virus (SFFV) release by interferon or azidothymidine. Exp. Cell. Res. **116:** 21–29.
8. LUFTIG, R. B., J. F. CONSCIENCE, A. SKOALTCHI, P. MCMILLAN, M. REVEL & F. RUDDLE. 1977. Effect of interferon on dimethsulfoxide-stimulated Friend erythroleukemic cells: Ultrastructural and biochemical study. J. Virol. **23:** 799–810.
9. STRAUCHEN, V. A., N. A. YOUNG & R. M. FRIEDMAN. 1977. Interferon-mediated inhibition of mouse mammary tumor virus expression in cultured cells. Virology **82:** 232–236.
10. BILLIAU, A., V. G. EDY, H. SOBIS & P. DESOMER. 1974. Influence of interferon on virus particle synthesis in oncornavirus carrier lines. II. Evidence for a direct effect on particle release. Int. J. Cancer **14:** 335–340.
11. FRIEDMAN, R. M., E. H. CHANG, J. M. RAMSEUR & M. W. MYERS. 1975. Interferon-directed inhibition of chronic murine leukemia virus production in cell cultures: Lack of effect on intracellular viral markers. J. Virol. **16:** 569–574.
12. PITHA, P. A., W. P. ROWE & M. N. OXMAN. 1976. Effect of interferon on exogenous, endogenous and chronic murine leukemia virus infection. Virology **70:** 324–338.
13. BILLIAU, A., V. G. EDY, E. DECLERCQ, H. HEREMANS & P. DESOMER. 1975. Influence of interferon on the synthesis of virus particles in oncornavirus carrier cell lines. III. Survey of effect on A-, B-, C-type oncornaviruses. Int. J. Can **15:** 947–953.
14. SHAPIRO, S. Z., M STRAND & A. BILLIAU. 1977. Synthesis and cleavage processing of oncornavirus proteins during interferon inhibition of virus particle release. Infect. Immun. **16:** 742–747.
15. CHANG, E. H., S. J. MIMS, T. J. TRICHE & R. M. FRIEDMAN. 1977. A morphologic study of interferon inhibition of murine leukemia virus release. Correlation with biochemical data. J. Gen. Virol. **34:** 363–367.
16. PITHA, P. A., S. P. STAAL, D. P. BOLOGNESI, T. P. DENNY & W. P. ROWE. 1977. Effect of interferon on murine leukemia virus infection. II. Synthesis of viral components in exogenous infection. Virology **77:** 1–13.
17. FAN, H., & P. MACISAAC. 1978. Virus-specific RNA synthesis in interferon-treated mouse cells productive by infected with Moloney murine leukemia virus. J. Virol. **27:** 449–452.
18. CHANG, E. H., M. W. MYERS, R. K. Y. WONG & R. M. FRIEDMAN. 1977. The inhibitory effect of interferon on a temperature-sensitive mutant of Moloney murine leukemia virus. Virology **77:** 99–101.

19. WONG, P. K. Y., P. H. YUEN, R. MACLEOD, E. H. CHANG, M. W. MYERS & R. M. FRIEDMAN. 1977. The effect of interferon on *de novo* infection of Moloney leukemia virus. Cell **10:** 245–252.
20. CHANG, E. H. & R. M. FRIEDMAN. 1977. A large glycoprotein of Moloney leukemia virus derived from interferon-treated cells. Biochem. Biophys. Res. Comun. **77:** 392-398.
21. BAXT, B., J. A. SONNABEND & R. BABLANIAN. 1977. Effect of interferon on vesicular stomatitis virus transcription and translation. J. Gen. Virol. **35:** 325–334.
22. MARCUS, P. I., D. L. ENGELHARDT, J. M. HUNT & M. J. SEKELLICK. 1971. Interferon action: Inhibition of vesicular stomatitis virus RNA synthesis induced by virion-bound polymerase. Science **174:** 593–598.
23. BALL, L. A & C. N. WHITE. 1978. Effect of interferon pretreatment on coupled transcription translation cell-free extracts of primary chick cells. Virology **84:** 496–508.
24. OGBURN, C. A., K. BERG & K. PAUCKER. 1973. Purification of mouse interferon by affinity chromatography on anti-interferon globulin-sepharose. J. Immunol. **111:** 1206–1218.
25. COLONNO, R. J. & A. K. BARERJEE. 1977. Mapping and initiation studies on the leader RNA of vesicular stomatitis virus. Virology **77:** 260–268.
26. WAGNER, R. R., T. C. SCHNAITMAN & R. M. SNYDER. 1969. Structural proteins of vesicular stomatitis viruses. J. Virol. **3:** 395–403.
27. PEACOCK, A. C. & C. W. DINGMAN. 1968. Molecular weight estimation and separation of ribonucleic acid by electrophoresis in agarose-acrylamide composite gels. Biochemistry **7:** 668–674.
28. LODISH, H. F. & R. A. WEISS. 1979. Selective isolation of mutants of vesicular stomatitis virus defective in the production of viral glycoproteins. J. Virol. **30:** 177–189.
29. CHANG, E. H., F. T. JAY & R. M. FRIEDMAN. 1978. Physical, morphological and biochemical alterations in the membrane of AKR mouse cells after interferon treatment. Proc. Nat. Acad. Sci. USA **75:** 1859–1863.
30. MAHESHWARI, R. K. & R. M. FRIEDMAN. 1979. Production of vesicular stomatitis virus with low infectivity by interferon-treated cells. J. Gen. Virol. **44:** 261–264.
31. KESSLER, S. W. 1975. Rapid isolation of antigens from cells with a Staphylococcal protein A-antibody adsorbent: Parameters of the interaction of antibody-antigen complexes with protein A. J. Immunol. **115:** 1617–1624.
32. DE LARCO, J. & G. T. TODARO. 1976. Membrane receptors for murine leukemia viruses: Characterization using purified envelope glycoprotein gp71. Cell **8:** 365–371.

THE INTERFERON SYSTEM AS A REGULATOR OF PERSISTENT INFECTION*

Margaret J. Sekellick and Philip I. Marcus

Microbiology Section
University of Connecticut
Storrs, Connecticut 06268

One of the most awesome effects of interferon (IF) is its capacity to spare cells from the lethal action of viruses. This attribute of IF action, while not generally appreciated as separate from its antiviral effects,[1] has been observed by numerous investigators (reviewed in ref. 2). Recently we have determined the quantitative relationship between IF dose and the sparing of cells from the lethal action of vesicular stomatitis virus (VSV).[3] From this study we concluded that the IF system conceivably might assume a critical role in the initiation and maintenance of persistent infection *in vitro* by regulating the expression of cell-killing by viruses. This manifestation of IF action would provide a mechanism for *cell persistence* in the presence of a lethal virus—a hallmark of persistent infection tacitly accepted though never explained.[4] In our approach to an understanding of persistent infection through IF action and cell-sparing we chose to examine separately the viral reactants implicated in persistent infection by others and to ascertain their role as potential inducers of interferon. We demonstrated that *rna*$^-$ *ts*mutants of VSV, the type universally selected during persistent infection,[5] were excellent inducers of IF,[6] as were a class of [±]RNA DI particles.[7,8] From the results of these experiments we proposed a model† for cell-virus persistence (persistent infection) in which IF induced by resident viral reactants (*ts*mutants and/or [±]RNA DI particles) acts to establish an equilibrium between cell sparing $\rightleftharpoons$ cell killing and virus inhibition $\rightleftharpoons$ virus replication.[4,6] The model predicts that the introduction of specific anti-IF serum into cultures manifesting virus-cell persistence would upset this equilibrium and precipitate a "crisis," namely, cell death and termination of infection. Such results have been reported in the virus-cell systems thus far challenged with anti-IF serum.[9,10] The data that follow constitute our evidence for a regulatory role of the IF system in persistent infection, and stress the importance of *cell persistence* in viral persistence.

Cell Sparing by Interferon Action

Interferon is the biological reagent *par excellence* for protecting cells from the lethal action of a virus once it has entered the cell. This effect was

*The authors' research described herein was supported by National Science Foundation Grants PCM 77-24875 and PCM 79-05429 and National Cancer Institute Grant CA 20882, and benefited from use of the Cell Culture Facility supported by National Cancer Institute Grant CA 14733.

†Obviously this model exclusively addresses virus-cell persistence in which the cell is fully competent for the IF system. Most types of cells display this characteristic and may be described phenotypically as *ifi*$^+$ (responds to inducers of interferon) and *ifa*$^+$ (responds to the action of interferon). Green monkey kidney-Vero and BHK-21 cells are exceptional and may be described phenotypically as *ifi*$^-$, *ifa*$^+$. Persistent infection in these cells clearly does not involve the IF system.[4,14]

0077-8923/80/0350-0545 $01.75/0 © 1980, NYAS

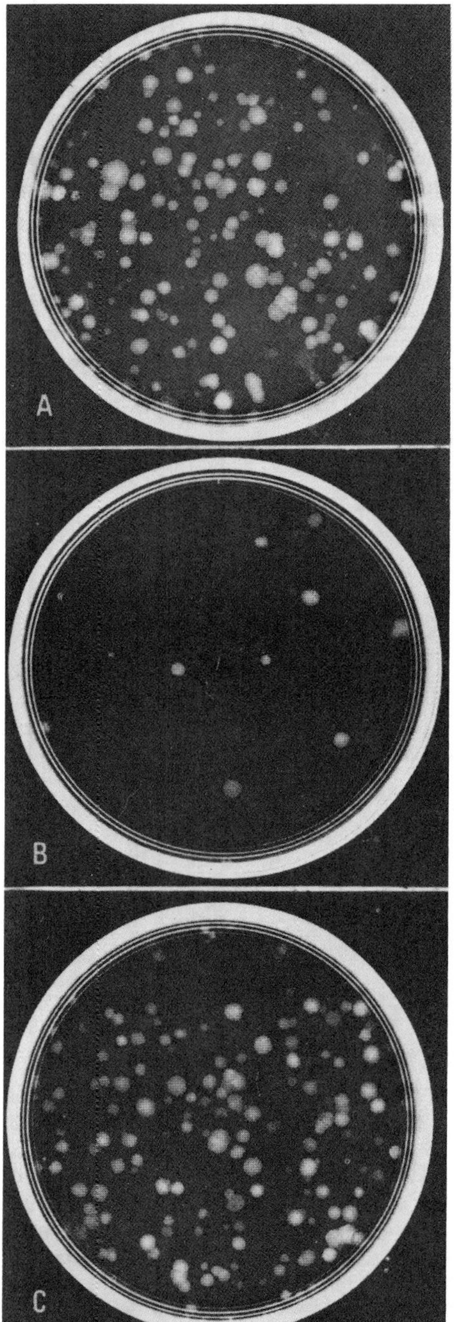

FIGURE 1. Colony formation by GMK Vero cells treated with human interferon (IF) and challenged with VSV *ts*G114(I). Photographs show colonies from surviving cells incubated for 20 hr at 30.0°C (pulse-infection) and 8 days at 40.0°C. All petri dishes (50 mm) were inoculated with 200 cells from monolayers treated with IF and challenged with VSV as follows: (A) 54 units/ml of IF, no virus; (B) no interferon, $m_{CKP} = 6$; (C) 54 units/ml of IF, $m_{CKP} = 6$. (From Marcus and Sekellick.[3])

documented quantitatively by exposing GMK-Vero cells to different concentrations of human IF and determining their capacity to resist the cell-killing particle activity[2,3,11–13] of vesicular stomatitis virus (VSV). The photographs of colonies in FIGURE 1 demonstrate that Vero cells treated with 54 units of IF, challenged with VSV at m_{ckp} = 6 and seeded as single cells, plate with about 100% efficiency (compare FIGURES 1A and 1C). Thus, these IF-treated cells are spared completely from the lethal action of the virus (FIGURE 1B). The quantitative relationship between IF dose and cell survival (sparing) is illustrated in FIGURE 2. From such

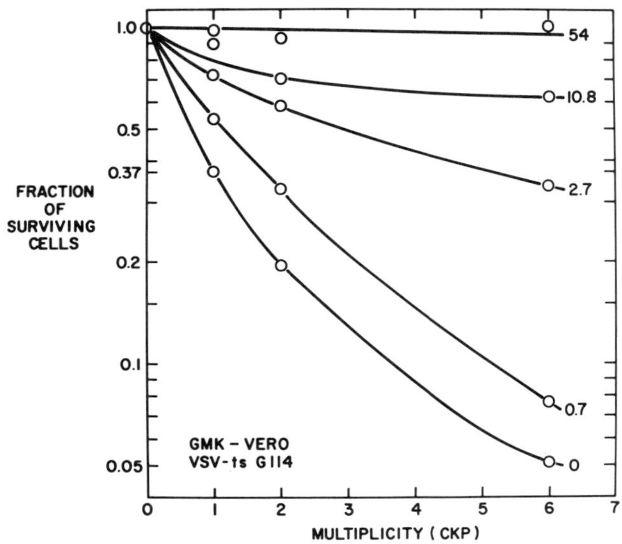

FIGURE 2. Survival curves of GMK Vero cells exposed to different concentrations of human interferon (IF) for 24 hr at 37.5°C and challenged with varying multiplicities of VSV tsG114(I). Following virus attachment and entry, infected and control cell monolayers were dispersed with trypsin, and the cells were counted and plated in growth medium containing VSV antiserum. All plates were held at 30.0° for 24 hr (pulse-infection) before shifting to 40.0°C for colony formation from surviving cells. The *abscissa* represents the CKP multiplicities calculated from the 37% survival level in mock-treated cells ("0" IF). The concentrations of IF, in PR_{50} (VSV) units/ml, are indicated to the right of each survival curve. Individual points represent the averages of duplicate plates and agreed within ±20% of the mean value. (From Marcus and Sekellick.[3])

data we calculated the fraction of surviving cell-killing particle activity as a function of IF concentration and generated the curve shown in FIGURE 3. These data reveal that only 1 or 2 units/ml of IF are required to prevent expression of 50% of the cell-killing (CK) particle activity of VSV, and that 10 units/ml of IF blocked about 90% of the CK particle activity. In this context, Ramseur and Friedman[9] reported that 2 units/ml of interferon completely inhibited the cytopathic effect of VSV (m_{PFP} = 10) on mouse L cells. Cell sparing is particularly effective when IF-treated cells are challenged by only a single virion.[3] These conditions of infection are characteristic of cultures persistently infected with

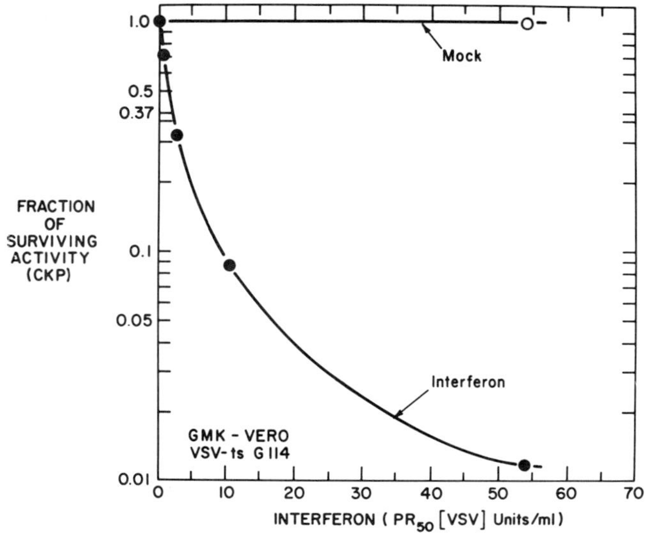

FIGURE 3. Surviving activity curve of VSV cell-killing particles (CKP) as a function of interferon (IF) concentration. The CKP titer for *ts*G114(I) was calculated, as previously described (Marcus. 1959. *Virology* **9:** 546–563), for each dose of IF used in the experiment of FIGURE 2 and was plotted relative to the activity in mock-treated GMK Vero cells. (From Marcus and Sekellick.[3])

VSV where the concentration of infectious virus in the medium bathing from 10^6 to 10^7 cells usually ranges from 10^3 to 10^6 PFP/ml.[5,9,15] Furthermore, the effective multiplicity may be even lower as a result of the distribution of infectious virus in a relatively large volume, and the latter's effect on virus attachment kinetics.[16]

INTERFERON IN CELL CULTURES PERSISTENTLY INFECTED WITH VESICULAR STOMATITIS VIRUS

If we are to invoke IF-mediated cell sparing as a mechanism for *cell persistence* in persistent infection of VSV, then IF or the manifestation of its action on cells, namely a heterologous antiviral state, must of necessity be demonstrable. In this regard we note reports demonstrating directly low levels of IF in cells persistently infected with VSV,[9,15,17] or the presence of IF inferred through a state of heterologous interference,[9,10,15] or the use of anti-IF serum.[9,10] Nishiyama[15] reported levels of 2 to 5 units of IF in VSV-mouse L cells as did Friedman[9] during prolonged infection of mouse L cells.

In assessing the contribution of IF action to cell sparing from viruses in a complex situation like persistent infection, it is perhaps prudent to consider the actual level of the antiviral state within the cell as a more accurate barometer of IF action than the concentration of *detectable* interferon. For example, while only a few units of IF were detected in the medium bathing human FS-4 cells infected with an IF-inducing DI particle, a significant antiviral state developed as measured by yield reduction of a heterologous virus.[7] Similar observations have been recorded in other virus-cell systems.[9,15,18]

These data suggest that cells persistently infected with VSV may produce enough IF, and develop an antiviral state, of sufficient magnitude to render feasible a model of *cell persistence* based on IF action. Consequently, we sought to determine the nature of the inducer(s) responsible for activating the IF system, keeping in mind that VSV generally is considered a poor inducer of interferon.[19] These experiments are described next.

Interferon Induction by Viral Reactants Implicated in Persistent Infection

[±]RNA Defective-Interfering Particles

Although DI particles of VSV seem to play a critical role in maintaining persistent infection in cells deficient in some aspect of the IF system,[14] they do not appear to serve a comparable role in IF-competent cells.[10] In the latter case DI particles may be important in the initiation of persistent infection and the transient state leading to a stable virus-cell relationship, but apparently are not required in the maintenance of prolonged[17] or persistent infection with VSV.[10] In IF-competent cells the function of DI particles in the initiation and establishment of persistent infection must go beyond the simple expedient of reducing the yield

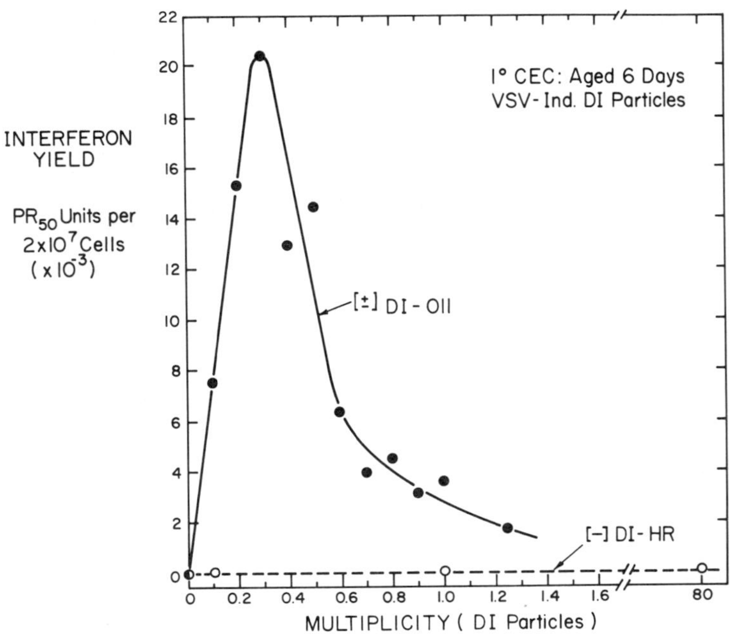

FIGURE 4. Interferon-inducing capacity of [±]RNA DI-011 and [–]RNA DI-HR particles. Primary chick embryo cells aged *in vitro* for 6 days[24] were infected with various multiplicities of DI particles obtained as thrice gradient-purified stocks. The infected cell monolayers were incubated at 40.5°C for 24 hr. The supernatant fluid was collected and assayed for interferon as described previously.[6] (From Marcus and Sekellick.[7])

of virus available for cell killing, for we have demonstrated that the CK particle activity of VSV is expressed fully in cells manifesting DI particle-mediated (homotypic) interference[11]—even when the yield of infectious virus is reduced to zero per cell.[21] For this reason it may be equally important to activate a mechanism for cell sparing.[3] Induction of IF by DI particles of VSV that possess covalently linked self-complementary [±]RNA[22,23] provide such a mechanism through their capacity to function as IF-inducing particles.[7] This capacity is demonstrated in FIGURE 4. A conventional [−]RNA DI-HR particle did not function as an IF-inducing particle under the same conditions. An analysis of the dose (multiplicity)-response (IF yield) curve shown in FIGURE 4 indicates that in "aged" chick embryo cells[24] a single particle of [±]DI-011 suffices to induce a quantum yield of IF and that every physical particle registers as an IF-inducing particle.[7] We also observed[6] IF-inducing particle activity in mouse L(Y) cells (TABLE 1), as have others.[20] Our analysis of the dose-response curve in this latter study by Frey *et al.*[20] indicates only 1 in about 500 physical particles appear to register as an IF-inducing particle—a difference in efficiency certainly warranting further investigation.

Temperature-Sensitive (Small Plaque) Mutants

Temperature-sensitive (*ts*) small-plaque mutants of VSV emerge as the viral reactant most consistently implicated in the maintenance of persistent infection in IF-competent cells,[5,10] and hence constitute the most likely inducer of interferon. We tested this possibility and found that *ts*mutants of the type commonly selected for in persistent infection,[5] i.e., *rna*⁻ from complementation group I, were excellent inducers of IF in both "aged" chick embryo cells and in mouse

TABLE 1

INTERFERON-INDUCING, PROTEIN SYNTHESIS-INHIBITING, AND CELL-KILLING PARTICLE ACTIVITY OF VESICULAR STOMATITIS VIRUS *ts*MUTANTS

			Interferon Yield†	
Phenotype*	Complementation Group	*ts*Mutant Designation	Chick Embryo Cells (units/10^7 cells) at 40.5°C	Mouse L (Y) Cells (units/5×10^6 cells) at 37.5°C
ts^{psi^-, ckp^-, ifp^+}	I	G114	8,700	480
		G11	17,400	3,600
		T1026	24,600	>12,000
	II	G22	12,000	3,750
	IV	G41	26,500	570
W^+		HR-C	300	<10
Non-*ts* revertant of T1026		R1	29,500	15,600
[−] RNA DI-HR *ifp*⁻ particle			<100	—
[±] RNA DI-011 *ifp*⁺ particle			32,100	2,700

*ts^{psi} phenotype = cellular *p*rotein *s*ynthesis *i*nhibition; ts^{ckp} phenotype = *c*ell-*k*illing *p*article activity; ts^{ifp} phenotype = *i*nter*f*eron-inducing *p*article activity.

†Experimental details and data in reference 6.

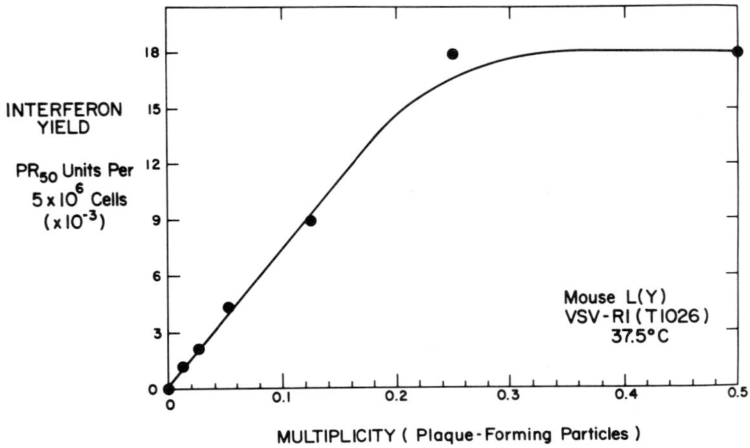

FIGURE 5. Dose (multiplicity)-response (interferon-yield) curve relating infection multiplicity of the VSV non-*ts* revertant R1 (T1026)[26] to the 24-hr yield of IF from mouse L(Y) cells at 37.5°C. The curve best fits a model in which maximal yields of IF are induced in cells infected with one or more IF-inducing particles.[25] This curve reveals there are about 5 IF-inducing particles for every 1 plaque-forming particle.[25] (From Marcus and Sekellick.[25])

L(Y) cells.[4,6,25] The results in FIGURE 5 illustrate the dose-response curve of a small-plaque non-*ts* revertant, R1 of *ts*T1026(I)[26] and demonstrate that there are about 5-times more IF-inducing particles in this preparation than plaque-forming particles (see calculations in Marcus and Sekellick).[25] Mutant *ts*G11(I) gave similar results.[25] These results are not surprising in light of evidence that only a small fraction of the VSV genome need be transcribed to produce an IF inducer moiety.[25] Conceivably, there is a comparable excess of IF-inducing particles in a culture of persistently infected cells contributing to the production of IF.

The data in TABLE 1 show that all mutants of VSV that fail to kill cells (ckp^-) or inhibit cellular protein synthesis (psi^-) at a non- or semipermissive temperature are excellent inducers of IF (ifp^+). These mutants also fail to amplify RNA synthesis (rna^-). Phenotypically these characteristics describe the type of *ts*mutant consistently isolated by Youngner *et al.*[5,10] from persistently infected mouse L cells.

These data establish that rna^-, psi^-, ckp^- *ts*mutants phenotypically similar to those isolated from persistently infected cells are excellent inducers of IF (ifp^+) at non- and semipermissive temperatures. We will demonstrate next the capacity of such mutants to spare cells through IF action.

CELL SPARING THROUGH THE ACTION OF INTERFERON INDUCED BY VIRAL REACTANTS IMPLICATED IN PERSISTENT INFECTION

[±]RNA Defective-Interfering Particles

The IF-inducing capacity of [±]DI-011 particles can function to spare cells from the lethal action of VSV. We demonstrated that preinfection of IF-competent cells [GMK-BSC or mouse L(Y)] with DI-011 particles rendered them

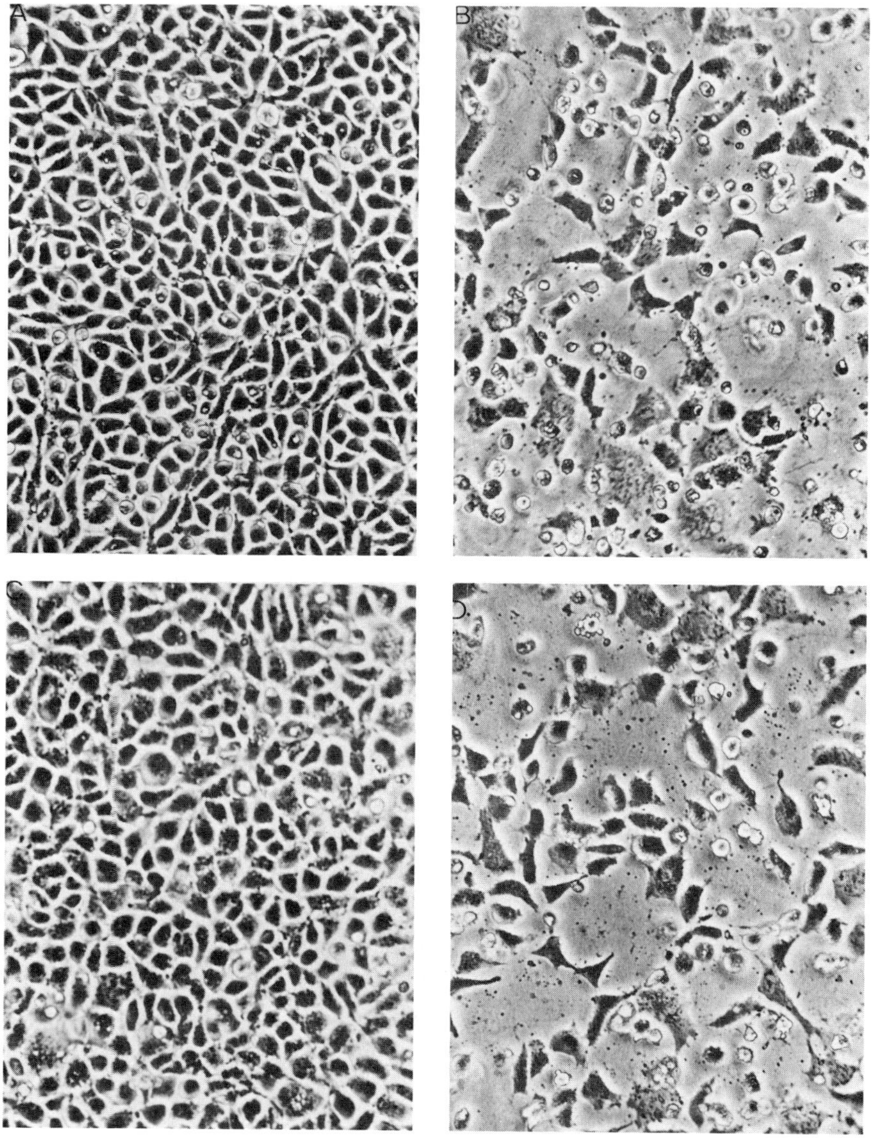

FIGURE 6. Photomicrographs of mouse L(Y) cells illustrating cell sparing against VSV induced by preinfection of cells with *ts*G11(I), and the prevention of this cell sparing by treatment with interferon (IF) antiserum. Confluent monolayers of cells were infected with *ts*G11(I) at $m_{pfp} = 1$. Antiserum to mouse IF was included in the growth medium at this time whenever appropriate. Following incubation at 37.5°C for 24 hr, the medium was removed by aspiration, and the cell monolayers were washed and then infected with wildtype VSV at $m_{pfp} = 5$. This challenge virus was allowed to adsorb for 30 min at 37.5°C. Unadsorbed virus was removed by aspiration, and the cell monolayers were washed prior to adding medium containing VSV antiserum (1:400 dilution) to each plate. Control plates were mock

totally refractory to the CK particle activity of VSV, and that the state of cell sparing was due to IF action, and not homotypic interference.[8] Since [±]RNA DI particles of the DI-011 prototype appear frequently in wildtype stocks of VSV,[22,23] but do not appear to be selected for during prolonged[17] or persistent infection[10] in IF-competent cells, we would relegate their role to the early stages of persistent infection for reducing the yield of infectious (cell-killing) virus through homotypic interference and their capacity to activitate the IF system. We suggest that this latter event may contribute to cell sparing and thus aid in the establishment of cell persistence.

Temperature-Sensitive (Small Plaque) Mutants

To determine whether an *ifp*$^+$ *ts*mutant of VSV could induce cell sparing through IF action, we exposed monolayers of mouse L(Y) cells to a low multiplicity of *ts*G11(I) [m_{pfp} = 1] at 37.5°C for 24 hr and then challenged the cells with wildtype VSV (m_{pfp} = 5) for 18 hr. FIGURE 6a shows the appearance of uninfected mouse L(Y) cells. Cells infected with *ts*G11(I) for 24 hr at 37.5°C were indistinguishable from uninfected cells, showing that the *ckp*$^+$ phenotype was not expressed under these conditions. However, we know that prolonged incubation at 37.5°C in an IF-incompetent cell would result in the eventual demise of that cell.[6] FIGURE 6b illustrates the extensive cytopathic effect brought on by infection of control cells with wildtype virus at m_{pfp} = 5 for 18 hr. In the test situation, cells infected with *ts*G11 for 24 hr at 37.5°C then were challenged with wildtype VSV and incubated for another 18 hr. FIGURE 6c demonstrates that the preinfection with *ts*G11 rendered the cells totally refractory to the cytopathic effect of the superinfecting wildtype VSV, showing that an *ifp*$^+$ *ts*mutant can spare cells from the lethal action of a virus.[6] Proof that this cell sparing was mediated by IF action came from an experiment in which anti-mouse IF serum was included in the medium during the 24-hr infection with *ts*G11. The photomicrograph in FIGURE 6d shows the results of that experiment and demonstrates that the cell sparing induced by *ts*G11 was mediated by interferon. This conclusion is based on the elegant demonstration by Vengris *et al.*[27] that the IF produced by a cell must be externalized in order to act on that cell. Further evidence for IF as the mediator of cell sparing derives from the heterologous nature of the cell sparing reaction: the *ts*G11 treated cells were also refractory to the cytopathic effect of Mengo virus.[6] Results similar to these were obtained when the mouse L(Y) cells were preinfected with the *ifp*$^+$ DI-011 particle.[8]

A study by Nishiyama *et al.*[28] provided direct evidence that *ts* (small plaque) mutants of VSV isolated from persistently infected L cells induced IF whereas the wildtype virus did not. Youngner and Preble have obtained similar results (personal communication).

---

infected but otherwise manipulated similarly. Cell monolayers were photographed following incubation at 37.5°C for 18 hr. *Conditions:* (A) uninfected cells (cells infected with only *ts*G11(I) at m_{pfp} = 1 were indistinguishable); (B) cells infected with VSV at m_{pfp} = 5; (C) cells preinfected with *ts*G11(I) at m_{pfp} = 1 and then challenged with VSV at m_{pfp} = 5; (D) cells preinfected with *ts*G11(I) at m_{pfp} = 1 in the presence of mouse anti-IF serum and then challenged with VSV at m_{pfp} = 5. Incubation for 2 to 3 days produced no change in the appearance of cells in A and C, whereas cells in B and D progressed to complete destruction. (From Sekellick and Marcus.[6])

A Model for the Regulatory Role of Interferon in Persistent Infection (Virus-Cell Persistence)

We have presented and reviewed evidence that certain prototypes of the viral reactants most common to persistent infection with VSV are capable of inducing IF[4,6–8] and that relatively low doses of IF can spare cells from the lethal action of this virus.[2,3] We propose that the induction of IF by these reactants and its subsequent action function in concert to produce cell persistence (sparing) during persistent infection.

DI particles of VSV do not appear to assume a significant role in the maintenance of prolonged[17] or persistent infection in cells with a fully functional IF system.[10] Consequently, we ascribe their function through homotypic interference, to that of reducing the load of infectious (cell-killing) virus and providing some measure of IF-mediated cell sparing during the early stages of persistent infection. Presumably selection for *ts*mutants with an *ifp*$^+$ phenotype then leads to a population of viruses better suited to maintaining virus-cell persistence. Also at the semipermissive temperatures of persistent infection such variants would be less efficient in producing or expressing the putative cell-killing factor of VSV.[2,11–13] Since IF-mediated interference does not appear to confer any selective advantage in the replication of *ts*mutants over that of wildtype VSV,[10] we suggest that the selection for *ts*mutants during persistent infection derives from their efficacy as IF-inducing particles and hence their capacity to spare cells—a reaction deemed critical for the maintenance of virus-cell persistence.

Figure 7 presents a simplified scheme of the equilibrium between cell sparing ⇌ cell killing and virus inhibition ⇌ virus replication which we contend is regulated by IF induction and its action during persistent infection. Note that any increase in the concentration of IF (due to induction by *ifp*$^+$ *ts*mutants) pushes persistent infection toward cell sparing and an inhibition of virus replication. However, suppression of virus replication in turn would lead to a decrease in the amount of IF inducer (*ifp*$^+$ *ts*mutants) produced and a subsequent decrease in the concentration of interferon. These events would lead to a waning of IF-mediated interference and push the reaction toward cell killing and virus replication. We suggest that the proper regulation of these events leads to persistent infection, which more accurately should be termed virus-cell persistence. The scheme presented in Figure 7 is certainly over-simplified; for example, we have observed an excess of IF-inducing particles over plaque-forming particles in stocks of *ts*mutants.[25] Should this situation pertain in virus-cell persistence, the IF-inducing potential of the virus population would be greater than anticipated from the plaque titer. On the other hand, we have observed that low doses of IF—of the magnitude reported in virus-cell persistence[9,15]—may influence the IF-inducing capacity of IF-inducing particles.[29,30] Conceivably, the production of IF by an excess of IF-inducing particles would be counter-balanced by an effect of IF action on the induction process. Thus, these two opposing reactions might contribute to a kind of fine tuning required to keep the normally lethal virus and susceptible cell in a state of concinnity—with the interferon system as the modulator.

Clearly, our model of virus-cell persistence predicts a critical regulatory role for interferon. Indeed, when Ramseur and Friedman[9] and Youngner *et al.*[10] added anti-IF serum to their persistently infected cultures a crisis was precipitated: they observed an increase in virus replication and cell killing, and the subsequent loss of the culture. Since anti-mouse IF serum is a highly specific reagent we interpret these results as direct evidence that IF plays a critical regulatory role in VSV-cell persistence. Our model also predicts a "cure" of virus persistence following the direct addition of sufficiently high concentrations of interferon. In this regard, Hallum *et al.*[31] reported the "cure" of mouse L cells persistently infected with Newcastle disease virus. A similar result has been reported for the VSV-L cell system.[15] As an extreme example of regulation by the IF system we observed that in mouse L(Y) cells infected with Sindbis virus the production of IF and its subsequent action on the same cell in which it was induced was so effective that the cell-killing activity of that otherwise lethal IF-inducing virus was aborted.[32]

The dramatic effects of interferon[33] and of interferon-antiserum[34] on the course of virus disease lead us to favor the interferon-inducing particle as an element of importance in the outcome of virus infection. The extraordinarily efficient interferon-inducing capacity[7] of the newly recognized class of [±]RNA

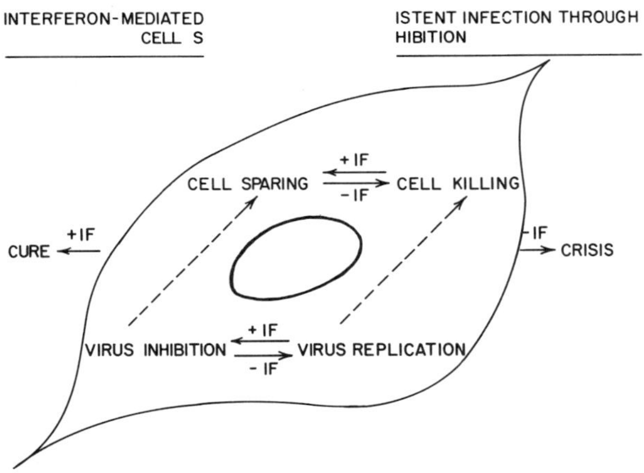

FIGURE 7. A scheme for interferon-mediated regulation of persistent infection (virus-cell persistence) through cell sparing and virus inhibition. "Cure," i.e., total cell-sparing, occurs when the concentration of IF is sufficiently high to inhibit all virus replication. "Crisis," i.e., total cell-killing, occurs when the concentration of IF is sufficiently low to permit virus replication and cell killing.

DI particles[22] and their apparent ubiquitous distribution[23] portend an important role for them in viral diseases. Temperature-sensitive and small plaque mutants with IF-inducing capacity exceeding that of parental virus may assume this same role. Thus, IF-inducing particles of viral origin emerge as potentially important reactants in virus disease. Their role, through the regulation of the IF system, appears critical in the maintenance, if not initiation of virus-cell persistence *in vitro;* their role *in vivo* remains a challenge to our investigative skills.

REFERENCES

1. STEWART, W. E., II. 1979. Non-antiviral actions of interferon. *In* The Interferon System.: 223. Springer-Verlag. Vienna, New York.
2. MARCUS, P. I. & M. J. SEKELLICK. 1980. Cell killing by vesicular stomatitis virus: The

prototype rhabdovirus. *In* Rhabdoviruses. D. H. L. Bishop, Ed. Vol. III, Chap. 2.: 13–49. CRC Press.

3. MARCUS, P. I. & M. J. SEKELLICK. 1976. Cell killing by viruses. III. The interferon system and inhibition of cell killing by vesicular stomatitis virus. Virology **69:** 378–393.
4. SEKELLICK, M. J. & P. I. MARCUS. 1980. Persistent infection by rhabdoviruses. *In* Rhabdoviruses. D. H. L. Bishop, Ed. Vol. III, Chap. 4.: 67–97. CRC Press.
5. YOUNGNER, J. S., E. J. DUBOVI, D. O. QUAGLIANA, M. KELLY & O. T. PREBLE. 1976. Role of temperature-sensitive mutants in persistent infections initiated with vesicular stomatitis virus. J. Virol. **19:** 90–101.
6. SEKELLICK, M. J. & P. I. MARCUS. 1979. Persistent infection. II. Interferon-inducing ts-mutants of vesicular stomatitis virus as mediators of cell sparing: Their possible role in persistent infection. Virology **95:** 36–47.
7. MARCUS, P. I. & M. J. SEKELLICK. 1977. Defective interfering particle with covalently linked [±]RNA induce interferon. Nature **266:** 815–819.
8. SEKELLICK, M. J. & P. I. MARCUS. 1978. Persistent infection. I. Interferon-inducing defective-interfering particles as mediators of cell sparing: Possible role in persistent infection by vesicular stomatitis virus. Virology **85:** 175–186.
9. RAMSEUR, J. M. & R. M. FRIEDMAN. 1977. Prolonged infection of interferon-treated cells by vesicular stomatitis virus: Possible role of temperature-sensitive mutants and interferon. J. Gen. Virol. **37:** 523–533.
10. YOUNGNER, J. S., O. T. PREBLE & E. V. JONES. 1978. Persistent infection of L cells with vesicular stomatitis virus: Evolution of virus populations. J. Virol. **28:** 6–13.
11. MARCUS, P. I. & M. J. SEKELLICK. 1974. Cell killing by viruses. I. Comparison of cell-killing, plaque-forming, and defective-interfering particles of vesicular stomatitis virus. Virology **57:** 321–338.
12. MARCUS, P. I. & M. J. SEKELLICK. 1975. Cell killing by viruses. II. Cell killing by vesicular stomatitis virus: A requirement for virion-derived transcription. Virology **63:** 176–190.
13. MARVALDI, J. L., J. LUCAS-LENARD, M. J. SEKELLICK & P. I. MARCUS. 1977. Cell killing by viruses. IV. Cell killing and protein synthesis inhibition by vesicular stomatitis virus require the same gene functions. Virology **79:** 267–280.
14. HOLLAND, J. J., L. P. VILLARREAL, R. M. WELSH, M. B. A. OLDSTONE, D. KOHNE, R. LAZZARINI & E. SCOLNICK. 1976. Long-term persistent vesicular stomatitis virus and rabies virus infection of cells *in vitro*. J. Gen. Virol. **33:** 193–211.
15. NISHIYAMA, Y. 1977. Studies of L cells persistently infected with VSV: Factors involved in the regulation of persistent infection. J. Gen. Virol. **35:** 265–279.
16. TOLMACH, L. J. 1957. Attachment and penetration of cells by viruses. *In* Advances in Virus Research. **4:** 63–110.
17. RAMSEUR, J. M. & R. M. FRIEDMAN. 1978. Prolonged infection by L cells with vesicular stomatitis virus. Defective-interfering forms and temperature-sensitive mutants as factors in the infection. Virology **85:** 253–261.
18. GLASGOW, L. A. 1974. Cytomegalovirus interference *in vitro*. Infect. Immun. **9:** 702–707.
19. MARCUS, P. I. 1980. The interferon system and rhabdoviruses. *In* Rhabdoviruses. D. H. L. Bishop, Ed. Vol. III, Chap. 1.: 1–12. CRC Press.
20. FREY, T. K., E. V. JONES, J. J. CARDAMONE & J. S. YOUNGNER. 1979. Induction of interferon in L cells by defective-interfering (DI) particles of vesicular stomatitis virus: Lack of correlation with content of [±] snap-back RNA. Virology. **99:** 95–102.
21. SEKELLICK, M. J. & P. I. MARCUS. 1980. Viral interference by defective particles of vesicular stomatitis virus measured in individual cells. Virology **104:** 247–252.
22. LAZZARINI, R. A., G. H. WEBER, L. D. JOHNSON & G. M. STAMMINGER. 1975. Covalently linked message and anti-message (genomic) RNA from a defective vesicular stomatitis virus particle. J. Mol. Biol. **97:** 289–307.
23. PERRAULT, J. & R. W. LEAVITT. 1977. Characterization of snap-back RNAs in vesicular stomatitis defective-interfering virus particles. J. Gen. Virol. **38:** 21–34.
24. CARVER, D. H. & P. I. MARCUS. 1967. Enhanced interferon production from chick embryo cells aged *in vitro*. Virology **32:** 247–257.

25. MARCUS, P. I. & M. J. SEKELLICK. 1980. Interferon induction by viruses. III. Vesicular stomatitis virus: Interferon-inducing particle activity requires partial transcription of gene N. J. Gen. Virol. **47:** 89–96.
26. STANNERS, C. P., A. M. FRANCOEUR & T. LAM. 1977. Analysis of VSV mutant with attenuated cytopathogenicity: Mutation in viral function, P, for inhibition of protein synthesis. Cell **11:** 273–281.
27. VENGRIS, V. E., B. D. STOLLAR & P. M. PITHA. 1975. Interferon externalization by producing cell before induction of antiviral state. Virology **65:** 410–417.
28. NISHIYAMA, Y., Y. ITO & K. SHIMOKATA. 1978. Properties of the viruses selected during persistent infection of L cells with VSV. J. Gen. Virol. **40:** 481–484.
29. FULLER, F. J. & P. I. MARCUS. 1980. Interferon induction by viruses. IV. Sindbis virus: Early passage defective-interfering particles induce interferon. J. Gen. Virol. **48:** 63–73.
30. MARCUS, P. I. & M. J. SEKELLICK. 1979. Unpublished observation.
31. HALLUM, J. V., H. R. THACORE & J. S. YOUNGNER. 1972. Effect of exogenous interferon on L cells persistently infected with Newcastle disease virus. Infect. Immun. **5:** 145–146.
32. SEKELLICK, M. J. & P. I. MARCUS. 1979. Virion-self-induced cell sparing through interferon action. Am. Soc. Microbiol., Abstract, p. 252.
33. KRIM, M. & F. K. SANDERS. 1977. Prophylaxis and therapy with interferons. *In* Interferons and Their Actions. W. E. Stewart II, Ed.: 153–201. CRC Press.
34. GRESSER, I., M. G. TOVEY, C. MAURY & M. T. BANDU. 1976. Role of interferon in the pathogenesis of virus disease in mice as demonstrated by the use of anti-interferon serum. II. Studies with herpes simplex, Maloney sarcoma, vesicular stomatitis, Newcastle disease, and influenza viruses. J. Exp. Med. **144:** 1316–1323.

INTERACTION BETWEEN INTERFERON AND HOST GENES IN ANTIVIRAL DEFENSE*

Otto Haller,† Heinz Arnheiter,† Michel A. Horisberger,‡
Ion Gresser,§ and Jean Lindenmann †

*†Institute for Medical Microbiology
Division of Experimental Microbiology
University of Zürich,
8028 Zürich, Switzerland*

*‡Research Department, Pharmaceutical Division
Ciba-Geigy Ltd.
4002 Basel, Switzerland*

*§Institut de Recherches Scientifiques sur le Cancer
94800 Villejuif, France*

INTRODUCTION

Inborn resistance of animals to certain viruses could be caused by barriers at several points in the virus-host interaction. Thus, invading viruses might get inactivated by factors in serum or secretions or might fail to infect cells for lack of appropriate receptors. Viruses might undergo abortive infection where no infectious progeny are produced. In addition, infection of a first line of target cells might lead to defective particles interfering with further spread. Furthermore, the interferon (IF) system of the host could be particularly efficient: IF could be formed more rapidly or in greater amounts than in susceptible animals, or potential virus target cells could be more sensitive to the general antiviral action of interferon. Moreover, scavenger cells such as macrophages might be able to act as a sort of dump until immunity becomes established. Finally, a highly efficient immune response might quench viral infection before symptoms become apparent. To make matters more complicated, all these factors might act in combination.

None of the above explanations satisfactorily accounts for specific resistance of mice to influenza virus as effected by the allele *Mx*.[1-3] The only manipulation that rendered *Mx*-bearing mice fully susceptible to the lethal action of influenza A virus was treatment with potent anti-IF type I serum.[4] This finding might have indicated that one of the above mechanisms involving IF was responsible for resistance. This seemed unlikely for two reasons: (1) The amount of IF produced after infection with influenza virus was found to be much lower in *Mx*-bearing mice than in susceptible controls.[4,5] (2) The *Mx*-related resistance was limited to orthomyxoviruses and did not affect susceptibility to numerous other viruses.[1] Interferon, however, is thought to inhibit the multiplication of all animal viruses more or less indiscriminately. An increase in the production of IF or an increase in the sensitivity to IF action would therefore be expected to result in a generally heightened ability to inhibit viral replication, but not in specific resistance

*This study was supported by the Swiss National Science Foundation, Grants No. 3.139–077 and 3.393.078 and the Directions de Recherches Moyens et Techniques, Contract 78–34–210.

0077-8923/80/0350-0558 $01.75/0 © 1980, NYAS

towards a narrow spectrum of viruses. Yet the results with the anti-IF serum suggested that IF somehow played an important part in this resistance. These seemingly contradictory observations are reconciled by the present findings, which show that the host resistance gene *Mx* influences sensitivity to IF action selectively for myxoviruses.

Results

Inhibition by Interferon of Influenza A Virus Growth in Macrophages of Different Genotypes

Macrophages proved a suitable adult cell type for virus growth studies *in vitro.*[6] When macrophages were tested within a few days of being harvested from the peritoneal cavity, macrophages from susceptible mice supported viral replication to high titers, whereas in machrophages from genetically resistant mice virus titers slowly declined (Figure 1). This initial observation led to a series of experiments based on the assumption that macrophages were causally related to virus resistance *in vivo*. Attempts at transferring resistance or susceptibility with corresponding macrophage populations failed.[3] We then learned that there were

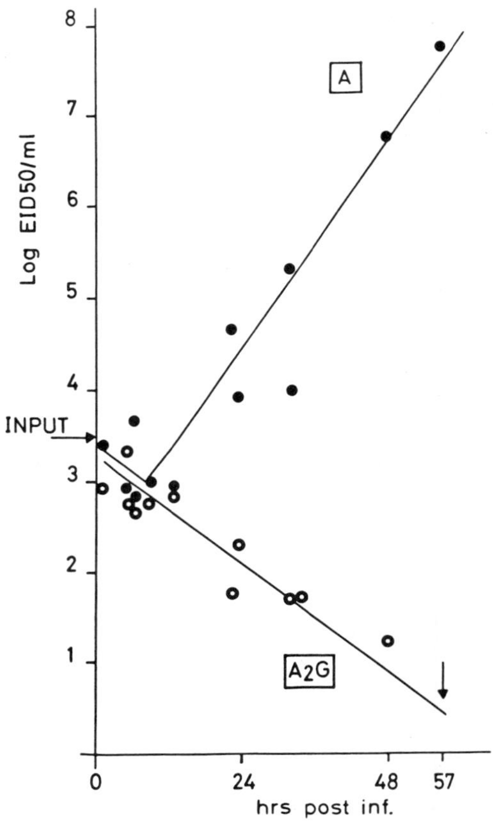

Figure 1. Growth of M-TUR virus in macrophages from genetically susceptible A/J mice (A) and in macrophages from genetically resistant *Mx/Mx* mice (A2G).

Macrophages were harvested from the peritoneal cavity of mice stimulated by thioglycollate medium 3 days previously. Cells were infected within the first days of cultivation as described.[6] M-TUR virus is an avian influenza A virus strain derived from A/Turkey/England/63 (Havl,Nav3) adapted to grow in mouse peritoneal macrophages *in vitro.*[6] (Reproduced from Lindenmann *et al.*[6] by permission of the publisher of *J. Exp. Med.*)

two ways of obtaining susceptible macrophages from resistant mice: We either had to pretreat the donor animals with anti-IF serum,[4] or we had to keep macrophages *in vitro* long enough for resistance to wane.[7] FIGURE 2 shows the growth of macrophage-adapted influenza A virus M-TUR in 3-week-old macrophages from genetically *Mx*/+ (*panel a*) or +/+ backcross mice (*panel b*). In the absence of exogenous IF virus growth in *Mx*/+ macrophages was comparable to that in macrophages from susceptible +/+ mice. Upon addition of 40 NIH reference units of IF, virus growth was only slightly delayed in +/+ macrophages, but so severly inhibited in *Mx*/+ macrophages that intial virus titers actually declined much as in FIGURE 1.

Infectivity of course is a complex measure of virus synthesis. To obtain some insight into the level at which viral maturation was arrested, we performed polyacrylamide gel electrophoreses of viral proteins in aged macrophages from either resistant (*Mx*/*Mx*) or susceptible (+/+) mice with or without pretreatment with interferon.

Anti-IF serum was added at the time of infection so that only the amount of IF used to pretreat the cells influenced the results shown in FIGURE 3. Synthesis of viral proteins was obvious in both types of macrophages in the absence of IF (lanes 7 and 10); addition of anti-IF serum at the time of infection did not alter

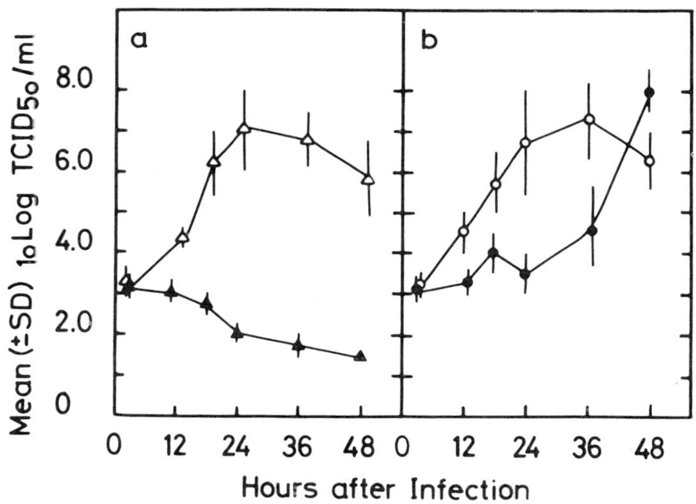

FIGURE 2. Inhibition by interferon of multiplication of M-TUR virus in macrophage cultures from backcross mice segregating for the allele *Mx*.

(A2G x C57BL/6J)F$_1$ (*Mx*/+) were backcrossed with C57BL/6J mice (+/+). The offspring were characterized as carriers (*Mx* +) or noncarriers (+/+) of the allele *Mx* as described.[6] After 3 weeks in culture, peritoneal macrophages obtained from individual *Mx*/+ or +/+ backcross mice where incubated for 18 hr with 40 reference units of mouse IF induced by NDV in mouse C-243 cells and partially purified to 1 x 10^7 reference units/mg protein.[16] Cells were then washed and infected with M-TUR virus at a multiplicity of 5. After incubation for 90 minutes at 37°C the virus inoculum was removed by repeated washings. Cell-free medium from individual cultures was titrated on primary chick embryo fibroblast (CEF) monolayers at the times after infection indicated. Titers represent mean values from three macrophage cultures of either resistant *Mx*/+ (*panel a*) or susceptible +/+ genotype (*panel b*).

△——△ (*Mx*/+) untreated; ▲——▲ (*Mx*/+) IF-treated; ○——○ (+/+) untreated; ●——● (+/+) IF-treated.

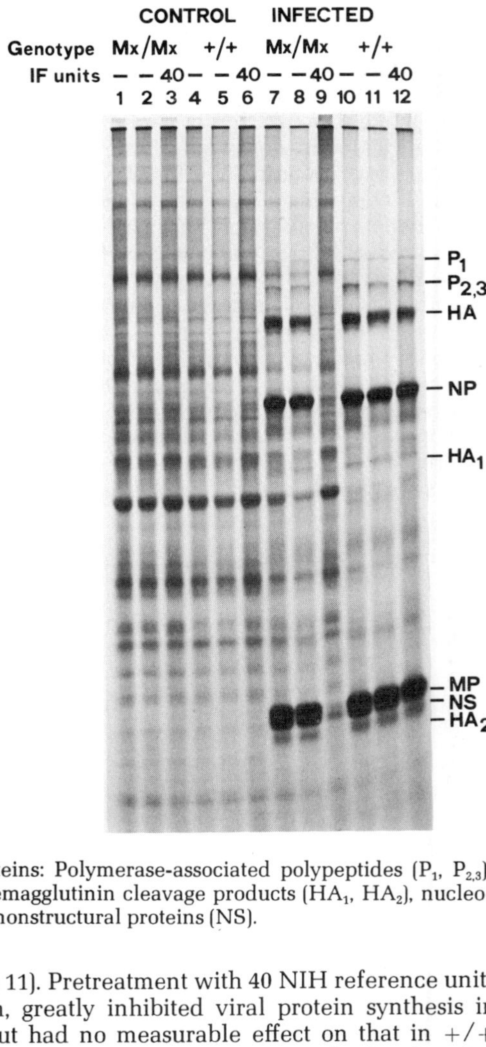

FIGURE 3. Effects of IF on synthesis of influenza virus proteins in aged macrophages from resistant A2G (*Mx/Mx*) or susceptible A/J (+/+) mice.

Peritoneal macrophages from mice genetically *Mx/Mx* (lanes 1–3 and 7–9) or +/+ (lanes 4–6 and 10–12) were kept for 3 weeks in culture and were then incubated for 18 hr with either 40 reference units/ml of partially purified mouse IF[16] (lanes 3,6,9,12) or normal control medium. Interferon pretreated and untreated cells were washed and infected with M-TUR virus at multiplicities of 5 (lanes 7–12). Sheep anti-mouse IF globulin[17] diluted to give a neutralizing titer of 1.2×10^{-3} was added at the time of infection to all but four culture wells to which normal sheep globulin was added (lanes 1,4,7,10). Infected and uninfected control cells were labeled for 30 min with [^{35}S]methionine at 7 hr after infection. Whole cell lysates were prepared and were subjected to electrophoresis on 11% polyacrylamide slab gels as described.[18] Autoradiography revealed the following viral proteins: Polymerase-associated polypeptides (P_1, $P_{2,3}$), uncleaved hemagglutinin (HA) and hemagglutinin cleavage products (HA_1, HA_2), nucleoprotein (NP), matrix protein (MP) and nonstructural proteins (NS).

virus protein patterns (lanes 8 and 11). Pretreatment with 40 NIH reference units of IF, followed by anti-IF serum, greatly inhibited viral protein synthesis in *Mx/Mx* macrophages (lane 9), but had no measurable effect on that in +/+ macrophages (lane 12). This gel pattern represents protein synthesis 7 hr after infection. All identifiable proteins appear to be similarly inhibited.

Specificity of Antiviral Action of Interferon in Cells of Different Genotypes

These experiments, while showing that *Mx*-bearing cells were more sensitive to the antiviral action of IF than their +/+ counterparts when challenged with influenza virus, failed to address the question of specificity. Two viruses capable of growing in macrophages, VSV (a rhabdovirus) and EMC (a picornavirus), were therefore compared with M-TUR (influenza A) for reduction of yields by graded doses of IF in aged *Mx/Mx*, *Mx*/+ and +/+ macrophages. FIGURE 4 shows that, whereas yields of VSV and EMC were similarly inhibited in all types of cells, yields of M-TUR were markedly reduced in homozygous (*Mx/Mx*) and heterozygous (*Mx*/+) cells from resistant animals, but much less reduced in cells from susceptible (+/+) mice. Yields of M-TUR virus in macrophages not pretreated with IF were not influenced by the presence or absence of the host resistance gene *Mx*.

To make sure that this was not some peculiarity of macrophages, we also used hepatocytes cultivated from resistant and from susceptible adult mice.[8] These could be used as hosts for a fourth virus, the DNA virus, HSV-1 (herpes simplex virus). A comparison of 24-hr yields of M-TUR, VSV and HSV-1 in *Mx*/*Mx* and +/+ hepatocytes treated with partially purified mouse IF is shown in TABLE 1. Untreated *Mx*/*Mx* hepatocytes were equally permissive for all three viruses as +/+ hepatocytes. However, 1000 reference units of IF severely impeded the growth of M-TUR virus in *Mx*-bearing hepatocytes (2.2 logs difference), but did not affect the same virus in ++ control cells. By contrast, IF had the same inhibitory power against VSV in both *Mx*-carrying cells and in controls (1.8 logs difference). Similarly, inhibition of HSV-1 multiplication was independent of the host cell genotype. Thus, in hepatocytes homozygous for *Mx*, M-TUR behaved as if it were a virus highly sensitive to IF action (in fact, as sensitive as VSV), whereas in +/+ cells it behaved as a virus extremely insensitive to IF (being the least sensitive of the three viruses tested).

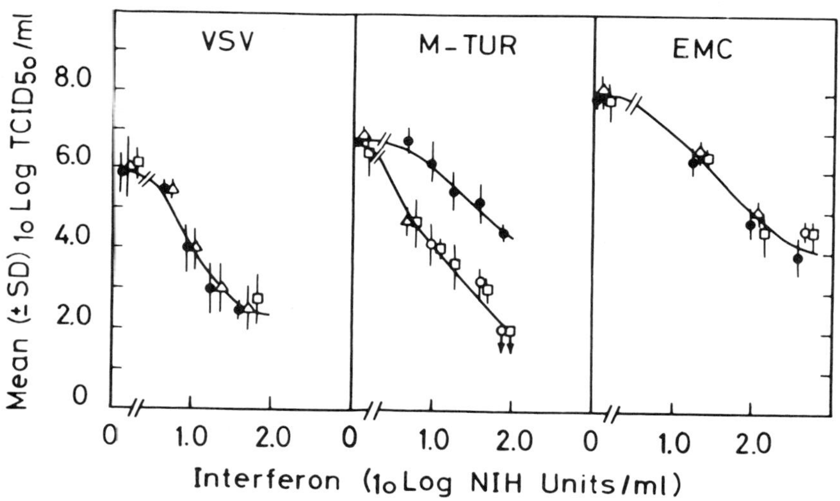

FIGURE 4. Effects of interferon on multiplication of VSV, M-TUR and EMC virus in macrophages from resistant or susceptible mice.

Peritoneal macrophages from resistant mice homozygous, (□——□), or heterozygous (Δ——Δ) for the allele *Mx*, and from susceptible +/+ mice (●——●) were cultured for 3 weeks and were then incubated for 18 hr with various doses of partially purified mouse interferon.[16] Thereafter, cultures were washed and infected at a multiplicity of 5 with either VSV, M-TUR or EMC virus. After an incubation period of 60 min at 37°C the virus inoculum was removed by repeated washings. The viral titer of cell-free medium from three individual cultures per IF dilution was determined 18 hr after viral infection (at the time of peak virus production in control cultures). VSV and EMC virus was titered in monolayer cultures of L_{929} cells and M-TUR virus in CEF. Mean $TCID_{50}$ values and standard deviations are indicated. The differences in yields of M-TUR virus between IF-treated +/+ and *Mx*-bearing macrophage cultures were statistically significant ($p < 0.01$ for all IF doses used).

TABLE 1

EFFECT OF INTERFERON ON VIRUS YIELD IN PRIMARY MONOLAYER CULTURES OF ADULT +/+ OR *Mx/Mx* HEPATOCYTES*

Type of Hepatocyte Culture	Interferon Reference Units	log_{10} $TCID_{50}$/ml		
		M-TUR	VSV	HSV-1
A/J (+/+)	0	7.5	7.1	7.0
	1000	7.3	5.3	5.5
A2G (*Mx/Mx*)	0	7.2	7.0	6.9
	1000	5.0	5.2	5.5

*Hepatocytes were isolated from genetically resistant or susceptible adult mice by a collagenase perfusion technique and primary monolayer cultures were established as described[8]. To avoid interference by spontaneously liberated IF (an unexplained property of mouse hepatocytes in culture[19,20]) anti-IF antibodies[17] (diluted to neutralize 10,000 reference units/ml) were added for the first 25 hr of culture. Antibodies were then removed by repeated washings and hepatocytes were incubated for 18 hr with either 1000 reference units of partially purified mouse IF (10^7 reference units/mg protein)[16] or normal control medium. Thereafter cells were infected with either M-TUR (at a multiplicity of 10) or with VSV (at a multiplicity of 10) or with HSV-1 (at a multiplicity of 0.1). Virus yield was determined 24 hr after infection as described.[19]

DISCUSSION

As an antiviral agent IF is thought to be largely nonspecific, except for differences in the amount of crossprotection of xenogeneic cells between IF preparations.[9,10] In the *Mx*-dependent resistance analyzed above, cooperation between a host gene and IF results in the establishment of an antiviral state that is particularly efficient in inhibiting the orthomyxo group. We could explain this by assuming either that essentially one antiviral state is created, but that its shape (the extent to which it trespasses on the biosynthetic demands of various viruses) is host gene dependent. This is schematically illustrated in FIGURE 5. Or we could envisage the overall antiviral state as being composed of several discrete antiviral sectors each specialized at inhibiting one particular group of viruses. This idea, which is perhaps not as different from the first one as might appear, is sketched in FIGURE 6. As the concentration of IF is increased, the areas inimical

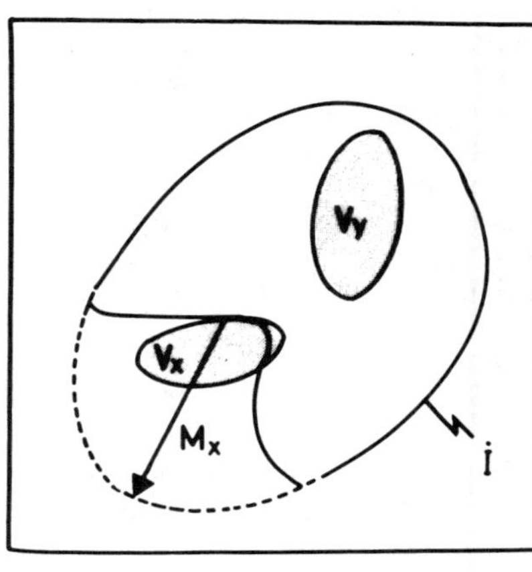

FIGURE 5. First working hypothesis based on the present findings.

A threshold amount of interferon (i) induces, in the absence of *Mx*, an antiviral state which is inhibitory to various groups of viruses (including e.g. the group V_y) but which is inefficient at inhibiting the orthomyxo group (V_x). In the presence of the resistance allele *Mx* the same amount of interferon creates a different antiviral state (dashed line) that is now also inhibitory to orthomyxo viruses. Thus, the host resistance gene *Mx* would either modulate the overall antiviral state induced by interferon or code for an additional antiviral mechanism activated by interferon.

to viral replication will enlarge and may eventually coalesce, thus increasing the resemblance between FIGURE 5 and FIGURE 6.

Although it may seem extravagant to postulate the existence of multiple antiviral states, the degree of complexity of IF action already brought to light and the likelihood that the *Mx* gene system is but one example of a whole family of resistance genes operating through IF mechanisms tend to make this an acceptable working hypothesis. Interferon appears to be a contributory if not a key factor e.g. in inborn resistance of mice to flaviviruses,[11] to mouse hepatitis virus,[12] and to herpes simplex virus.[13] We are currently investigating the extent to which IF plays a role in natural resistance against these and other unrelated viruses.

CONCLUSIONS

A prominent character of the IF system has been its absence of virus specificity. Nevertheless, it would now appear that, in the mouse, a certain degree of specificity may occur both at the level of IF production and at the level of IF action. Thus, De Maeyer and his coworkers have shown that inbred mouse strains differ significantly in their ability to produce IF in response to a given virus. Several *If* loci have been found to control the amount of circulating IF that is produced after injection of mice with different viruses.[14,15] Here, we have presented evidence for a genetic control of sensitivity to IF action resulting in virus-specific host resistance.

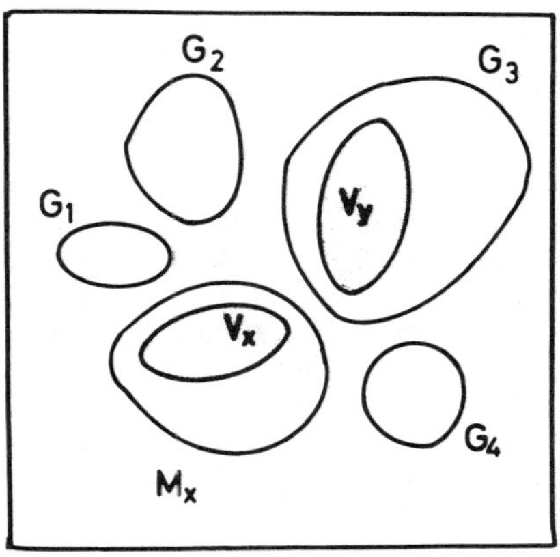

FIGURE 6. Second working hypothesis based on the present findings.

The host resistance gene *Mx* belongs to a number of gene loci (G_1 to G_4) each controlling a discrete antiviral state effective against one particular group of viruses (V_y, V_x). The co-expression of multiple antiviral states would explain the seemingly nonspecific antiviral action of interferon. Allelism at such loci would account for various degrees of protection induced by interferon.

If generally applicable, the present results and the observations of De Maeyer and associates might provide a clue to the better understanding of individual variations in susceptibility to viral diseases. It is conceivable that similar interactions between IF and host genes could be important not only in pathogenesis of viral infections but also with respect to nonantiviral effects of interferon.

ACKNOWLEDGMENTS

The expert technical and secretarial assistance of Mrs. M. Acklin, Mr. G. Barmettler, and Miss R. Leemann is gratefully acknowledged.

REFERENCES

1. LINDENMANN, J., C. A. LANE & D. HOBSON. 1963. The resistance of A2G mice to myxoviruses. J. Immunol. **90:** 942–951.
2. HALLER, O. & J. LINDENMANN. 1974. Athymic (nude) mice express gene for myxovirus resistance. Nature **250:** 679–680.
3. HALLER, O., H. ARNHEITER & J. LINDENMANN. 1979. Natural, genetically determined resistance toward influenza virus in hemopoietic mouse chimeras. J. Exp. Med. **150:** 117–126.
4. HALLER, O., H. ARNHEITER, I. GRESSER & J. LINDENMANN. 1979. Genetically determined, interferon-dependent resistance to influenza virus in mice. J. Exp. Med. **149:** 601–612.
5. FISKE, R. A. & P. A. KLEIN. 1975. Effect of immunosuppression on the genetic resistance of A2G mice to neurovirulent influenza virus. Infect. Immun. **11:** 576–587.
6. LINDENMANN, J., E. DEUEL, S. FANCONI & O. HALLER. 1978. Inborn resistance of mice to myxoviruses: Macrophages express phenotype in vitro. J. Exp. Med. **147:** 531–540.
7. HALLER, O., H. ARNHEITER, J. LINDENMANN & I. GRESSER. 1980. Host gene influences sensitivity to interferon action selectively for influenza virus. Nature **283:** 660–662.
8. ARNHEITER, H. 1980. Primary monolayer culture of adult mouse hepatocytes—A model for the study of hepatotropic viruses. Arch. Virol. **63:** 11–22.
9. STEWART, W. E. II, W. D. SCOTT & S. E. SULKIN. 1969. Relative sensitivites of virsuses to different species of interferon. J. Virol. **4:** 147–153.
10. YOUNGNER, J. S., H. R. THACORE & M. E. KELLY. 1972. Sensitivity of ribonucleic acid and deoxyribonucleic acid viruses to different species of interferon in cell cultures. J. Virol. **10:** 171–178.
11. HANSON, B., H. KOPROWSKI, S. BARON & C. E. BUCKLER. 1969. Interferon-mediated natural resistance of mice to arbo B virus infection. Microbios **1B:** 51–68.
12. VIRELIZIER, J.-L. & I. GRESSER. 1978. Role of interferon in the pathogenesis of viral diseases of mice as demonstrated by the use of anti-interferon serum. V. Protective role in mouse hepatitis virus type 3 infection of susceptible and resistant strains of mice. J. Immunol. **120:** 1616–1619.
13. ZAWATZY, R., J. HILFENHAUS & H. KIRCHNER. 1979. Resistance of nude mice to herpes simplex virus and correlation with *in vitro* production of interferon. Cell. Immunol. **47:** 424–428.
14. DE MAEYER, E. & J. DE MAEYER-GUIGNARD. 1969. Gene with quantitative effect on circulating interferon induced by Newcastle disease virus. J. Virol. **3:** 506–512.
15. DE MAEYER, E., J. DE MAEYER-GUIGNARD, W. T. HALL, & D. W. BAILEY. 1974. A locus affecting circulating interferon levels induced by mouse mammary tumor virus. J. Gen. Virol. **23:** 209–211.
16. TOVEY, M. G., J. BEGON-LOURS & I. GRESSER. 1974. A method for the large scale production of potent interferon preparation. Proc. Soc. Exp. Biol. Med. **146:** 809–815.
17. GRESSER, I., M. G. TOVEY, M.-T. BANDU, C. MAURY & D. BROUTY-BOYE. 1976. Role of interferon in the pathogenesis of virus diseases in mice as demonstrated by the use of anti-interferon serum. I. Rapid evolution of encephalomyocarditis virus infection. J. Exp. Med. **144:** 1305–1315.
18. HORISBERGER, M. A., O. HALLER & H. ARNHEITER. 1980. Interferon-dependent, genetic resistance to influenza virus in mice: Viral replication in macrophages is inhibited at an early step. J. Gen. Virol. In press.
19. ARNHEITER, H., O. HALLER & J. LINDENMANN. 1980. Host gene influence on interferon action in adult mouse hepatocytes specificity for influenza virus. Virology **103:** 11–20.
20. RENTON, K. W., L. B. DELORIA & G. J. MANNERING. 1978. Effects of polyriboinosinic acid·polyribocytidylic acid and a mouse interferon preparation on cytochrome P-450-dependent monooyxgenase systems in cultures of primary mouse hepatocytes. Mol. Pharmacol. **14:** 672–681.

CLOSING REMARKS

Thomas C. Merigan

Division of Infectious Diseases
Department of Medicine
Stanford University School of Medicine
Stanford, California 94305

During recent years and especially at this meeting, interferons have achieved a new status. They no longer just loosely defined factors, but are rather a group of full-fledged glycoprotein hormones, each one of which, within a given animal species, has a somewhat different structure, and they are now awaiting our precise definition of their individual functions. Such definition may allow practical applications as yet undreamed of. Unfortunately for those who must purify them, however, these hormones are not the products of a specific gland from which they may be extracted in bulk. Each interferon is capable of producing a plethora of specific changes within cells, even when they are purified to homogeneity. For those of us who are trying to use them as crude materials clinically, this latter point is reassuring in that we now can expect any beneficial effects we observed will also be seen with the pure material which will be used as a drug in the future.

Very efficient and simplified methods for interferon purification have been presented. New standards for characterization of interferon have been set at this meeting. Fortunately, this sometimes just represents a verification of the original investigator's impression. Some interferons are now very well defined structurally, with partial amino acid sequences having been determined. The structural homology between one pair of mouse and human interferons is reassuringly in keeping with the expected extent of evolutionary divergence from a common primordial parental form mediated by point mutations associated with single base changes. In addition, the homology should reassure the skeptics that contaminants are not being sequenced. Furthermore, for the genetic engineer with a DNA synthetic bent—the homology somewhat restricts the possible triplets for each amino acid codon. Finally, I believe that with complete structural definition, many rational pharmacological innovations will be possible—even possibly targeting of delivery within certain tissues.

Now, virtually no one can have doubts about the significance or existence of the interferon system. Its importance for the whole animal is underscored by the difficulties in identifying natural deficiency mutants and the presence of this mechanism in virtually all vertebrate species in which it has been sought.

The development of several quite reproducible *in vitro* translation systems has been facilitated by the great potency of interferon's biological activity. As with globin, such systems will be of great assistance in isolation of an interferon gene. The information on chromosomal location of interferon production presented at this meeting also should be helpful in genetic engineering efforts to produce interferon. For example, an appropriate synthetic cDNA or mRNA might be used to locate an interferon gene within the DNA of a specific chromosome. Because of the great interest and many laboratories working the recombinant DNA approach to interferon, we undoubtedly will begin to hear of results in this area in the near future.

Several biological roles of interferons have been defined, for example by use of neutralization with specific anti-interferon serum. We know interferon is but one component of what is fortunately a multi-tiered host defense system against viruses, other intracellular parasites, and tumor cells. In order to maintain their pathogenicity, all such agents have developed mechanisms to elude host defenses. Therefore, there can be no one single critical defense mechanism, which some investigators would have preferred for simplicity.

Considering the demands on cell differentiation, it is also critical that the regulatory effects of interferon not be simplistic, whether it is examined in the immune or hemopoietic systems, or for its action on other normal or neoplastic cells. In fact, the need for very stringent control of all regulation demands multiple regulatory and feedback mechanisms.

The molecular level mechanism of interferon's action is also better understood. Now, it is not defined just through its application to each advance in definition of viral replicative cycles, but, instead interferons are now revealing the existence of new intracellular regulatory pathways such as the (2′5′) oligo A system. This situation is analogous to work done with insulin in the past. That hormone has been utilized to discover new metabolic pathways for the utilization of carbohydrates, lipids, and proteins as fuels. So, interferon appears to be revealing pathways for the regulation of genetic expression. As these must be closely regulated, it should not be surprising that "too much of a good thing is bad."

The molecular biologists forte is the separation, isolation, and *in vitro* reconstitution of genetic elements. The mechanism by which DNA is expressed and RNA and protein are synthesized has now been clarified by such approaches in the least complex systems. Currently, the mechanism for expression of eukaryotic genes is under intense study, and I would not be surprised at all if the pathways that interferon plays upon turn out to be critical controlling elements. For example, the finding that heme controls globulin synthesis through phosphorylation of Initiation Factor 2 suggests their generality. Of course the final results of such regulation may be expressed on the cell's surfaces as well as within the cell.

As we have seen, mouse immunogenetics provides many powerful methods for taking apart the complexity of immunoregulation. However, a multiplicity of soluble factors other than interferon as well as direct cell-to-cell interactions have been identified for certain well-defined immunoregulatory functions such as suppressor T-cell actions. On the other hand, as demonstrated at this meeting, I do believe that now, most immunologists are quite interested in interferon and we can expect much more activity in this area by them as well. In fact, considering all the new faces, the significant advances, and the high quality of the work presented at this meeting, we can expect much progress in defining interferon's regulatory actions at the molecular, cellular, and whole animal levels.

MINIMAL INTERFERON INDUCTION IN DOGS AFTER USE OF A POTENT INDUCER

Jean S. Smith, Pamela A. Yager, and George M. Baer

Viral Zoonoses Branch, Virology Division
Bureau of Laboratories, Center for Disease Control
Public Health Service
Lawrenceville, Georgia 30246

Because of its nuclease resistance, poly I Eg poly C complexed with poly-L-lysine and carboxymethylcellulose (PICLC) induces high levels of interferon (IF) in normally resistant primates.[1] The effective dose in rhesus monkeys, however, is far above the lethality and tolerated toxicity range in dogs. Intravenous (i.v.) injection of 1 mg/kg of PICLC-induced IF in only 2 of 3 dogs and was extremely toxic to all 3. One animal died 4 hr after injection. The maximum response (expressed as the dilution of serum that reduces by 50% the vesicular stomatitis virus (VSV) plaque count on Madin-Darby canine kidney (MDCK) cell cultures) was 1:100 3 hr after injection of 1 mg/kg of PICLC. No IF was detectable by 24 hr after injection. Lower doses of PICLC were less toxic but were less successful in inducing IF.

Approximately the same toxicity was seen after intrathecal (i.t.) administration of smaller doses of PICLC, although the ultimate IF response was slightly better per milligram of PICLC. Twenty-four hours after i.t. injection of 0.4 mg/kg of PICLC, both injected animals had a cerebrospinal fluid (CSF) IF titer of 1:100. Serum IF was detectable in parallel blood samples in only one of the two animals injected i.t. and the titer (1:10) was lower than the CSF titer. As was found after i.v. injection, lower doses of PICLC produced less toxicity but also lower IF responses. The *in vitro* interfering effect of the CSF samples was shown not to be due to residual PICLC, since treatment of the CSF samples with RNAase A did not reduce the IF titer.

Intravenous injection of 8 ml of live Newcastle disease virus produced only barely detectable levels of IF, and injection of smaller amounts produced no response.

Assay of IF-positive serum samples on primary neonatal canine kidney (PNCK) failed to increase the titer obtained by assay on MDCK.

No IF was detected in PNCK or primary neonatal canine lung cultures pretreated with poly I · poly C or PICLC when the supernates were assayed on PNCK or MDCK. Despite this fact, a 24-hr pretreatment of these monolayers with as little as 200 μg/ml of PICLC protected them from infection with VSV. Treatment of the PICLC with RNAase A for 30 min destroyed this protective effect.

Several investigators have suggested that the low levels of IF in dogs after induction with a variety of inducers is due to the lack of sensitivity of the assay system used. However, because heterologous IF can be assayed on MDCK cells[2,3] and because we could protect these monolayers from VSV infection with only small amounts of PICLC, we believe that the low levels of IF induced in dogs by PICLC is not the result of an insensitive assay system but the result of a natural refractoriness of dogs to IF induction.

REFERENCES

1. LEVY, H. B., G. BAER, S. BARON, C. E. BUCKLER, C. J. GIBBS, M. J. IADAROLA, W. T. LONDON & J. RICE. 1975. A modified polyriboinosinic-polyribocytidylic acid complex that induces interferon in primates. J. Infect. Dis. **132:** 434–439.
2. SELLERS, R. F. & M. FITZPATRICK. 1963. Multiplication, interferon production and interferon sensitivity of viruses in dog kidney tissue cultures. Res. Vet. Sci. **4:** 151–159.
3. JAMESON, P., M. A. DIXON & S. E. GROSSBERG. 1977. A sensitive interferon assay for many species of cells: Encephalomyocarditis virus hemagglutinin yield reduction. Proc. Soc. Exp. Biol. Med. **155:** 173–178.

INTERFERON-INDUCED ENHANCEMENT OF LYMPHOCYTE CYTOTOXICITY: PRELIMINARY STUDIES OF LYMPHOCYTE SUBPOPULATIONS

Michael J. Droller

Johns Hopkins Hospital
Baltimore, Maryland

Hakan Borg

Kabi AB
Stockholm, Sweden

Introduction

Recent studies have documented an enhancement effect by interferon (IF) of both natural and antibody-dependent lymphocyte cytotoxicity against a variety of target cells *in vitro*. Since only certain subpopulations of lymphocytes may be involved in these cytotoxic mechanisms, we thought it of interest to examine whether the enhancement effect of IF was directed specifically on these populations of cells or whether other lymphocyte subpopulations not directly involved in either natural or antibody-dependent lymphocyte cytotoxicity might play a role in the enhancment effects of IF in these mechanisms.

Materials and Methods

Human peripheral blood lymphocytes were purified by gelatin sedimentation, elimination of monocytes by carbonyl iron incubation, and Ficoll-Hypaque centrifugation. These preparations were fractionated on columns of Sepharose gel coupled to the hemagglutinin A of the snail *Helix pomatia*. Briefly, neuraminidase-treated lymphocytes placed on the column either passed directly through the gel (fraction I) or were eluted with 0.1 mg/ml α-*N*-acetyl-D-galactosamine (D-Gal*N*Ac; fraction II) or 1.0 mg/ml D-Gal*N*Ac (fraction III). Fractions I and II were enriched in cells with F_c receptors (approximately 45–50% of cells in these fractions), as determined by formation of EA rosettes, and fraction III, having fewer F_c receptor-bearing cells (only ~10% of cells), was enriched in cells forming rosettes with sheep erythrocytes (approximately 65% of cells).

Cytotoxicity of these fractions was assessed by incubating lymphocytes with ^{51}Cr-labeled target cells (T_{24} and HCV_{29}) in the presence or absence of anti-T_{24} antiserum, and calculating the percent ^{51}Cr release after 16 hr at 37°C. Human leukocyte- or fibroblast-derived IF preparations (PIF, courtesy of the Finnish Red Cross and Dr. Kari Cantell, and preparation 563-Kabi) were tested in these assays for their direct effect on cytotoxicity. In other experiments, lymphocyte fractions generally not cytotoxic in this system (fraction III), especially when antibody-dependent lymphocyte cytotoxicity was examined, were preincubated with interferon and then recombined with nonpreincubated lymphocyte fractions ordinarily cytotoxic in this system (fractions I or II) in order to detect possible indirect IF-induced enhancement effects.

Results

Both leukocyte- and fibroblast-derived IF preparations were found to enhance natural and possibly antibody-dependent lymphocyte cytotoxicity. Parallel preparations of "mock" IF did not enhance cytotoxicity. Examination of these effects on fractionated lymphocytes demonstrated IF-induced enhancement only of cytotoxicity of fractions I and II in this system. Minimal or no enhancement of either the natural or antibody-dependent cytotoxicity mechanism by IF could be demonstrated with fraction III lymphocytes.

When fraction III lymphocytes were preincubated with IF and then added to nonpreincubated fractions I or II lymphocytes, no enhancement of cytotoxicity was seen. In these experiments, enhancement only occurred when IF was present for the duration of incubation during the cytotoxicity assay.

Discussion

Interferon appeared to enhance natural and possibly antibody-dependent lymphocyte cytotoxicity in the present system by direct action on lymphocyte fractions enriched in cells with F_c receptors. In contrast, lymphocyte fractions that ordinarily appeared to express minimal or no antibody-dependent cytotoxicity did not demonstrate enhancement of natural cytotoxicity when incubated with interferon.

If these same lymphocytes were preincubated with IF, fraction III cells did not enhance cytotoxicity by fractions I or II lymphocytes that had not been preincubated when recombined fractions were tested in the cytotoxicity assay. It therefore appeared that cells not ordinarily involved in antibody-dependent lymphocyte cytotoxicity did not respond to incubation with IF by enhancing the expression of either the natural or the antibody-dependent cytotoxicity mechanism by other lymphocyte fractions.

DIFFERENT SUSCEPTIBILITY OF K AND NK CELLS TO MODULATION BY INTERFERONS

H. Rumpold, D. Kraft, O. Scheiner, P. Meindl, and G. Bodo

Institute of General and Experimental Pathology
University of Vienna and
Ernst-Boehringer Research Institute
Vienna, Austria

Two different interferons (IFs) derived either from a human lymphoblastoid cell line (Namalva) or from human fibroblasts were tested for their ability to modulate NK- or K-cell activity.

The lymphoblastoid IF (LIF) was purified by ion exchange chromatography on SP-Sephadex C-25 and gel filtration on Sephadex G-100. The fibroblast-derived IF (FIF)was purified by chromatography on porous glass beads. The specific activity was 3×10^6 IU/mg protein for LIF and 1.2×10^5 IU/mg protein for FIF.

Various tissue culture cells (HeLa, K 562, T 56) showing different susceptibility to lysis by NK cells were used as targets. With any of these target-cells NK cell activity was enhanced by LIF or FIF in a dose-dependent manner; both IFs were active to a similar extent. Augmentation of cytotoxicity was observed at IF concentrations as low as 33 IU/ml. Kinetic studies of the response of NK cells to interferons revealed peak activity after 2 hours preincubation time with LIF or FIF.

Since most tissue culture cells which are used in K-cell studies are also susceptible to lysis by NK cells, the influence of IF on K-cell activity can hardly be estimated, and different results have been reported so far showing either unchanged (Trinchieri *et al.* 1978. J. Immunol. **120:** 1849) or enhanced (Herberman *et al.* 1979. Nature **277:** 221) K-cell activity by IF. Therefore we used a K-cell assay that allows us to measure K-cell activity alone: autologous lymphocytes or erythrocytes were coated with bencylpenicilloyl (BPO) groups and an affinity chromatographically purified rabbit anti-BPO IgG was used at a concentration of 3 μg/ml. In this experimental setup no NK-cell activity is found with or without the addition of LIF or FIF. However, these hapten-coated autologous cells served as good targets for measurement of K-cell activity. Addition of LIF or FIF caused no change in K-cell activity. It can be concluded from our results that only NK-cell activity is modulated by IF.

EFFECT OF HUMAN LEUKOCYTE INTERFERON ON NATURAL KILLER ACTIVITY AND GROWTH INHIBITORY ACTIVITY OF HUMAN PERIPHERAL BLOOD LYMPHOCYTES AGAINST TUMOR CELLS*

Takashi Amagai,† Masakazu Kita, Jiro Imanishi, and Tsunataro Kishida

Department of Microbiology
Kyoto Prefectural University of Medicine
Kyoto, Japan

Sigeru Muramatsu

Department of Zoology, Faculty of Science
Kyoto University
Kyoto, Japan

It is becoming clear that interferon (IF) preparations have not only a direct inhibitory effect on tumor cells but also indirect tumoricidal or tumorstatic effects by the activation of lymphoid cells and macrophages. We investigated the effect of human leukocyte interferon (HLIF) on two types of inhibitory activities of human peripheral blood lymphocytes (PBL) against tumor cells, i.e., natural killer cell (NK) activity and tumor cell-growth inhibitory activity *in vitro*.

PBL were prepared from healthy donors by the method of Ficoll-Hypaque, and used as effector cells. Specific activity of partially purified HLIF was 3×10^5 IU/mg-protein. NK assay was done by ^{51}Cr-release test for 9 hr, and growth-inhibitory activity was assayed by viable cell counting of adherent tumor cells 1 and 3 days after culture initiation.

HLIF at the concentration of 50 IU/ml or more enhanced the NK activity only against NK-sensitive target cells (BALL, Daudi, Molt-4, and Namalva). Raji cells were not suceptible even to HLIF-treated PBL. HLIF at the concentration of 1.7 IU/ml or more also augmented the growth inhibitory activity of PBL against HeLa, KB, HEp-2, FL, and U cells. No correlation was found between the HLIF-stimulated tumor-inhibitory activities and the sensitivity of target cells to the direct action of HLIF in either assay. Anti-HLIF serum-treated HLIF did not cause enhancement in either assay.

NK and growth inhibitory activities of PBL was not clearly separated by fractionation using AET-E rosetting. Both activities did not depend on the presence of phagocytic cells in PBL preparation: moreover, in the case of NK activity, the enhancing effect of HLIF was rather increased after depletion of phagocytic cells. By fractionation with nylon wool column, though original NK activity was found in the nylon-passed fraction of PBL, both nylon-passed and nylon-retained cells were activated by HLIF to express tumoricidal activity against BALL. On the other hand, nylon-wool-adherent cells were responsible

*Supported by a grant-in-aid for cancer research from the Ministry of Education, Science, and Culture of Japan.

†*Present address:* Institute of Immunology, Medical Sciences Building, University of Toronto, Toronto, Ontario, Canada.

for the original and HLIF-stimulated growth inhibitory activity of PBL against HeLa cells.

X-irradiation (2000 rad) of PBL did not affect original and enhanced tumor inhibitory activities in either assay. Cycloheximide or actinomycin-D treatment caused suppression of HLIF-stimulated NK activity. The suppression of original NK activity by these drugs was rather weak. Furthermore, the enhancement of NK activity by HLIF was also shown in the cytotoxic assay that was started with calcium-free medium, with the medium containing calcium and cytochracin A being added 1 or 2 hours after the initiation of incubation.[1]

Our results suggest that at least two different types of tumor-inhibitory activities of human PBL are enhanced by the addition of HLIF without proliferation of effector cells. In the case of NK activity, the treatment of PBL with HLIF caused an increase in the number of effector cells. This suggests that IF may act as a promotor of cell differentiation without mitosis.

Reference

1. Thorn, R. N., & C. S. Henny. 1976. Enumeration of specific cytotoxic T cells. Nature **265:** 75–76.

ON THE EXPEDIENCY OF USING AS A THERAPEUTIC METHOD THE REMOVAL OF LYMPHOCYTES (AS SOURCES OF INTERFERON PRODUCTION) FROM THE BLOOD OF PATIENTS WITH RHEUMATOID ARTHRITIS (RA)

Semyon V. Skurkovich

261 Congressional Lane #709
Rockville, Maryland 20852

It has been suggested that each antigen or substance that might be an antigen determinant can induce interferon (IF).[1,2] It is considered that hyperproduction of IF plays an important role in mechanisms of the development of the allergic and autoimmune diseases (AAID) in man. Excessive amounts of IF are produced by immune lymphocytes and target cells which will be later involved in the pathology of AAID, and interferon accumulates in the blood.[2,3] Interferon causes target cells to become more sensitized to autoantibodies[4]; and immmune lymphocytes become more cytotoxic to the antigens.[5-7] Also, the possibility must not be ruled out that target cells which produce IF become sensitized to the circulating natural antibodies (against these target cells); and natural killer cell cytotoxicity of lymphocytes to the target cells in augmented by IF (produced in excessive quantities).[7] Impairment of the regulation of IF production by lymphocytes and nonlymphoid cells leads to the distortion of the integral immunity.[2] It is possible that hyperproduction of IF can also lead to the removal of the immunological tolerance to some autoantigens[2] and can disturb the immunosurveillance of lymphocytes. Circulating autoantigens, autoantigen complexes (especially complexes of viruses with cell antigens), denaturated DNA, immune complexes and other agents, may become important factors in the stimulation of interferon development. In our earlier studies[2] and many further observations, IF was found in the blood of patients with AAID. These data were confirmed by J. J. Hooks *et al.*[8] The treatment of immune lymphocytes with anti-IF antibodies decreases their specific cytotoxicity.[9] We think that one possible method of the treating AAID or diseases connected with the harmful action of IF could be removal of IF from the patient's body, or its disintegration.[2,3] Earlier we successfully used anti-IF immunoglobulin for the treatment of patients with RA and several other AAID.[10] Because lymphocytes are the main source of immune IF we suggested[10] that AAID be treated by periodic removals of lymphocytes from the blood of the patients by lymphocytopheresis. Jointly with Drs. N. Dubrovina and E. Eremkina, repeated removals of lymphocytes from the blood of 5 RA patients were made. Our preliminary data showed therapeutic effects. The patients showed a tendency for the IF level in their blood to change. We believe that the IF level in the sera of patients with AAID can be one of the criteria for evaluating their clinical course. We think that it is important to find chemical and biological agents which might inhibit IF. It is possible that biological substances isolated from malignant cells or from products of the metabolism of oncogenic viruses may be a probable source of such agents. Also, new drugs, especially drugs used for the therapy of AAID, should be checked for their possible IF-producing or IF-disintegrating activity. It is of great importance to develop an efficient method for the determination of IF levels in sera of patients with AAID for diagnostic and prognostic purposes.

REFERENCES

1. SKURKOVICH S. V., E. G. KLINOVA, I. M. ALEXANDROVSKAYA, N. V. LEVINA, N. A. ARKHIPOVA & T. I. BULICHEVA. 1973. Stimulation of transplantation immunity and plasma cell reaction by interferon in mice. Immunology **25:** 317–322.
2. SKURKOVICH S. V. & E. I. EREMKINA. 1975. The probable role of interferon in allergy. Ann. Allergy **35:** 356.
3. SKURKOVICH S. V., E. G. KLINOVA, E. I. EREMKINA & N. V. LEVINA. 1974. Immunosuppressive effect of anti-interferon serum. Nature **217:** 551.
4. SKURKOVICH S. V., I. A. KALININA, E. I. EREMKINA & T. I. BULICHEVA. 1976. Increased sensitivity of leukemic cells incubated in interferon to the action of immune serum. Byull. Eksp. Biol. Med. **12:** 1459 (in Russian). English translation Russian: Bexban **82**(12): 1761–1930, 1976, Consultants Bureau, New York.
5. LINDHAL P., P. LEARY & I. GRESSER. 1972. Enhancement by interferon of the specific cytotoxicity of sensitized lymphocytes. Proc. Nat. Acad. Sci. USA **69**:3: 721.
6. SVET-MOLDAVSKY G. J., B. M. NEMIROVSKAJA, T. B. OSIPOVA, E. G. SLAVINA, S. N. ZINZAR, N. B. KARMANOVA & L. F. MOROZOVA. 1973. Interferon, immunologicheskoe raspoznavanie i zitotoksichnost' limfozitov. Vopr. Virusol. **5:** 541 (in Russian).
7. SKURKOVICH S. V., A. S. SKORIKOVA & E. I. EREMKINA. 1978. Enhancement by interferon of lymphocyte cytotoxicity in normal individuals to cells of human lymphoblastoid lines. J. Immunol. **121:** 1173–1176.
8. HOOKS J. J., H. M. MOUTSOPOULOS, S. A. GEIS, N. I. STAHL, J. L. DECKER & A. L. NOTKINS. 1979. Immune interferon in the circulation of patients with autoimmune disease. New Engl. J. Med. **301:** 5–8.
9. SKURKOVICH S. V., A. S. SKORIKOVA, N. V. OL'SHANSKAJA, A. J. OL'SHANSKY & E. G. KLINOVA. 1976. Decreases of cytotoxic activity of immune lymphocytes after their treatment with antiinterferon globulin. Personal communication. Interferon Scientific Memoranda, October.
10. SKURKOVICH S. V., A. S. SKORIKOVA, N. A. DUBROVINA, T. V. RIABOVA, E. I. EREMKINA, V. N. GOLODNANKOVA, E. G. KLINOVA, A. J. OL'SHANSKY & N. F. SHURLAPOVA. 1977. Lymphocytes' cytotoxicity towards cells of human lymphoblastoid lines in patients with rheumatoid arthritis and systemic lupus erythematosus. Ann. Allergy **39:** 344–350.

RELEASE OF HUMAN LEUKOCYTE INHIBITORY FACTOR (LIF) BY BLOOD MONONUCLEAR CELLS IN THE PRESENCE OF INTERFERON (IF) AND ANTIGEN

I. Suslov, J. L. McCoy, and R. B. Herberman

Laboratory of Immunodiagnosis
National Cancer Institute, National Institutes of Health
Bethesda, Maryland 20205

The ability of IF to affect host immune systems is now widely recognized. Somewhat dependent on dosage levels, IF has both stimulatory and inhibitory actions on a variety of immune parameters including antibody production,[1-5] allograft rejection responses,[6,7] graft-versus-host reactions[8,9] and augmentation of cytotoxicity by natural killer lymphocytes[10-13] and macrophages.[14-17] This study was designed to determine the possible stimulation of antigen-triggered production of the lymphokine, leukocyte-inhibitory factor (LIF)[18] from human mononuclear (MN) cells in the presence of IF. LIF may be produced by either T and B lymphocytes,[19] with the aid of monocyte accessory tells (McCoy, unpublished data).

MN cells from tuberculin skin test negative individuals were incubated with purified protein derivative (PPD) for 2 hr with or without IF, washed and then cultured for 24 hr in the presence of media without PPD or IF. Culture supernatants were harvested and assayed for LIF activity by the inhibition of migration of human polymorphonuclear cells from agarose droplets. In the absence of IF none of 22 tuberculin skin-test-negative donors produced LIF in response to PPD. In contrast, 18/23 (78%) of tuberculin-negative individuals released LIF following PPD stimulation in the presence of IF. LIF was also produced by MN cells that were exposed for only 5 min to IF, washed, and then incubated with PPD. LIF was detectable after the exposure of MN cells from some individuals with as little as 33 units of IF, and 100–333 units was sufficient with most of the other donors. Higher doses of IF (10^3–10^5 units) usually failed to stimulate LIF release. Further, antisera against IF completely abolished the effect of IF on LIF production.

Stimulation of LIF production in the presence of IF was also detected after exposure of MN cells of normal donors to another antigen: a 3M KC1 extract of lung carcinoma tissue (7661) known to be antigenic in LIF assays with lung cancer patients but not in normal donors. None of 30 normal donors reacted to the 7661 extract alone whereas 13/30 (43%) produced LIF in response to the extract in the presence of IF.

MN cells of normal donors were also incubated with a third antigen, keyhole limpet hemocyanin (KLH), in the presence of IF. A total of 10/12 (82%) KLH-nonsensitive normal donors produced LIF following exposure to KLH in the presence of IF, as compared to none of 12 normal donors tested without IF. The data with the KLH antigen largely excluded the possibility that the individuals with positive LIF responses in the presence of IF with the PPD and lung cancer antigens might be due to a low level presensitization, with *in vitro* IF treatment augmenting the usually undetectable immune responses to these antigens.

Studies with subpopulations of MN cells using G-10 Sephadex column separation techniques, suggested that IF augmentation of LIF production occurred at the level of the monocyte. When separated monocytes were treated with IF and then added into T and B lymphocytes depleted of monocytes, LIF was released following exposure to antigen. In contrast, IF-treated T and B lymphocytes depleted of monocytes, followed by addition of untreated monocytes, failed to produce LIF in the presence of antigen.

In summary, the results show that low concentrations of IF stimulate production of the lymphokine, LIF. IF stimulation is apparently antigen-dependent, and it appears to trigger or accentuate the ability of monocytes to react with antigen prior to an interaction of these monocytes with T and B lymphocytes. IF may actually facilitate or accelerate *in vitro* induction of a primary immune response to these antigens.

References

1. Johnson, H. M., B. G. Smith & S. Baron. 1975. Inhibition of the primary *in vitro* antibody response by interferon preparations. J. Immunol. **114:** 403.
2. Brodeur, B. R. & T. C. Merigan. 1975. Mechanism of the suppressive effect of interferon on antibody synthesis *in vivo*. J. Immunol. **114:** 1323.
3. Gisler, R. H., P. Lindahl & I. Gresser. 1974. Effects of interferon on antibody synthesis *in vitro*. J. Immunol. **133:** 438.
4. Brown W. & H. B. Levy. 1972. Interferon preparations as modifiers of immune responses. Proc. Soc. Exp. Biol. Med. **141:** 769.
5. Stannegard, Ö, I. Larsson, E. Lundgren, H. Miörner & H. Persson. 1978. Modulation of immune responses in new-born and adult mice by interferon. Infect. Immun. **20:** 334.
6. Hirsh, M. S., D. A. Ellis, M. R. Proffit, P. H. Back & M. A. Chirigos. 1973. Effects of interferon on leukemia virus activation in graft versus host disease. Nature New Biol. **244:** 102.
7. Skurkovich, S. V., E. G. Klinova, I. M. Alexandrovskaya, N. V. Levina, N. A. Arkhipova & T. I. Bulicheva. 1973. Stimulation of transplantation immunity and plasma cell reaction by interferon in mice. Immunology **25:** 317.
8. DeMaeyer, E. & J. DeMaeyer-Guignard. 1977. Effect of interferon on cell-mediated immunity. Tex. Rep. Biol. Med. **35:** 370.
9. Levy, H. B., R. Adamson, P. Carlone, V. DeVita, A. Gazdar, J. Rhim, A. Weinstein & F. Riley. 1971. Studies of the antitumor action of poly I:poly C. *In* Biological Effects of Polynucleotides. R. F. Beerds & W. Brown, Eds.:55. Springer-Verlag.
10. Herberman, R. B., J. R. Ortaldo & G. D. Bonnard. 1979. Augmentation by interferon of human natural and antibody-dependent cell-mediated cytotoxicity. Nature **277:** 221.
11. Herberman, R. B., J. Y. Djeu, H. D. Kay, J. R. Ortaldo, C. Riccardi, G. D. Bonnard, H. T. Holden, R. Fagnani, A. Santoni & P. Puccetti. 1979. Natural killer cells: Characteristics and regulation of activity. Immunol. Rev. **44:** 43.
12. Senik, A., I. Gresser, C. Maury, M. Gidlund, A. Örn & M. Wigzel. 1979. Enhancement of mouse NK cells by interferon. Transplant. Proc. **11:** 993.
13. Einhorn, S., H. Blomgren & H. Strander. 1979. Interferon and spontaneous cytotoxicity in man. Cancer Letters **7:** 1.
14. Huang, K. Y., R. M. Dunahoe, F. B. Gordon & H. B. Dressler. 1971. Enhancement of phagocytoses by interferon containing preparations. Infect. Immun. **4:** 581.
15. Dunahoe, R. M. & K. Y. Huang. 1976. Interferon preparations enhance phagocytosis *in vivo*. Infect. Immun. **13:** 1250.
16. Hamburg, S. I., R. E. Manejias & M. Rabinovitch. 1978. Macrophage activation: Increased injestion of IgG-coated erythrocytes after administration of interferon-inducers in mice. J. Exp. Med. **147:** 593.

17. DEGRÉ, M. & M. ROLLAG. 1979. Influence of interferon on the *in vivo* phagocytic activity of reticuloendothelial system cells. J. Reticuloendothel. Soc. **25:** 489.
18. ROCKLIN, R. E. 1974. Products of activated lymphocytes: Leukocyte inhibitory factor (LIF) distinct from migration inhibition factor. J. Immunol. **112:** 1461.
19. CHESS, L., R. E. ROCKLIN, D. MACDERMOTT, JR. & S. F. SCHLOSSMAN. Leukocyte inhibitory factor (LIF). Production by purified human T and B lymphocytes. J. Immunol. **115:** 315.

IN VIVO ADMINISTRATION OF INTERFERON TO MAN: STUDIES ON THE IMMUNE SYSTEM.

Stefan Einhorn,* Henric Blomgren,* Kari Cantell,†
Hans Strander,* and Marita Troye‡

**Radiumhemmet*
Karolinska Hospital
Stockholm, Sweden
†Department of Virology
Central Public Health Laboratory
Helsinki, Finland
‡Department of Immunology
University of Stockholm
Stockholm, Sweden

Introduction

Clinical trials in man for the evaluation of the antitumor effect of human leukocyte interferon (IF) therapy have been going on in Stockholm since 1969. To date more than 200 patients with a variety of tumors have been included in these studies. Although IF has been shown to exert antitumor effects in animals and, at least in some tumors, also in man, the mechanism behind these effects is not fully understood. One possibility could be an IF effect on the immune system. We have therefore studied the effect of *in vivo* administration of IF on some functions of the immune system.

Natural Killer Activity

Certain nonsensitized lymphocytes have the capacity to spontaneously kill allogeneic tumor cells *in vitro*. When the lymphocytes are treated with IF this natural killer (NK) activity is enhanced. Since, it has been suggested that the NK system plays a role in the host's defense against tumors, we studied the effect of *in vivo* administration of IF on the NK activity of peripheral lymphocytes in 40 patients with a variety of tumors (mainly myeloma, osteosarcoma, and melanoma). In 5 of these, NK activity was tested before and 6, 12, 24 and 48 hr after the first injection of IF (3 million units). After a slight decrease in NK activity 6 hr after the injection this activity increased and reached a peak activity 24 hr after the injection. Thereafter NK activity decreased, but was still above preinjection level 48 hr after the injection. Of the patients tested, 39 exhibited an enhanced NK activity 24 hr after the injection. This effect was statistically significant ($p < 0.001$).

In 5 patients NK activity was measured before and after 1 day, 1 week, 3 months and 6 months of IF therapy (3 million units daily). After the initial increase of NK activity after the first IF injection, the enhanced NK activity was maintained during prolonged IF therapy. In 15 patients tested before and after 3 months of IF therapy, 14 exhibited enhanced NK activity during *in vivo* administration of IF. This effect was statistically significant ($p < 0.001$).

Lymphocyte Subpopulations: In Vivo *Studies*

The frequency of lymphocytes forming E-(T-cells), EA-(Fc-receptor bearing cells) and EAC-rosettes (C'3 receptor-bearing cells) was studied in 20 tumor patients before and after an injection of IF (3 million units). Six hr after the injection a statistically significant reduction in the proportion of E-rosette forming lymphocytes was seen, followed by a statistically significant increase 24 hr after IF injection. No major change in the frequency of lymphocyte formation of EA- and EAC-rosettes was seen after the IF injection.

Lymphocyte Subpopulations: In Vitro *Studies*

The frequency of lymphocyte formation of E-, EA- and EAC-rosettes after treatment with IF was also studied *in vitro*. After pretreatment of the lymphocytes with IF the frequency of E-rosette-forming lymphocytes increased whereas the proportion of lymphocytes forming EA-rosettes decreased. In 12 experiments performed, the mean increase in percent E-rosettes was 11 ± 2 (S.E.) and the mean decrease in percent EA-rosettes was 5 ± 1 (S.E.). These effects were statistically significant ($p < 0.001$). The proportion of lymphocytes forming EAC-rosettes was not altered to any measurable extent by IF treatment *in vitro*.

Mitogens

In 20 patients with osteosarcoma the response of peripheral lymphocytes to the mitogens PHA, PWM and Con A was studied before, during, and after IF therapy (3 million units 3 times weekly for 18 months). The response of the lymphocytes to these mitogens remained essentially unchanged during as well as after completion of IF therapy.

Conclusion

Some functions of the immune system are affected by *in vivo* administration of human leukocyte IF. We do not know if these effects are of benefit for the tumor patients.

EFFECT OF MURINE INTERFERON ON PHAGOCYTOSIS *IN VITRO* AND *IN VIVO*

M. Degré and H. Rollag, Jr.

Captain Wilhelmsens Institute of Bacteriology
University of Oslo
Rikshospitalet
Oslo, Norway

Phagocytosis is considered to be one of the key defense factors against infections. The particles in the first step attach to one of the several functional surface receptors on the phagocytic cell before ingestion. The three types of receptors are: the Fc receptor, the complement receptor, and the nonspecific receptor.[1] The receptor chosen in a system is dependent on the nature of the particles and the presence of some external factors. Several phases of the phagocytic process, including attachment, can be influenced by external factors, e.g. by interferon (IF).[2,3]

Earlier studies on the effect of IF on phagocytosis have been done with crude methods and usually employed inert particles like latex or carbon particles. We have reexamined the problem employing the naturally occurring object of phagocytosis, bacteria, using improved methods, and defining the uptake by the nonspecific attachment pathway as the object of the study.

Peritoneal macrophages were obtained from unstimulated mice and cultured in Leighton tubes. The cells were treated with L-cell IF in various concentrations and for various time periods. Suspensions of ^{32}P-labeled *E. coli* were presented to the macrophages in Krebs-Ringer buffer with 10 μM glucose, without serum. The phagocytosis period was usually 90 min. Uptake of bacteria was registered by several parameters. Monolayers were light-microscopically quantitated for the proportion of macrophages containing bacteria and the number of bacteria per macrophage. The distribution of the radioactive label was determined by liquid scintillation.[4]

Interferon treatment dose-dependently enhanced uptake of bacteria, up to ca. 10^3 units per ml. Very high concentrations (i.e. over 10^4 units per ml) depressed the uptake. The active factor was characterized as IF by the standard physicochemical treatments. Specific anti-IF serum neutralized the phagocytosis-enhancing effect. The development of the phagocytosis-enhancing effect was time-dependent, and it was similar to the development of the antiviral effect of IF. Only a slight effect was observed after 2 hr of treatment. With prolonged treatment the effect increased until the maximal effect was obtained after 24 hr of treatment.

In another series of experiments we examined whether the phagocytosis can be influenced by IF *in vivo*. Mice were injected intraperitoneally with various concentrations of IF. The phagocytic effect was measured by the clearance of intravenously injected collidal carbon particles.[5]

The phagocytic index was calculated on the basis of spectrophotometrically measured concentration of carbon particles in paired blood samples. The IF effect was dose and time dependent. No effect was observed 4 hr after injection. Significant enhancement was seen 24 hr later by 5×10^4 units of IF. This effect was diminishing but still present 48 hr after injection. Interferon could be demonstrated in the serum for ca. 4 hr in concentrations 100–150 units per ml. Mock IF had no effect. Currently we are investigating the localization of the IF effect on the various phases of phagocytosis, the possible mechanism of the action, and a similar effect on other types of phagocytic cells.

References

1. Schroit, A. J. & R. Gallily, 1977. Immunology **33:** 121–127.
2. Huang, K. Y., R. M. Donahoe, F. B. Gordon & H. R. Dressler. 1971. Infect. Immunol. **4:** 581–588.
3. Imanishi, J., Y. Yokota, T. Kishida, T. Mukainaka & A. Matsuo, 1975. Acta Virol. **19:** 52–58.
4. Rollag, H., Jr 1979, Acta Pathol. Microbiol. Scand. Sect. C **87:** 99–105.
5. Biozzi, G., B. Benacerraf & B. N. Halpern, 1953. Br. J. Exp. Pathol. **34:** 441–457.

BIOLOGICAL CHARACTERIZATION OF TUBERCULIN-INDUCED HUMAN LYMPHOCYTE INTERFERON-LIKE SUBSTANCE (PPD-IF)

Spencer H. S. Lee and Kenneth R. Rozee

Department of Microbiology
Dalhousie University
Halifax, Nova Scotia, Canada

We described (1) an *in vitro* PPD-induced interferon (IF) system using human peripheral lymphocytes producing acid-labile (type II) human IF; (2) the immunocyte origin of this IF and (3) the antiviral and the cell-multiplication-inhibitory activities of type II IF compared to classic acid-stable (type I) human leukocyte IF (Leu-IF) in various cell cultures.

Leukocytic cell suspensions were prepared from peripheral blood obtained from groups of healthy Mantoux positive (PPD-POS) and negative (PPD-NEG) adults. PPD sensitivity, assessed by skin test reactivity, was correlated with the donors' lymphocyte antigenic response to PPD (2-25 μg/ml), using uptake of H^3-TdR into DNA[1] on day 6 of culture.

Peripheral blood mononuclear cells (PBMC) were isolated from 50–100 ml of heparinized venous blood by Ficoll-Hypaque (F/H) gradient centrifugation.[2] PBMC were further separated by repeated rosetting with neuraminidase-treated sheep erythrocyte (E) followed by F&H centrifugation into E-rosette-forming (E-RF) (T-enriched) and non-E-RF (B-enriched + monocyte) cell populations.[3] Monocytes were separated from the B-enriched cell fraction by adherence to plastic surface (Falcon dish) and by subsequent recovery with a rubber policeman. The purity of T-enriched, B-enriched and monocyte populations was assessed by E-RF, representing T cells; by immunofluorescence staining of surface immunoglobulin and by EAC rosette formation,[4] a characteristic of B cells; and by peroxidase staining reactivity, a property of monocytes.[5]

Cell viability was assayed by trypan blue exclusion and was greater than 98%. The functional capacity of T cells was monitored by their 3-day mitogenic response to PHA, and of B cells by their 3-day mitogenic response to PWM when cultured together with puromycin-treated T cells.[3,6]

IF production experiments were done in 1 ml volume of McCoy's 5a medium plus 15% heat-inactivated fetal calf serum and antibiotics in 16 × 150 mm plastic tubes (Falcon 2045) containing 2 × 10^6 lymphocytes; 0.1 ml amounts of PPD (Central Veterinary Laboratory, Weybridge, Surrey, England) were added to each culture at the desired concentration. IF assay was performed on B-SC-1 cells grown in 24-well Cluster plates (Costar). The IF assay was performed on B-SC-1 cells grown in 24-well Cluster plates (Costar). The IF titer was expressed as the reciprocal of that dilution of sample, which, in 0.5 ml volume, resulted in 50% reduction of plaques produced by bovine vesicular stomatitis virus (PRD_{50} unit) (U).

The results of experiments using PBMC from two PPD-POS donors with PPD at different concentration revealed a concentration-dependent IF response. Cultures incubated with PPD at 50, 100, 250, 500 and 1000 μg/ml, produced a significant IF response (12-270 U) throughout a 6-day period. Peak IF response (270 U) on day 3 occurred in cultures exposed to 250 μg of PPD without an obvious mitogenic or antigenic response. In contrast, cultures incubated with 10 and 25 μg of PPD produced no detectable IF until day 6 and the amount produced was low (10-15 U). These cultures also showed 4–8-fold increase in H^3-TdR uptake characterizing an antigenic response.

The 3-day optimal IF response following stimulation with 250 μg of PPD was not reliably predicted by the donor Mantoux status. Using PBMC from 10 PPD-POS and 7 PPD-NEG donors, we observed an overall PPD-IF response ranging from 38-729 U (mean-234.5 ± 183.6) and from 32-334 U (mean = 139 ± 111.9) from these donors, respectively.

We determined also the cell type involved in IF production. In 6 experiments, the mean IF response was 179 ± 105 for unseparated PBMC, 9 ± 8 U for T-enriched lymphocytes, 314 ± 41.5 U for B-enriched lymphocytes and <5 U for monocytes. We noted that the amount of IF produced by B-enriched cells (317 U) was not assisted when cultured together with varying proportions of T cells. On the other hand, the presence of monocytes enhanced IF production; B-enriched cell populations containing 9–15% monocytes produced 4–10-fold more interferon. The significance remains unclear, since the separation method used yielded B-enriched cell population contaminated routinely with an average of 3.3 ± 2.3% monocytes.

Characteristically, PPD-IF was sensitive to trypsin treatment (1 mg/ml, 1 hr at 37°C), to heating (1 hr at 56°C) and to acid treatment (pH 2, 24 hr at 4°C). It had similar range of antiviral activity as Cantell's type 1 human Leu-IF when assayed in human diploid foreskin, in simian B-SC-1, and in porcine PK15 cells. In contrast to Leu-IF, which was superactive in bovine EBTr cells, PPD-IF exhibited a modest activity similar to that in B-SC-1 cells. Both types of IF were inactive in canine MDCK cells. In addition, PPD-IF like Leu-IF had pronounced antiproliferative effects on HeLa and on SV-40-transformed human 2RA cells. The multiplication of these cells in culture was inhibited by 50% or more when cultured in the presence of 50 U and higher of either interferon.

In conclusion, the observations described and enhanced our understanding of a potentially useful source of high-titered type II human interferon.

References

1. Rozee, K. R., S. H. S. Lee & J. Ngan. 1973. Nature New Biol. **245:** 16–15.
2. Boyum, A. 1968. Scand. J. Clin. Invest. Suppl. **21:** 8 31–50.
3. Han, T. & B. Dadey. 1978. Immunology **34:** 625–629.
4. Tachibana, T. & M. Ishikawa. 1973. Japan. J. Exp. Med. **43:** 227–230.
5. Lee, S. H. S. & L. B. Epstein. 1980. Cell. Immun. **50:** 177–190.
6. Rasanen, L. 1979. Immunology **37:** 715–721.

Acknowledgments

This work was supported by grant from Medical Research Council of Canada. We are indebted to Mrs. M. DeCoste for skilled technical assistance.

SUPPRESSION OF ANTIGEN-INDUCED INTERFERON SYNTHESIS IN HUMAN LYMPHOCYTES BY COTTON-ADHERENT MONONUCLEAR CELLS*

F. Volvovitz, E.A. Havell,† H. Bartfeld,‡ and J. Vilček

New York University School of Medicine
New York, New York 10016
†Trudeau Institute
Saranac Lake, New York 12983
‡St. Vincent's Hospital
New York, New York 10011

Interferon (IF) synthesis in cultures of antigen-stimulated human mononuclear white blood cells varied according to the method used to purify these cells from the peripheral blood leukocyte population. Heparinized blood was obtained by venipuncture from healthy BCG-immunized donors. Erythrocytes were gravity-sedimented and purified lymphocytes were obtained from the white blood cell-rich plasma by removing adherent cells either on a cotton column or on a Ficoll gradient. The purified lymphocytes were suspended in culture medium and tested for the ability to produce IF following induction with the specific antigen, tuberculin PPD. Cells obtained by separation on the cotton column alone or subjected to cotton column treatment following Ficoll gradient purification were good IF producers. However, cells processed only on a Ficoll gradient were poor IF producers, and when such cells were mixed with those obtained from the cotton column there was a significant suppression of IF synthesis in the resultant culture. Our observations support the notion that a Ficoll-buoyant, cotton-adherent suppressor lymphocyte may play a role in regulating antigen-induced IF synthesis. This suppressor activity is partially reversed at high PPD concentrations, suggesting that the suppressor cell may play a role in antigen presentation of processing.

The bulk of the IF induced in PPD-stimulated nonadherent lymphocytes was distinct from the *LE* and *F* types of human IF in antigenic, physicochemical, and biological properties. Antibody affinity chromatography and neutralization experiments employing monospecific anti-*Le* and anti-*F* sera revealed the presence of variable amounts of *Le*-like IF in the PPD-induced samples. The contaminating *Le* species could be removed with immobilized anti-*Le* serum; the resulting IF activity was unstable at pH 2 or upon heating to 56°C for 1 hr, retaining 1% and <1% of the original activity after each treatment, respectively. The antiviral state induced by this IF (referred to as immune, type II, or *T* interferon) appeared to be more transient than that induced by the *Le* and *F* IF; cells exposed to this IF demonstrated a prolonged lag phase in the development of antiviral resistance. In addition, removal of this IF species from the culture medium after maximum antiviral resistance was allowed to develop resulted in a more rapid loss of antiviral resistance when compared to the *Le* and *F* types. These data clearly imply that "immune" IF is a distinct entity and suggest possible differences in the mechanism of its antiviral action as compared with the *Le* and *F* species.

*This work was supported by United States Public Health Service Grants 5PO1 NS 11605 and 2RO1 AI 07057.

STUDIES OF THE PRODUCER CELL OF INTERFERON IN HUMAN AND MURINE LYMPHOCYTE CULTURES

H. Kirchner, H. H. Peter, R. Zawatzky, and H. Engler

Institute of Virus Research
German Cancer Research Center
Heidelberg, Federal Republic of Germany

Initially, our interest in interferon (IF) was triggered by the observation that *Corynebacterium parvum*, an immunostimulant widely used in immunotherapy of experimental tumors, effectively protected mice against infection with Herpes simplex virus (HSV).[1] We have then shown that *C.parvum* represented a potent inducer of IF *in vivo* in mice[2] and also *in vitro* in spleen cell cutures of mice and in human peripheral leukocytes.[3,4] In the latter cultures we have attempted to define the producer cell of HSV and *C.parvum*-induced IF.[5] This cell was not a B cell or a macrophage since IF production was demonstrable in cultures containing 1% phagocytic cells and <1% of cells positive for surface immunoglobulin markers. When rosetting with sheep erythrocytes was performed, the producer cell of IF was in the nonrosetting fraction. Our studies have therefore suggested that IF production was a function of a nonrosetting T cell or a null cell, possibly a cell type related to the natural killer (NK) cell.

In mouse spleen cell cultures we have studied IF induction by allogeneic spleen cells (mixed lymphocyte culture, MLC), by HSV, and by the T-cell mitogens phytohemagglutinin (PHA) and concanavalin A (Con A) (refs. 6, 7, and unpublished data). Interferon production induced by PHA, Con A, or in the MLC was T-cell-dependent and was abolished by pretreatment of the spleen cells by anti-theta serum plus complement. We have been able to confirm the interesting observation of Wietzerbin *et al.*[8] that spleen cells of homozygous nude mice responded to PHA with IF production to the same degree as spleen cells of their heterozygous littermates. However, spleen cells of nude mice did not respond to Con A or allogeneic cells with IF production, suggesting that different subsets of T cells respond to the latter two stimuli than the subpopulation that responds to PHA.[9,10]

HSV-induced (type 1) IF production was T-cell independent since it was not abolished by pretreatment of spleen cells with anti-theta serum and since spleen cells of nu/nu mice were fully reactive. In addition, the producer cell of HSV-induced IF was not removed by nylon wool columns, or by adherence to plastic and was not inactivated by treatment with silica. It was not removed by a consecutive series of treatments including plastic adherence plus nylon wool column passage plus two cycles of treatment with anti-theta serum plus complement. The resulting cell population consisting of 5% of the starting population of unseparated spleen cells was fully active in NK-cell activity against YAC lymphoma cells and produced high titers of type I IF. Our tentative conclusion is that type I IF in mouse spleen cells is produced by a cell type which may be closely related to NK cells.

REFERENCES

1. KIRCHNER, H., H. M. HIRT & K. MUNK. 1977. Protection against herpes simplex virus infection in mice by Corynebacterium parvum. Infect. Immun. **16:** 9–11.

2. KIRCHNER, H., H. M. HIRT, H. BECKER & K. MUNK. 1977. Production of an antiviral factor by murine spleen cells after treatment with Corynebacterium parvum. Cell. Immunol. **31:** 172–176.
3. HIRT, H. M., H. BECKER & H. KIRCHNER. 1978. Induction of interferon production in mouse spleen cell cultures by Corynebacterium parvum. Cell. Immunol. **31:** 168–175.
4. HIRT, H. M., M. SCHWENTECK, H. BECKER & H. KIRCHNER. 1978. Interferon production and lymphocyte stimulation in human leukocyte cultures stimulated by Corynebacterium parvum. Clin. Exp. Immunol. **32:** 471–476.
5. KIRCHNER, H., H. H. PETER, H. M. HIRT, R. ZAWATZKY & P. BRADSTREET. 1979 Studies of the producer cell of interferon in human lymphocytes cultures. Immunobiology **156:** 65–75.
6. KIRCHNER, H., R. ZAWATZKY & V. SCHIRRMACHER. 1979. Interferon production in the murine mixed lymphocyte reaction. I. Interferon production caused by differences in the H-2K and H-2D region but not by differences in the I region or the M locus. Eur. J. Immunol. **9:** 97–99.
7. ZAWATZKY, R., J. HILFENHAUS & H. KIRCHNER. 1979. Resistance of nude mice to herpes simplex virus and correlation with in vitro porduction of interferon. Cell. Immunol. **47:** 424–428.
8. WIETZERBIN, J., S. STEFANOS, R. FALCOFF, M. LUCERO, L. CATINOT & S. E. FALCOFF. 1978. Immune interferon induced by phytohemagglutinin in nude mouse spleen cells. Infect. Immun. **21:** 966–972.
9. KIRCHNER, H., R. ZAWATZKY, H. ENGLER, V. SCHIRRMACHER, H. BECKER & P. v. WUSSOW. 1979. Production of interferon in the murine mixed lymphocyte culture. II. Interferon production is a T cell dependent function, independent of proliferation. Eur. J. Immunol. **9:** 824.
10. KIRCHNER, H., H. FENKL, R. ZAWATZKY, H. ENGLER & H. BECKER. 1980. Dissociation between interferon production induced by phytohemagglutinin and concanavalin A in spleen cell cultures of nude mice. Eur. J. Immunol. **10:** 224.

PRODUCTION OF INTERFERON IN LYMPHOCYTE CULTURES FROM PATIENTS WITH ABNORMAL IMMUNE FUNCTION

Ö. Strannegård,* J. Björkander,† S. Hermodsson,* E. Lundgren,¶ I.-L. Strannegård‡, and G. Westberg§

*Departments of *Virology, †Allergy, ‡Pediatrics, and §Medicine*
University of Göteborg
Göteborg, Sweden
¶Department of Pathology
University of Umeå
Umeå, Sweden

Lymphocytes of both the T-cell and B-cell lineage as well as macrophages take part in the production of interferons (IFs). Therefore, one might expect that patients with immunological diseases involving disturbed function of any of these cells would display an altered ability to produce IF. In the present investigation we have studied the production of IF by cultured mononuclear cells from patients with common variable hypogammaglobulinemia (hypo-γ), systemic lupus erythematosus (SLE), and atopic disease. Since IF activates natural killer (NK) cells we have also studied the activity of such cells in the patients.

Interferon production in lymphocyte cultures was determined 4 days after stimulation with Sendai virus or phytohemagglutinin (PHA). Sendai virus-induced IF was subjected to treatment at pH 2 before being assayed in microplates. NK-cell activity was determined using 18-hr incubations with Cr^{51}-labeled target cells with an effector-target cell ratio of 25:1. To minimize the effect of methodological variation on the results, all NK-cell tests were performed on matched pairs of patients and controls. Statistical evaluation of the results was performed with Wilcoxon's nonparametric test.

The production of Sendai virus-induced interferon was significantly higher in hypo-γ patients than in controls ($p < 0.01$), whereas patients with SLE and 9–17 year-old children with atopic disease produced less IF than the controls ($p < 0.05$ and $p < 0.01$, respectively). The production of PHA-induced IF, which was determined in hypo-γ patients only, was higher in patients than in controls ($p < 0.01$).

NK cell activity was determined using one suspension-growing cell line (P 3HR1) and one line of anchored cells (GMK or human embryonic lung) as target cells. In hypo-γ patients there was a tendency to increased NK-cell activity against P 3HR1 cells ($p < 0.1$) but not against GMK cells. SLE patients had significantly subnormal activity against both these cell types ($p=0.05$ and $p=0.02$, respectively). The children with atopic diseases had increased activity against P 3HR1 cells ($p < 0.01$) but not against human embryonic lung cells.

It is not possible to establish from the present results whether the abnormalities observed are primary or consequences of treatment or manifestations of the diseases. However, the hypo-γ patients received no treatment other than gammaglobulin, and their high ability to produce IF and their possibly increased NK-cell activity may help to explain why they have a much better defense against viral than against bacterial infections. The subnormal IF production and

NK-cell activity in SLE patients, on the other hand, may be consistent with the observations of possibly increased susceptibility to viral infections and increased incidence of certain tumors in these patients.

The parallelism between IF-producing ability and NK activity in hypogammaglobulinemia and SLE patients is striking in view of the well-documented stimulatory effect of interferon on NK activity. However, there did not seem to be a clearcut correlation between the two activities, as exemplified by the results obtained with lymphocytes from atopic children. A possible explanation for this could be that antibody-dependent cellular cytotoxicity contributed to the results.

It is interesting to note that type I IF production was high in patients (hypo-γ) considered to have high suppressor cell activity and subnormal in patients (SLE and atopy) thought to have suppressor cell deficiency. In hypo-γ patients, production of type II IF, which is considered to be a mediator of suppressor cells, was above normal limits. It is therefore possible that IF production in the patient groups studied is in some way related to disturbance of suppressor cell function.

HUMAN LYMPHOBLASTOID INTERFERON CAN INHIBIT THE GROWTH OF HUMAN BREAST CANCER XENOGRAFTS IN ATHYMIC (NUDE) MICE

F. Balkwill,* J. Taylor-Papadimitriou,* K.H. Fantes,‡ and A. Sebesteny*

*Imperial Cancer Research Fund
Lincoln's Inn Fields
London, WC2 England
†Wellcome Research Laboratories
Langley Court
Beckenham, Kent, England

Clinical trials to test the antitumor effect of interferons (IFs) in man have been limited by the availability of human IFs prepared from blood bank leukocoyte, fibroblast or lymphoblastoid cell-line sources. Thus, information on the sensitivity of human tumors to IFs would help determine the most suitable tumors for clinical trial. The failure of many human tumor cells to grow in the tissue culture systems currently available has led us to use human tumor xenografts in athymic (nude) mice as a model system to test sensitivity to interferons. We have established 3 primary human breast carcinomas as transplantable tumors in nude mice.[1] These tumors are slow growing, retain their original morphology and surface phenotype, and like the cells from the original carcinoma, the cells from the xenografts do not grow *in vitro*. We have found that the development of these tumors can be inhibited by a human IF prepared from human lymphoblastoid (Namalwa) cells which will soon be available for clinical trials in man (N. Finter personal communication).

All experiments used random bred nu/nu female mice of mixed genetic background, housed in a negative pressure isolator. Tumors were cut into cubes of 1–8 mm and 4 such fragments loaded into Bashford needles and implanted subcutaneously into 4 ventral sites per animal. Mice were subsequently dosed daily with a subcutaneous injection of IF or placebo, the tumors recorded weekly and at the end of the experiment the mice were killed and the tumors excised and weighed. Preliminary work showed that a subcutaneous injection of 1×10^4 U of human lymphoblastoid interferon, HLyIF, resulted in serum levels of 300–400 U/ml 2–6 hr post-injection and that repeated doses of HLyIF were not antigenic.

In the first experiment the growth of tumor code no: 630 in 18 mice was followed for 13 weeks with daily doses of 2×10^4 U HLyIF (sp. act. 5.6×10^7 u/mg protein) or placebo. At the end of the experiment 3 tumors developed in the HLyIF group and 19 in the control group, and the development of tumors in the HLyIF group was delayed. The difference between control and HLyIF groups was highly significant ($p < .001$ as assessed by the log rank test). In a second experiment tumor code no: 534 was implanted into 18 mice and then the mice treated daily with 1×10^4 U of the HLyIF or placebo. Once again a strong inhibitory effect was noted. After a period of 12 weeks, 11 tumors developed in 9 mice in the HLyIF group and 29 tumors in 9 mice in the control group. This was statistically significant $p < .005$ as assessed by the log rank test. In both these experiments there was no significant difference in the mean weight of individual tumors. Further experiments with these 2 tumors showed that the growth inhibition could be abrogated by preincubation of the IF by a specific antiserum.

The growth and development of a third tumor, code no: 236, was not significantly inhibited by daily doses of 2×10^4 HLyIF over 12 weeks. Thirty-two tumors developed in 8 mice in the HLyIF group and 38 tumors in 7 mice in the control group.

The mechanisms by which IFs exert an antitumor effect are not yet clear. Interferons may act by inhibiting viral oncogenesis and tumor cell growth, or by enhancing host responses against the tumor.[2,3] Two lines of preliminary evidence indicate that HLyIF in this system is acting directly on the tumor cells and inhibiting their growth. Firstly, the mouse immune system, as measured by natural killer cell activity, can be stimulated by mouse L-cell IF but not by HLyIF; and secondly a mouse IF did not inhibit the growth of the human tumors.

REFERENCES

1. SEBESTENY, A., J. TAYLOR-PAPADIMITRIOU, R. CERIANI, R. MILLIS, C. SCHMITT & D. TREVAN. 1979. Primary human breast carcinomas transplantable in the nude mouse. J. Nat. Cancer Inst. **63:** 1331.
2. GRESSER, I. & M.G. TOREY. 1978. Antitumour effects of interferon. 1978 Biochem Biophys. Acta **515:** 231–247.
3. BALKWILL, F. R. 1979. Interferons as cell regulatory molecules. 1979. Cancer Immunol Immunother. **7:** 7–14.

RARE EARTH SALTS STABILIZE INTERFERONS

J. J. Sedmak and S. E. Grossberg

Department of Microbiology
Medical College of Wisconsin
Milwaukee, Wisconsin 53226

The addition of rare earth salts at a concentration of 0.002 M or greater to partially purified interferons (IFs) prepared in human fibroblasts, human leukocytes, and mouse L cells increases the original antiviral potency of the preparation by a factor of two or more. At these concentrations the salts completely stabilize human fibroblast IF at pH 7 for at least 4 days against inactivation at 37°C and protect against mechanical inactivation in a vortical agitational test, whereas control samples lose 95% and 90%, respectively. Human leukocyte IF was also stabilized against thermal inactivation but to a lesser extent than fibroblast interferon. The addition of these salts to low pH buffers negates the stabilizing effects of these buffers against thermal inactivation of interferons. The ionic radius of the rare earth ions did not seem to be important in stabilizing the IFs since all of the rare earths tested were effective. The low toxicity of rare earths indicates that these salts might be valuable in preparing IFs for clinical use as well as in the preparation and handling of purified interferons.

THE COMPLETE PURIFICATION OF HUMAN LEUKOCYTE INTERFERON

Kurt Berg, Kurt Osther, and Iver Heron

The Institute of Medical Microbiology
University of Aarhus
DK-8000 Aarhus C, Denmark.

INTRODUCTION

Human leukocyte interferon (HuLeIF) has now, for the first time, been completely purified into two major species (Mv 18,400 and 20180 D) representing 85% of the antiviral activity. Three more species (Mv 19,500, 20900, and 22,130 D) representing 15% of the antiviral activity were also found. Each IF species was identified as a stainable protein. All five species of HuLeIF exhibited anticellular activity when tried in the Daudi cell system (inhibition of [$_3$H]thymidine uptake) as well as potentiating activity on the NK system, etc.

RESULTS

The starting material was obtained from crude HuLeIF (2% human serum, Sendai virus induction) which was first concentrated by means of 0.5 M KSCN (pH 4.5) and, thereupon, dialyzed vs. 20 mM phosphate buffer, pH 7.2 (PB), 1 M NaCl, and 25% ethylene glycol. The first step involved a gel filtration using Ultrogel AcA 5/4 in a 100 cm long column (4°C) starting out with 4×10^6 IFU (interferon units) in 10 ml containing more than 400,000 μg of proteins. After gel filtration the IF fractions were pooled; specific activity was close to 10^6 IFU/mg proteins, the recovery close to 85 percent. This pool was then, in turn, purified on a Cu-chelate column (8 ml) according to Sulkowski (personal communication) using the same buffers as during the gel filtration. The bound IF was eluted at pH 4.5; purification factor varied 3–5-fold and the recovery was about 75 percent. The eluate was dialyzed very thoroughly vs. 20 mM PB (recovery 60%) before loaded to a Blue dextran column (size 5–6 ml). After washing with 20 mM PB, the outlet of the Blue dextran column was connected to the inlet of a highly absorbed antileukocyte interferon immunoglobulin column, and the washing was continued with 10–20 ml of additional buffer.* Thereafter, the two columns were disconnected and the antibody column was washed further wtih 0.1 M NaOAc/0.3 M NaCl, pH 7.2 until the background was negligible.

The IF was eluted into plastic tubes by means of 0.1 M HOOAc/0.3 M NaCl, pH 2.4, including a small amount of citric acid, enough to keep pH firmly at pH 2.4, subsequent to addition of 100 μl of 0.1% SDS to each tube. The IF-containing fractions were pooled and concentrated before subjected to SDS-PAGE (20–25 cm long gels, gradient varied from 12–20%). The pooled fractions contained about 2×10^6 IFU with about 0.5 μg of proteins as determined by comparing the intensity of the stained IF bands with known markers but different concentrations. If SDS was omitted during the collection of the IF, more than 80% of the IF activity was lost. The concentrated IF preparation was subjected to an SDS-

*20 mM PB/0.6 M NaCl.

PAGE. After staining in Coomassie Blue, only two proteins were seen at 18,400 and 20,180 daltons together with a minor one at 22,130. In another experiment the amount of IF-loaded to the SDS-PAGE was increased 2–3-fold and the same bands, but at higher intensity, were noted. In one of the experiments a parallel slot was also loaded with IF and, after electrophoresis, cut into 1 mm pieces and minced with a Teflon rod before being eluted for IF activity and titrated on the same day. It turned out that the two major proteins each had a distinct IF activity. Three more peaks of IF activity were seen. When increasing the IF load further to the SDS-PAGE, barely detectable proteins were also seen at the exact same location as the three extra IF peaks. Thus it can now be stated that human leukocyte interferon exists as five separate species which all have been demonstrated by staining with Coomassie Blue. In a separate experiment the stained IF bands were cut separately according to the location of the five protein bands, minced with a Teflon rod, and eluted for IF activity. It turned out that all five stained protein bands contained a distinct IF activity which was detectable even after treatment with a staining solution. All five species were able to neutralize rabbit antileukocyte IF raised against PIF. None of the five species were able to neutralize rabbit antifibroblast interferon.

Le INTERFERON PRODUCTION BY HUMAN FIBROBLASTS

Teresa G. Hayes, Y.K. Yip, and Jan Vilček

Department of Microbiology
New York University School of Medicine
New York, New York 10016

Earlier experiments[1] showed that the amount of *Le* interferon (IF) produced by two human fibroblast strains depends on the nature of the inducing agent. We now demonstrate that both the cell type and the inducer determine the proportion of *Le* and *F* IFs produced by human fibroblast strains. Of 8 strains tested, GM-258 cells (with trisomy 21) produced the highest absolute and relative amounts of *Le* IF after NDV inoculation. There was no correlation between *Le* production and number of copies of chromosome 21. Only *F* IF was detectable in GM-258 cells induced with poly(I)·poly(C) under 5 different conditions (simple induction, induction after priming with IF, induction in the presence of DEAE-dextran or hypertonic medium, and superinduction). In GM-258 cells induced with NDV, it was possible to manipulate the relative proportion of *F* and *Le* interferons and the time at which they were made by altering the induction conditions. The percentage of *Le* was increased by decreasing the multiplicity of infection or irradiating the virus with UV light. Kinetics of *F* and *Le* production after different modes of NDV inoculation paralleled each other closely. The Komarov strain of NDV induced a pattern of IF production similar to that of the Hickman strain.

Interferons produced by NDV-induced GM-258 cells were physically separated by affinity chromatography on immobilized anti-*Le* and anti-*F* globulins. On SDS-PAGE, the *Le* IF component formed two separate peaks (with molecular weights of approximately 18,000 and 25,000), closely resembling a control *Le* IF preparation made by Sendai virus-induced buffy coat cells. Similar to control *F* interferon [made by FS-4 cells induced with poly(I)·poly (C)], the *F* interferon moiety made in GM-258 cells formed a single peak with a molecular weight of approximately 26,000.

A more detailed description of these experiments will soon be published.[2]

REFERENCES

1. HAVELL, E.A., T.G. HAYES & J. VILČEK. 1978. Synthesis of two distinct interferons by human fibroblasts. Virology **89:** 330–334.
2. HAYES, T.G., Y.K. YIP & J. VILČEK. 1979. *Le* interferon production by human fibroblasts. Virology **98:** 351–363.

SEPARATION OF HUMAN LEUKOCYTE INTERFERON COMPONENTS BY CONCANAVALIN A–AGAROSE AFFINITY CHROMATOGRAPHY AND THEIR CHARACTERIZATION

Peter M. Grob and Kailash C. Chadha

Department of Viral Oncology
Roswell Park Memorial Institute
Buffalo, New York 14263

Human leukocyte interferon (HL-IF) contains two molecular weight components: a 16,000 dalton and a 21,000 dalton component in the approximate ratio of 7:3. The relative extent of glycosylation of these two molecular components is apparently responsible for the molecular weight heterogeneity of HL-IF. Treatment of HL-IF with glycosidases (Bose *et al.*[1]) or periodate (Stewart *et al.*[2]) has been shown to cause a reduction in its molecular weight and when HL-IF is produced in the presence of inhibitors of glycosylation, only a single component corresponding to 16,000 daltons is observed (Chadha *et al.*[3]). We have utilized lectin affinity chromatography to further investigate the glycoprotein nature of HL-IF.

HL-IF was resolved into three distinct fractions when chromatographed on Concanavalin A-agarose. The major portion (70–75%) of the IF activity appeared in the break-through (BT fraction). The bound IF (25–30%) was displaced from the column as two fractions: the first fraction was eluted with 0.1 M α-methyl-D-mannoside yielding 15–20% of the IF activity (α-MM fraction) and the second fraction by including 70% ethylene glycol in the eluant yielding the remaining 5–15% of the IF activity (EG fraction). Each fraction has distinct physicochemical and biological properties. The molecular weights of interferon contained in the BT, α-MM and EG fractions were determined by sodium dodecyl sulfate polyacrylamide gel electrophoresis. The BT fraction contained exclusively the 16,000 dalton component. The α-MM fraction contained predominantly (~90%) the 21,000 dalton component. However, the EG fraction contained both the 16,000 dalton component and 21,000 dalton component in essentially equal proportions. HL-IF produced in the presence of the glycosylation inhibitors, tunicamycin or 2-deoxy-D-glucose, contain a single molecular weight component (16,000 daltons, Chadha *et al.*[3]), and this IF was not retained when chromatographed on Com A-Sepharose (Grob & Chadha[4]). These results demonstrate that the majority of bound IF has a molecular weight of 21,000 and is apparently the glycosylated component of HL-IF. The 16,000 dalton component is either nonglycosylated or is deficient in specific sugar residues and consequently is unable to bind to Con A-Sepharose.

It is well documented in the literature that HL-IF exhibits heterologous antiviral activity (Gresser *et al.*,[5]). We have observed that IF in the BT and α-MM fractions has significant levels of antiviral activity on heterologous (bovine) cells, whereas the EG fraction interferon showed insignificant heterologous activity. This result suggests that the majority of IF present in the EG fraction is fibroblast type IF which is present in all HL-IF preparations (Havell *et al.*[6]). This conclusion was further strengthened by utilizing specific antisera in neutralization experiments. The interferon in the BT and α-MM fractions was selectively neutralized by HL-IF antiserum, whereas the EG fraction IF was preferentially neutralized (~70%) by antiserum to human fibroblast interferon.

Con A-Sepharose affinity chromatography of HL-IF resolves the two molecular weight components and in addition separates the fibroblast type IF into a separate fraction. Since no SDS was used in our approach to separate the two molecular weight components of HL-IF, the technique will enable us and others to accurately assign the biological significance of each of the two components. Studies on the antiviral, antitumor and other nonantiviral properties of apparently glycosylated and nonglycosylated components of HL-IF are now in progress in our laboratory.

References

1. Bose, S. *et al.* 1976. J. Biol. Chem. **251:** 1659.
2. Stewart W. E. *et al.* 1977. Proc. Nat. Acad. Sci. USA **74:** 4200.
3. Chadha, K. C. *et al.* 1980. Arch. Virol. **64:** 109.
4. Grob, P. M. & K. C. Chadha. 1979. Biochemistry. **18:** 5782.
5. Gresser, I. *et al.* 1974. Nature **251:** 543.
6. Havell, E. A. *et al.* 1975. Proc. Nat. Acad. Sci. USA **72:** 2185.

LARGE-SCALE PURIFICATION OF HUMAN FIBROBLAST INTERFERON FOR ANTIVIRAL AND ANTIPROLIFERATIVE STUDIES

James E. Whitman, Jr., Chia-ling Hung, and Gavin M. Crowley

Electro-Nucleonics Laboratories, Inc.
Viral Science Laboratory
Silver Spring, Maryland 20904

Human fibroblast interferon (HF-IF) is now being produced and purified, on a large scale basis, in our laboratory to determine the feasibility of producing enough HF-IF, with high antiproliferative activity, for clinical trials in human cancer patients. Human foreskin (HFS) cell strains, isolated and characterized in our laboratory, are regularly superinduced with Poly IC, cycloheximide, and actinomycin-D to yield average crude titers of 2×10^4 international reference units (IRU)/ml. Interferon is assayed by the dye uptake method (Finter) in HFS cells (FS-7) against the NIH HF-IF standard G 023-902-527, using vesicular stomatitis virus (VSV) as the challenge virus. Current methods, using roller bottle culture vessels, allow for a total weekly production of $1.2–1.6 \times 10^8$ IRU. Purification steps include use of controlled pore glass beads and hydrophobic affinity chromatography. Recently a zinc precipitation step was added to the purification scheme in order to compare the biological characteristics and overall percent recovery of IF by two diverse purification methods. Method A consisted of a tandem two-step hydrophobic affinity chromatography procedure (Concanavalin-A/Phenyl-Sepharose CL-4B) as described by Carter *et al.*[1] Method B is also a two-step tandem procedure using controlled pore glass (CPG-350) chromatography, with elution at pH 2, and zinc precipitation of interferon (Edy, modified[2,3]). Using method A overall recoveries of HF-IF are usually 10–14% (occasionally 25%) with specific activities of $1.0–1.5 \times 10^7$ μ/mg protein. Method B yields overall recoveries of approximately 30% with specific activities of 3.2×10^6 μ/mg protein. Final preparations of the purified HF-IF (2,000–3,000 μ/ml) from either method A or B, had a marked antiviral effect for 5–7 days on herpes simplex virus type 1 and varicella-zoster virus, even when diploid HFS cells were infected prior to treatment with interferon. The antiproliferative activity of purified HF-IF was demonstrated against human cancer cells (A204 rhabdomyosarcoma) where 80–90% of the cells were destroyed or inhibited by cytotoxic effects, while $\leq$10% of the normal diploid cells (MRC-5 or HFS) were inhibited by equal quantities (2,000–3,000 μ/ml) of purified IF in serial cell passages. The AP activity was demonstrated to be inhibitory and transient rather than cytocidal, and the inhibited cells grew back following removal of the interferon after a few-day lag phase. The present antiviral and antiproliferative data suggest that sufficient high quality purified HF-IF can now be prepared to expand human clinical trials in selected cancer patients, while continuing to search for even more efficient ways to mass produce and purify human fibroblast interferon. However, recent reports suggesting the need for as much HF-IF as 18×10^6 μ/day/60 kg patient[4] make it imperative to search for much more economical methods of production and better purification recovery yields than now exist. Beyond the problem of high cost for patient treatment rises the specter that HF-IF may not even be effective for treatment of cancer patients because of its instability or rapid clearance from the host.[4,5] In spite of the above-mentioned concerns regarding inadequate availability and modest effectiveness in treating cancer patients, it is imperative that the scientific community continue work on all forms of IF until sufficient experimental and clinical data are accumulated to answer the question of whether HF-IF or any other known interferon is really an effective antitumor agent.

REFERENCES

1. CARTER, W. & J. HOROSZEWICZ. Production, purification and clinical application of human fibroblast interferon. J. Pharmacol. Ther. In press.
2. EDY, V., I. BRAUDE, E. DECLERCQ, A. Billiau & P. DESOMER. 1976. Purification of interferon by adsorption chromatography on controlled pore glass. J. Gen. Virol. **33:** 517.
3. EDY, V., A. BILLIAU & P. DESOMER. 1977. Purification of human fibroblast interferon by zinc chelate affinity chromatography. J. Biol. Chem. **252:** 5934–5935.
4. BILLIAU, A., P. DESOMER, V. EDY, E. DECLERCQ & H. HEREMANS. 1979. Human fibroblast interferon for clinical trials: Pharmacokinetics and tolerability in experimental animals and humans. Antimicrob. Agents Chemother. **16:** 56–63.
5. HANLEY, D., M. WIRANOWSKA-STEWART & W. STEWART II. Pharmacology of interferons. I. Pharmacologic distinctions between human leukocyte and fibroblast interferons. Int. J. Immunopharmacol. In press.

SELECTIVE INHIBITION OF GLYCOPROTEIN AND MEMBRANE PROTEIN CONTENT OF VESICULAR STOMATITIS VIRUS RELEASED BY INTERFERON-TREATED CELLS

Radha K. Maheshwari, Francis T. Jay, and Robert M. Friedman

Laboratory of Experimental Pathology
National Institute of Arthritis, Metabolism, and Digestive Diseases
National Institutes of Health
Bethesda, Maryland 20205

Interferon (IF) has been shown to inhibit the replication of a wide variety of viruses. In most systems studied, virus directed translation or transcription was inhibited[1]; however, an unusual inhibitory effect of IF treatment on the replication of RNA tumor viruses has been described. Inhibition of virus production did not correlate with inhibition of the accumulation of viral RNA[2] or of viral proteins.[3] These results suggested that in these systems the release of virus from the plasma membrane or the production of infectious virus particles was inhibited by IF treatment.

One important question about this work is whether such findings are restricted to RNA tumor virus systems. We have studied the effect of low concentrations of IF (3-30 units/ml) on vesicular stomatitis virus (VSV) infection of Ly cells, in contrast to previous studies, which employed much higher IF concentration and reported inhibition of VSV-directed transcription or translation.[4] Our results indicated that in Ly cells treated with 30 reference units/ml of IF, there was an approximately 200-fold reduction in the titer of infectious VSV particle production; however, virus particle production as measured by virion-associated transcriptase, virion RNA, or N protein (the structural protein present in VSV in the highest concentration) was inhibited by a maximum of 10-fold at this concentration of IF. However, we observed a marked inhibition in glycoprotein (G) and membrane or matrix (M) protein content of VSV released from IF-treated cells. The migration of the protein was similar in both of the samples. These findings suggested that in the presence of IF not only is the production of infectious virus particles inhibited, but also the production of noninfectious virus particles is disproportionately enhanced. The results in many respects resemble those previously reported in IF-treated cells infected with MLV. We concluded that such findings are not limited to murine RNA tumor virus systems.

The inhibition of membrane-associated virus yields by treatment with low concentrations of IF may be closely related to functional abnormalities in the protein incorporated into the virion or to absence of specific protein in the noninfectious virions produced. Since many studies[5] have demonstrated that VSV particles with reduced amount of glycoproteins are low in infectivity, it is likely that at least some of the reduced infectivity of VSV particles produced by IF-treated cells may be due to the reduced amount of this protein incorporated into such particles. It is possible that induced changes which have been reported to occur in the plasma membrane of IF-treated cells[6] may account for the alteration in infectivity of both VSV and murine RNA tumor viruses, since these viruses bud from the cell surface as a terminal step in the replication process.

The noninfectious particles produced by IF-treated cells appear to contain only 42S viral RNA; they do not interfere with the growth of wild-type VSV, nor do they produce IF in culture. They are, therefore, unlikely to be defective interfering forms of VSV. Such noninfectious forms may, however, play a role in the initiation of chronic infections by VSV in IF-treated cells.[7]

References

1. Friedman, R. M. 1977. Bact. Rev. **41:** 543-567.
2. Pitha, P. M., S. P. Staal, D. P. Bolognesi, T. P. Denny & W. P. Rowe. 1977. Virology **79:** 1-13.
3. Friedman, R. M. & J. M. Ramseur. 1974. Proc. Nat. Acad. Sci. USA **71:** 3542–3544.
4. Marcus, P. I., D. L. Engelhardt, J. M. Hunt & M. J. Sekellick. 1971. Science **174:** 593–598; Baxt, B., J. A. Sonnabend & R. Bablanian. 1977. J. Gen. Virol. **35:** 325–334.
5. Chang, E. H., S. J. Mims, T. J. Triche & R. M. Friedman. 1977. J. Gen. Virol. **34:** 363–367; Lodish, H. F. & R. A. Weiss. 1979. J. Virol. **30:** 177–178.
6. Lindahl, P., P. Leary & I. Gresser. 1973. Proc. Nat. Acad. Sci. USA **70:** 2785–2788; Chang, E. H., F. T. Jay & R. M. Friedman. 1978. Proc. Nat. Acad. Sci. USA **75:** 1859–1863.
7. Ramseur, J. M. & R. M. Friedman. 1977. J. Gen. Virol. **37:** 523–533.

2′,5′-OLIGOADENYLATE SYNTHETASE: A NEW ASSAY AND PRELIMINARY STRUCTURE-ACTIVITY RELATIONSHIPS FOR ENZYME ACTIVATION BY NUCLEIC ACIDS

Margaret I. Johnston, Robert M. Friedman, and Paul F. Torrence

Laboratories of Chemistry and Experimental Pathology
National Institute of Arthritis, Metabolism, and Digestive Diseases
National Institutes of Health
Bethesda, Maryland 20205

To date, 2′,5′-oligoadenylate synthetase has been assayed by two different methods: (1) in solution[1]; (2) bound to dsRNA attached to an insoluble support.[2,3] Although the latter method offers some degree of enzyme purification, it is extremely cumbersome if different nucleic acids are to be evaluated as enzyme activators. The former method may not always permit synthesis of maximal concentrations of active 2′,5′-oligoadenylates, since some cell extracts may contain high levels of inactivating enzymes.[4] We report here a new assay method based on adsorption of the oligoadenylate synthetase to 2′,5′-ADP-Sepharose.

S100 extracts were prepared from mouse L cells pretreated overnight with 30 units/ml of mouse interferon. In a typical experiment, 100 μl of S100 was mixed at 0–4°C for 2–18 hr with an equal volume of packed 2′,5′-ADP-Sepharose equilibrated in a buffer of 20 mM HEPES, pH 7.5, 50 mM KCl, 1.5 mM $Mg(OAc)_2$, 7 mM β-mercaptoethanol, 20% v/v glycerol. The resin was washed with buffer and then incubated at 30°C for 2–6 hr with 100 μl of the fresh buffer made 90 mM KCl, 10 mm $Mg(OAc)_2$, 5 mM ATP and 10^{-3} to 10^{-7} M nucleic acid. The supernatants were removed, heated at 95°C for 15 min and centrifuged to provide 2′,5′-$(Ap)_n$A-containing supernatants that were then assayed for their ability to inhibit protein synthesis in an EMC viral RNA-directed mouse L cell-free system.

The heat stable inhibitor was formed in concentrations similar to those obtained using the $(I)_n \cdot (C)_n$-Sepharose method under identical conditions. Radiolabeled inhibitor, prepared from [^{3}H]ATP, was characterized as 2′,5′-ppp$(Ap)_n$A by chromatography on a Tener column and by thin-layer chromatography, before and after digestion with bacterial alkaline phosphatase. Under our experimental conditions at 30°C, the bound murine enzyme was relatively stable over a period of three days. Inhibitor synthesis was linear for at least 5 hr, and was dependent on $(I)_n \cdot (C)_n$, ATP, Mg^{2+}, and K^+ concentrations and on the amount of S100 bound to the resin. Synthetase activity was substantially increased in extracts from cells pretreated with interferon.

This assay was used to investigate the ability of various nucleic acids to activate the 2′,5′-oligoadenylate synthetase of mouse L cells. All single-stranded, triple-stranded, and double-stranded polymers that contained sugar modifications were negative. Other polymers varied over 1000-fold in their ability to activate the enzyme. $(I)_n \cdot (s^2C)_n$, $(A)_n \cdot (U)_n$ and its analogues containing a $(c^7A)_n$ strand were weak activators of the enzyme. In order of decreasing potencies, the stronger activators were *P. chrysogenum* dsRNA ≈ $(I)_n \cdot (C)_n$ > $(c^7I)_n \cdot (C)_n$ > $(I)_n \cdot (br^5C)_n$ ≈ $(c^7I)_n \cdot (br^5C)_n$ > bacterophage Qβ RNA.

The availability of this assay now makes possible a detailed comparison of the abilities of various dsRNAs to activate the 2′,5′-oligoadenylate synthetase with their abilities to inhibit protein synthesis in extracts from interferon-treated cells and to induce interferon.[5]

References

1. Hovanessian, A. G. & I. M. Kerr. 1978. Synthesis of an oligonucleotide inhibitor of protein synthesis in rabbit reticulocyte lysates analogous to that formed in extracts from interferon-treated cells. Eur. J. Biochem. **84:** 149–159.
2. Hovanessian, A. G., R. E. Brown & I. M. Kerr. 1977. Synthesis of low molecular weight inhibitor of protein synthesis with enzyme from interferon-treated cells. Nature **268:** 537–540.
3. Stark, G. R., W. J. Dower, R. T. Schimke, R. E. Brown & I. M. Kerr. 1979. 2-5A Synthetase: Assay, distribution and variation with growth or hormone status. Nature **278:** 471–473.
4. Williams, B. R. G., I. M. Kerr, C. S. Gilbert, C. N. White & L. A. Ball. 1978. Synthesis and breakdown of pppA2′p5′A2′p5′A and transient inhibition of protein synthesis in extracts from interferon-treated and control cells. Eur. J. Biochem. **92:** 455–462.
5. Torrence, P. F. & R. M. Friedman. 1979. Are double-stranded RNA-directed inhibition of protein synthesis in interferon-treated cells and interferon induction related phenomena? J. Biol. Chem. **254:** 1259–1267.

INHIBITION BY DOUBLE-STRANDED RNA OF A PHOSPHOPROTEIN PHOSPHATASE PRESENT IN INTERFERON-TREATED CELLS

David A. Epstein, Paul F. Torrence,* and Robert M. Friedman

*Laboratories of Experimental Pathology and *Chemistry*
National Institute of Arthritis, Metabolism,
and Digestive Diseases
National Institutes of Health
Bethesda, Maryland 20205

Previously reported work from this laboratory showed that polynucleotides varied greatly in their ability to induce interferon (IF) and to inhibit protein synthesis in the cell-free system from L-cells.[1] These studies have now been extended to include the effect of these polynucleotides on the phosphorylation of the 67,000 dalton protein P_1. Under conditions that approximate those of protein synthesis (EMC-virus RNA and [^{3}H]-L-leucine are omitted), polynucleotides that inhibited protein synthesis generally stimulated the phosphorylation of P_1 present in the 100,000 × g pellet of extracts of IF-treated cells (P100-IF). In general, polynucleotides that did not inhibit protein synthesis did not stimulate phosphorylation of P_1 under these conditions. However, this rule does not apply to poly (A) · (2′-fluoro-2′-deoxyuridylic acid), which had been shown previously not to inhibit protein synthesis.[1] This polynucleotide enhanced the phosphorylation of P_1 without inhibiting protein synthesis in a 10,000 × g supernatant of an extract from IF-treated L cells. This finding was observed during the simultaneous labeling of P_1 with ^{32}P from γ-[^{32}P]-ATP and of EMC-virus RNA directed incorporation of ^{3}H from [^{3}H]-L-leucine into TCA-insoluble material.

We have also found that the phosphorylation of P_1 in the presence of a given polynucleotide may be dependent on experimental conditions. For example, poly (I) · (br^{5}C), which had been shown not to inhibit protein synthesis, stimulated the incorporation of ^{32}P-label into P_1 present in the P100-IF if the incubation were carried out in buffer A (20 mM K HEPES, pH 7.5, 10 mM KCl, 60 mM. KOAc, 26.5 mM $Mg(OAc)_2$, and 0.5 mM DTT). However, there was no enhancement of ^{32}P-incorporation into P_1 during protein synthesis in the presence of poly (I) · (br^{5}C). By contrast, poly (I) · (C) enhanced the phosphorylation of P_1 under both conditions.

The role that experimental conditions play in determining whether or not poly (I) · (br^{5}C) could stimulate phosphorylation of P_1 became clear when P100-IF fractions were labeled in buffer A in the presence of either poly (I) · (C) or poly (I) · (br^{5}C) and then transferred to buffer B, which was identical in composition to those of protein synthesis conditions except that no EMC-virus RNA or [^{3}H]-L-leucine were present. The dsRNA, poly (I) · (C), but not poly (I) · (br^{5}C), stabilized the ^{32}P-label incorporated into P_1. When ^{32}P-labeled P100-IF fractions was transferred to conditions which lead to ATP depletion in buffer A, poly (I) · (C), but not poly (I) · (br^{5}C), stabilized the label in P_1. When poly (I) · (C) was added to P100-IF fractions ^{32}P-labeled in the presence of poly (I) · (br^{5}C), the P_1 was stabilized. These results show the strong inhibition by poly (I) · (C) of a phosphoprotein phosphatase. This inhibition of P_1 dephosphorylation may be very specific. A partial proteolytic digest by *Staph. aureus* protease V8 of P_1

labeled in the absence of dsRNA or in the presence of either poly (I) · (C) or poly (I) · (br^{5}C) gave rise to very similar fingerprints. It is likely, therefore, that the sites of phosphorylation are equally accessible to the phosphatase.

Reference

1. Torrence, P. F. & R. M. Friedman. 1979. Are double-stranded RNA-directed inhibition of protein synthesis in interferon-treated cells and interferon induction related phenomena? J. Biol. Chem. **254:** 1254–1267.

STRUCTURAL REQUIREMENTS OF dsRNA FOR THE ACTIVATION OF 2′5′OLIGO(A) POLYMERASE OF INTERFERON-TREATED HeLa CELLS

Michael A. Minks, Susan Benvin, and Corrado Baglioni

Department of Biological Sciences
State University of New York
Albany, New York 12222

Treatment of HeLa cells with human fibroblast interferon (IF) induces an enzymatic activity which polymerizes ATP into oligoadenylate by forming 2′-5′ phosphodiester bonds. We have designated this enzyme 2′5′oligo(A) polymerase and have proposed that it plays a role in the antiviral state. Presumably, upon activation by double-stranded RNA (dsRNA) of viral origin, this enzyme synthesizes 2′5′oligo(A), which in turn activates an endonuclease. To define the viral structures which may be responsible for the activation of the 2′5′oligo(A) polymerase, we have investigated the features of dsRNA recognized by this enzyme *in vitro*.

Polymers of known C and G content were synthesized from CDP and GDP with polynucleotide phosphorylase. The resultant poly(C_nG) was annealed to poly(I) to form a mismatched duplex in which base pairing is interrupted at each G residue. When tested for activation of the 2′5′oligo(A) polymerase, duplexes formed from poly(C_nG) of C/G ratio greater than 35 were fully active whereas those with lower ratios exhibited decreasing activity; the duplex containing poly(C_7G) was inactive.

The C_nG copolymers were digested with ribonuclease T_1, which cleaves C-G bonds, to produce poly(C) fragments terminating in a G residue. These fragments were separated by chromatograpy on Sephadex columns and their size determined from the C/G ratio. This method yields direct estimates of polymer sizes, which are unaffected by polymer conformation unlike those determined by most physical methods. The sized polymers were annealed with high mw poly(I) ($S_{20,w} = 9.4$) and assayed for activation of the polymerase. With 20 mM magnesium, the concentration optimal for 2′5′oligo(A) synthesis, $(I)_n \cdot (C_{35})_n$ had low activity, $(I)_n \cdot (C_{55})_n$ was active and larger polymers were fully active relative to $(I)_n \cdot (C)_n$. The minimum size required for activity increased slightly when the magnesium concentration was lowered. Similar results were obtained with sized poly(A) and poly(U); $(A_{33})_n \cdot (U)_n$ was inactive, $(A_{55})_n \cdot (U)_n$ partially active and $(A)_n \cdot (U_{120})_n$ fully active. The slightly higher apparent size requirement for the $(A_x)_n \cdot (U_y)_n$ series relative to the $(I)_n \cdot (C)_n$ series may be due to lower stability of the duplexes or may be explained by a less precise method of size determination by velocity centrifugation. The 2′5′oligo(A) polymerase, therefore, requires for activation a relatively long stretch of base pairs uninterrupted by mismatches or discontinuities in either strand of the duplex.

The similarity of this structural requirement to that for induction of interferon by dsRNA led us to investigate the effect of 2′-O-methylation of the ribose moieties of poly(I) · poly(C). Complete methylation of either strand resulted in total loss of activity. Partial methylation of the C strand had a greater effect than a corresponding methylation of the I strand. As little as 20% methylation of poly(C) resulted in loss of activity, whereas 60% methylation of the poly(I) strand was required before significant loss of activity was observed. The activity of the various substituted duplexes appeared to correlate with the probability of occurrence of discrete size clusters of unsubstituted nucleotides. At 20 mM magnesium clusters of three unmodified residues may suffice, but this size increases as the magnesium concentration falls.

These results are compatible with a biphasic activation of the polymerase in which the enzyme binds to a relatively large segment of perfectly matched dsRNA, followed by an activation step which requires only a small segment of the dsRNA to be in the correct conformation. The behavior of the polymerase toward the various polymers is similar to that observed in the induction of IF by dsRNA, indicating that the two processes may recognize similar features in dsRNA and that both may occur *via* a biphasic activation mechanism.

DISCRIMINATION BETWEEN VIRAL AND HOST mRNA IN INTERFERON-TREATED CELLS

Timothy W. Nilsen and Corrado Baglioni

Department of Biological Sciences
State University of New York
Albany, New York 12222

Treatment of animal cells with interferon (IF) results in the induction of an enzymatic activity which, in the presence of double-stranded RNA (dsRNA), polymerizes ATP into pppA(2'p5'A)$_{1\text{-}6}$. These oligonucleotides have been designated 2,5A and the enzyme 2,5A polymerase. The levels of this enzymatic activity in IF-treated cells correlate with the inhibition of virus replication, as measured for example by the reduction in encephalomyocarditis virus (EMCV) RNA synthesis. This suggests that the 2,5A polymerase plays a role in the establishment of the antiviral state.

The 2,5A activates a single-strand specific endoribonuclease present in both IF-treated and untreated cells. This nuclease cleaves both viral and cellular mRNA in the presence of 2,5A. This fact must be taken into account in proposing a role for the 2,5A polymerase/endonuclease system in the antiviral state, since in IF-treated cells the accumulation of viral transcripts is specifically inhibited while host mRNA remains intact. Two properties of the 2,5A-activated endonuclease suggest a possible mechanism for the preferential degradation of viral mRNA: (1) the endonuclease activity is dependent on 2,5A concentration; (2) the endonuclease reverts to an inactive state in the absence of 2,5,A. If the 2,5A polymerase were activated by dsRNA present in viral replicative complexes (RC), there would be a locally high concentration of 2,5A. The endonuclease could then be effectively activated only near the site of 2,5A synthesis and this localized activation could result in the preferential degradation of nascent viral mRNA.

To test this working hypothesis, we constructed model substrates that share with RC one common feature: ssRNA is covalently linked to dsRNA. These substrates were cellular and viral poly(A)-containing mRNA, in which the poly(A) was annealed with poly(U), and EMCV RNA, in which a poly(C) tract was annealed with poly(I). These substrates were mixed with ssRNA labeled with a different isotope, which served as an internal control, and incubated in extracts of control and IF-treated cells. In all cases the ssRNA linked to dsRNA was preferentially cleaved relative to the unlinked ssRNA in extracts of IF-treated cells but not in extracts of control cells. The preferential degradation of ssRNA linked to dsRNA was not due to a nuclease that cleaves dsRNA, nor to binding to ribosomes and protection of mRNA not linked to dsRNA. This preferential degradation takes place regardless of the location of the dsRNA at the 3'-or near the 5'-terminus of RNA and of the base composition of the dsRNA linked to ssRNA. The preferential degradation requires Mg^{2+} and ATP, but is abolished by high concentrations of 2,5A or dsRNA. In this latter case all ssRNA is degraded. Moreover, the dsRNA linked to ssRNA has to be at least 60 base pairs long.

We have also examined the degradation of labeled EMCV replicative intermediate (RI) in extracts of control and IF-treated cells. The RI is preferentially degraded in extracts of IF-treated cells; only ssRNA is cleaved and an RNase resistant "core" is produced. This degradation is explained by the activation of the 2,5A polymerase by the dsRNA present in RI and by the localized activation of the 2,5A-dependent endonuclease.

These experiments have defined the conditions under which ssRNA linked to dsRNA can be preferentially degraded in extracts of IF-treated cells. Several lines of evidence indicate that this degradation is due to the 2,5A polymerase/endonuclease system. Finally, these results suggest a possible mechanism for the IF-mediated inhibition of viral RNA synthesis in cells infected by viruses which replicate through a dsRNA-containing intermediate.

ANTICELLULAR AND ANTIVIRAL EFFECTS OF PPPA(2′P5′A)N

A. G. Hovanessian, J. Wood, E. Meurs, and L. Montagnier

Unité d'Oncologie Virale
Département de Virologie, Institut Pasteur
Paris, 15ème, France

PppA (2′p5′A)n, the 2′5′ linked oligoadenylic acid triphosphate commonly known as 2-5A, is synthesized by an enzyme fraction from interferon-treated cells and rabbit reticulocyte lysates.[1,2] It is effective at subnanomolar concentrations in cell-free systems prepared from control cells and their effect seems to be mediated at least in part, by a nuclease that degrades mRNA.[3] By the use of a calcium phosphate coprecipitation technique[4] we show here that treatment of cells with 2-5A results in the inhibition of *in vivo* protein, RNA and DNA synthesis. In addition to these effects, treatment of vesicular stomatitis virus (VSV)-infected cells with 2-5A results in the inhibition of viral RNA synthesis. It is possible therefore to suggest that 2-5A plays a role at least in part in the antiviral action of interferon.

2-5A is a potent inhibitor of protein synthesis in intact cells of different origins: human, monkey, hamster and mouse. At a concentration of 10 nM (in AMP equivalents), protein synthesis is inhibited by 50 to 85 percent. There is also a secondary effect on the total RNA and DNA synthesis that becomes evident several hours after inhibition of protein synthesis. These inhibitory effects of 2-5A are transient at low concentrations of 2-5A (<20 nM). At higher concentrations, however, the inhibition of protein, RNA and DNA synthesis continue with an apparent effect on cell growth. In the virus-infected cell, although virus production is inhibited by <90%, the total shut down of cellular metabolic processes is not reversed after treatment with 2-5A (<20 nM). The VSV-infected cell dies with or without treatment with 2-5A. By 2-5A treatment, however, viral replication is eliminated or limited to a certain extent.

A nuclease activity is detected in cells following treatment with 2-5A, both total and polyadenylated RNA measured by ^{3}H-counts were reduced by 50 and 60–70%, respectively. In accord with this, electrophoretic profiles of total RNA indicated an apparent degradation of 28S and 18S ribosomal RNA into several small molecular weight components. Moreover, polyadenylated RNA was also degraded giving rise to a wide spectrum of products that were detectable as a smear on electrophoresis in polyacrylamide gels. Contrary to these results tRNA did not seem to be degraded in cells treated with 2-5A. Some minor degradation or modification of tRNA species, however, cannot be excluded. These results are difficult to explain on any other basis than an enhanced level of nuclease activity, since they represent degradation of previously labeled RNA. Accordingly, extracts from 2-5A-treated cells manifested an enhanced nuclease activity *in vitro* on viral and cellular RNAs.

REFERENCES

1. HOVANESSIAN A. G., R. E. BROWN & I. M. KERR. 1977. Nature **268:** 537–540.
2. HOVANESSIAN, A. G. & I. M. KERR. 1978. Eur. J. Biochem. **84:** 149–159.
3. CLEMENS, M. J. & B. R. WILLIAMS. 1978. Cell **13:** 565–572.
4. GRAHAM, F. L. & A. J. VAN DER EB. 1973. Virology **52:** 456–467.

INTERFERON-INDUCED SYNTHESIS OF SPECIFIC PROTEINS IN HUMAN FIBROBLASTS AND THE DEVELOPMENT OF THE ANTIVIRAL STATE

Berish Y. Rubin and Sohan L. Gupta

Interferon Laboratories
Memorial Sloan-Kettering Cancer Center
New York, New York 10021

The development of the antiviral effect of interferon (IF) is blocked by inhibitors of RNA and protein synthesis and by enucleation of cells, thus indicating that the expression of certain cellular gene(s) is required to be induced. We showed recently[1] that IF treatment induced the synthesis of at least three proteins in mouse Ehrlich ascites tumor cells and five proteins in human fibroblasts. Studies carried out with human cells are summarized here.

Human fibroblasts (FS-4, GM258, etc) were labeled with [^{35}S]methionine for 16–18 hr in the absence or presence of human leukocyte IF (400 reference units/ml), their extracts (200,000 × g supernatants) prepared and analyzed by sodium dodecyl sulfate (SDS)-polyacrylamide gel electrophoresis in slab gels. These experiments revealed four bands of proteins whose synthesis was markedly induced by IF treatment. These proteins had molecular weights of 88,000, 80,000, 67,000, and 56,000 (referred to as $P88_H$, $P80_H$, $P67_H$ and $P56_H$, respectively).[1] Extracts of IF-treated cells contain two enzymes, a protein kinase(s) and a 2′-5′-oligoadenylate synthetase, which are strongly activated by double-stranded RNA. Therefore, we fractionated these [^{35}S]methionine-labeled extracts on poly I · poly C-agarose columns, and after extensive washing, the material retained on the columns was extracted with SDS and analyzed on slab gels. These experiments revealed two protein bands (apparent molecular weights 120,000 and 80,000) which were detected strongly in samples derived from IF-treated cells but poorly, if at all, in similar samples obtained from untreated cells. Thus at least five proteins were found to be induced in human fibroblasts by IF treatment. Knight and Korant[2] have also detected four new proteins that were synthesized in human fibroblasts after treatment with interferon.

The characteristics of the induction of $P88_H$, $P80_H$, $P67_H$ and $P56_H$ by IF have been studied as they can be easily quantitated. The experiments indicate that the induction of these proteins by IF treatment has features in common with the development of the antiviral state thus suggesting a correlation between the two. For example: (1) it was blocked by actinomycin D (2 μg/ml) and cycloheximide (50 μg/ml) when added together with IF, thus indicating a requirement for *de novo* transcription and translation; (2) the induction of these proteins as well as the establishment of the antiviral state became resistant to inhibition by actinomycin D within 2 hr after the addition of IF, thus indicating that under the conditions employed, the transcription event induced by IF is essentially completed within 2 hr; (3) in agreement with the known species specificity, these proteins were induced by human leukocyte and human fibroblast IFs but not by mouse interferon[1]; and (4) the induction of these proteins and the establishment of the antiviral state show a similar dependence on the concentration of interferon.

Labeling for 2-hr periods at various times intervals after the addition of IF revealed that the synthesis of these proteins was induced within a few hours, peaked at different time intervals, and was soon followed by a marked decline, suggesting that the messenger RNAs for these proteins have short half-lives. Moreover, this decline occurred despite the fact that the cells were continuously exposed to IF, and there was no measurable loss of IF activity in the medium. This suggests that the induction of these proteins is transient and is apparently subject to further control.

References

1. Gupta, S. L., B. Y. Rubin & S. L. Holmes. 1979. Interferon action: Induction of specific proteins in mouse and human cells by homologous interferons. Proc. Nat. Acad. Sci. USA **76:** 4817–4821.
2. Knight, Jr., E. & B. D. Korant. 1979. Fibroblast interferon induces synthesis of four proteins in human fibroblast cells. Proc. Nat. Acad. Sci. USA **76:** 1824–1827.

INTERFERON-INDUCED mRNAs AND PROTEINS IN EHRLICH ASCITES TUMOR AND HeLa CELLS

Paul J. Farrell, Robert J. Broeze, and Peter Lengyel

Department of Molecular Biophysics and Biochemistry
Yale University
New Haven, Connecticut 06511

We are interested in the regulation and activation of various cytoplasmic enzymes in mouse Ehrlich ascites tumor (EAT) and human HeLa S3 cells by interferon (IF) and have looked at changes which occur in the protein and mRNA populations of these cells after IF treatment.

In EAT cells we previously found[1] one mRNA to be clearly induced by highly purified mouse IF; this mRNA is translated *in vitro* into a protein of MW 14,500 and pI 7.5. This protein is found in increased amounts in EAT cells after IF treatment and its synthesis is maximal after 8 hr of IF treatment.

More recently we have examined proteins and mRNAs induced in HeLa cells by human interferon. HeLa cell monolayers were treated with 500 U/ml of partially purified human leukocyte IF (specific activity 5×10^6 U/mg; a kind gift of Dr. K. Cantell) in the presence or absence of 2 μg/ml actinomycin D, or were not treated with IF (control cells). At various times after IF treatment, the cells were pulse labeled with [^{35}S]methionine for 1 hour, lysed, and the extracts analyzed by SDS-PAGE. One protein band (MW 53,000) was enhanced in the IF-treated cells. Synthesis of this protein occurred maximally 7–8 hr after IF treatment.

To determine whether this change was mirrored by a change in the mRNA population of the cells, poly A$^+$ mRNA was extracted from either cells treated with 500 U/ml IF for 8 hr, cells treated with 500 U/ml IF and 2 μg/ml actinomycin D for 8 hr or control cells. When the products of translation of these mRNAs in a wheat germ system were analyzed by SDS-PAGE, the mRNA from IF-treated cells yielded increased amounts of the 53,000 dalton protein compared with the mRNA from control cells. The mRNA from the actinomycin-treated cells gave only the control amount of the 53,000 dalton protein.

To examine more closely the populations of mRNAs and proteins, we analyzed the cell extracts and mRNA translation products by two dimensional gel electrophoresis.[2] Compared with control cells, two proteins (both MW 50,000 and pI approx 7) and one protein (MW 53,000, pI approx 6.5) accumulated in increased amounts in HeLa cells pulse-labeled for 1 hr with [^{35}S]methionine after 7 hr of IF treatment. The same three proteins were found to be enhanced in the *in vitro* translation products of mRNA from IF-treated HeLa cells as compared with those derived from control cell mRNA. Further analyses were done by nonequilibrium pH gradient electrophoresis.[3] One additional enhanced protein was observed in the translation products of mRNA from IF-treated HeLa cells. However, this protein was not observed in IF-treated HeLa cells by this method of analysis so is of doubtful significance. No additional enhanced proteins or mRNAs were detected by this method in the EAT cells treated with mouse interferon.

We have not yet been able to correlate any of these induced proteins with the enzyme activities known to be induced in IF-treated cells. Although we have purified preparations of the pppA(2′p5′A)$_n$ synthetase and the eIF-2 protein kinase (both dsRNA dependent) as markers in the EAT cell system, we have not yet visualized these in cell extracts by the above procedures. It is possible that these enzymes are present in very low amounts even in IF-treated cells and are beyond our limit of detection in the unfractionated ^{35}S-labeled extracts. It may be that the proteins we have observed to be enhanced are made in substantially larger amounts after IF treatment than the known induced enzymes and it will be interesting to try to determine their function.

References

1. Farrell P. J., R. J. Broeze & P. Lengyel. 1979. Nature **279:** 523–525.
2. O'Farrell, P. H. 1975. J. Biol. Chem. **250:** 4007–4021.
3. O'Farrell P. Z., H. M. Goodman & P. H. O'Farrell. 1977. Cell **12:** 1133–1142.

A NEW PROTEIN SYNTHESIS IS REQUIRED IN PRIMING BY INTERFERON

Takashi Fujita, Sakura Saito, and Seiya Kohno

Department of Measles Virus
National Institute of Health of Japan
Tokyo 190-12, Japan

Previous exposure of animal cells to an appropriate concentration of interferon (IF), priming, often converts them to better producers when they are stimulated for IF afterwards.[1-4] This facet of the biological functions of IF has been said to be distinguishable from the antiviral activity, mainly because development of the primed state in the cells was reported to be far less sensitive to cycloheximide than that of antiviral state.[1]

The priming of mouse L cells renders them responsive to the IF-inducing stimulus of live GD-7 virus infection,[3] or improves by some 10- to 30-fold the yield of poly(rI) · poly(rC)-induced IF synthesis.[4] In earlier communications, we reported that the enhancement in both systems is preceded by a distinct increase of its messenger RNA (mRNA) activity extractable from these cells. We presumed accordingly, that there was an acceleration of the transcription of the IF gene, or inhibition of the process(es) inactivating the IF mRNA, in primed cells.

These results encouraged us to re-investigate an involvement of *de novo* protein synthesis in the establishment of the primed state. Although this possibility had been once ruled out by Stewart II *et al.*[1] for mouse cells in the development of a primed state, we thought that the alteration induced by priming appears to be more extensive and profound than that which can be ascribed merely to a physical modification of cell membrane.

We now report two findings: (1) the induction for, and the synthesis of the IF mRNA in primed and poly(rI) · poly(rC)-treated cells are insensitive to the presence of cycloheximide (50 μg/ml, more than 99% of radioactive leucine incorporation into acid insoluble material is inhibited); and (2) the presence of this inhibitor during the priming period completely abolishes IF mRNA synthesis, hence, the priming effect.

CCL strain of mouse L cells were employed as a sole substrate for IF synthesis. Cell cultivation, poly(rI) · poly(rC) treatment, and the titration and the standardization of IF potencies were described elsewhere.[4] Cytoplasmic RNA was extracted from denucleated cells by the method described by Penman.[5] It was further fractionated into adenine-rich molecules by oligo-dT-cellulose chromatography[6] before being injected into oocytes of *Xenopus laevis*.[4,7] Conditions in correlating IF mRNA amount to the IF activity produced in the oocyte culture were detailed in our preceding paper.[4]

FIGURE 1 depicts result of an experiment in which the time courses of appearance of IF were studied in primed and in mock-IF-treated cultures after exposure to poly(rI) · poly(rC). At the times indicated in the figure, the cytoplasmic RNA extracts were determined for their IF mRNA amounts, which were plotted as the open (primed) and filled (unprimed) blocks. Results summarized in FIGURE 1 show that the priming *does* enhance the yield of, but *does not* advance or alter the time of the appearance of interferon. It is also evident from the figure

0077-8923/80/0350-0617 $01.75/0 © 1980, NYAS

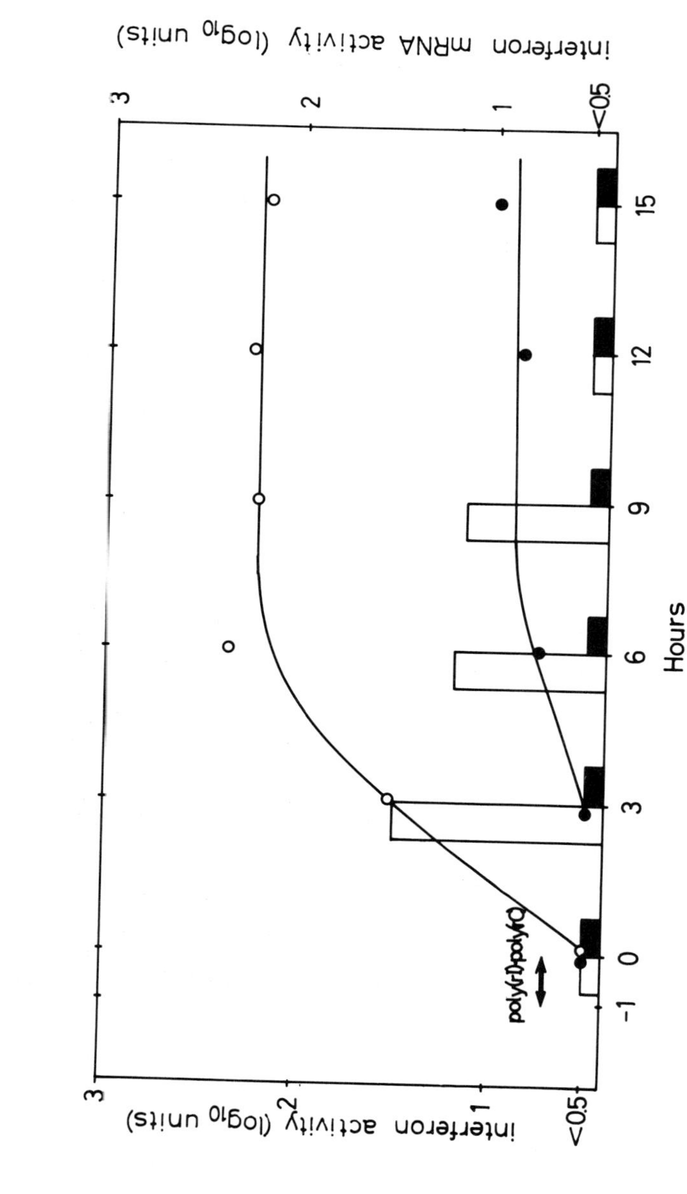

FIGURE 1. Quantification of cytoplasmic IF mRNA in L cells during primed and unprimed IF production. Open and filled circles denote potencies of IF in culture media of primed and unprimed L cells, respectively. Open and filled blocks represent the IF mRNA activity in RNA extracts from primed and unprimed cells, respectively.

that the priming increases the amount of cytoplasmic IF mRNA. In spite of an extensive search, in which the time of RNA extraction was carefully examined, we were unable to detect IF mRNA activity in the cytoplasmic RNA preparations obtained from unprimed cells.

Put together, these results imply that the level of primed state in mouse L cells can be estimated by determining either the yield of IF in the culture medium, or the accumulation of intracytoplasmic IF mRNA, provided that the cells were

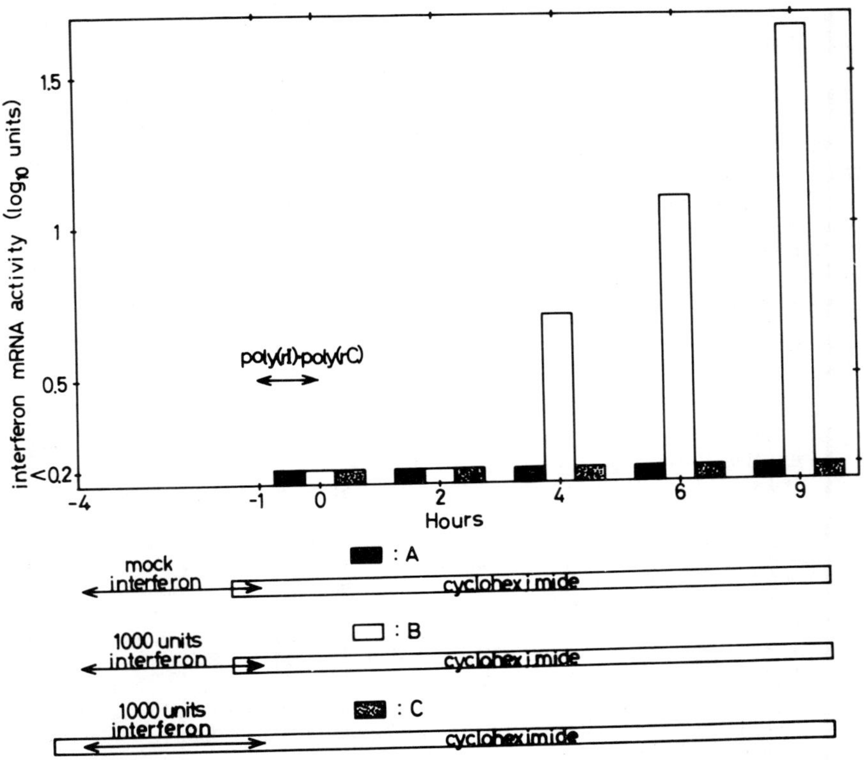

FIGURE 2. Effect of 50 μg/ml of cycloheximide on the priming by interferon. L-cell cultures were divided into three groups (A, B, and C) according to the schedule of cycloheximide treatment as shown in the bottom of the figure (see also text). The levels of primed state were estimated as a function of time by measuring cytoplasmic IF mRNA.[4]

properly induced. Consequently, we measured IF mRNA as a parameter of primed state in the experiment to elucidate a role of protein synthesis during the priming by interferon. A typical result of such experiments is illustrated in FIGURE 2.

L cells grown in 750 ml Roux bottles were divided into three groups (A, B, C in FIGURE 2). Cells of group C were under a constant exposure to 50 μg/ml of cycloheximide, starting 30 min before initiation of priming by 1,000 units of interferon. Cells of groups A and B were either mock-IF-treated (A), or primed

(B) in the absence of the inhibitor, which is introduced to the culture fluids of these cells at 30 min before the induction and made to remain in the culture thereafter. At 0 (immediately after the induction), 2, 4, 6, and 9 hr. five bottles of L cells of each group were collected, disrupted and extracted for interferon mRNA.

As can be seen clearly in FIGURE 2, the cells which were primed normally and induced for IF by poly(rI)·poly(rC) in the presence of overwhelming concentration of cycloheximide produced the mRNA which continued to accumulate cytoplasmically until 9 hr (group B). On the other hand, in the cells that were not primed (group A), or primed in the presence of cycloheximide (group C), the IF mRNA activity did not show up.

The presence of a high concentration of cycloheximide in the culture medium, arresting cellular protein synthesis in general, was thought to protect the mRNA from degradation by controlling hydrolytic enzymes.[8] Our failure to observe a leveling off of interferon mRNA activity in cells of group B, FIGURE 2, may be explained by assuming this stabilization.

The implication of these results presented here is the requirement of *de novo* synthesis of protein(s) for the cells to be primed by interferon. It is out of harmony with the earlier conclusion of others,[1] but quite reminiscent of a growing body of knowledge on the cellular processes involved in the expression of the antiviral activity of interferon.[9]

REFERENCES

1. STEWART II, W. E., L. B. GOSSER & R. Z. LOCKART, JR. 1971. Priming: A nonantiviral function of interferon. J. Virol. **7:** 792–801.
2. ABREU, S. L., F. C. BANCROFT & W. E. STEWART II. 1979. Interferon priming effects on interferon messenger RNA. J. Biol. Chem. **254:** 4114–4118.
3. SAITO, S., T. MATSUNO, T. SUDO, E. FURUYA & S. KOHNO. 1976. Priming activity of mouse interferon: Effect of interferon messenger RNA synthesis. Arch. Virol. **52:** 159–163.
4. FUJITA, T. S. SAITO & S. KOHNO. 1979. Priming increases the amount of interferon mRNA in poly(rI) · poly(rC)-treated L cells. J. Gen. Virol. **45:** 301–308.
5. PENMAN, S. 1969. Preparation of purified nuclei and nucleoli from mammalian cells. *In* Fundamental Techiques in Virology. K. Habel & N. P. Salzman, Eds.: 35–48. Academic Press. New York, London.
6. AVIV, H. & P. LEDER. 1972. Purification of biologically active globin messenger RNA by chromatography on oligo thymidylic acid-cellulose. Proc. Nat. Acad. Sci. USA **69:** 1408–1412.
7. GURDON, J. B. 1976. Injected nuclei in frog oocytes: Fate, enlargement and chromatin dispersal. J. Embryo. Exp. Morphol. **36:** 523–540.
8. VILČEK, J., E. A. HAVELL & M. KOHASE. 1976. Superinduction of interferon with metabolic inhibitors possible mechanisms and practical applications. J. Infect. Dis. **133** (Suppl): A22–A-29.
9. KIMCHI, A., L. SHULMAN, A. SCHMIDT, Y. CHERNAJOVSKY, A. FRADIN & M. REVEL. 1979. Kinetics of induction of three translation-regulatory enzymes by interferon. Proc. Nat. Acad. Sci. USA **76:** 3208–3212.

DISTINCT INTERFERON RESPONSES IN CULTURED MAMMALIAN CELLS

Lee H. Kronenberg

Calbiochem-Behring Corporation
La Jolla, California 92037

A series of studies tested the effects of antimetabolites, ultraviolet irradiation or interferon pretreatment (priming) on production of interferon (IF) by mouse (L929), rabbit (RK13), and diploid human cell strains. Cultures were induced with poly I:poly C ("IC"), poly I:poly C:DEAE-dextran complex ("ICD") or Newcastle disease virus (NDV) and IFs were assayed as described previously.[1,2]

Rates of accumulation of IF were measured by assaying culture fluids changed at 2 hr intervals. As reported[3,4] IC induces an early response followed by a rapid "shutoff" of IF accumulation; NDV and ICD induced later responses without a marked shutoff.

The effects of priming 15 hr with 0.01–100 ref. unit/ml on subsequent IF yields were tested. Enhanced IF yields were evident for induction by IC, but not ICD or NDV.

Preirradiation with UV (254 nm) showed that induction by NDV is radiosensitive at all doses and that the curve is biphasic. The more- and less-radiosensitive portions of the curve (I and II respectively) have a ratio of slopes I/II of about 2.5 to 1. Induction by ICD is also radiosensitive at all UV doses with a slope similar to I. However, induction by IC is markedly enhanced by UV doses up to ca. 500 erg/mm^2 but is inactivated at higher doses, confirming earlier reports.[5,6] For the inactivation portion of the IC curve, the slope is indistinguishable from II for NDV. This suggests that NDV induces two IF responses with different target sizes for inactivation, one of which is also induced by IC, and the other by ICD.

Treatment with antimetabolites followed procedures of Tan[7] and Vilček[8] with minor modifications. Whether cultures were "superinduced" with actinomycin D alone or with actinomycin plus cycloheximide, only IF yields induced by IC were enhanced by treatment with antimetabolites.

Human IFs were assayed on both human fibroblasts and bovine kidney (MDBK) cultures.[9] It was found that NDV-induced IFs contain 5–15% IF-L by this criterion, whereas no detectable IF-L was induced by IC or ICD, as reported by Havell *et al.*[10]

Previous studies by Montagnier *et al.*[11] and in this laboratory indicate that different forms of IF mRNA can be extracted from mouse cells induced with NDV or IC. Erickson and Paucker[12] have recently shown that different populations of IF species are produced by L929 cells in response to NDV and ICD, and preliminary evidence in our laboratory suggests that human fibroblasts produce different populations of IF species in response to each of the three inducers described above.

The foregoing suggests that a pattern of two IF responses appears ubiquitous in mammalian cell lines, distinguishable at several stages of the response: (1) the transcriptional unit, as suggested by the UV data; (2) susceptibility to priming by IF; (3) susceptibility to superinduction by antimetabolites; (4) kinetics of accumulation and shutoff of IF synthesis; (5) IF mRNAs; and (6) IF gene products. Finally, since polycations have been used widely to enhance IF yields, it is of interest that DEAE-dextran converts the regulation from an IC-type to an NDV-type response.

Induction of IF by viruses may be a combination of two mechanisms among various cell/virus combinations. The secondary structure in viral mRNAs or replicative products may be responsible for an IC-type response, and to this extent amenable to enhancement by priming or superinduction. On the other hand, some aspect of the virion or of viral nucleoprotein may stimulate the alternate response, typified here by NDV and ICD.

References

1. BRYSON, Y. J. & L. H. KRONENBERG. 1977. Antimicrob. Agents Chemother. **11:** 299.
2. KRONENBERG, L. H. 1977. Virology **76:** 634.
3. BAUSEK, G. H. & T. C. MERIGAN. 1970. Proc. Soc. Exp. Biol. Med. **133:** 982.
4. VILČEK, J., S. L. BARMAK & E. A. HAVELL. 1972. J. Virol. **10:** 614.
5. MOZES, L. W. & J. VILČEK. 1974. J. Virol. **13:** 646.
6. LINDNER-FRIMMEL, S. J. 1974. J. Gen. Virol. **25:** 147.
7. TAN, Y. H., J. A. ARMSTRONG, Y. H. KE & M. HO. 1970. Proc. Nat. Acad. Sci. USA **67:** 464.
8. VILČEK, J. & M. H. NG. 1971. J. Virol. **7:** 588.
9. GRESSER, I., M. T. BANDU, D. BROUTY-BOYE & M. G. TOVEY. 1974. Nature **251:** 543.
10. HAVELL, E. A., T. G. HAYES & J. VILČEK. 1978. Virology **89:** 330.
11. MONTAGNIER, L., H. COLLANDRE, J. DE MAEYER-GUIGNARD & E. DE MAEYER. 1974. Biochem. Biophys. Res. Commun **59:** 1031.
12. ERICKSON, J. S. & K. PAUCKER. 1979. J. Gen. Virol. **43:** 521.

INTERFERON REGULATES CELL MOTILITY

John Wérenne,* Xavier Emonds-Alt, and Jacques Bartholeyns†

International Institute of Cellular and Molecular Pathology (ICP)
Brussels, Belgium

We showed recently (J. Wérenne, M. Revel and D. Wallach, unpublished) that interferon (IF) decreases cell migration in wounded monolayers of human cells, and using the L1210 cell system we attempted to determine if IF also regulates other aspects of cell motility.

It is well established that IF treatment causes a modification of a number of cell membrane characteristics. For example, we observed that IF decreases in L1210 cells the level of plasminogen activator. The glucocorticoid hormone dexamethasone exerts a synergistic action with IF on this enzyme. This action is expressed similarly on the adhesion of the cells to glass. They adhere less loosely when treated by IF and dexamethasone, which is probably indicative of the recovery of a more normal phenotype. We postulated that the effect of IF on plasma membrane results from a modification of their dynamic properties. As a recycling process of plasma membrane constituents has been recently proposed[1] we could expect that IF also affects the properties of intracellular organelles.

Indeed, we have shown previously[2] that the lysosomes of the murine leukemic L1210 R, an IF-resistant variant of our cell system kindly donated by I. Gresser, are much more stable than those of the sensitive parent line. A modification by IF of the properties of the lysosomes of murine fibroblasts has been independently observed by others.[3]

We showed here that relatively high amounts of IF (3000 U/ml) and a long treatment (48 hr) of the cells by this agent are necessary in order to detect a significant increase in the fragility of the lysosomes.

We propose that this increase of the lysosomal fragility is the final consequence of the effect of IF on the dynamic flow of membrane constituents. As membrane internalization leading to the formation of intracellular vesicles is accompanied by pinocytosis of exogeneous material, to test our hypothesis we studied the uptake of horse radish-peroxidase (HRP, 1 mg/ml) as a marker for cellular loading by the endocytic process. No significant difference in uptake of the exogeneous enzyme is observed with IF treatment (24 hr of 300 U/ml of a 10^6 U/mg preparation of IF-induced in L929 cells by NDVo) during the 4 hr of incubation necessary to obtain the steady state of HRP trapping.

After washing the cells, a progressive decrease of the activity of the trapped enzyme resulting in either exocytosis or degradation (with a half-life time of about 3 hr) was observed in the IF-treated cells; the fate of HRP is different. A bimodal phenomenon characterizes the unloading of the enzyme activity. Part of the trapped enzyme (about 50%) is first released very rapidly (in less than 10 min). As a secondary process, the remaining activity appears in the extracellular fluid, but much more slowly than in the control. We may conclude from our data that compared to the control, in the IF-treated cells, a higher proportion of the

**Present address:* Université Libre de Bruxelles, Laboratoire de Chimie Générale I, Faculté des Sciences, B-1050 Brussels, Belgium.

†*Present address:* Centre de Recherches Merrell-International, 16, Av. d'Ankara, F-67084 Strasbourg, France.

exogeneous material remains trapped in uncompletely closed vacuoles and is therefore released by a simple washing of the cells. Less enzyme must be therefore completely internalized. After washing, this internalized HRP is more slowly released from the IF-treated cell in the extracellular milieu. As this exocytosis process is accompanied by the recycling of membrane components associated with the internalized phagocytic vesicles towards the plasma membrane, we may interpret our data as showing a slowing of the transit of membrane in IF-treated cell constituents between the intracellular organelles and the membrane.

According to this interpretation, both membrane internalization and recycling would be affected by interferon. This effect would be characterized by a more rigid membrane structure, which could explain the observed reduction of cell mobility.

Acknowledgments

Part of this work was supported by a NATO Grant.

References

1. Schneider, Y. J., Tulkens, C. de Duve & A. Trouet. 1979. J. Cell. Biol. **82:** 466–474.
2. Wérenne, J. & J. Bartholeyns. 1977. Biochem. Soc. Trans. **5:** 1176–1178.
3. Halbach, M., K. Koschel & C. Jungwirth. 1978. J. Gen. Virol. **39:** 387–390.

INTERFERON INHIBITS CELL FUSION BY SENDAI VIRUS

Y. Tomita and T. Kuwata

Department of Microbiology
School of Medicine, Chiba University
Chiba 280, Japan

Interferon (IF) causes gradual biochemical effects on cultured cells and some of the effects have been attributed to alteration of the plama membrane. Recently, we found that UV-inactivated RD-114 virus, a type C virus from the domestic cat, induced fusion of human transformed cells RSa and IF^r, as well as KC cells, and that the fusion was prevented by the treatment of cells with human IF prior to the addition of UV-inactivated RD-114 virus.[1] In view of these observations, we have studied the effect of IF on cell fusion by UV-inactivated Sendai virus (Sendai virus-UV). We report here that treatment with human leukocyte interferon (Le-IF) or fibroblast interferon (F-IF) produces alteration of cells and inhibits cell fusion by Sendai virus-UV.

Monolayers of human cell lines RSa, RSb, IF^r, RD-114 and SV40-transformed VA were treated with Le-IF or F-IF for 16 to 20 hr, then washed with fresh medium without IF and fused with Sendai Virus-UV for an additional 16 hr. Cell fusion was estimated by the number of syncytia per dish. Interferon treatment reduced cell fusion in every cell line. The effect of IF increased according to its concentration. At 200 to 500 U/ml of Le-IF or F-IF, the number of syncytia per dish was reduced to less than 13% relative to the untreated control. Le-IF, which is not anitviral for mouse cells, did not inhibit fusion of mouse L cells by Sendai virus-UV. A fusion-inhibitory state of the cells persisted for about 50 hr after the cells were treated with Le-IF at 250 U/ml. Anti-Le-IF serum (250 U/ml), which was supplied by Dr. K. Cantell, neutralized the IF activity. Mock IF prepared in the same manner as Le-IF had no apparent effect on cell fusion. To demonstrate that the inhibition of RSa cell fusion was not due to the suppression of replication of residual infectious Sendai virus, RSa or HeLa-S3 cells suspended at 2×10^7 cells per ml were fused by Sendai-UV during 45 min at 37°C according to the methods described by Okada *et al.*[2] Fusion of untreated cells depended on the dose of Sendai-UV. Pretreatment of cells with Le-IF (250 U/ml) or F-IF (500 U/ml) for 16 hr decreased cell fusion to less than 12% of untreated controls. Simultaneous treatment of cells with cycloheximide at 1 to 5 μg/ml blocked the activity of Le-IF (250U/ml). In this case, cell fusion was 81 to 98% of the control without cycloheximide and Le-IF. All these data suggest that the antifusion activity is a function of IF and for the development of antifusion state in cells, macromolecular synthesis is required.

References

1. Tomita Y. & T. Kuwata. 1979, J. Gen. Virol **43:** 111–117.
2. Okada, Y. & J. Tadokoro. 1963. Exp. Cell Res. **32:** 417–430.

HUMAN FIBROBLAST AND HUMAN LEUKOCYTE INTERFERON: THEIR DIFFERENCES IN CELL GROWTH INHIBITION ACTIVITIES ON LYMPHOBLASTOID CELLS

J. Hilfenhaus and R. Mauler

Research Laboratories of Behringwerke AG
D-3550 Marburg, Federal Republic of Germany

Besides their antiviral activity interferons (IFs) show several other biological activities of which the capability to inhibit cell growth, particularly that of tumor cells *in vitro*, has been extensively studied. We determined the cell growth inhibitory activity of human fibroblast interferon (F-IF) and human leukocyte interferon (Le-IF) on various human lymphoblastoid cell lines. Among these cell lines, all of which except the cell line MOLT-4 were carriers of the Epstein-Barr virus genome and were characterized as B-type lymphoblasts, the cell line Daudi was the most sensitive to F-IF as well as to Le-IF.[1] We therefore established a growth-inhibitory-activity assay of human interferon using Daudi cells.[2] In this assay the inhibitory effect of human IF in a 5-day Daudi cell culture in microtiter plates is measured by the [^{14}C]thymidine uptake during the last 18 hours. The [^{14}C]thymidine uptake is directly correlated to the final cell count per culture.

Using this assay on Daudi cells we found that (1) F-IF as well as Le-IF preparations were active whereas respective mock-IF preparations were inactive and that (2) IF preparations of different purity, including the international F-IF and Le-IF standard preparations showed almost the same ratio of cell growth-inhibitory to antiviral activity. In this assay 50% inhibition of Daudi cell growth was caused by 43 i.u. of F-IF (range 21–89 i.u., 17 determinations) or by 25 i.u. of Le-IF (range 13–52 i.u., 51 determinations). Antiviral activity titers in international units (i.u.) refer to the NIH F-IF and Le-IF standard preparations. F-IF obtained from human diploid foreskin fibroblast cell strains alpha-1 or FS4 revealed the same ratio of cell-growth-inhibitory to antiviral activity. Although based on the antiviral activity of F-IF and Le-IF preparations both types of human IF inhibit Daudi cell propagaation to nearly the same extent, the dose response curves of both human IFs on these cells differ, however, in their slopes. Consequently, we conclude that separate standard preparations of F-IF and Le-IF should be used in order to standardize cell-growth-inhibitory assays of human interferons.

Einhorn and Strander[3] previously reported that human lymphoblastoid and osteosarcoma lines differed in their sensitivities to the growth-inhibitory activity of F-IF and Le-IF. When studying the growth inhibitory activity of F-IF and Le-IF preparations, we compared various lymphoblastoid cell lines. We found a considerably higher sensitivity of the T-type lymphoblastoid cell MOLT-4 to F-IF than to Le-IF while the sensitivities of seven other human B-type lymphoblastoid cell lines (highly sensitive: Daudi; moderately sensitive: Diehl I and P3HR1; insensitive: Kaplan, Namalva, RPMI 1788, SKL 1) were within the range of error comparably sensitive to both type-I human interferons. Whether human B-type and T-type lymphoblastoid cell lines generally differ in their affinities to the cell-growth-inhibitory activity of F-IF and Le-IF needs further investigation.

REFERENCES

1. HILFENHAUS, J., H. DAMM & R. JOHANNSEN. 1977. Sensitivity of various human lymphoblastoid cells to the antiviral and anticellular activity of human leukocyte interferon. Arch. Virol. **54:** 271–277.
2. HILFENHAUS, J., H. DAMM, H. E. KARGES & K. F. MANTHEY, 1976. Growth inhibition of human lymphoblastoid Daudi cells in vitro by interferon preparations. Arch. Virol. **51:** 87–97.
3. EINHORN, S. & H. STRANDER. 1977. Is interferon tissue-specific? Effect of human leukocyte and fibroblast interferons on the growth of lymphoblastoid and osteosarcoma cell lines. J. Gen. Virol. **35:** 573–577.

COMPARATIVE STUDY ON THE EFFECTS OF FIBROBLAST AND LEUKOCYTE INTERFERON ON SHORT-TERM CULTURES OF LEUKEMIC CELLS

E. Lundgren, W. Hillörn, D. Holmberg, P. Lenner, G. Roos, and Ö. Strannegård.

University of Umeå
Umeå, Sweden

University of Göteborg
Göteburg, Sweden

In mouse models hematopoetic neoplasms are often successfully treated with interferon (IF). Some studies have been initiated in man. To evaluate the mechanism of IF effects in human leukemia, an *in vitro* test was developed with the aim to analyze the inhibition of cell proliferation.

Leukemic cells were isolated from peripheral blood and cultivated for 24 hr in the presence of varying IF concentrations. The [^{3}H]TdR incorporation after 24 hr was determined as a measurement of the rate of DNA synthesis. The relevance of this method was tested on some established neoplastic hematopoetic cell lines.

When tested on four different leukemic hematopoetic cell lines, IF had to be present at least 24 hr to express its effect on cell growth. This was observed both when cell number and thymidine incorporation was quantitated. After 72 hr IF had fully expressed its effect. In the clinical material there was a progressive cell death if the culture time was more than 24 hr and hence this time of incubation with IF was used throughout the study. This means that IF sensitivity could not be detected in cells responding later than 24 hours.

Most leukemic cells were sensitive to interferon. When antiviral titers were compared, fibroblast IF seemed to be a more efficient suppressor of DNA synthesis. There was a marked difference in IF sensitivity between cells from different individuals. The IF concentration necessary to suppress DNA synthesis by 50% was usually higher than the concentration achieved in serum after injection of therapeutic doses. It is not known if IF exerts its effect mainly by cell growth inhibition or by the immune system (e.g. NK cells). The possible value of the present method for prediction of a therapeutic effect of IF can only be evaluated by clinical trials.

EFFECT OF INTERFERON ON SYNTHESIS OF VIRAL AND CELLULAR PROTEINS BY CHRONICALLY INFECTED MOUSE CELLS

Marc De Ley, Alfons Billiau, and Pieter De Somer

Rega Institute
Katholieke Universiteit Leuven
B-3000 Leuven, Belgium

The release of infectious C-type particles from chronically infected human and mouse cells is drastically but reversibly inhibited by interferon (IF) treatment. Evidence exists suggesting that this inhibition is due to a defect in late stages of virus formation.[1] A threefold accumulation of virus particles at the cell surface (trapping effect) was observed.[2] With respect to structural proteins the relative enhancement of a 85,000 dalton glycoprotein[3] and a defective complex between p30 and the viral reverse transcriptase have been shown.[4]

It has been observed that the establishment of the IF-induced antiviral state coincides with the induction of several enzymatic activities: a phosphodiesterase, an adenylate cyclase, a membrane-bound alkaline ribonuclease, a protein kinase and a (2′–5′)A_n synthetase. Interferon-induced proteins in human[5] and chick cells[6] have recently been visualized by autoradiography.

We have used SDS-PAGE and 2-dimensional electrophoresis to detect IF-induced changes in cellular as well as in viral proteins: both radioactively labeled virus particles and cell lysates of chronically infected JLSV5 cells were analyzed.

The cells were labeled with L-[^{35}S]-methionine and treated with 0 and 10^3 U/ml of mouse interferon. After 24 hr, virus was isolated from the supernatant fluids and lysates were prepared from the cells. SDS-PAGE of the sucrose gradient-purified virus particles showed that, as a consequence of IF treatment, the relative amount of a 69,000-dalton protein decreased while that of an 84,000-dalton protein increased. The latter was shown by 2-dimensional electrophoresis to have a pI of 5.5. The glycoprotein nature of both the 69,000- and the 84,000-dalton protein was demonstrated by [^{14}C]glucosamine labeling. The 84,000-dalton glycoprotein could not be precipiated with either anti-gp69/71 or with anti-p30.

Examination of L-[^{35}S]-methionine-labeled lysates revealed a 63,000-dalton protein, only present in IF-treated cells. The induction of this protein started at an IF concentration of 100 U/ml. The induction of a similar protein in mouse embryo fibroblasts from NMRI mice was a strong indication for its cellular rather than its viral origin. A pI of 6.3 for the induced protein was determined by 2-dimensional electrophoresis. The 63,000-dalton protein was shown to bind the poly(I) · poly(C)-Sepharose and could only be eluted with 1 M KCl. In this respect it behaved like the (2′–5′)A_n synthetase and the protein kinase described by others.[7]

REFERENCES

1. BILLIAU, A., H. HEREMANS, P. T. ALLEN, S. BARON, & P. DE SOMER. 1978. Arch. Virol. **57:** 205–220.

2. BILLIAU, A., H. HEREMANS, P. T. ALLEN, J. DE MAEYER-GUIGNARD & P. DE SOMER. 1976. Virology **73:** 537–542.
3. CHANG, E. H., & R. M. FRIEDMAN. 1977. Biochem. Biophys. Res. Commun. **77:** 392–398.
4. BANDYOPADHYAY, A. K., E. H. CHANG, C. C. LEVY & R. M. FRIEDMAN. 1979. Biochem. Biophys. Res. Commun. **87:** 983–988.
5. KNIGHT, E., JR., & B. D. KORANT. 1979. Proc. Nat. Acad. Sci. USA **76:** 1824–1827.
6. BALL, L. A. 1979. Virology **94:** 282–296.
7. HOVANESSIAN, A. G., & I. A. KERR. 1979. Eur. J. Biochem. **93:** 515–526.

INHIBITION OF MURINE MAMMARY TUMOR VIRUS PRODUCTION BY INTERFERON TREATMENT OF MAMMARY TUMOR CELLS *IN VITRO*

Ganes C. Sen and Nurul H. Sarkar

Memorial Sloan-Kettering Cancer Center
New York, New York 10021

Murine mammary tumor virus (MuMTV), a type B retrovirus, is the only viral agent known to cause mammary carcinoma in mice. Cell lines have been established from the mammary tumors of mice of different strains. A cell line established from the mammary tumor of a GR mouse, produces MuMTV upon treatment with dexamethasone, a synthetic steroid hormone. We report here the effects of treating the dexamethasone-stimulated GR cells with mouse interferon (IF). A partially purified mouse IF preparation with a specific activity of about 10^7 units/mg protein was used for most of the experiments described here. The dose of IF was 50 units/ml. We found that extracellular MuMTV production was inhibited by about 80% when the cells were treated with interferon. The amount of virus production was measured either by measuring the virus-associated reverse-transcriptase activity or by metabolic labeling of the virus with [^{3}H] uridine or [^{14}C] amino acids. There was no inhibition of cellular RNA or protein synthesis under these conditions. When pure homogeneous mouse IF was used instead of the partially purified IF preparation the same inhibitory effects on MuMTV production were observed. This demonstrated that the effects were due to IF itself. Moreover, it also established that the observed antiviral effects on the replication of retroviruses and other viruses are caused by the same IF molecule although the molecular mechanisms of these inhibitions seem to be entirely dissimilar.

The extracellular MuMTV particles produced by the IF-treated cells contained all the proteins present in a normal MuMTV. There was also no extra protein present in such viruses. Though the IF-treated cells produced less extracellular virus particles, the intracellular level of viral RNA as measured by hybridization analyses and the intracellular levels of the major viral envelope protein gp52 and the major viral core protein p27 as measured by radioimmuno-competition assays were not lower in the IF-treated cells as compared to the untreated cells. Electron microscopy of thin sections from the control and IF-treated cells revealed no gross differences in any subcellular structures including those of the budding viruses. Scanning electron microscopy of the control and IF-treated cells showed an increased number of virus particles on the cell surface of the IF-treated cells. These results suggest that the impairment of extracellular MuMTV production by IF-treatment of GR cells is caused by an IF-induced block at a very late stage of virus morphogenesis.

PRIMING EFFECT OF INTERFERON ON THE PRODUCTION OF ENDOTOXIN-INDUCED INTERFERON IN RABBITS AND RABBIT LYMPHOID CELLS

Yasuhiko Kojima, Hiroshi Hashimoto, and Nobuyuki Shibukawa

The Kitasato Institute
Tokyo, Japan

In previous reports, we indicated that the *in vitro* production of endotoxin-induced interferon (IF) in rabbit lymphoid cell cultures could be enhanced by pretreatment with IF.[1] It turned out that when 10–30 units/ml of rabbit IF was given for pretreatment and incubated for 6 hr the maximal priming effect was attained. Occasional lymphoid cells naturally showing a noninducible state, or lymphoid cells rendered noninducible by incubation at 37°C for 1 day could produce IF after priming with IF.[2] These results suggested occurrence of a similar priming *in vivo* after injection of IF.

The present study was undertaken to test this possibility in rabbits. Spleen, bone marrow, lymph nodes, thymus, liver and blood leukocytes were primed with IF *in vitro*. In control unprimed cell cultures, IF produced by these cells averaged 115, 16, 61, 22, 20, and 15 units, whereas in primed cell cultures it averaged 1700, 1285, 403, 79, 110, and 10 units, respectively. Spleen and bone marrow cells were the most sensitive tissues to the priming effect of IF, but blood leukocytes did not respond to the priming effect. To test the priming effect in rabbits, 11 rabbits were injected intravenously with 10^6 or 2×10^5 units of IF or phosphate buffered saline (PBS). After 6 hr, spleen and bone marrow cells from these rabbits were exposed to 1 μg of endotoxin *in vitro*. The cells from the rabbits pretreated with 10^6 or 2×10^5 units of IF or PBS produced IF averaging 970, 170, or 35 units, respectively, in the case of spleen cells, and 530, 275, or 66 units, respectively, in the case of bone marrow cells.

An attempt was then made to test the *in vitro* priming and *in vivo* production of endotoxin-induced IF. Eight rabbits were injected with 10^6 units of IF or PBS and after 6 hr these rabbits were injected with 100 μg of endotoxin. After 2 hr, the primed and unprimed rabbits produced IF that averaged 4925 and 938 units, respectively, in circulation. These results show that a priming effect *in vivo* occurred after an injection of 10^6 units of IF.

When lymphoid cells from rabbits receiving 100 μg of endotoxin 48 or 24 hr previously were primed with IF *in vitro*, these otherwise poorly responding or noninducible cells could produce an appreciable amount of endotoxin-induced IF.

These facts would suggest the efficacy of a combination-therapy using IF and IF inducers *in vivo*.

References

1. Hashimoto, H., N. Shibukawa & Y. Kojima. 1978. The mode of production of endotoxin-induced interferon in rabbit tissue cells. I. Development of priming by pretreatment with interferon. Microbiol. Immunol. **22:** 673–681.
2. Hashimoto, H., N. Shibukawa & Y. Kojima. 1979. The mode of production of endotoxin-induced interferon in rabbit lymphoid cell cultures. II. Priming effect of interferon on apparently noninducible cells. Microbiol. Immunol. **23:** 1033–1036.

EFFECT OF MULTIPLICITY OF INFECTION ON THE ANTIVIRAL ACTION OF INTERFERON *IN VITRO*

L. W. Stitz

Primate Center TNO, Virology Section
Rijswijk, the Netherlands

H. Schellekens

Department of Virology
Erasmus University
Rotterdam, the Netherlands

Early reports on the influence of the multiplicity of infection (MOI) on the antiviral state induced by interferon (IF) *in vitro* are conflicting. Results supporting dependence as well as independence on the MOI have been both reported. In all of these studies a MOI of much less than 1 was used. These early results are, however, difficult to compare, because it is not always clear what was the exact MOI and whether the antiviral activity was mediated by interferon.

This study was done to determine the influence of the MOI on the protection of cells of different species provided by the appropriate IF both DNA and RNA as well as positive- and negative-strand viruses were included. In our study the antiviral activity of IF was found to be dependent on the MOI. Cells of different species could not be protected by IF against the cytopathogenic effect of vaccinia, herpes, ECHO or vesicular stomatitis virus (VSV) at an MOI > 1. Protection could only be achieved at a MOI ≤ 1. The amount of IF necessary was inversely related to the MOI and the protection was only transient. The duration of the antiviral effect of IF was also inversely related to the MOI. The dependence of the antiviral effect of IF on the MOI could not be explained by assuming the viruses to be mixtures of subtypes with different IF sensitivity. This we have shown by the similar sensitivity of clones of VSV against the protective effect of interferon. Neither could a selection by IF treatment of IF-insensitive subtypes be shown. VSV passaged at high MOI in IF-treated cells showed no difference in sensitivity to IF compared with the parental strain. By prechallenging cells at a low MOI before IF treatment and the final challenge we could show that the enhanced antiviral effect of IF at low MOI was probably not caused by IF induction by the infecting virus. There was no obvious difference between preinfected cells and cells that were not prechallenged. Neither a direct inactivation by the virus of the antiviral effect of IF could be established. No protection could be achieved by additional IF treatment during the incubation period after infection.

These results indicate that when IF-treated cells are infected these cells will not survive the infection. The only result of the IF treatment will be the inhibition of viral replication to some extent leading only to a delay in cell death.

APPLICATION OF TYPE I MOUSE INTERFERON IN VIRUS-INDUCED ERYTHROID LEUKEMIA

J. Trapman and R.A.C.P. Hekman

Department of Pathology
Erasmus University
Rotterdam, the Netherlands

Interferons (IFs) possess, by definition, antiviral activity. Besides this, other biological properties have been described, such as inhibition of cell growth and modulation of the immune system. Therefore, IFs promise to be efficient antitumor agents.

From earlier studies it is known that IF preparations are able to retard the development of Rauscher murine leukemia virus (R-MuLV)-induced erythroid leukemia in BALB/c mice.[1] We have extended these observations, using high dosages of interferon. The IF preparation used in this study (pIC-IF) was produced by induction of mouse L-929 cells by poly (I)·poly (C).[2] This preparation has a specific activity of about 10^6 (pIC-IF-C) to 4×10^6 (ammonium sulfate purified, pIC–IF–AS) u/mg protein. Thus far we have studied the effect of short-term treatment (two weeks) starting 6 hr after i.p. inoculation of large amounts of R-MuLV. Under the conditions applied R-MuLV-infected mice (female animals, 4 to 5 weeks old) normally die within 3 to 4 weeks after virus infection.

In our first series of experiments we have demonstrated, using both pIC-IF-C and pIC-IF-AS, that moderate doses of this type of IF (3 to 5×10^4 u/day) are able to retard the development of Rauscher disease in BALB/c mice. Histological and cytological examination of spleen and liver revealed a better conserved morphological structure with fewer Rauscher cells and a diminished infiltration by erythroid cells of the liver in IF-treated infected animals as compared to infected untreated mice. These results are essentially similar to those obtained by others using IF preparations from different sources (see refs. in 1).

Subsequently, we have investigated the effect of daily i.p. injections of high dosages of IF (3.2×10^5 u). IF-treated infected mice showed after 13 days no or only minimum signs of Rauscher disease. That is:

1. Spleen weights of IF-treated R-MuLV infected mice are comparable to those of mice treated with IF alone.
2. Absence of virus from the serum as determined by reverse transcriptase assay.
3. No infiltration of the liver by erythroid cells.
4. No or only slight indications for the presence of Rauscher cells in the spleen.

Pharmacokinetic studies demonstrated that 1 to 2 hour(s) after injection (i.p.) of 3×10^5 units IF, serum IF levels are 5 to 10×10^3 u/ml. After 24 hours less than 50 u/ml IF could be detected in the serum.

We tentatively conclude from our data, that high doses of IF are able and necessary to obtain an almost complete inhibition of viral induced leukemia in mice. We are presently investigating the effect of further purified IF preparations on Rauscher disease.

Moreover, our results suggest that the antiviral activity of IF plays an important role in inhibiting viral induced leukemia. Whether other IF properties are also of significance in this system remains to be established.

References

1. Gresser, I. & M. G. Tovey. 1978. Biochim. Biophys. Acta **516:** 231–247.
2. Trapman, J. 1979. FEBS Lett. **98:** 107–110.

INTERFERON STUDIES IN CHILDREN: A NEW ASSAY OF INTERFERON PRODUCTION AND ACTIVITY

Thalia Hahn and Stanley Levin

The John Askin Pediatric Research Department
Kaplan Hospital
Rehovot, Israel

The interferon (IF) system consists of IF production on the one hand and the response to IF on the other. The purpose of this study is to try to evaluate both these aspects of the IF system by simultaneously assessing serum and cells from children and attempting to correlate the findings with their clinical status.

The parameters evaluated were: (1) *in vivo* serum IF levels; (2) *in vitro* production of types I and II IF by peripheral blood mononuclear cells (PBMC) following stimulation with poly-IC and PHA as well as with no extrinsic stimulation; (3) the ability of PBMC to promote viral replication, and (4) their sensitivity, *in vitro*, to the antiviral effect of exogenous human IF. We have assessed these parameters in healthy children and in those with viral, neoplastic, and immunodeficiency diseases.

Materials and Methods

Using micromethods, 2–5 ml of blood was sufficient for these studies which were done on 23 normal children, 17 children with viral illnesses, 12 with varied immunodeficiency diseases, and 9 with neoplasms.

The assay is based on the cytopathic effect (CPE) of vesicular stomatitis virus (VSV) on the human IF-sensitive fibroblast line MDBK, and its inhibition by IF. Ficoll-Hypaque separated PBMC are suspended in wells of microtiter test plates in tissue culture medium with and without phytohemagglutinin and poly-IC (for IF production) and with and without several concentrations of human leukocyte IF (for viral replication studies). After 24 hr of incubation, the cells that have been incubated with and without IF are infected with VSV while the IF-producing cells are left to incubate for an additional 24 hr. Twofold dilutions are then made of the supernatant tissue culture media of the PHA and poly-IC-stimulated as well as the nonstimulated cells. Serum that had previously been separated from the original blood sample is also serially diluted as well as a standard IF preparation. Fibroblasts are then seeded into the dilution-containing wells and into additional wells to be used for virus titration. The fibroblast monolayers are then infected with VSV and tenfold dilutions are made of the VSV-infected PBMC suspended in their supernatants on MDBK fibroblast monolayers. CPE is determined when control VSV-infected fibroblasts show confluent CPE.

Results

In normal healthy children blood serum IF was very low with a mean of <4 u/ml. Their PBMC responded well to stimulation with PHA and poly-IC with a mean IF value of 205u/ml. in each case. There was no IF production by nonstimulated PBMC, and in 90% of these normal cases, PBMC promoted good viral replication with a mean $TCID_{50}$ of 10^4, and going as high as 10^7. Eighty percent of these latter were inhibited by 64u of exogenous IF, and 100 by 128u.

The findings in children with viral diseases were reversed. Here, 82% had serum IF values greater than 16u/ml. with a mean of 80u/ml. IF production by stimulated lymphocytes was less than in normals, particularly so with PHA, while viral growth on PBMC was markedly inhibited, occurring in only 1 of 17 cases.

In a mixed group of cases with various types of immunodeficiency including several cases of Down's syndrome, the trend seems to be intermediate between normal and those with viral diseases.

In the small group of neoplastic diseases, mainly leukemia and neuroblastoma, the serum IF levels and the PHA and poly-IC-stimulated PBMC response resembled those seen in viral infections. Of interest is that ⅓ of the neoplastic cases and immune deficiency patients showed spontaneous IF production by lymphocytes without stimulation. This could be a possible indication of some intrinsic viral or antigenic stimulant being present in lymphocytes in neoplasia and ID cases, and could hint at possible etiology. This finding is being further investigated.

Discussion

Overall, these preliminary studies are interesting because of the finding of an inverse relationship between *in vivo* plasma IF values, and the ability of PBMC to promote viral replication. The marked difference between normal children and those with viral infections is most striking.

In two patients treated with human leukocyte IF, one an immunosuppressed child with neuroblastoma and progressive herpes zoster infection, and the other a comatose pregnant woman with fulminant hepatitis B infection, the results of this IF assay system paralleled very closely the clinical condition of the patients, and the findings helped in the clinical management of the cases, and in particular was useful in determining when to terminate IF therapy.

The information obtained from our assay system in the diagnosis and prognosis of cases suspected of viral etiology, as well as in the assessment of cases which may benefit from IF therapy should prove of great benefit to the clinician.

Index of Contributors